Quality Care
in the
Nursing Home

Quality Care
in the
Nursing Home

John N. Morris, PhD

Lewis A. Lipsitz, MD

Katharine Murphy, RN, MS

Pauline Belleville-Taylor, RN, CS, MS

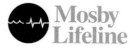

St. Louis Baltimore Boston Carlsbad Chicago Naples New York Philadelphia Portland
London Madrid Mexico City Singapore Sydney Tokyo Toronto Wiesbaden

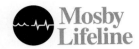

Vice President and Publisher: David Dusthimer
Managing Editor: Susan Cole
Developmental Editor: Michael Rogers
Production Manager: Chris Baumle
Production Editor: Susie Coladonato
Manufacturing Manager: Bill Winneberger
Cover Design: Nancy McDonald

Printed in the United States of America
Printing/binding by Maple-Vail Binghamton

Library of Congress Cataloging-in-Publication Data

Quality care in the nursing home / John Morris ... [et al.]
            p.   cm.
        Includes bibliographical references and index.
        ISBN 0-8151-4222-6
        1. Geriatric nursing. 2. Nursing home care   I. Morris, John,
    1941-   .
        [DNLM: 1. Geriatric Nursing–methods. 2. Nursing Homes. 3. Homes
    for the Aged.   WY 152 Q11 1996]
        RC954.Q345   1996
        610.73´65–dc20
        DNLM/DLC
        for Library of Congress   96-17375
                                                         CIP

Mosby-Year Book, Inc.
11830 Westline Industrial Drive
St. Louis, MO 63146

ISBN 08151-4222-6

96 97 98 99 00 / 9 8 7 6 5 4 3 2 1

To the residents and staff of the Hebrew Rehabilitation Center for Aged

Contributors

Sonia Ancoli-Israel, PhD
VA Medical Center, V116A
3350 La Jolla Village Drive
San Diego, CA 92161

Jerry Avorn, MD
Brigham and Women's Hospital
Program for Analysis of Clinical Strategy
221 Longwood Avenue Room 309
Boston, MA 02115

Craig Barth, PhD
Hebrew Rehabilitation Center for Aged
1200 Centre Street
Roslindale, MA 02131

Margaret Baumann, MD
VA Medical Center
820 South Damen Avenue
Chicago, IL 60612

Pauline Belleville-Taylor, RN, MS, CS
Hebrew Rehabilitation Center for Aged
1200 Centre Street
Roslindale, MA 02131

Kathryn Bowers, MD
Beth Isreal Hospital
330 Brookline Avenue
Boston, MA

Gary Brandeis, MD
Edith Nourse Rodgers VAMC
200 Springs Road
Bedford, MA 01730

Sarah Greene Burger, RN, MPH
National Citizens Coalition
1424 16th Street, Suite 202
Washington, DC 20036

Adam Burrows, MD
Hebrew Rehabilitation Center for Aged
1200 Centre Street
Roslindale, MA 02131

Jane Carlson, ACC
RR #1, Box 450
Ilion, NY 13357

Carter Catlett Williams ACSW
287 Dartmouth Street
Rochester, NY 14607

Donna Colpitts, CRTT
Hebrew Rehabilitation Center for Aged
1200 Centre Street
Roslindale, MA 02131

Robert S. Crausman, MD, MMS
Building A, Apartment 306
2575 South Syracuse Way
Denver, CO 80231

Kenneth M. Davis, MD, MS
Vice President, Medical Office
North Mississippi Medical Center
830 South Gloster Street
Tupelo, Mississippi 38801

Marie Eckler, MS, RN, CS, GNP, CRRN
Hebrew Rehabilitation Center for Aged
1200 Centre Street
Roslindale, MA 02131

Nancy Emerson-Lombardo, PhD
Hebrew Rehabilitation Center for Aged
1200 Centre Street
Roslindale, MA 02131

Maria Fiatarone, MD
Hebrew Rehabilitation Center for Aged
1200 Centre Street
Roslindale, MA 02131

Loretta Fish, RN, MS, CS
Hebrew Rehabilitation Center for Aged
1200 Centre Street, Roslindale, MA 02131

Elliot Finkelstein, MD
1371 Beacon Street
Brookline, MA 02146

Christy Flory, RN, MA
Beth Isreal Hospital
330 Brookline Avenue
Boston, MA

Barry Fogel, MD
Center for Gerontology and
    Health Care Research
85 Brown Street, Bio Med Science Building
Providence, RI 02912

Carol Frattali, PhD
Director of Health Services Division
American Speech, Language, Hearing
Association
10801 Rockville Pike
Rockville, MD 20852

Terri Fried, MD
Division of Geriatrics
Rhode Island Hospital
593 Eddy Street
Providence, RI 02903

Ann Gallagher, RD, LD
11413 Dell Loch Way
Fort Wayne, IN 46804

Claire Gerstein, MSW
Hebrew Rehabilitation Center for Aged
1200 Centre Street
Roslindale, MA 02131

Marsha Goodwin-Beck, RN-C, MA, MSN,
    Director
Geriatrics, Grants and Management Service
Mail Code 114
810 Vermont Avenue, NW
Washington, DC 10420

Michael Griffiths, DMD, MSPH
Institutional Dental Care
3100 20th St, NE
Washington, DC 20018

Jerry H. Gurwitz, MD
Program for Analysis of Clinical Strategy
221 Longwood Avenue, Room 309
Boston, MA 02115

Lisa Gwyther, MSW
Duke Family Support Program
Duke South, Blue Zone Third Floor
Duke University Medical Center
Trent Drive, 3508 Duke Hospital South
Durham, NC 27710

Danielle Harari, MD
Massachusettes General Hospital
Geriatric Medicine Unit
100 Charles River Plaza, 5th Floor
Boston, MA 02114

Susan Hartery, MS, RD
Hebrew Rehabilitation Center for Aged
1200 Centre Street
Roslindale, MA 02131

Simon Helfgott, MD
Hebrew Rehabilitation Center for Aged
1200 Centre Street
Roslindale, MA 02131

Liz Kass, MD
55 Louders Lane
Jamaica Plain, MA 02130

Amy Katzew, DPM
Hebrew Rehabilitation Center for Aged
1200 Centre Street
Roslindale, MA 02131

Kate Kelley, RN, CS, MS, GNP
85 Lancaster Terrace
Brookline, MA 02146
Nurse Practitioner, Urban Medical Group,
Boston, MA

Margaret Kelley-Gagnon, RN
Hebrew Rehabilitation Center for Aged
1200 Centre Street
Roslindale, MA 02131

Douglas P. Kiel, MD, MPH
Hebrew Rehabilitation Center for Aged
1200 Centre Street
Roslindale, MA 02131

Linda Kilburn, MSSS
125 Hunt Valley Circle
Berwyn, PA 19312

Claire A. LeVesque, MD
280 Manning Street
Needham, MA 02192

David A. Levine, PhD
1419 West Street
South Attleboro, MA 02703

Sue Levkoff, ScD
Geriatric Education Center
643 Huntington Avenue
Boston, MA 02115

Lewis A. Lipsitz, MD
Hebrew Rehabilitation Center for Aged
1200 Centre Street
Roslindale, MA 02131

Steven Littlehale, MS, RN, CS
Hebrew Rehabilitation Center for Aged
1200 Centre Street
Roslindale, MA 02131

Rosemary Lubinski, EdD
Department of Communicative Disorders
and Sciences
State University of New York at Buffalo
109 Park Hall
Buffao, NY 14260

Nancy Mace, MA
100 Master Court #1
Walnut Creek, CA 94598

Patricia McGuinn, RN
VA Medical Center, V116A
3350 La Jolla Village Drive
San Diego, CA 92161

Kenneth L. Minaker, MD
MGH Beacon Hill Geriatrics Health Practice
100 Charles River Plaza, CPZ-502
Boston, MA 02114

Susan Mitchell, MD
Hebrew Rehabilitation Center for Aged
1200 Centre Street
Roslindale, MA 02131

Mark Monane, MD
Brigham and Women's Hospital
221 Longwood Avenue
Boston, MA 02115

Susan Monane, RN, MSN
Hebrew Rehabilitation Center for Aged
1200 Centre Street
Roslindale, MA 02131

Vincent Mor, PhD
Center for Gerontology and Health Care
Research
85 Brown Street, Bio Med Science Building
Providence, RI 02912

John N. Morris, PhD
Hebrew Rehabilitation Center for Aged
1200 Centre Street
Roslindale, MA 02131

Katharine Murphy, RN, MS
Hebrew Rehabilitation Center for Aged
1200 Centre Street
Roslindale, MA 02131

Sue Nonemaker, RN, MS
7 Crawford Court
New Freedom, PA 17349

Anne Nastasi, MD
Sepulveda VA
16111 Plummer Street
Mail Station 117
Sepulveda, CA 91343

Thomas Perls, MD
New England Deaconess
Deaconess Eldercare
185 Pilgrim Road
Boston, MA 02215

Ruth Perschbacher, RMT-BC, ACC
Bristlecone Consulting Company
15 Overbrook Road
Asheville, NC 28805

David Pilgrim, MD
Hebrew Rehabilitation Center for Aged
1200 Centre Street
Roslindale, MA 02131

Kathleen Pintell, RD
11413 Dell Loch Way
Fort Wayne, IN 46804

Julia Powell, RN
Vice President of Patient Services
National Health Corp
100 East Vine Street
Murfreesboro, TN 37130

Neil Resnick, MD
Chief, Geriatrics
Brigham & Women's Hospital
75 Francis Street
Boston, MA 02115

Gretchen Robinson, RD
11413 Dell Loch Way
Fort Wayne, IN 46804

Joanne Sandberg Cook, RN, C, MS
Route 113
Thetford Centre, VT 05075

Andrew Satlin, MD
McLean Hospital
115 Mill Street
Belmont, MA 02178

Hilary Siebens, MD
Cedars Sinai Medical Center
Department of Rehabilitation Medicine
8700 Beverly Boulevard MGBR M-600
Los Angeles, CA 93348-1869

Gail Schober, RN
Hebrew Rehabilitation Center for Aged
1200 Centre Street
Roslindale, MA 02131

Myles N. Sheehan, MD
315 North Grove Avenue
Oak Park, IL 60302

Heike Tuplin, CTRS, ACC
Hebrew Rehabilitation Center for Aged
1200 Centre Street
Roslindale, MA 02131

Michael Westerman, CTRS
Hebrew Rehabilitation Center for Aged
1200 Centre Street
Roslindale, MA 02131

Denise Williams Jones, MA
VA Medical Center, V116A
3350 La Jolla Village Drive
San Diego, CA 92161

Thomas T. Yoshikawa, MD
Professor and Chair
Department of Internal Medicine
Martin Luther King Jr./Charles Drew Medical
   Center
12021 South Wilmington Avenue
Los Angeles, CA

NURSING ADVISORY GROUP
AT THE HEBREW REHABILITATION
CENTER FOR THE AGED

Robert Baseman, RN, MS
Steven Littlehale, RN, MS, C, CS
Sharon Gallagher, RN, MS
Carole Stolzenbach, RN, MSN, CNA

PREFACE

There is general public confidence that nurses and physicians have been properly trained to deal with the problem of acute illnesses requiring medical attention. Unfortunately, when elderly people develop chronic and disabling illnesses that require care in a nursing facility, their health care professionals may not be adequately prepared to treat these conditions. Preparing health professionals to address the long-term care needs of persons in nursing homes has not been a priority in our society's educational system. Since over 40% of individuals 65 years of age or older can expect to spend some time in a nursing home, there is a need for information about the management of disabling conditions in the real-world setting of the nursing facility. There is a significant body of relevant information, and many professionals have a high level of expertise in treating chronic illness. Therefore, it is our goal to disseminate this information within the medical and nursing communities. This volume provides care professionals with information on the latest technologies, research, and clinical approaches to meet the difficult challenges in caring for residents of nursing facilities.

In 1986, the prestigious Institute of Medicine of the National Academy of Sciences released a report calling for better nursing home resident assessment and care planning. In response to this report, the Nursing Home Reform Act, a part of the Omnibus Budget Reconciliation Act of 1987 (OBRA 87) called for the development of a standardized resident assessment instrument to facilitate care planning aimed at helping residents achieve their highest level of function and well-being. This resident assessment instrument was developed under contract from the Health Care Financing Administration (HCFA), after extensive consultation and testing, by a team of clinicians, educators, and researchers from the Hebrew Rehabilitation Center for the Aged, Research Triangle Institute, Brown University, and the University of Michigan. Development of this system was under the direction of two of the editors of this volume. In 1990, the instrument was mandated for use in all Medicare-and Medicaid-supported nursing facilities. It establishes a minimum data set (MDS) for every nursing home resident, which can be used to identify problems and plan appropriate interventions. The MDS has since been revised and Version 2.0 has been in use throughout the United States since January

1996. The MDS represents an important step toward improving nursing home care, but this instrument cannot achieve its full potential unless health care professionals are also armed with the information they need to develop and implement a comprehensive plan of care. This book is dedicated to addressing that need. Our goal is to assist health care professionals in their complex, challenging, and demanding practice in the nursing home setting.

There is a need for a practical, clinically relevant, scientifically grounded guide to treating the common medical and functional problems of nursing home residents. Information should be relevant to both traditional long-term care residents as well as residents in the more recent subacute and even acute categories. The editors, working in an Academic Nursing Home setting, aim to generate new knowledge to improve the care of disabled elders, and disseminate that knowledge to long-term care settings that are not affiliated with academic centers of geriatrics and gerontology. Our institution is a major setting for the education of physicians and nurses in the latest of geriatric practice models. Dr. Lipsitz has been responsible for the geriatric medical education fellowship program at Harvard University. Two of the editors (John Morris and Katharine Murphy) have had lead responsibility for the development of both the original and more recent Version 2.0 of the MDS. We have worked with professionals in nursing homes in the United States and abroad, and sense the excitement among professionals, families, and advocates as they look to an even brighter future of quality care in nursing home settings. With this text, we have created a companion to the MDS, providing a guide to care planning based on the findings of each resident's assessment. Evaluation guidelines from the Resident Assessment Protocols (RAPs) in the HCFA Resident Assessment Instrument system are elaborated in this text, and will enable health professions to complete the MDS and RAP process in the manner in which it was intended. In addition, we cover a variety of additional topics for which RAPs have not yet been constructed: Infection, discharge planning, bowel care, foot care, arthritis, and stroke.

This book is made possible by the growth and development of geriatric medicine and nursing in academic centers over the past decade, as well as the emergence of a body of practical knowledge that has not yet been widely disseminated. Since appropriate care requires an interdisciplinary approach, integrating the skills of medical, nursing, rehabilitation, and other disciplines, we have made an effort to include at least one physician and nurse as authors of most chapters. Each author is familiar with the MDS, and many participated in the design of the RAPs.

The material presented in this book goes beyond the logic of the RAPs. RAPs were designed to help professional staff identify a problem and its causal factors, with the hope that an appropriate care plan would follow. RAPs do not explain fully why causal factors are important, nor is there any attempt to prescribe a responsive program of care. In this book, treatment strategies are explained relative to key causal factors to increase understanding of possible treatment strategies. Most chapters include case examples to illustrate key concepts.

The chapters are organized under three broad categories—Assessment, Geriatric Syndromes, and Therapeutic Approaches. Each chapter is written to stand on its own. The intended audience is nurses and physicians, although other health professionals should be able to use the material in most chapters. You may wish to look at chapters that cover areas that have been more problematic at the nursing facilities with which you are affiliated, e.g., Behavior Management, Delirium, Dehydration, or Oral Care. You could also start by reviewing the chapters that cover the RAP areas in

HCFA's MDS system. If the nursing facility has or is about to embark on serving a new population (e.g., dementia special care or subacute care), you may find it useful to review chapters relevant to those populations. For the dementia population, it may be useful to review the chapters on Cognitive Loss, Activities Programming, Behavioral Symptoms, Communication, Depression, and Psychosocial Well-Being. To examine the special needs of the subacute population, you may wish to review the chapters on Activites of Daily Living, Hip Fracture, Falls, Skin Disorders, Delirium, Stroke, AIDS, Dehydration, Feeding Tubes, Infection, and Nutrition. In general, this text can serve as an active companion as you approach careplanning responsibilities.

We realize that it is not easy to get people of different disciplines to work together and speak a common language. Moreover, it is difficult to appeal to professionals from different backgrounds within a single book. Nevertheless, to deliver appropriate care to elders in residential settings, it is crucial that the community of nurses and physicians develop skills in interdisciplinary teamwork, simultaneously addressing the medical, functional, emotional, and social needs of the residents. The authors have referenced a scientifically sound knowledge base derived from multiple disciplines. Treatment recommendations are based on research findings whenever possible. However, high quality research in long-term care is still relatively sparse. Therefore, the authors also rely on empirical data from experts with extensive experience in long-term care settings. We intend to continuously update this text as new information becomes available.

The editors hope this book will serve as a valuable reference for care planning in all nursing homes, as well as a text for the teaching of long-term care in medical and nursing schools. We invite comments and suggestions from our readers, who can help improve the practical value of this work through their experience. Finally, we wish to thank each of the authors who proved to us that professionals from many diverse backgrounds can effectively work together to help improve the quality of life and dignity of the frail elderly.

John N. Morris, PhD
Lewis A. Lipsitz, MD
Katharine Murphy, RN
Pauline Belleville-Taylor, RN

Acknowledgments

The publication of this book could not have been accomplished without the effort and support of many people whose names do not appear as authors. We specifically acknowledge the enormous support given to us by Mr. Maurice May, President, and Mr. John Cupples, Senior Vice-President of the Hebrew Rehabilitation Center for Aged. Their creation of a high-quality long-term care environment inspired the vision behind the textbook and their generous support of our work made it possible to put the vision into action. We would like to especially thank the members of our Nursing Advisory Group at the Hebrew Rehabilitation Center for Aged: Robert Basemen, RN, MS; Sharon Gallagher, RN, MS; Steven Littlehale, RN, MS, C, CS; and Carole Stolzenbach, RN, MSN, CNA. Their time spent reviewing each chapter and sharing their insights helped us strengthen the clinical relevance of the material. We also appreciate the meticulous efforts of our secretarial staff, Yvonne Anderson, Bernice MacLean, and Romanna Michajiw.

Contents

1   Vital Signs 1

2   Polypharmacy 13

3   Infection... 26

4   Pulmonary Rehabilitation 35

5   AIDS and HIV Infection 47

6   Sleep Disorders 64

7   Stroke 74

8   Arthritis 97

9   Parkinson's Disease 106

10 Cognitive Loss 116

11 Delirium 145

12 Behavioral Symptoms.................................... 157

13 Depression... 172

14 Psychotropic Drugs 186

15 Psychosocial Well-Being 212

16 Communication 224

17 Vision 239

18 Falls 258

19   Hip Fractures 268

20   Foot Care 278

21   Skin Disorders 289

22   Pressure Ulcers 303

23   Nutritional Status 315

24   Dehydration 332

25   Oral Status 347

26   Feeding Tubes 358

27   Urinary incontinence 377

28   Bowel Disorders 408

29   Activities of Daily Living Rehabilitation 421

30   Activities Programming 444

31   Restraint Reduction 465

32   Advanced Directives 473

33   Terminal Care 483

34   Discharge Planning 513

Bibliography   522

Glossary   541

Appendix A   564

Index   567

1
Vital Signs

Lewis A. Lipsitz, MD
Margaret Kelley-Gagnon, RN, BS

Vital signs provide essential data for the acute assessment of nursing home residents. Traditionally, four vital signs are taken: blood pressure, pulse, respiratory rate, and temperature. Two additional evaluations are also recommended: weight and overall appearance. Any significant change from baseline in weight or overall appearance may be the first indication of a serious illness, and, coupled with abnormalities in other vital signs, should trigger a careful search for an underlying cause.

This chapter describes how to measure and evaluate the vital signs in an infirm, elderly nursing home population. Suggestions are given regarding proper use and maintenance of equipment, and standardized procedures are offered to minimize errors in measurement.

OVERVIEW

As their name implies, vital signs provide essential data for the acute assessment of nursing home residents. Traditionally, the four vital signs include blood pressure, pulse, respiratory rate, and temperature. To these, two additional evaluations should be added to the initial assessment of a geriatric patient: weight and overall appearance. Often, the first mani-

festation of serious illness is that the "resident just does not look right." This observation, particularly when coupled with abnormalities in any of the other vital signs, should prompt a careful search for an underlying acute illness.

For the nurse who first suspects that a resident is acutely ill, and the physician who must assess the urgency of medical intervention, the vital signs provide critical information to guide an appropriate response. Therefore, any assessment of the nursing home resident should begin with a careful documentation of the vital signs.

GENERAL APPEARANCE

Primary care nursing staff and relatives who are accustomed to the usual appearance of a resident are generally the first to be aware that the resident just does not look right. Triggering their concern may be a decreased level of alertness in the resident, sudden confusion, lethargy, a pale complexion, decreased appetite, or any number of other subtle observations that are often important clues to the development of an acute illness.

It is common for such reports to be dismissed or ignored, however, particularly if they do not conform to the typical presentations of

1

illness or if they come from a demanding or anxious family member. Yet any observation that a resident's general appearance has changed should be taken seriously by clinicians, since a change in general appearance may be the first outward sign of one of the following problems:

- Urinary tract infection
- Early pneumonia
- Congestive heart failure (CHF)
- Silent myocardial infarction (MI)
- Dehydration with azotemia
- Hyperglycemia or hypoglycemia in the diabetic resident
- Hyponatremia
- Anemia
- Fecal impaction
- A neurologic problem (e.g., stroke or subdural hematoma)

In response to a reported change in general appearance, examine the other vital signs, perform a physical examination, and, if the etiology is not readily apparent, obtain an electrocardiogram and blood studies, including a complete blood count, electrolytes, blood urea nitrogen, creatinine, and glucose.

BLOOD PRESSURE

Systemic arterial blood pressure represents the product of cardiac output (the heart's ability to pump blood) and systemic vascular resistance (the ability of the blood vessels to dilate or constrict in order to maintain vascular tone). Table 1-1 lists the common causes of decreased cardiac output in an infirm elderly nursing home population.

Vascular resistance is commonly affected by vasodilators, which reduce blood pressure, and vasoconstrictors, which raise blood pressure. Too much salt in the body may raise blood pressure, while too little salt may have the opposite effect. Medications such as nonsteroidal antiinflammatory drugs (NSAIDs) (e.g., ibuprofen, naproxen), which cause the body to retain salt, may increase blood pressure, while medications such as diuretics (e.g.,

Table 1-1. Common Causes of Decreased Cardiac Output

Cardiac Output May Decrease if	Possible Causes
There is inadequate blood volume	Dehydration
	Bleeding
	Obstruction of blood return to the left ventricle (LV) as in mitral stenosis or constrictive pericarditis)
The heart muscle is weak	Myocardial infarction
	Cardiomyopathy
The heart is stiff and does not fill well with blood	Diastolic dysfunction
The heart rate is too slow	Sinus bradycardia
	Heart block
The heart rate is too fast	Sinus tachycardia
	Ventricular tachycardia
	Supraventricular tachycardia

furosemide, and thiazides), which cause the kidneys to excrete salt, may lower blood pressure. Table 1-2 describes the physiologic determinants of normal blood pressure and common abnormalities that may result in hypotension or hypertension.

High Blood Pressure

Diastolic blood pressure above 95 mm Hg and/or systolic blood pressure above 160 mm Hg are considered hypertensive and are known to be associated with increased cardiovascular morbidity and mortality. In younger patients (i.e., younger than 65 years

Table 1-2. Physiologic Determinants of Normal Blood Pressure and Abnormalities Resulting in Hypo- or Hypertension

Physiologic Determinant	Abnormalities Resulting in Hypotension	Abnormalities Resulting in Hypertension
Cardiac Output		
Blood volume	Dehydration; renal salt-wasting (nephropathy and diuretics); bleeding	Excessive salt intake; renal failure (salt retention); Cushing's syndrome; NSAIDs, steroids; systemic shunts, Paget's disease
Blood return to LV	Decreased due to mitral stenosis, pulmonic stenosis, constrictive pericarditis	
Blood ejection into systemic circulation	Decreased due to mitral regurgitation, ventricular septal defect	
Cardiac muscle function	Muscle weakness (MI, cardiomyopathy) Muscle stiffness (diastolic dysfunction, ventricular hypertrophy)	Increased sympathetic activity (stress, CHF, hyperthyroidism, pheochromocytoma, sympathomimetic drugs [e.g., amphetamines, cocaine, alpha and beta agonists])
Heart rate	Sinus bradycardia; heart block; sinus tachycardia; atrial fibrillation; ventricular or supraventricular tachycardia	Moderate tachycardia associated with causes of increased sympathettic activity (see previous listing)
Vascular Resistance	Decreased due to vasodilators (low-dose alcohol, calcium channel blockers, nitrates, prazosin, terazosin, alpha-methyldopa, reserpine, clonidine, hydralazine)	Increased due to high dose of alcohol or withdrawal, Neosynephrine, pseudoephedrine, phenylephrine, thyroid hormone, amphetamines

of age), elevations in diastolic blood pressure are more common; in elderly nursing home residents, elevations in systolic blood pressure are encountered more frequently.

Studies have confirmed that isolated systolic hypertension is a risk factor for stroke and MI in the elderly, and that treatment is associated with a significant reduction in these events among active, community-dwelling elderly people. It is not clear, however, whether the treatment of systolic hypertension has the same positive effect in people over 80 years of age, particularly in a population of multiply impaired nursing home residents. For these residents, the risks of hypertension and the degree of associated damage to the heart (LV hypertrophy or cardiac ischemia), brain (strokes or transient ischemic attacks), kidneys (chronic renal insufficiency), or blood vessels (retinopathy, carotid or coronary atherosclerosis) must be balanced against the risks of adverse antihypertensive drug effects (see Table 1-3).

Interpreting Blood Pressure in an Acute Situation

To interpret the meaning of blood pressure during an acute situation, it is important not to rely on a single value at one point in time, but rather to look for a persistent change from baseline over several measurements. Blood pres-

Table 1-3. Antihypertensive Drug Effects.

Drug Type	Possible Adverse Effect
Diuretics	Dehydration Urinary Incontinence Electrolyte disturbances Arrhythmias Glucose intolerance Gout
Calcium blockers	Constipation Bradyarrhythmias
Angiotensin-converting enzyme inhibitors	Renal insufficiency Hyperkalemia
All antihypertensives	Confusion Syncope Hypotension

sure is extremely labile in elderly nursing home residents. It is common to observe declines after meals, posture changes, or medication administration, and to observe increases during periods of exercise or emotional stress. Treatment of elevated blood pressure before breakfast may result in profound hypotension and syncope after eating.

When a blood pressure elevation is due to the stress of an acute illness, treatment of the illness is usually sufficient to control the blood pressure, and more aggressive medical intervention may be detrimental. For example, acute blood pressure elevation is commonly seen at the onset of stroke. Aggressive blood pressure lowering in this situation may critically reduce cerebral blood flow, which increases the degree of brain damage. However, sustained elevations of blood pressure may result in symptoms of stroke, in which case blood pressure should be lowered gradually to moderate ranges. The appropriate response to each situation requires knowledge of the resident's previous blood pressure during relative good health and repeated measurements over time during an acute event.

Nursing staff commonly encounter an isolated elevation in blood pressure during their routine recording of the vital signs in an otherwise stable resident. This situation may be either a warning to the insidious development of an acute illness or a transient event with no clinical significance. The appropriate response is to examine the other vital signs, including the resident's overall appearance, for confirming evidence that something is awry, and to retake the blood pressure at appropriate intervals (usually one-half hour) if other indicators of disease are unchanged.

Low Blood Pressure

The problem of hypotension is commonly responsible for falls and syncope in the elderly nursing home resident. Hypotension is defined as a decline of 20 mm Hg or greater in systolic blood pressure from the usual baseline, or a decline of 10 mm Hg or greater in diastolic blood pressure from the usual baseline. Decline is usually detected within 1 to 3 minutes of sitting or standing from the supine position, or within 30 to 60 minutes after eating a meal.

An absolute systolic blood pressure value of less than 90 mm Hg is also considered hypotension. However, relative hypotension may be present at much higher values, particularly if the resident's usual blood pressure is in the hypertensive range. Physiologically, it is important that blood pressure be at a level that permits optimal cerebral perfusion. The physiologic process of cerebral autoregulation maintains 100% cerebral blood flow until blood pressure drops below a certain threshold (usually about 90 mm Hg systolic), and then cerebral blood flow begins to fall. In hypertension, the threshold is shifted to higher blood pressure levels, so the hypertensive resident may experience a fall in cerebral blood flow and associated symptoms of cerebral ischemia at blood pressure levels much higher than that in the normotensive resident.

Understanding the variability of cerebral autoregulation is especially important in the treatment of hypertensive residents with multi infarct dementia, who, as studies have shown, perform best when systolic blood pressure is lowered to a range between 135 and 150 mm Hg. In such cases, systolic blood pressure values below 135 mm Hg may be relatively hypotensive. In a resident whose systolic blood pressure usually ranges between 150 and 170 mm Hg during monthly recordings, a value of 130 mm Hg deserves attention. The nurse should note time of day and any circumstances that may be impacting the value recorded. For example, did it occur before breakfast (suggesting early morning dehydration)? Did it occur after breakfast (suggesting postprandial hypotension)? Did it occur after the resident received a medication (suggesting an adverse

drug effect)? Were there associated symptoms? Was it reproducible during repeated measurements at the same time, or on different days during similar circumstances? Such information can make a major impact on the care of a nursing home resident, and will greatly reduce the risk of a subsequent fall, stroke, or syncopal event.

Measurement of Blood Pressure

The indirect measurement of blood pressure with a sphygmomanometer and stethoscope is susceptible to several sources of error, that may seriously compromise the accuracy of recorded data. Inexact measurement may result from:
- Defective equipment or improper cuff size
- Observer errors
- Failure to standardize the measurement technique

The recommendations in the subsections that follow will help to minimize these problems.

Defective or Improperly Sized Equipment

According to the American Heart Association, the mercury gravity manometer and the aneroid manometer provide accurate and reproducible results when functioning properly. To prevent errors in measurement using this equipment, the following process is recommended:

1. Observe the level of mercury (or needle in the aneroid manometer) without applying pressure to the cuff. The edge of the mercury meniscus or aneroid dial should be precisely at zero. If necessary, add mercury to the reservoir or adjust the dial of the aneroid manometer.

2. Regularly inspect the column of the mercury gravity manometer for dirt and signs of oxidation. A clogged air vent or filter at the top of the manometer column will cause the mercury to respond sluggishly to declining pressure in the bladder, resulting in

a erroneous measurement. Service the filter and vent at least once a year to ensure accuracy.

3. Mercury that does not rise easily or that bounces noticeably when the valve is closed indicates that the pores in the kidskin diaphragm are clogged.
4. The stethoscope should be a standard one in good condition. A bell soundpiece gives better sound reproduction; a diaphragm is easier to secure with one hand and covers a larger area.
5. Choose the correct cuff size. Measure the arm circumference and multiply it by 2.5 cm. This need be done only initially with each person, unless there is significant weight change. If the bladder is too wide, the pressure may be underestimated. If the bladder is too narrow, the pressure may be overestimated. The bladder width and length should be 40% and 80%, respectively, of the arm circumference.

Observer Errors

The following are potential sources of observer error in measuring blood pressure:
- Improper application and use of equipment
- Expectation bias
- Terminal digit preference
- Failure to recognize an auscultatory gap
- Failure to recognize pseudo hypertension
- Cardiac arrhythmias

Improper Application and Use of Equipment. When measuring blood pressure, the resident's arm should be bare, with the palm facing upward. After selecting the proper cuff size, locate the brachial artery. Wrap the cuff smoothly and snugly around the arm, centering the cuff bladder over the brachial artery, 2.5 cm above the antecubital space. Failure to apply the cuff snugly will result in falsely elevated readings. Failure to center the cuff bladder over the brachial artery may result in an elevated

reading. Hold the arm at heart level during measurement.

Expectation Bias. Expectation bias results from the tendency of the observer to be influenced by prior knowledge of a resident's blood pressure readings. Values are often assigned according to the preconceived bias.

Terminal Digit Preference. Terminal digit preference results from the tendency of an observer to record certain numbers in preference to others, or to round off measurements to a terminal 5 or 10. For example, if the blood pressure is 123/72 mm Hg, the observer may record 120/70.

Failure to Recognize an Auscultatory Gap. In some residents, particularly hypertensives, Korotkoff sounds disappear as the pressure is reduced, then reappear at some lower level. This gap can extend over a range as great as 40 mm Hg, which can seriously underestimate systolic pressure or overestimate diastolic pressure. Estimate the systolic pressure by palpating the radial or brachial artery during cuff inflation. Disappearance of the radial (or brachial) pulse indicates the level of systolic pressure.

Failure to Recognize Pseudohypertension. Older persons can have sclerotic and calcified vessels. The stiff, thick, hard vessel wall may resist compression by the inflated bladder. Therefore, more pressure may be needed to occlude the artery, resulting in a spuriously high estimation of systolic pressure.

The technique used to identify residents at risk of pseudo hypertension is known as Osler's maneuver, which is performed by inflating the cuff above systolic pressure and carefully palpating the brachial artery. When the artery remains clearly palpable (despite being pulseless), then the person is Osler-positive and susceptible to pseudo hypertension.

Cardiac Arrhythmias. An irregular cardiac rhythm or premature ectopic beats may increase or decrease the time interval between beats when the heart normally fills with blood. As a result, a transient increase in systolic pressure may occur during a long interval with increased ventricular filling, or a decrease in systolic blood pressure may occur during a short interval with decreased filling. The blood pressure will vary depending on the beat-to-beat time interval when Korotkoff sounds were heard. In this situation, the clinician must rely on an average blood pressure from at least three measurements.

Standardized Procedure for Measuring Blood Pressure

The following procedure is the standard used to measure blood pressure:

1. Explain the procedure to put the resident at ease. Be sure the resident is free from anxiety, bladder distension, pain, and other symptoms before continuing.
2. The resident may be supine, seated, or standing. Be sure the environment is quiet and comfortable.
3. The resident's arm should be bare and unrestricted by clothing, with the palm upward and the arm relaxed at heart level.
4. The resident should be comfortable and remain at rest for 5 minutes before baseline measurements are obtained. (Postural measurements are taken 1 and 3 minutes after sitting or standing.)
5. Place the manometer at eye level and sufficiently close to read the calibrations marking the mercury column or aneroid dial.
6. Place the correct cuff size on the arm. Note the arm being used and size of the cuff.
7. Locate the brachial artery in the antecubital fossae.
8. Wrap the cuff smoothly and snugly around the arm, centering the cuff bladder over the brachial artery with the lower margin 2.5 cm above the antecubital space.
9. Determine the level for maximal inflation by observing the pressure at which the radial pulse is no longer palpable as the cuff is rapidly inflated (palpated systolic). Check for a palpable artery after pulselessness (Osler's maneuver). Note the presence of an irregular pulse.
10. Rapidly and steadily deflate the cuff, then wait 15 to 30 seconds before reinflating.
11. Position the stethoscope over the brachial artery. The ear pieces should be pointed forward.
12. Rapidly and steadily inflate the cuff to the maximal inflation level as determined in step 9.
13. Release the air in the cuff so that the pressure falls at a rate of 2 to 3 mm Hg per second.
14. Note the systolic pressure at the onset of at least two consecutive beats (phase 1). Note diastolic pressure at the cessation of sound (phase 5). Listen for 10 to 20 mm Hg below the last sound to confirm disappearance and then deflate completely.
15. To obtain postural blood pressure changes, ask or assist the resident to stand up from the supine position. Do not remove the cuff.
16. When both of the resident's feet touch the floor, begin timing.
17. Support the resident's arm with your arm to keep it relaxed and at heart level.
18. Take the first standing blood pressure at 1 minute, following the procedure above (steps 12 to 14). Verbally check with the resident to determine if there are symptoms of dizziness, lightheadedness, or weakness.
19. At 3 minutes, repeat this blood pressure measurement in the same manner.
20. Record blood pressure results for the rela-

tive supine, 1 minute standing and 3 minutes standing, with the date and time of day. Document any symptoms.

PULSE

The heart rate, or pulse, is another important indicator of acute illness in the elderly. Key diagnostic features are the rate, rhythm, quality, and responsivity of the pulse.

Pulse Rate

The pulse is generally considered abnormal if it is less than 60 or greater than 100 bpm. Since many healthy elderly people develop sinus bradycardia with heart rates below 60 bpm, a slow pulse must be interpreted in light of blood pressure and associated symptoms. If blood pressure is abnormally low, or the resident has symptoms of chest pain, dizziness, syncope, confusion, or postural instability, the presence of bradycardia may be an urgent, potentially life-threatening medical problem. Obtain an electrocardiogram to determine the cause of bradycardia (e.g., heart block and slow junctional or ventricular rhythms). In the resident taking digoxin, beta blockers, or calcium-channel blockers, a slow pulse may indicate drug toxicity. Bradycardia may also be a sign of hypothyroidism.

Tachycardia is almost always a sign of underlying illness. By itself, a rapid heart rate may cause:

- Cardiac ischemia (by increasing cardiac oxygen utilization and reducing coronary blood flow)
- Systemic hypotension (by decreasing diastolic ventricular filling)
- Embolic events, particularly if due to atrial fibrillation

Tachycardia may be caused by any acute illness (e.g., fever, dehydration, CHF, pericarditis, pulmonary embolism, pneumonia, thyrotoxicosis, acute anxiety), or by medications, particularly those with adrenergic properties (e.g., cold medications) or anticholinergic effects (e.g., antidepressants, neuroleptics, and antihistamines). The evaluation of a rapid heart rate requires an electrocardiogram to determine the nature of the cardiac arrhythmia, and a careful physical examination and laboratory studies to search for underlying illness. This may require transfer to the hospital for a brief period.

Rhythm

Evaluate the pulse for its regularity or irregularity. An irregular cardiac rhythm may represent frequent atrial or ventricular premature beats, atrial fibrillation, or intermittent conduction abnormalities. A regular tachycardia is most likely due to sinus or supraventricular tachycardias. Noting the rhythm of the pulse during an acute medical problem can give important clues to the etiology that may no longer be present by the time an electrocardiogram is obtained. For example, syncope commonly occurs in elderly nursing home residents at the onset of atrial fibrillation. This arrhythmia may revert to normal sinus rhythm before an electrocardiogram can be obtained. If the caregiver who first attends the resident notes the rhythm of the pulse, the diagnosis is readily made by the irregularity that is characteristic of atrial fibrillation.

Quality

The quality of the pulse can also provide important diagnostic information. The carotid pulse is most useful for this purpose. Normally, the pulse of an older person has a brisk quality with a rapid early portion prior to its peak (the upstroke) due to an increase in arterial rigidity in advanced age. A very weak, low-amplitude pulse suggests that cardiac output and blood pressure are low, which commonly occurs during hypotensive episodes or in aortic stenosis. Hemodynamically significant aortic stenosis also results in a delay in the upstroke of the pulse, which delays the time from onset of a palpable pulsation to the point of its greatest amplitude. A bounding pulse with a fast upstroke and downstroke is characteristic of hypertension, thyrotoxicosis, and aortic regurgitation.

Responsivity

It is also important to note the heart rate response to stress, particularly the stress of posture change. The baroreflexes guard against hypotension by causing an increase in heart rate during activities such as standing up or eating a meal, which tend to reduce blood pressure by pooling blood in the legs or gut. Baroreflexes also prevent excessive hypotension from medications that reduce blood pressure.

A small or absent increase in pulse on standing or taking an antihypertensive medication is indicative of baroreflex impairment, and strongly suggests that the resident is at risk of developing hypotension when exposed to situations or medications that reduce blood pressure.

An excessive heart rate response to stress is also meaningful. It may suggest that a resident is becoming dehydrated in response to diuretic therapy, or that the resident is in pain following an accident or procedure. In a demented resident who may not be able to express pain, fear, or anxiety during a particular situation, an increase in pulse provides an important clue.

Examination of the Pulse

Count the pulse at the radial artery for a full minute while the resident is lying, sitting, or standing quietly. Be sure it is the resident's pulse you are feeling and not your own, which is always a possibility if the resident is experiencing hypotension. Avoid any confusion by simultaneously feeling your own radial pulse with your other hand. Note whether the resident's pulse feels the same at the radial, carotid, and (if peripheral vascular disease is suspected) femoral, popliteal, and dorsalis

pedis or posterior tibial arteries. Listen for bruits over areas where the pulse is diminished to detect atherosclerotic narrowing of the vessel.

Respiratory Rate

Respiratory rate is another sensitive sign of acute illness, but of all the vital signs it is susceptible to the greatest error in measurement. For example, it is common to see the numbers 16 or 20 recorded unvaryingly on vital sign sheets, reflecting the examiner's counting of 4 or 5 respirations over a 15 second period, then multiplying by 4. A preferable method is to count excursions of the chest, unmasked by clothing or resident movement, for a full minute.

Respirations can be quite variable, ranging in healthy young individuals between 8 to 16 breaths per minute, and in chronically impaired elderly people between 16 and 25 breaths per minute. In the nursing home setting, any respiratory rate over 25 breaths per minute (tachypnea) should evoke a prompt evaluation for underlying acute illness. Tachypnea may represent not only cardiopulmonary disease but also any condition that results in metabolic acidosis, requiring a rapid breathing rate to remove carbonic acid from the body.

When observing respiration, several breathing patterns and associated findings can provide valuable diagnostic information. Observe the resident for cyanosis, which suggests hypoxemia. Also, note the depth and regularity of the resident's breathing. Table 1-4 lists various breathing pattern characteristics and suggests possible diagnostic associations.

TEMPERATURE

Body temperature may be too high (fever) or too low (hypothermia) in the acutely ill nursing home resident. In contrast to younger patients, geriatric patients are less given to fever and more so to hypothermia. To be able

Table 1-4. Breathing Pattern Characteristics and Suggested Associations

Pattern	Suggested Diagnosis
Rapid, shallow breathing	Restricive lung disease Pleuritic chest pain Pneumothorax Elevated diaphragm Metabolic acidosis
Deep breathing (Kussmaul's respirations) Slow breathing	Diabetic coma Drug-induced respiratory depression (e.g., benzodiazepine overdose) Increased cranial pressure
Progressively increasing, then decreasing depth of respiration with regularly recurring periods of apnea (Cheyne-Stokes respiration)	CHF Coma resulting from affection of the nervous centers
Ataxic breathing (Biot's breathing), irregular and unpredictable	Medullary brain damage
Prolonged expiratory phase during each breath	Obstructive lung disease

to detect both of these conditions, it is important to have thermometers capable of reading low temperatures (i.e., below 91°F [32.8°C]) as well as elevated temperatures. Since rapid respiratory rates and a resident's inability to follow instructions during acute illnesses make it difficult to obtain accurate oral temperatures, rectal temperatures should be standard prac-

tice in the nursing home setting. Ear thermometers soon will be available as well. If a mercury thermometer is used, the staff should be careful to shake the mercury column down to its lowest point in order to be able to detect hypothermia. Keep the thermometer in the rectum for a full 3 minutes to obtain an accurate reading.

Fever

Rectal temperatures above 100°F (38°C) are considered clinically significant fevers and should prompt a search for the underlying etiology. Most fevers are caused by infectious or inflammatory processes, but in the nursing home resident other problems (e.g., fecal impaction, pulmonary atelectasis, and drug reactions) are also common causes.

Immediately treat temperature elevation because it can rapidly lead to dehydration, delirium, and associated falls. It is common practice in some acute settings to withhold antipyretic medications in order to follow the fever curve, but this is unwise in the nursing home, where complications of the fever itself are likely to occur. Give residents ample fluids at the onset of fever, and temporarily withhold diuretic medications.

Hypothermia

A reduction in core body temperature to below 95°F (35°C) commonly occurs in frail, multiply impaired nursing home residents, even in environments where ambient temperatures are quite comfortable. There are many possible causes of hypothermia in this population:

- Impairments in vasoconstriction, shivering, and basal metabolic rate
- Exposures to medications that effect thermoregulation
- Reduced lean (muscle) body mass
- Low levels of physical activity

It is not unusual for a nursing home resident to develop hypothermia in an air-conditioned nursing unit in the middle of the summer. Other risk factors include diabetes, hypothyroidism, malnutrition, stroke, Parkinson's disease, alcohol, and medications such as tranquilizers, sedatives, and antidepressants. Other common causes of hypothermia to consider include sepsis (where a low, rather than high, temperature may develop) and hypoglycemia.

Hypothermia is often overlooked because of the unavailability of low-reading thermometers (conventional thermometers read only to 94°F (34.4°C), and the fact that hypothermia presents with nonspecific signs and symptoms such as lethargy, dysarthria, ataxia, and confusion. Associated findings typically include a lack of shivering, bradycardia, and cool, dry skin. The blood glucose level may be high (if hypoglycemia is not the cause) because of reduced insulin action in the cold, and the electrocardiogram often shows a very fine baseline tremor and characteristic J wave (Osborne wave) in the ST segment.

If the body temperature is higher than 90°F (32.2°C), the treatment of choice is slow spontaneous rewarming at a rate of 1°F (0.6°C) per hour with blankets and a warm environment. Below this temperature, life-threatening arrhythmias, including ventricular fibrillation, and CHF may develop, necessitating a more aggressive approach. This requires a quick transfer to the hospital. Additional rewarming measures include ventilation with warm, humidified air and gastric or peritoneal lavage with warm fluids. Carefully monitor the resident for aspiration pneumonia and cardiac arrhythmias. Do not treat hyperglycemia with insulin until the temperature rises to normal, since insulin is ineffective at low temperatures and may result in hypoglycemia as rewarming occurs.

WEIGHT

A recent change in body weight, rather than its absolute value, is such an important indicator of underlying illness in the nursing home resident that it deserves to be designated a vital sign. An increase in weight over several days or weeks may be a warning to the insidious development of CHF long before the classic symptoms develop. Similarly, unexpected weight loss may be an early sign of depression, an occult malignancy, hyperthyroidism, or chronic inflammatory disease. Body weight can be used to guide the course of diuretic therapy for CHF or the nutritional rehabilitation of a resident following an acute illness or injury such as hip fracture.

When evaluating a recent change in a resident's clinical or functional status, and when reviewing current medications or choosing the appropriate dose of a new medication, carefully consider the body weight. For example, a 1 to 2 pound increase in weight in a resident who has suddenly become lethargic or confused often signals the development of CHF. Alternatively, the development of similar symptoms in a resident taking digoxin who has lost 5 to 10 pounds over the past 6 months may represent digoxin toxicity. If a resident becomes acutely ill with a life-threatening gram-negative pneumonia, use body weight to determine the initial dosage of aminoglycoside antibiotic therapy. It is important to have a recent body weight recorded in the medical record in order to detect vital changes and to influence current therapy.

Measure body weight in a consistent fashion, at the same time of day and with the resident wearing the same amount of clothing each time. Check the scale for proper zero calibration before each reading. Compare only readings from the same scale. When residents are moved to different nursing units or transferred to and from the hospital, weight measurements may differ considerably as a result of the different scales used in these locations. Therefore, it is important to obtain a baseline reading whenever a resident is relocated.

CASE EXAMPLE

Mrs. G. is an 89-year-old woman who has been residing in a nursing home for the past year. She is independent in activities of daily living and uses a walker for ambulation following a fall that resulted in a hip fracture last year. Her past medical history includes angina, CHF, osteoarthritis, occasional insomnia, and gait impairment. Her current medications are isosorbide dinitrate (Isordil), 5 mg orally three times a day, furosemide (Lasix), 40 mg orally every day, acetaminophen (Tylenol), 500 mg orally four times a day, and temazepam (Restoril), 15 mg as needed for sleep.

After her usual weekly overnight visit with her family, Mrs. G.'s daughter reported to the nurse that her mother just did not seem like herself during the visit. She stated that Mrs. G. did not sleep well overnight and got out of bed several times during the night to sit in a chair in her room. Mrs. G. also refused to wear her shoes and insisted on wearing her slippers back to the nursing home. Her grandson noted that her gait appeared to be slower than normal.

The nurse found Mrs. G. sitting in a chair in her room. She denied any symptoms. She was not wearing her dentures, which was unusual. Her vital signs were as follows: blood pressure 148/90 mm Hg, pulse 108 bpm and regular, respiration 24 breaths per minute, and rectal temperature 99.2°F. Her weight was 105.5 pounds. She had some swelling in both ankles and dyspnea when lying flat in bed.

Careful review of Mrs. G.'s medical record revealed her usual blood pressure readings to be 130-138/72-76 mm Hg, pulse rate between 70 and 76 bpm, and respirations 16 to 18 per minute. Mrs. G.'s weekly weights had been stable at 103 pounds for 3 months.

The observations made by Mrs. G.'s family members are important clues to consider in the overall evaluation of this resident. For example, Mrs. G. may have experienced dyspnea during her overnight visit, making it more comfortable for her to sit in a chair than be in bed and causing her gait to be slower. In addition, she may have had difficulty putting on her shoes due to the swelling in her ankles.

Mrs. G. was diagnosed with CHF and was treated effectively with diuretic therapy. This case shows the importance of careful evaluation of vital signs, including weight changes and overall appearance, in the acute assessment of an elderly, multiply impaired nursing home resident.

2
Polypharmacy

Jerry H. Gurwitz, MD
Mark Monane, MD
Susan Monane, RN, MSN
Jerry Avorn, MD

The nursing home setting is characterized by some of the most complex and challenging pharmacotherapeutic issues in all of medicine. Use of multiple concurrent drug therapies is frequently necessary and appropriate in the care of the elderly nursing home resident with multiple medical problems in order to optimize physiologic, social, and functional status. However, the excessive and unnecessary use of medications brings with it the risk of adverse drug reactions and serious drug-drug interactions. In addition, at a time of increasing concern about rising financial expenditures for nursing home care, the optimal use of drugs in this clinical setting represents an important opportunity for containing health-care costs.

OVERVIEW

Residents in long-term care facilities receive more medication than noninstitutionalized older persons. A study of 12 nursing homes in the greater Los Angeles area reported that the 1106 residents were prescribed an average of 7.2 medications each. In a study of more than 800 residents of 12 representative intermediate-care facilities in Massachusetts, residents were prescribed an average of 8.1 medi-

cations. Table 2-1 lists the most commonly prescribed medications in this study.

There are concerns about the suboptimal use of a variety of specific medication classes in the nursing home, including antibiotics, H_2 blockers, NSAIDs, laxatives, and digoxin. However, the potentially excessive use of sedatives and antipsychotic medications has attracted the greatest attention. In a 1980 study of Medicaid patients residing in Tennessee facilities, 43% were reported to have had an order for antipsychotic medication. Some researchers have observed a direct relationship between the use of sedative and antipsychotic medications and the size and staffing levels of facilities. Such findings indicate that these drugs may sometimes be used as behavioral management or crowd control strategy rather than therapeutically.

Many factors can contribute to inappropriate drug use in the nursing home setting. The education of physicians and nurses generally does not include adequate training or experience in geriatric medicine, nursing, or pharmacology. Events that are perceived to require an immediate pharmacotherapeutic decision frequently occur when there is no physician present. Using telephone orders can accelerate

13

Table 2-1. Most Commonly Prescribed Medications to Residents (n=823) of 12 Intermediate-Care Facilities in Massachusetts

Medication Category	Orders per 100 Residents	Medication Category	Orders per 100 Residents
Gastrointestinal Medications		**Psychoactive Medications**	
Laxatives/enemas	179	Sedatives/hypnotics§	29
Acid-peptic*	36	Antipsychotics	28
Other†	41	Antidepressants	16
Analgesic Medications		Diphenhydramine (Benadryl)	9
Acetaminophen	96	**Antibiotics and Antifungals**	20
Aspirin	26	**Endocrine/Metabolic Medications**	
Opioids	15	Hypoglycemic agents	12
NSAIDs	12	Thyroid replacement	8
Cardiovascular Medications		**Respiratory Medications**	
Digoxin	27	Theophylline	7
Loop diuretics	26	Beta-sympathomimetics	6
Nitrates	23	**Neurologic Medications**	
Thiazide diuretics	15	Antiseizure	8
Beta-blockers	10	Antiparkinsonian	5
Calcium channel blockers	5	**Anticoagulant/Antiplatelet Medications**	
Antiarrhythmic agents	3	Dipyridamole (Persantine)	6
Other‡	9	Warfarin (Coumadin)	4
Vitamins and Supplements		**Ophthalmic Medications**	
Multivitamins	45	Artificial tears	6
Potassium	19	Glaucoma	4
Iron	15	**Steroids**	4
Calcium	4	**Urinary Medications**	1

*Antacids, H_2 blockers, sucralfate (Carafate).

†Antidiarrheals, simethicone, metoclopramide (Reglan).

‡Includes angiotensin-converting enzyme inhibitors and potassium sparing diuretics.

§Excluding diphenhydramine.

the provision of therapy to a resident, but these orders can also serve to intensify a pattern of episodic care without adequate evaluation or follow-up. Approximately 50% of all medication orders for nursing home residents are written with directions for administration as needed, so the nursing staff is left with the primary responsibility for a substantial proportion of clinical decision-making regarding drug therapy.

The occurrence of potentially avoidable adverse drug reactions is the most serious consequence of polypharmacy in the nursing home setting. These reactions can cause confusion, falls, and hip fractures relating specifically to antipsychotic medication and sedative use. Incontinence, constipation, blurred vision, and dry mouth are potential side effects of anticholinergic medications including some of the tricyclic antidepressants. Renal impairment and upper gastrointestinal bleeding are well recognized adverse effects of NSAID therapy. A very troubling negative consequence of the excessive use of antibiotics is the development of increasingly virulent bacterial strains, forcing reliance on potentially more toxic and expensive antibiotic regimens.

A balanced discussion of the topic of drug therapy in the nursing home cannot ignore the fact that some categories of medication are also underused. One prominent example is antidepressant therapy. Significant clinical depression is common among residents of nursing homes, much of which is undiagnosed and untreated. The symptoms of depression can be dismissed inappropriately as reasonable reactions to chronic illness and an understandable response to institutionalization. This is particularly unfortunate, since depres-

sion in the elderly often responds well to therapy. By contrast, untreated depression is associated with increased mortality as well as an obvious decrement in quality of life.

PHARMACOLOGY IN AGING: PHARMACOKINETICS AND PHARMACODYNAMICS

The following sections discuss the topics of pharmacokinetics and pharmacodynamics and their relation to elderly nursing home residents.

Pharmacokinetics

Pharmacokinetics is defined as what the body does to a drug. Of the traditional components of pharmacokinetics—absorption, distribution, and clearance (drug removal from the body)—only absorption appears to be unaffected by age. For certain medications,

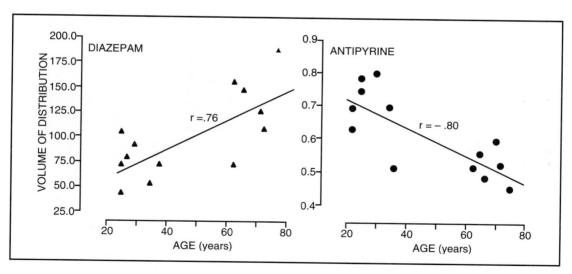

Figure 2-1. *Changes in volume of distribution with age for diazepam and antipyrine in healthy male volunteers. Because of an age-related increase in body fat, highly lipid-soluble drugs such as diazepam are distributed more extensively in elderly patients. By contrast, the volume of distribution of water-soluble agents such as antipyrine decreases with advancing age. From: Greenblatt DJ, et al.: "Drug disposition in old age." Reprinted by permission of* The New England Journal of Medicine, *306:1081-1088, 1982.*

drug distribution can vary importantly in the elderly. An age-related increase in body fat at the expense of muscle leads to a greater volume of distribution for lipid-soluble medications (e.g., many of the benzodiazepines). *See* Fig. 2-1 for more information.

Additionally, important pathways of drug metabolism in the liver and drug excretion by the kidney may be impaired in elderly patients. Such age-related changes in pharmacokinetics can have important implications for dosing of medications in this population.

The liver represents the major site of metabolism for many drugs. Hepatic biotransformation of drugs is categorized into phase I (preparative) and phase II (synthetic) reactions. Phase I reactions lead to intermediate products (often with their own drug effects) that then undergo transformation to pharmacologically inactive, polar, water-soluble metabolites by phase II reactions. Phase I reactions include oxidation, reduction, and hydrolysis. Phase II reactions involve conjugation reactions (glucuronidation, acetylation, and sulfation). The efficiency of phase I reactions is reduced somewhat with advancing age, while aging has little impact on phase II metabolic pathways.

Elimination

An increase in the volume of distribution and/or a reduction in clearance will cause a prolongation of elimination half-life, which might prolong the duration of action of a single dose of a drug. This relationship is expressed as the following equation: half-life (T°) is proportional to volume of distribution (Vd) divided by clearance (Cl).

$$T° \propto Vd/Cl$$

Selected agents in the benzodiazepine class show the impact of aging on drug elimination half-life. Because diazepam (Valium) is very fat soluble, it has an increased volume of dis-

tribution in older patients. It is metabolized initially by phase I reactions in the liver. The elimination half-life of diazepam in a young person is approximately 24 hours compared with 75 hours in the elderly. In contrast, oxazepam (Serax) is substantially less fat soluble than diazepam and is metabolized only by a phase II reaction. The elimination half-life of oxazepam is unchanged with advancing patient age (approximately 10 hours).

It is frequently assumed that the duration of clinical action of a drug is related to its half-life. Under this assumption, a long elimination half-life implies a long duration of action, and a short elimination half-life implies a short duration of action. This is not always a correct interpretation, but epidemiologic data do support an association between the use of

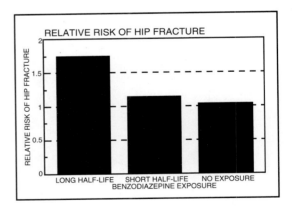

Figure 2-2. *Risk of hip fracture associated with use of benzodiazepines with different elimination half-lives. Elderly patients treated with agents having short (less than or equal to 24 hours) elimination halflives (e.g., oxazepam) had no increased risk. A significantly increased risk was associated with use of long elimination half-life agents (e.g., diazepam). Adapted from: Ray WA, et al.: "Benzodiazepines of long and short elimination half-life and the risk of hip fracture," JAMA, 262:3303-3307, 1989.*

agents with a long elimination half-life and the occurrence of drug side effects in the elderly. *See* Fig. 2-2 for more information.

The Cockcroft-Gault formula is often used to estimate renal function in older patients who are to receive potentially nephrotoxic drugs (e.g., aminoglycosides) or drugs that are excreted primarily by the kidneys (e.g., digoxin). The formula to estimate renal function is as follows:

Creatinine clearance (mL/min) =

$$\frac{(140 - age\ [yr])(body\ wt\ [kg])}{(72)(serum\ creatinine\ (mg/dL])}$$

The value is 15% less in women

Estimates of creatinine clearance based on this formula are valid only for residents whose renal function is in a steady state, and who are not taking medications that directly alter renal function or affect creatinine excretion. While the formula has some utility in assessing renal function in healthy ambulatory older individuals, it has only limited utility in severely ill or clinically unstable elderly nursing home residents.

Repeated Drug Dosing: Steady-State Drug Levels

Most medications are administered repeatedly rather than as a single dose. In this case, the major goal of pharmacotherapy is to achieve and maintain a therapeutic steady-state concentration of a medication. This concentration is frequently an important determinant of clinical outcome. The steady-state drug concentration (Css) is proportional to the medication dosing rate (dose/dosing interval) and inversely proportional to drug clearance. The equation for steady-state drug concentrations is as follows:

$$Css \propto (Dose/Dosing\ Interval)/Clearance$$

With chronic dosing, reduced clearance without a change in the dosing interval will lead to an increased Css.

Understanding the implications of the equation for Css can help guide prudent prescribing of medications. Drug clearance is a biologically determined variable in each individual resident, over which the health care provider has no control, but the medication dose and the dosing interval can be adjusted. To prevent the excessive accumulation of a drug when its clearance is reduced (as may be the case in the elderly person), the prescriber can reduce the medication dose, increase the interval between doses, or both, depending on the medication and the clinical setting.

Interpreting Serum Drug Levels

One aspect of drug distribution that is frequently raised in relation to the elderly is the binding of drugs to serum or plasma proteins. Albumin and alpha$_1$ acid glycoprotein are the two most important proteins in this regard. In large populations of healthy elderly, clinically meaningful reductions in serum albumin have not been observed with advancing age, but there is a modest (albeit statistically significant) downward drift in albumin. Studies that have purported to show an age-related decline in serum albumin levels have probably been marred by the problem of confounding illness with aging. Nonetheless, marked reductions in serum protein levels often do occur in older patients suffering from malnutrition or advanced disease.

One of the more important risks of diminished binding proteins is an iatrogenic one, resulting from misinterpretation of serum drug levels. Most assays measure the total amount of drug present in serum (i.e., both protein-bound and unbound [*free*] drugs). The unbound drug concentration is more clinically relevant than the total concentration because

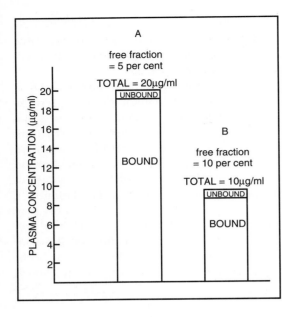

***Figure 2-3.** Example of how differences in protein binding can influence interpretation of drug concentrations. Patients A and B are receiving the same daily dose of phenytoin, yet the total plasma concentration of phenytoin in patient A is 20 μg/mL compared with 10 μg/ml in patient B. However, patient B has a reduced serum albumen level due to malnutrition, leading to an increase in the fraction of the total drug concentration that is unbound to plasma proteins (i.e., free)—from 5% to 10%. Despite having different total plasma concentrations of phenytoin, patients A and B both have the same concentration of pharmacologically active unbound drug. Therefore, it is not appropriate to increase the daily dose of phenytoin in patient B. From: Greenblatt DJ, Shader RI: Pharmokinetics in Clinical Practice, page 99, Philadelphia, 1985, WB Saunders Company.*

only unbound drug is pharmacologically active. For a resident with hypoalbuminemia or another deficiency in binding protein, any given serum drug level will reflect a greater concentration of unbound drug than the same

level would signify in a resident with normal binding capacity. This is due to an increase in free drug fraction (Fig. 2-3).

A hypoalbuminemic resident with a normal total serum drug level may have an unbound drug concentration that is unacceptably high. In contrast, the same resident with a slightly lower than normal total serum concentration may have an unbound drug concentration that is in a very reasonable range. Phenytoin (Dilantin), which is highly bound to albumin, and lidocaine, which is highly bound to alpha-1 acid glycoprotein, are two examples of drugs for which the interpretation of serum levels reflecting total drug concentration (rather than free concentration) can be problematic in malnourished elderly persons.

Pharmacodynamics

In the elderly, the clinical response to a drug may be enhanced due to higher drug concentrations and increased accumulation after repeated dosing (i.e., an age-related pharmacokinetic change). Alternatively, older residents may be intrinsically more sensitive to a medication. Therefore, at any particular serum concentration, the clinical response is greater than in younger patients (i.e., an age-related pharmacodynamic change).

Pharmacodynamics is defined as what a drug does to the body. Pharmacodynamic changes with aging have been more challenging to describe than pharmacokinetic changes. One of the first studies describing age-related changes in pharmacodynamics involved a group of patients between the ages of 30 and 90 years of age undergoing elective cardioversion who were medicated with intravenous diazepam. The clinical endpoint used was the patient's inability to respond to vocal stimuli, with preservation of response to a painful stimulus. The serum level of diazepam at which this central nervous system effect occurred was significantly lower in elderly patients (Fig. 2-4).

Similar findings have emerged from other studies involving benzodiazepines and the opioids. A recent study also suggested that increasing patient age is associated with an increased sensitivity to the effects of warfarin therapy. By contrast, the elderly have been shown to be *less sensitive* to the effects of some medications, including beta-adrenergic agonists and antagonists.

Be careful when drawing conclusions from the results of studies examining age-related changes in pharmacodynamics and applying these findings to clinical practice. For example, while older patients have been shown to be *more sensitive* to the effects of opioid analge-

sics, such as morphine, this research finding should never limit the provision of adequate analgesic therapy to treat an elderly patient in pain. While older persons may be *less sensitive* to the effects of beta-adrenergic antagonists, do not use this observation to formulate general dosing guidelines for beta-blocker therapy in elderly residents. However, age-related changes in pharmacokinetics and/or pharmacodynamics of some benzodiazepine sedatives and hypnotics do suggest a need to reduce dosage in the elderly (e.g., with triazolam and diazepam). Furthermore, the increased sensitivity to warfarin therapy in the elderly may indicate a need to intensify monitoring of anticoagulant therapy.

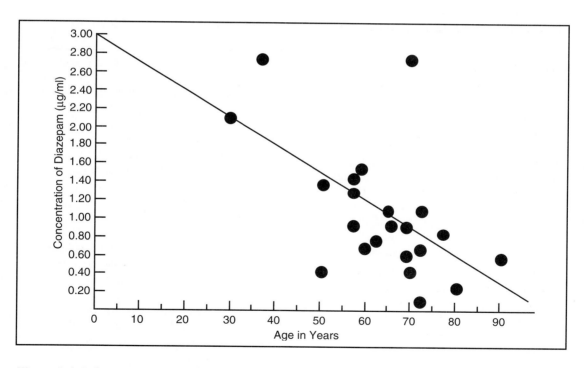

Figure 2-4. Relationship between age and serum diazepam concentration that causes failure to respond to vocal but not painful stimuli. Modified from: Reidenberg MM, et al.: "Relationships between diazepam dose, plasma level, and central nervous system depression." Clinical Pharmacology and Therapeutics, 23:371-374, 1978.

DEFINING INAPPROPRIATE MEDICATION USE

Inappropriate medication use includes excessive use, underuse, and improper dosing or duration of therapy. Defining inappropriate therapy is not always straightforward. Ideal or acceptable treatment goals are often controversial or poorly understood (e.g., the treatment of hypercholesterolemia in the elderly), and what is "appropriate" for a middle-aged patient may be undesirable for the nursing home resident.

The challenges of defining criteria for inappropriate medication use in nursing home residents have been underscored by the re-

sults of a recent study that employed a national panel of experts to reach a consensus on published guidelines for the use of medication in the elderly population. Table 2-2 lists the selected criteria for inappropriate medication. The panelists were able to reach consensus on many aspects of medication use, but they could not reach an agreement on a wide range of pharmacotherapeutic issues, including:

- The appropriateness of antipsychotic medication use in nonpsychotic patients
- The use of diphenhydramine as a hypnotic agent, and the safety of cimetidine relative to other H_2-receptor antagonists

Table 2-2. Selected Criteria for Inappropriate Drug Use in the Nursing Home

Drug Name or Class	Statement
Sedative-hypnotics	
Long-acting benzodiazepines: chlordiazepoxide, diazepam, flurazepam	Avoid all use; use short-acting benzodiazepines if needed
Meprobamate	Avoid use except in those already addicted
Oxazepam	Avoid any dose greater than 30 mg
Short-acting benzodiazepines	Avoid use for more than 4 weeks
Short-duration barbiturates: phenobarbital, secobarbital	Avoid all use except in those already addicted; safer sedative-hypnotics are available
Triazolam	Avoid any single dose greater than 0.25 mg
Antidepressants	
Amitriptyline	Avoid all use; use a less anticholinergic antidepressant if needed
Combination antidepressants-antipsychotics, e.g., amitriptyline-perphenazine (Triavil)	Avoid all use; if needed, prescribe individual components at proper geriatric doses; avoid amitriptyline
Antipsychotics	
Haloperidol	Avoid oral doses greater than 3 mg/day; residents with known psychotic disorders may require higher doses
Thioridazine	Avoid doses greater than 30 mg/day; residents with known psychotic disorders may require higher doses
Antihypertensives	
Hydrochlorothiazide	Avoid doses greater than 50 mg/day
Methyldopa	Avoid all use; safer antihypertensives are available
Propranolol	Avoid use except if used to control violent behaviors; other beta-blockers offer less CNS penetration or more beta selectivity

Table 2-2. Selected Criteria for Inappropriate Drug Use in the Nursing Home–*Cont'd*

Drug Name or Class	Statement
NSAIDs	
Phenylbutazone	Avoid all use; other NSAIDs are less toxic
Oral Hypoglycemics	
Chlorpropamide	Avoid all use; other hypoglycemics have shorter half-lives and do not cause SIADH
Analgesics	
Propoxyphene	Avoid all use; other analgesics are safer and more effective
Pentazocine	Avoid all use; other analgesics are safer and more effective
Platelet Inhibitors	
Dipyridamole	Avoid all use; effectiveness at low doses is in doubt; toxic reaction is high at higher doses; aspirin is a better alternative
H2 Blockers	
Cimetidine	Reevaluate doses greater than 900 mg/day and therapy beyond 12 weeks
Ranitidine	Reevaluate doses greater than 300 mg/day and therapy beyond 12 weeks
Antibiotics	
Oral antibiotics	Avoid therapy for more than 4 weeks except when treating osteomyelitis, prostatitis, tuberculosis, or endocarditis
Decongestants	Avoid daily use for more than 2 weeks
Iron	Avoid doses greater than 325 mg/day; does not substantially increase iron absorption and increases side effects
Muscle relaxants-antispasmodics	
Cyclobenzaprine, orphenidrate, methocarbamol, carisoprodol	Avoid all use; the potential for toxic reaction is greater than the potential benefit
GI antispasmodics	Avoid all long-term use; the potential for toxic reaction is greater than the potential benefit
Antiemetics	Avoid all use

CNS–central nervous system; GI–gastrointestinal; SIADH–syndrome of inappropriate antidiuretic hormone secretion.

RECOGNIZING AND PREVENTING ADVERSE DRUG EFFECTS IN ELDERLY NURSING HOME RESIDENTS

Adverse drug effects can mimic almost any clinical syndrome in geriatric medicine. While clinicians are most familiar with mental status changes as adverse effects of psychoactive drugs in the elderly, equally important are the somatic side effects that can be caused by many drugs. For example, anticholinergic toxicity can be responsible for numerous symptoms apparently unrelated to the indication for which the drug was prescribed (Table 2-3). Drugs with strong anticholinergic properties range from antiarrhythmics to allergy medications to antipsychotic drugs.

The diagnosis of drug-induced illness in elderly residents is sometimes complicated by

Table 2-3. Anticholinergic Toxicity in Elderly Patients*

Mechanism	Symptom	Possible Misinterpretation or Adverse Consequences
Reduction in salivation	Dry mouth	Loss of appetite, trouble swallowing food, ill-fitting dentures
Reduction in gastrointestinal motility	Constipation	Gastrointestinal tract workup, overuse of laxatives
Disordered acetylcholine in transmission in central nervous system	Confusion	Unnecessary dementia workup, mislabeling as senility, treatment of symptoms with another drug
Reduction of impulses needed to contract detrusor muscle of bladder	Urinary retention with or without overflow	Diagnosis of prostatic obstruction or urinary incontinence, unnecessary treatment with prostatectomy or drug therapy, continuation of urinary symptoms

*Drugs with anticholinergic potential include disopyramide; antipsychotic medications, particularly low-potency drugs such as chlorpromazine and thioridazine; tricyclic antidepressants; and belladonna-type drugs (e.g., atropine).

the tendency of residents, families, and even health care providers to mislabel new symptoms as signs of just growing old. As a result, drug-induced incontinence, confusion, fatigue, depression, and many other remediable sufferings are misattributed to the aging process, when they may well be amenable to appropriate diagnosis through a careful review of the resident's medication regimen. A useful antidote to these problems is a very high index of suspicion for drug-induced illness in nursing home residents. A principle of geriatric clinical pharmacology that is of great clinical use and forms an excellent starting point for the evaluation of the older patient may be stated as follows: "Any symptom in an elderly patient may be a drug side effect until proved otherwise."

CLINICAL STRATEGIES

Admission to a nursing home facility presents an ideal opportunity for a comprehensive drug regimen review. The elderly in general are at risk for accumulating many layers of drug therapy as they go through life, often from physician to physician. The setting from which they are admitted must be considered during their medication review:

From the hospital. The need for careful scrutiny of the medication regimen is probably greatest for residents who enter the nursing home following hospitalization, where additional medications have been added to treat acute problems, even though their indication may not persist beyond the hospital stay.

From the community. For residents entering a nursing home from the community, a different, potential problem exists in that as many as 50% have not adhered to medication regimens as prescribed. The administration of every medication dose that the resident was thought to be taking conscientiously before admission can result in toxicity in those who in fact had been noncompliant.

Therapeutic Untrial

One maneuver with a very useful diagnostic as well as therapeutic potential is the therapeutic untrial of a medication of dubious value that is currently in a resident's regimen. Medications used for symptomatic relief (e.g., for insomnia) are fairly easy to taper because their removal does not usually put the resident at any significant medical risk. However, even this must be done carefully, as chronic benzodiazepine users are at risk for withdrawal symptoms that can occur after acute discontinuation of the drug.

More challenging is the reassessment of medications that may be vital to the resident's health or, alternatively, may be presenting a risk of toxicity with no therapeutic benefit; examples include digoxin, diuretics, antiarrhythmics, antihypertensives, and anticonvulsants. Very often, these agents will have been prescribed many years previously for reasons that were either poorly documented or transitory (e.g., digoxin for mild congestive heart failure following a myocardial infarction or phenytoin for a poorly described seizure). Some clinicians will argue that if a resident is stable and in no overt distress, it is too risky to change a regimen by removing drugs that may not be needed. However, it often is not appreciated that any chronically administered medication with no continuing indication poses the risk of potential toxicity to the resident.

The stable, supervised setting of the nursing home allows slow, cautious withdrawal of medications from residents in whom no clear ongoing indication is evident. It is possible to observe closely for simple clinical signs

that the drug may indeed be necessary and should be restored to the regimen. (Examples include weight gain indicating the development of congestive heart failure, suggesting the need to restore a diuretic, or a progressive increase in blood pressure, indicating the need to reinstitute an antihypertensive.) Table 2-4 summarizes the guidelines for prescribing drug therapy to nursing home residents.

CASE EXAMPLE

Mr. P. is an 83-year-old man who was transferred to a nursing home following a hospital admission for exacerbation of congestive heart failure. His past medical history is significant for degenerative joint disease involving the knees and hips, and open-angle glaucoma. Reasons for nursing home admission include increasing functional difficulties relating to osteoarthritis and the need for increased su-

Table 2-4. Guidelines for Prescribing Drugs to Nursing Home Residents

— On admission take a careful drug history, including any use of over-the-counter medications.

— Become familiar with the effects of age on the pharmacology of the drugs prescribed.

— Strive to make a diagnosis before treatment.

— In general, use smaller initial doses in the elderly.

— Adjust the dose according to the resident's response.

— Review the drugs in the treatment plan regularly and simplify the therapeutic regimen whenever possible.

— Be alert to the possibility of drug-induced illness and that of interactions between disease states and drugs.

pervision with prescribed cardiovascular medications. Prescribed medications as summarized in the hospital discharge summary include: digoxin 0.25 mg; furosemide, 40 mg; and KCl elixir, 20 mEq (each taken orally every day); ibuprofen, 600 mg orally four times a day; misoprostol, 200 mcg four times a day; timolol, 0.25% one drop to each eye twice a day; oxazepam, 15 mg orally every night; and dioctyl sodium sulfosuccinate, 100 mg orally twice a day. Careful questioning of the resident indicates that he is receiving many more medications than he had ever taken in the past. Before hospitalization, he was receiving only digoxin, furosemide, KCl elixir, ibuprofen, and the timolol eye drops. He reports no history of peptic ulcer disease. He has had recent difficulties with sleeping and loose stools, but did not experience these problems before hospitalization. When asked about his glaucoma therapy, Mr. P. stated that he often instilled two to three drops in each eye once a day to avoid the inconvenience of twice daily administrations.

The case of Mr. P. makes several important points regarding pharmacotherapy in nursing home residents. It is not uncommon for elderly patients to accumulate many new drug treatments during the course of an acute hospitalization. At the time of nursing home admission, carefully scrutinize the treatment plan with a goal of simplification whenever possible. Based on Mr. P.'s history and the complaint of loose stools in the absence of fecal impaction, it is obvious that he does not require a stool softener and this treatment can be discontinued. In addition, another medication in this resident's drug regimen (misoprostol) may be contributing to this complaint.

Although the choice of oxazepam (a short elimination half-life benzodiazepine) as a hypnotic is a good choice for elderly patients due to its favorable pharmacokinetic profile, avoid long-term use for any hypnotic therapy. Try nonpharmacologic approaches to improve sleep before resorting to drug therapy. A program to promote good sleep hygiene should include the limitation of daytime napping and maintenance of regular bedtimes. Environmental strategies include the use of a bed only for sleeping and a comfortable bedroom temperature. Other nonpharmacologic strategies include the omission of caffeine-containing beverages after midday, gentle exercise, and a light evening snack (see Chapter 6, Sleep Disorders).

When drug therapy is deemed absolutely necessary, there are sometimes safer alternatives to the medications that a newly admitted resident has been receiving. Mr. P. has been treated with chronic NSAID therapy with ibuprofen. In some patients, NSAID therapy can produce damage to the gastric mucosa ranging from superficial erosions to ulcer craters and severe hemorrhage. Many NSAIDs have topical irritative effects on the mucosa, but their ulcerogenic effects are more likely the result of systemic inhibition of prostaglandin production. The elderly may be at a particularly increased risk for the development of gastrointestinal toxicity following NSAID therapy. The inhibition of renal prostaglandin synthesis by NSAIDs can also place residents at risk for impairment of renal function and exacerbation of CHF.

Because of the iatrogenic nature of these disorders, the most prudent approach is to limit NSAID therapy to those clinical situations in which it is absolutely required and to prescribe the lowest feasible dose for the shortest time necessary to achieve the desired therapeutic effect. Alternative safer analgesic therapies are available and effective for many residents. These include acetaminophen and nonacetylated salicylates (e.g., Disalcid). One study comparing the analgesic effects of acetaminophen (4 g/day) to ibuprofen (1.2 g and 2.4 g/day) in patients with osteoarthritis found no difference in pain relief in patients treated with acetaminophen compared with those given NSAID therapy.

For the rare situation in which continued NSAID therapy is required despite a history of documented NSAID-associated ulceration, prophylactic treatment with misoprostol, an analogue of prostaglandin E_1, may be indicated. In the United States, misoprostol is approved for the prevention of NSAID-induced gastric ulcers in patients at high risk. It is costly as a primary preventive therapy for NSAID-induced gastrointestinal bleeding, and routine clinical prophylaxis with this agent is not justified. It may be cost-effective as secondary prevention in patients with a history of documented peptic ulcer disease who must be maintained on NSAID therapy. Diarrhea is very frequent with full-dose treatment with misoprostol (as was the case for Mr. P.) and can limit the ability of patients to tolerate this prophylactic therapy.

For residents entering a nursing home from the community, a potential problem exists in that as many as half have not adhered to medication regimens as prescribed. Mr. P.'s history indicates a problem with nonadherence in relation to the topical beta blocker therapy prescribed for treatment of glaucoma (timolol).

Glaucoma is an insidious and disabling disease that affects over 4% of patients 80 years of age or older. (Prevalence is probably even higher in the nursing home population.) Used properly, topical therapy reduces intraocular pressure and reduces the risk of visual impairment and eventual blindness. Although topical agents used to treat glaucoma are used for their local effect on the eye, considerable systemic absorption may occur with consequent systemic side effects. The drug enters the systemic circulation by drainage into the lacrimal ducts with subsequent absorption through the vascular mucosa of the nasopharynx.

Systemic absorption of ophthalmic beta blockers affects the cardiovascular system through beta-1 blockade. Such a blockade can lead to a reduction in cardiac contractility and potentially an exacerbation of congestive heart failure. The risk of such adverse effects is reduced by using the medication according to the prescribed dosage and by occluding the lacrimal puncta with gentle finger pressure for 5 minutes after application of the drug to limit systemic absorption.

3
Infection

Marsha Goodwin-Beck, RNC, MA, MSN
Thomas T. Yoshikawa, MD

Infection refers to the invasion and multiplication of microorganisms in body tissues, which may be clinically inapparent or may result in local cellular injury due to competitive metabolism, toxins, intracellular replication, or antigen-antibody response. The infection may remain localized, subclinical, and temporary if the body's defensive mechanisms are effective; or it may persist and spread by extension to become an acute, subacute, or chronic clinical infection or disease state. A local infection may also become systemic when the microorganisms gain access to the lymphatic or vascular system.

Age-related changes in the immune system, in concert with chronic disease, place the frail elderly nursing home resident at great risk for infection. A complicating factor is institutionalization, which may encourage the acquisition and spread of infectious disease.

It is estimated that 5% to 10% of nursing home residents have some type of infection at any given time (prevalence), and that five to 15 new infections develop for every 1000 resident-days (incidence). In 75% of cases, the urinary tract, respiratory tract, or skin/soft tissue will be the infection site.

The responsibility of the clinician is to evaluate the resident's clinical status and type of infection to determine whether the situation can be treated successfully in the nursing home setting or if acute care hospitalization is required.

OVERVIEW

The types and causes of infection among nursing home residents are well documented. Approximately 75% of all infections are attributable to urinary tract infection (UTI), pneumonia, or skin/soft tissue infection, with the distribution by site as follows:

- Urinary tract (25% to 50%)
- Respiratory tract (20% to 40%)
- Skin/soft tissue (10% to 20%)
- Gastrointestinal (5% to 15%)
- Other sites (5% to 10%)

Because most infectious diseases occurring among nursing home residents are acute illnesses, they generally cause a rapid change in the resident's status. Initial manifestations may include changes in functional performance, delirium (an acute confusional state), or various nonspecific complaints.

Infection is characteristically, but not always, accompanied by fever. Twenty-five percent to 30% percent of frail, elderly residents with a serious infectious disease do not run a temperature, so the absence of fever does not preclude the possibility of infection. Older persons—especially thin, frail, debilitated individuals—also often have lower body temperatures (e.g., 96°F to 97°F). When they become infected and respond with a significant temperature rise (≈2.4°F), the recording still falls short of the range usually associated with fever (100°F to 101°F). Therefore, given the lower baseline body temperature of many nursing home residents, if an unexplained temperature rise of at least 2.4°F occurs, or if a body temperature higher than 100°F is recorded on more than one occasion, proceed on the assumption that a serious infection is present until clinical evidence proves otherwise.

CONFIRMING THE PRESENCE OF INFECTION

The following sections describe how to confirm the presence of infection in nursing home residents.

Initial Evaluation Results

Infection may be present if the initial evaluation reveals any of the following conditions:

- A rise in body temperature of at least 2.4°F from baseline or a body temperature higher than 100°F
- The presence of delirium (acute confusional state)
- Rapid major change (worsening) in function in activities of daily living (ADLs)
- Loss of appetite, new or worsening acute urinary incontinence, cough, increased respiratory rate, falls, loose stools
- A fall in blood pressure or a rise in pulse rate
- A fall with no previous history of falling
  In addition, also consider infection if a resi-

dent has a stage 2, 3, or 4 pressure ulcer and develops a fever, decline in cognitive status, or a decline in ADL function.

Physical Examination Results

The presence of infection is strongly suggested if physical evaluation reveals any of the following conditions:

- Postural hypotension, a rise in pulse rate from baseline, or a respiratory rate increase
- Change (worsening) in cognitive patterns
- Lung consolidation or rales or wheezes or sputum production
- New heart murmur, or peripheral signs of endocarditis or splenomegaly
- Abdominal guarding, rigidity, or tenderness
- Rectal tenderness, or a scrotal mass
- Pressure ulcer (change in drainage, odor, or color); skin inflammation (redness, tenderness, edema and/or heat)
- New focal neurologic findings (e.g., seizure, neck rigidity)

Laboratory Test Results

Pursue laboratory examination according to the resident's symptoms and signs. The presence of infection is supported or confirmed if any of the following conditions are met:

- Elevated peripheral white blood cell (WBC) count and a left shift of WBC differential count
- WBCs and bacteria on urinalysis
- Infiltrate and effusion on chest radiograph
- Low oxygen saturation on arterial blood gas
- Blood cultures growing organisms
- Fecal WBCs on Gram's stain of stool
- New positive (or conversion of) tuberculin skin test

TREATING THE INFECTION

In any nursing home resident with suspected infection, the first responsibility is to determine whether the resident's clinical status and type of infection warrant acute care hospitalization. The decision-making process requires the caregivers to do the following:

- Determine any change in the resident's vital signs
- Assess the overall clinical appearance of the resident (toxic, diaphoretic [profuse perspiration], shivering, agitated, confused, dyspneic [labored breathing], and other signs)
- Examine the resident for evidence of sepsis, pneumonia, acute UTI, soft tissue infections, infective endocarditis, etc.
- Obtain a chest radiograph, urinalysis, complete blood count (CBC), serum electrolytes, renal function tests, electrocardiogram (ECG), and oxygen saturation or arterial blood gas, if available or obtainable

Indications for Acute Care Hospitalization

Consider evaluation for infection in the acute care hospital if any of the following indications are present and are not responsive to routine protocols:

- Unstable vital signs
- Resident appears toxic, diaphoretic, more confused, dyspneic, or cyanotic
- Presence of new gross purulence or moderate to severe cellulitis at site of pressure ulcer
- Most cases of pneumonia (see the section on Managing Pneumonia for those strains treatable in nursing homes)
- Discovery of new heart murmur consistent with infective endocarditis (e.g., diastolic murmur, conjunctival petechiae, Roth's spots [small retinal hemorrhages with central white areas], Osler's nodes, splenomegaly)
- Possible intraabdominal sepsis with abdominal pain, tenderness, guarding, and vomiting
- New focal neurologic findings consistent with central nervous system (CNS) infection
- Unexplained fever with indwelling bladder catheter
- Infection associated with evidence of cardiovascular disease on ECG (e.g., arrhythmia, ischemia) or significant renal impairment
- Radiographic evidence of active pulmonary tuberculosis

Infections Treatable in the Nursing Home

The following infections are generally treated with excellent results in the nursing home setting:

- UTI in a clinically stable resident (stable vital signs; nontoxic; no active underlying illness)
- Pneumonia in a clinically stable resident if:
  - 24-hour licensed nurse monitoring is available
  - A physician is available on short notice at all times
  - The resident is able to eat and drink adequately to maintain nutrition and hydration or parenteral/tube feeding/hydration can be administered in the nursing home
  - The resident is not bacteremic by blood culture
  - Laboratory support and radiography are readily available
  - There is no serious hypoxemia ($PO_2 < 60$ mm Hg), hypercapnia ($PCO_2 > 40$ mm Hg), or acidosis (pH<7.35)
  - There is oxygen, suctioning, and other supportive and emergency equipment available
  - The infection can be treated with oral/intramuscular antibiotics or parenteral therapy can be administered in the nursing home
- Infected pressure ulcers that require little or no surgical debridement, are not grossly purulent, or do not have associated osteomyelitis, large amounts of drainage, or extensive cellulitis
- Localized cellulitis without clinical evidence of sepsis or toxicity
- Mild gastroenteritis
- Tuberculin skin test conversion without ac-

tive pulmonary tuberculosis

MANAGING URINARY TRACT INFECTION

Use the procedures in the following sections to govern disease management of UTIs.

Specimen Collection

To collect specimens from noncatheterized residents:

- In men who are circumcised, first-voided urine is adequate. In uncircumcised men, cleanse the glans penis before collecting a first-voided specimen. (*Note:* A clean-catch midstream urinary specimen is not necessary for uncircumcised men. Uncircumcised men should have the penile foreskin retracted and glans penis cleansed.)
- In women, cleanse the perineum and obtain a midstream urine sample.
- For residents who have dementia, are unable to follow directions, or are uncooperative, consider catching the specimen in a sterile urine hat or bedpan after cleansing the perineum.
- Insert a catheter to obtain a specimen only if absolutely necessary.

To collect specimens from catheterized residents:

- Replace the old catheter and tubing if they have been in place for more than 30 days. However, many experts do not recommend changing catheters for diagnostic specimens until 30 days have elapsed. Obtain a urine specimen from the newly inserted catheter. (*Note:* Catheters that are in place for more than 2 to 3 weeks will quickly become colonized with organisms, contaminating any urine obtained from the bladder.)

Diagnostic Criteria

The diagnostic criteria to manage UTIs are:

- Urinalysis showing on Gram's stain more than one bacteria per field in almost every field on high-power or oil-immersion objective. Pyuria (more than five WBCs per high-power field) supports the diagnosis.
- Urine culture yielding 100,000 or more colonies/mL of an organism consistent with a uropathogen (e.g., *Escherichia coli, Klebsiella* sp., *Proteus* sp., *Enterococcus faecalis*). (*Note:* There is a 75% to 80% correlation between the presence of more than one bacteria per field on smear and 100,000 or more colonies of bacteria/mL urine by culture. Urine obtained from freshly inserted catheters may have significant bacteriuria with bacterial counts of less than 100,000/ mL.)
- Urine culture yielding less than 100,000 or more colonies/mL of an organism consistent with a *uropathogen.* In order to be considered an infection, this should be accompanied by fever, burning when urine passes, increased frequency of urination, or the feeling of a constant need to void.

Treatment

Follow these guidelines to treat UTIs:

- Based on sensitivity data, use an antibiotic to treat women for 7 to 10 days and men for 10 to 14 days. One of the following will be an effective agent:
  - Trimethoprim-sulfamethoxazole (Bactrim or Septra), one double-strength tablet (160 mg/800 mg) twice daily (for renal function with creatinine clearance of 30 mL/min or more)
  - An oral cephalosporin (e.g., cefadroxil [Duricef], 500 mg daily)
  - Amoxicillin-clavulanic acid (Augmentin), 250 mg/250 mg (one tablet) three times a day
  - A quinolone (e.g., ciprofloxacin [Cipro], 250 to 500 mg [one tablet] twice daily)
- If urgent therapy is indicated before culture data are available, start treatment with any one of the these agents. Start residents with

recurrent UTI or those on recent antibiotics on a quinolone (e.g., Cipro) because of the high probability of finding drug-resistant uropathogens.

Notes: Because men may have a coexisting occult prostate infection, a slightly longer duration of therapy is recommended (10 to 14 days), although the efficacy of this regimen has not been documented. Treat acute bacterial prostatitis with antibiotics for at least 3 to 4 weeks; chronic bacterial prostatitis requires a minimum of 4 weeks of antibiotics, and occasionally for periods up to 3 months. Following empiric therapy, use culture and sensitivity data to make any necessary changes in drug therapy. For residents with an indwelling catheter, treat for 10 days.

Pyridium (phenazopyridine hydrochloride) exerts a topical analgesic effect on the mucosa of the urinary tract. In conjunction with antibiotic treatment of a UTI, Pyridium may reduce the discomfort and pain during the period before the antibiotic controls the infection. However, the benefit of Pyridium for treating a UTI lasts for *no more than 2 days*. Because it is not recommended for more than 2 days, the value of Pyridium must be questioned. This drug also has undesirable side effects, such as orange discoloration of urine (may stain fabric); it may interfere with spectrometry or color reactions of tests on urine; and it tends to accumulate in patients with renal dysfunction (especially elderly patients) and may cause methemoglobinemia.

Monitoring and Follow-Up

To monitor and follow up on the progress of a UTI:

- Nursing staff should assess for improvement in vital signs, mentation, functional status, appetite, urinary symptoms, and general well-being. Increased assistance in ADLs during the period of infection may be required as well as safety measures to prevent falls (*see* Chapter 18, Falls).

- If a catheter is in place, note any changes in the appearance of urine (e.g., less cloudy).
- With clinical improvement within 24 to 48 hours, repeat urine culture can be delayed for 2 or 3 days following completion of antibiotic therapy.
- If the resident fails to improve in 24 to 48 hours, reassess for other potential infections and obtain a repeat urinalysis and culture.
- Measures that reduce bacterial replication or hasten bacterial removal from the urinary tract may decrease the duration of symptoms and improve the therapeutic outcome in noncatheterized residents with UTI. These measures include urinary acidification (e.g., with cranberry juice), hydration, and frequent voiding.

Note: To be effective in acidifying the urine, large amounts of ascorbic acid (vitamin C) or cranberry juice must be ingested. The antibacterial effect of cranberry juice may be due to production of benzoic acid from quinic acid by bacteria in the gut. Benzoic acid is then absorbed from the bowel and converted to hippuric acid by conjugation with glycine in the liver. The antibacterial effect of cranberry juice may be more related to volume of fluid intake. In addition, components of cranberry juice may prevent adherence of bacteria to uroepithelium.

- Residents *without catheters* or major genitourinary tract abnormalities (e.g., renal calculi or atonic bladder) who experience recurrent UTI may be similarly treated with urinary acidification (including vitamin C), hydration, regular bladder emptying, and good personal hygiene (in women). If these measures fail, try a daily bedtime dosage of an appropriate antibiotic (e.g., half a tablet of trimethoprim [Trimpex] 50 mg), or try half a tablet of trimethoprim-sulfamethoxazole (Bactrim or Septra), 40 mg/200 mg for 3 to 6 months.
- Chronically catheterized residents will *always* be bacteriuric, regardless of any inter-

ventions including instilling urinary antiseptics and administering systemic antibiotics (which sterilize urine transiently for only 2 to 4 weeks).

- Residents with chronic *asymptomatic* bacteriuria do not always require treatment, but should be monitored carefully for the development of fever or other symptoms of UTI.

MANAGING PNEUMONIA

Use the procedures in the following sections to govern disease management of pneumonia.

Diagnostic Criteria

The criteria for diagnosing pneumonia are:
- A chest radiograph showing new infiltrate with or without effusion.
- A sputum Gram's stain showing more than 25 WBCs and less than 10 epithelial cells per lower-power field (x10 objective, x100 magnification), which indicates that the expectorated specimen is more likely to be lower respiratory tract secretions than saliva.
- A sputum Gram's stain showing predominantly one type of organism (e.g., gram-positive coccus or gram-negative bacillus), and sputum culture yielding a respiratory pathogen.
- A negative purified protein derivitive (PPD) tuberculin skin test (if positive, order sputum for mycobacterial studies).
- Leukocytosis and/or a left shift of the WBC count.

Notes: Sputum is often difficult to obtain in nursing home residents because of disability or the inability to cooperate. Expectorated specimens are often primarily saliva and contaminated by mouth flora, so they are of limited diagnostic value. Aggressive diagnostic maneuvers, such as transtracheal aspiration or bronchoscopy, are not indicated for these residents. Frail elderly residents may fail to show leukocytosis, but a left shift of the white blood cell count is consistently present with serious bacterial infections.

Treatment

Follow these guidelines to treat pneumonia:
- If the sputum smear is adequate, select an antibiotic based on Gram's stain findings and any underlying illness that may impact on etiology or treatment of pneumonia (e.g., chronic obstructive lung disease), as well as drug allergies (e.g., to penicillins).
- If the sputum smear is not available or is nondiagnostic, begin empiric therapy based on the most likely etiology, underlying disease factors, and drug tolerance by the resident. Oral drug regimens to consider include one of the following:
  - Cefuroxime axetil (Ceftin), 250 to 500 mg twice daily
  - Amoxicillin, 500 mg, with clavulanic acid, 250 mg (Augmentin), one tablet three times a day
  - Ciprofloxacin (Cipro), 500 to 750 mg twice daily (or other equivalent quinolone, such as ofloxacin [Floxin] or lomefloxacin [Maxaquin] with or without amoxicillin, 500 mg three times a day
  - Trimethoprim-sulfamethoxazole (Bactrim DS, Septra DS), one double-strength (160/800 mg) tablet twice daily
- If parenteral drugs can be administered, consider one of the following drug regimens:
  - Cefonicid (Monocid), 1 g every 12 hours
  - Ceftriaxone (Rocephin), 1 g every 12 hours
  - Cefoperazone (Cefobid), 1 g every 12 hours
  - Supplemental oxygen
  - Adequate fluid and nutrition intake.
- Encourage coughing with deep breathing to remove secretions. The value of chest physiotherapy is inconclusive; however, if the resident has large volumes of sputa, and

is able to tolerate chest percussion and dependent drainage, try this intervention.

- Encourage residents to begin gradual levels of exercise (e.g., chair to ambulation) during day hours. Position the residents to minimize aspiration.
- Residents with certain types of highly resistant bacteria causing their pneumonia (or any other infection) should be managed using careful infection control measures (i.e., regular hand washing, wearing gloves to examine residents and handle specimens). The most serious organisms are multidrug-resistant *Pseudomonas aeruginosa* and methicillin-resistant *Staphylococcus aureus*. Respiratory isolation is generally unnecessary for these pathogens since transmission is primarily by contact and not inhalation.

Monitoring and Follow-Up

To monitor and follow up on the progress of residents with pneumonia:

- Assess the clinical status, functional status, feeling of well-being, and respiratory function (chest examination, respiratory rate).
- Determine daily intake and output and weigh the resident every other day to maintain good hydration and adequate nutrition. Daily intake should exceed total output (in urine, feces, sputum) by at least 1000 mL. *Any weight loss* during pneumonia therapy is cause for alarm, indicating either poor nutrition, dehydration, or both.

Note: Normal daily insensible water loss (through breathing, sweating, and evaporation) averages approximately 1000 mL. Residents with pneumonia can expect to lose more than 1000 mL/day if they are febrile, breathing rapidly, or coughing. Infection also raises the metabolic rate and pneumonia (inflammation, tissue necrosis) can result in a catabolic state.

- Repeat a chest radiograph 2 to 3 days after

starting antibiotics and after completion of therapy.

If the clinical status deteriorates or fails to improve in 48 to 72 hours, or a repeat chest radiograph shows significant progression of pneumonia, hospitalize the resident.

MANAGING INFECTED PRESSURE ULCERS

Use the procedures in the following sections to govern management of infected pressure ulcers.

Diagnostic Criteria

The criteria for diagnosing infected pressure ulcers are:

- Classify the ulcer based on the extent of tissue involvement; note the presence of purulence, devitalized tissue, and cellulitis; measure the size of the lesion. *See* Chapter 22, Pressure Ulcers, for a discussion on how to complete classification and measurement.
- All open wounds are contaminated with bacteria as a result of losing protection from the skin covering. Therefore, *surface swabs for culturing have little diagnostic value*. Obtain specimens for culture if there is an indication for antibiotic treatment, i.e., purulence, cellulitis, osteomyelitis, and sepsis. With purulence or cellulitis, suitable specimen collection techniques include aspiration of drainage material or needle aspiration of the ulcer margin through intact skin. These procedures are performed easily by the attending physician or nurse practitioners. If osteomyelitis is suspected, consult an infectious disease specialist and surgeon for a biopsy of deep tissue or bone. All specimens should be Gram's stained and cultured for anaerobes and aerobes.

Treatment

Follow these guidelines to treat infected pressure ulcers:

- Gram's stain results of purulent drainage or

ulcer margin, or tissue or bone biopsy will be useful to guide initial antimicrobial therapy. However, in the absence of such a specimen or if the Gram's stain is nondiagnostic, it can be anticipated that infected *chronic* pressure ulcers of stage 2 or greater severity will be infected with a mixture of anaerobes and aerobes. Start empiric antibacterial therapy and continue for at least 2 weeks' duration for ulcers associated with purulence, cellulitis, and sepsis. If osteomyelitis is documented, extend the therapy for a minimum of 4 to 6 weeks depending on the extent and severity of the bone infection.

- Oral antibiotic therapy for early stage 1 or 2 lesions associated with cellulitis, or stage 2 lesions associated with purulence will often include one of the following:
  ○ Amoxicillin-clavulanic acid, 500 mg/250 mg, (Augmentin), one tablet three times a day
  ○ Clindamycin (Cleocin), 150 to 300 mg three times a day
  ○ A cephalosporin (e.g., cephalexin [Keflex], 500 mg three times a day) or a quinolone (e.g. ciprofloxacin [Cipro], 500 to 750 mg twice a day)
- With deeper ulcers (Stage 3 or 4 lesions) mixed anaerobic-aerobic organisms are highly likely. Empiric oral therapy for these ulcers that are associated with gross purulence (often abscess), cellulitis, or osteomyelitis may be treated with combination regimens, e.g., clindamycin (Cleocin), 150 to 300 mg three times a day or metronidazole (Flagyl), 500 mg four times a day, plus a quinolone, e.g., ciprofloxacin (Cipro), 500 to 750 mg twice a day.

Note: If osteomyelitis is suspected or documented, avoid therapy until a bone biopsy for culture can be done. A definitive etiologic diagnosis may avoid 4 to 6 weeks of two antibiot-

ics, which may cause superinfection, antibiotic-associated colitis, and adverse drug reactions.

- Appropriate local treatment of pressure ulcers (*see* Chapter 22, Pressure Ulcers).
- Adequate nutrition with supplemental enteral alimentation as well as multivitamins and zinc.
- Relieve pressure; eliminate moisture and contamination (urine, feces); avoid friction and shear forces.

Monitoring and Follow-Up

To monitor and follow up on the progress of residents with infected pressure ulcers:

- Assess the resident for any systemic symptoms, functional status changes, or changes in vital signs (especially temperature).
- Examine the ulcer daily and note any changes in size, drainage, purulence, heat, redness, and other changes. Continue local ulcer care.
- Watch for antibiotic side effects, particularly diarrhea and antibiotic-associated colitis. Notify the physician if any of these effects appear. Stop the antibiotics if the diarrhea is severe.

Note: Send stool samples to the lab for a *Clostridium difficile* culture and toxin assay if diarrhea develops.

CASE EXAMPLE

Mrs. Lydia P. is an 81-year-old resident who has moderate short-term memory impairment. She requires limited assistance with bathing, dressing, toileting, and ambulating, but eats independently. On occasion she is incontinent of urine. Her medical diagnoses include adult-onset diabetes mellitus, osteoarthritis, peripheral vascular disease, and dementia. Medications are glyburide (Micronase), 5 mg daily, and sulindac (Clinoril), 150 mg twice daily. Her skin is dry and flaky on both legs, but her overall skin condition is good. Vital signs are normally: temperature (T) 97.2°F; blood pressure (BP) 130/80 to 140/88 mm Hg; pulse (P) 70 to 80 beats per minute and regular; respiration (R) 12 to 16 breaths per minute.

One morning at breakfast, a nurse's aide noticed that Mrs. P. was not eating and seemed somewhat drowsy. She offered her a small amount of juice, which Mrs. P. took with assistance but she refused the rest of the meal. During the morning Mrs. P. became very confused, had difficulty walking even with assistance, and was incontinent of urine. A registered nurse recorded the following findings:

Mental Status
Less alert, confused
Vital Signs
Temperature: 99.2°F
Blood Pressure: 110/70
Pulse: 90 regular
Respirations: 18
Skin: warm to touch
No diaphoresis
Color: normal
No redness or breakdown
Chest: no rales or rhonchi
Abdomen: soft, no tenderness

The consulting physician ordered a urinalysis, urine culture, and blood work. Because Mrs. P. could not provide a clean catch urine sample, the registered nurse inserted a urethral catheter to obtain the urine specimen for analysis and culture. The catheter was then removed.

While awaiting the results of the urine and blood tests, the nursing staff monitored and recorded Mrs. P.'s vital signs and mental status every 4 hours and her fluid intake and output were measured during each shift. Increased fluid intake was encouraged. The nursing staff also provided additional supervision and assistance in order to prevent her from falling or becoming dehydrated. She was placed on an every-2-hour toileting program to manage incontinence and was reassured that her symptoms were probably temporary. Because she was a diabetic, her food intake and blood sugar levels were also monitored closely.

The laboratory test results showed a urinalysis with more than 25 WBCs/mm^3 in the urine and bacteria on Gram's stain smear, a normal WBC count, normal renal function tests, and blood glucose within normal range. The urinalysis findings suggested a UTI, and Mrs. P. was started on an oral antibiotic (cefadoxil, 500 mg daily for 7 days). Urine culture results 2 days later confirmed the presence of *E. coli* bacteriuria. The nursing staff continued to reassess Mrs. P.'s vital signs, mental status, ADL function, nutrition and fluid intake, and urinary output and continence on a daily basis. Her status improved in all areas within 2 days. Three days after she finished the antibiotic therapy, a midstream clean-catch urine sample was obtained for a repeat culture. The test results were negative.

4
Pulmonary Rehabilitation

Donna Colpitts, CRTT
Robert S. Crausman, MD, MMS
Pauline Belleville-Taylor RN, CS, MS
Lewis A. Lipsitz, MD

With advancing age, a person's respiratory system changes, and there is a need to distinguish between age-related decline and disease-related dysfunction. Some residents will have a long history of chronic respiratory problems. Others will have acute episodes of respiratory distress that require prompt and effective management; and still others will develop chronic respiratory problems during their stay, requiring long-term management.

In each instance, the goal is to develop a care plan that minimizes the morbidity associated with these pulmonary disorders and the untoward side effects of medical treatment. This chapter describes the assessment of respiratory distress, the diagnosis of pulmonary disease, and the appropriate therapeutic interventions to maximize the quality of life for the resident with respiratory illness.

OVERVIEW

The primary function of the lungs is to oxygenate blood and eliminate carbon dioxide. With aging, alterations occur in pulmonary mechanics, in lung tissue characteristics, and in the control of breathing.

The usual age-related changes are relatively complex. The rib cage slowly stiffens and the respiratory muscles can become deconditioned, limiting chest expansion. However, age-related loss of inward lung elastic recoil (an increase in lung compliance) generally balances these effects, so that there is probably no significant change in the maximum volume of air the lung can hold, which is referred to as *total lung capacity*. There is also a rise in the volume of air remaining in the lungs after a full expiration, and this is referred to as *residual volume*. This reduces the volume of air that can be exchanged during deep breathing—referred to as *vital capacity*. This reduction in vital capacity also limits coughing and the ability to clear airway secretions. There seems to be a gradual loss of pulmonary functional reserve, which, in combination with stresses from an acute illness, can limit one's ability to deliver adequate amounts of oxygen (O_2) to the blood and clear carbon dioxide (CO_2) from the body.

The volume of air that can be forcibly exhaled in 1 second is the *forced expiratory volume* in 1 second (FeV_1). This volume decreases at a rate of 20 to 30 mL per year after the third decade of life. The effects of smoking are dramatic, accelerating the decline in FeV_1 by three- to fourfold. The FeV_1 is a reproducible test that can be used to follow response to treatment in asthma and *chronic obstructive pulmonary disease* (COPD).

The connective tissue attachments within the pulmonary parenchyma that act to tether open the small airways at low lung volumes in youth are altered with aging so that the airways are relatively collapsible. This can result in ventilation/perfusion mismatching, atelectasis, and air trapping.

With aging, there is also a reduction in the volume of a normal breath, which is referred to as *tidal volume*. This reduction is associated with an increase in respiratory rate to maintain normal ventilation.

The concentration of O_2 achievable in the blood while breathing room air is also reduced (increased A-a gradient). Despite this reduction, the elderly resident should still maintain an O_2 hemoglobin saturation of greater than 90%. CO_2 elimination is not significantly changed in advanced age.

Finally, it is unclear what effects aging has on the control of breathing. In many elderly persons, there is a blunting of hypoxic and hypercarbic drives. Therefore, the elderly resident may not have a normal response to either hypoxia (PaO_2 levels associated with an hemoglobin saturation less than 90%) or hypercarbia (elevated $PaCO_2$ levels usually greater than 45 Torr). As a result, the subjective symptoms of dyspnea may not be present until the development of severe, late-stage disease.

COMMON MEDICAL DISEASES THAT CONTRIBUTE TO CARDIOPULMONARY LIMITATION

The high prevalence of chronic cardiac and pulmonary disease among the elderly makes it difficult to discern what is a consequence of normal aging and what is the result of concurrent disease. A variety of acute and chronic diseases may be involved in deconditioning the cardiopulmonary system. When combined with the usual age-related decline in pulmonary function, the result can be marked impairment in independent performance of activities of daily living (ADLs). Table 4-1 lists the types of respiratory problems and common acute causal factors among elderly nursing home residents.

TREATING CARDIOPULMONARY DISEASE

The following sections describe some of the treatments of cardiopulmonary diseases in elderly residents.

Smoking Cessation

All cardiopulmonary conditions are exacerbated by cigarette smoking. Fortunately, even after a lifetime of smoking, an improved airflow and decreased mucous production can be expected in the months following cessation.

Bronchodilator Therapy

Asthma responds to bronchodilator therapy, which can reduce airflow limitation, decrease the work of breathing, and improve oxygenation. Occasionally, bronchitis and emphysema (both often referred to as a COPD) have a reversible bronchospastic component that also responds. The following medications can be dispensed as handheld multidose inhalers, as nebulized solutions, and as oral tablets or time-release preparations:

- Beta-agonists (e.g., albuterol, metaproterenol, isoproterenol, and terbutaline) and anticholinergics (ipatropium bromide; Atrovent) can be very effective when administered in 2 to 4 puffs four times a day.
- Use of a spacer device with a metered dose inhaler (MDI) assists in coordinating drug administration with breathing and enhances deposition of medication in the lungs. If a

Table 4-1. Types of Respiratory Problems and Common Acute Causal Factors

Common Respiratory Problems	Typical Clinical Findings	Causal Factors
Acute-Onset		
Upper respiratory infection	Fever, coryza, dry cough, myalgias	Viral illness, influenza
Bronchitis	Productive cough, fever, dyspnea, pulmonary rhonchi, no infiltrate on CXR	Viral or bacterial illness (pneumococcal, haemophilus influenzae are most common organisms)
Asthma	Nonproductive cough, wheezing, dyspnea, decreased FeV1, that improves with a bronchodilator	Allergy, environmental exposures, infection, CHF (cardiac asthma)
Congestive heart failure	Dyspnea, orthopnea, urinary frequency, weight gain, wheezing, Hb-O_2 desaturation, pulmonary rales, and cardiac S3 gallop	Acute MI, angina, rapid arrhythmia (e.g., atrial fibrillation), cardiomyopathy, aortic stenosis, mitral regurgitation
Pneumonia	Fever, productive cough, tachypnea, Hb-O_2 desaturation, decreased breath sounds, egophony, focal rales and rhonchi on exam, pulmonary consolidation on CXR	Viral, (e.g., influenza) or bacterial (pneumococcal, Legionella pneumophila, staphylococcal, gram-negatives, or anaerobes) illness often related to aspiration, and TB

Continued

resident cannot tolerate or coordinate use of an MDI, switch to a handheld nebulizer for bronchodilators. Periodic observation of a resident's technique is important to ensure appropriate use.

- Oral theophylline preparations, despite a narrow therapeutic window, are also very effective. Monitor theophylline blood levels to ensure that they do not reach toxic ranges.
- Corticosteroids (oral or inhaled) act to decrease inflammation within the airways and can markedly improve pulmonary function in the setting of an acute exacerbation of asthma, bronchitis, or emphysema. The chronic effects of steroids are much less impressive and benefit only the minority of patients. Due to their many untoward side effects (osteoporosis, hyperglycemia, muscular weakness, depression and psychosis), reserve oral steroids as a last resort.

Consider treating residents who are being given chronic oral steroids with calcium and vitamin D to minimize osteoporosis. Inhaled

Table 4-1. Types of Respiratory Problems and Common Acute Causal Factors–*Con't*

Common Respiratory Problems	Typical Clinical Findings	Causal Factors
Chronic-onset		
Emphysema	Dyspnea on exertion, minimal cough, irreversible reduction in FeV_1, use of accessory muscles to breathe, hyperinflation of lungs (low, flattened diaphragm, bullous changes on CXR), "pink puffers" with normal or small reduction in PaO_2	Tobacco smoke, genetic predisposition, alpha-$_1$-antitrypsin deficiency, toxic gas exposure
Chronic bronchitis	Productive cough with copious sputum at least 3 months per year, often overweight and cyanotic (blue bloater) with hypoxemia and CO_2 retention, an increased hematocrit and right ventricular heart failure often develop, irreversible decline in FeV1, increased bronchovesicular markings on CXR	Smoking, familial predisposition
Bronchiectasis	Widening and destruction of segmental and subsegmental airways causing recurrent infections, chronic cough with copious purulent sputum, occasional hemoptysis, clubbing, right ventricular heart failure, hypoxia	Childhood pneumonias, severe pneumonia, TB, fungal infections, aspirations, rare immunodeficiency states, secondary hypogamma-globulinemia, rare congenital syndromes (e.g., Kartagener's, Young's syndromes)
Diffuse interstitial lung disease	Insidious development of dyspnea on exertion progressing to dyspnea at rest, minimal physical findings at outset, ground glass haziness and reticulonodular patterns on CXR, decreased lung volumes (vital capacity and TLC), and increased alveolar-arterial O_2 difference	Over 100 causes including occupational exposures (silicosis, asbestosis, berylliosis), carcinoma, irradiation, idiopathic fibrosis, vasculitis, hypersensitivity pneumonitis, sarcoidosis, drug reactions (e.g., hydralazine, busulfan, nitrofurantoin, methylsergide, cyclophosphamide, and procainamide), and pulmonary emboli

CHF, congestive heart failure; CXR, chest radiography; MI, myocardial infarction; TB, tuberculosis; TLC, total lung capacity.

steroid preparations are generally not associated with these systemic effects and are the preparations of choice. However, there is a strong relationship between inhaled steroid use and the development of oral thrush, but using a spacer device with the inhaler and good oral hygiene greatly decreases the incidence of thrush.

Residents with adequate physical dexterity and cognitive abilities can be taught to use inhalers. Inhalers (metered dose) or aerosol therapy equipment needs to be kept clean and properly stored. Nurses need to consult with the pharmacist about specific administration instructions for the various inhalants. Most residents can be taught to shake the container before administration, exhale through the nose as completely as possible, administer aerosol while breathing deeply inward through the mouth, and then hold their breath about 10 seconds before exhaling slowly. If a resident is receiving more than one inhalant, consult the package insert and pharmacist to determine the optimum timing and spacing of doses.

While controversial, many respiratory therapists recommend sequencing of inhaled medications to enhance their delivery. To do this, administer beta-agonists 10 minutes in advance of steroid or anticholinergic preparations. Theoretically, this allows the airways to dilate and improves distribution of the steroids or ipatroprium bromide subsequently given.

Chest Physiotherapy and Incentive Spirometry

Bronchiectasis and *mucous plugging* are probably the only firm indication for chest physiotherapy and postural drainage. Using incentive spirometry is a helpful adjunct to cough and deep-breathing exercises. The following sections describe chest physical therapy and the techniques to help clear secretions.

Chest Physical Therapy

Use chest physical therapy for retained secretions if the resident can tolerate it. Tolerance can often be increased by modifying the positioning or changing the percussion and vibration intensity. However, never use chest physical therapy if the resident has metastatic cancer, tuberculosis, severe osteoporosis, pulmonary embolus, degenerative spinal disease, rib fracture, hemoptysis, or chest wounds, or if anticoagulant therapy is being given. Also, do not attempt any head-down postural drainage because of general cardiac complications and the possibility of aspiration in an elderly population.

The following technique for chest physical therapy is recommended, as appropriate:

- *Positioning:* Position the resident according to the location of the infiltrate or retained secretions as follows:
  - For lower and middle lobe areas: Have the resident lay flat on his or her side in bed, or use a pillow under the head if necessary. Extend the exposed arm overhead. Lay the resident on the right side for left lung infiltrates and on the left side for right lung infiltrates.
  - For upper lobe areas: Have the resident sit in an armchair, feet flat on the floor, leaning forward with arms, upper chest, and head resting on a pillow on a bedside table.
- *Percussion and Vibration:* Percuss the affected area for a full 5 minutes as follows:
  - Vary the intensity according to resident tolerance, but too light an intensity will not be effective. Follow with two to three vibration maneuvers.
  - Percussion is performed by cupping the hands and tapping firmly on the chest wall.
  - Vibration is performed by placing one hand on top of the other and tensing the

shoulders, keeping the arms straight and performing a vibrating motion from shoulder to hand.

When the therapy is concluded, have the resident sit up and end the session with a good cough and deep-breathing exercise. Use iodine preparations to thin thick secretions and hydrate the resident by increasing fluid intake or using humidification through a nebulizer.

Clearing Secretions

The following treatment is recommended to clear secretions:

- Ask the resident to sit in a high Fowler's position in bed or, preferably, out of bed in a chair with feet on the floor.
- Have the resident take three consecutive deep breaths with good chest expansion. If necessary, have the resident imitate you, or place your hands on the resident's rib cage and instruct him or her to cause your hands to move by taking deep breaths.
- Ask the resident to take as deep a breath as possible and to expel all the air at once in a coughing maneuver, demonstrating if necessary. If the resident is unable to cough effectively, try a huffing maneuver (expelling short blasts of air, two or three times per breath).

Antibiotics

Respiratory illness is complicated frequently by pulmonary infection. Determine the choice of antibiotics by obtaining a culture and Gram's stain of sputum. However, a good empiric choice can be made and instituted in advance of receiving the results of these tests through thoughtful consideration of the likely causative organisms, institutional microbiology, and the resident's medical history. Modify this empiric choice when Gram's stain and culture results are available or as a resident's clinical status dictates. Chronic bronchitis sometimes requires continuous or cyclic suppressive therapy with broad-spectrum antibiotics, such as trimethoprim-sulfamethoxazole, amoxicillin, or a cephalosporin.

Nutritional Treatment

Nutritional considerations are very important in the resident with cardiopulmonary disease. Dyspnea can make eating a difficult task and nutritional demands difficult to meet. Residents with COPD and flat diaphragms are placed at a further mechanical disadvantage after a large meal, which can increase the work of breathing. Most residents with COPD, even when overweight, are malnourished. These residents frequently do better with several small meals composed of nutritionally dense foods. Five small meals with a high-fat, low-carbohydrate content (to lower the respiratory quotient) and vitamin supplementation are preferable to three large ones. This approach reduces the work of breathing and helps the resident gain weight, both of which may improve functional capacity.

Oxygen

Oxygen is an expensive therapy, but when properly prescribed can dramatically improve the quality of life, increase exercise tolerance, and reduce mortality. Pulse oximetry with an ear or finger oximeter is a fairly accurate noninvasive method for assessing hemoglobin oxygen saturation. A saturation of less than 90% should lead to blood gas testing and consideration of supplemental O_2. Any resident on a good medication regimen with a PaO_2 less than 50 Torr or a PaO_2 less than 55 Torr with associated polycythemia, pulmonary hypertension, or myocardial ischemia may benefit from continuous O_2 therapy. Further, those who desaturate to less then 85% with exercise or sleep may also benefit from supplemental O_2 with those activities. These residents often have normal resting measurements.

After pneumonia or a COPD exacerbation, it is not uncommon for a resident to require temporary supplemental O_2 for several weeks.

It is important to reassess these residents because they often improve and no longer require such treatment.

Any asymptomatic resident with a normal respiratory rate and saturation greater then 90% may not benefit from supplemental O_2 and need not be assessed further.

Carbon dioxide retention in a patient with COPD and decreased hypercarbic drive can occur during supplemental oxygen therapy. Normally, the body responds to elevated $PaCO_2$ by increasing the respiratory rate in order to remove excess CO_2, usually when the PCO_2 is over 45 Torr. However, in residents with chronically elevated $PaCO_2$ levels, the body responds instead to low levels of oxygen (hypoxia). If the oxygen level is increased, the stimulus to breathe is reduced and further CO_2 retention can result.

Carbon dioxide retention has potentially serious consequences. If oxygen is given to a resident who is retaining CO_2, thereby raising the oxygen level above the threshold for hypoxic drive, the respiratory rate decreases, and even though the resident appears comfortable and well oxygenated, dangerous levels of CO_2 may be building. Rising CO_2 levels act as a narcotic, slowing respiration further and eventually resulting in respiratory arrest.

For the CO_2 retainer, a further increase in $PaCO_2$ may occur during exercise. Physical exertion causes increased oxygen consumption, greater oxidative metabolism in muscles, and CO_2 production. If pulmonary disease is sufficiently severe, the lungs will be unable to ventilate off the excess CO_2, and the resident will be unable to tolerate sustained activity in the form of pulmonary rehabilitation. Fortunately, this condition usually exists only in very severe, end-stage pulmonary disease. Most residents diagnosed with a significant degree of pulmonary disease can tolerate some levels of exercise even if they are CO_2 retainers.

Carbon dioxide retention is much less common in chronic disease than with acute exacerbation. Further, it is never adequate justification to tolerate hypoxia. Prescribe the minimal amount of supplemental O_2 needed to achieve a saturation of 90%. Slowly make changes in oxygen flow in 0.5 to 1 L increments.

Exercise Cardiopulmonary Rehabilitation Programs

Exercise cardiopulmonary rehabilitation programs are well established for treating residents with chronic pulmonary disease. However, the weight of evidence indicates that the improvement in functional performance observed is more the result of cardiovascular and skeletal muscle conditioning than of any improvement in pulmonary mechanics or gas exchange. It appears that a wide range of nursing home residents may benefit from a well-planned exercise program. It is critical to screen candidates for medical illness and treat them accordingly. Exercise rehabilitation, when implemented in concert with prudent medication prescription, holds the promise of markedly improving a resident's performance status and subjective quality of life. Chapter 29, ADL Rehabilitation includes an extensive discussion of this topic. The following discussion is limited to issues relevant to cardiopulmonary function.

Exercise Screening

For the preliminary screening, evaluate the resident to ensure medical stability and the absence of any acute cardiopulmonary illness, particularly ongoing myocardial ischemia. Be alert to side effects and possible interactions of respiratory medications, cardiac medications, and antidepressants.

Initially, when approaching a potential candidate, describe the program goals and solicit feedback. Determine the resident's desire to participate. Will the resident come to sessions routinely? Did the resident ever walk regularly for exercise or ride a bicycle? Directly assess whether the resident is able to follow simple instructions or mimic movement. What is the resident's perception of the degree of disability? What are the resident's desired goals from a rehabilitative exercise program?

Recommended Equipment

In structuring a rehabilitative exercise program, the following equipment is recommended:

- Stationary cycle—recumbent style with adjustable tension, timer, and odometer
- Table-top arm ergometer with adjustable tension
- Portable oxygen saturation monitor which should be sensitive enough for elderly residents with peripheral vascular problems, yet not overly sensitive to motion artifact
- Blood pressure cuff and stethoscope

Exercise Program

Assess the resident's physical condition before developing an individualized exercise program. Obtain the resting vital signs by following this procedure:

1. Measure the resident's blood pressure while he or she is sitting at rest in a chair. A blood pressure greater than 190/100 mm Hg is considered too hypertensive for safe exercise; a blood pressure less than 80/50 mm Hg is too hypotensive.
2. Note the heart rate and presence of any irregularities. An irregular rhythm or resting tachycardia or bradycardia may signify underlying pathology and indicate an unsafe condition for exercise.
3. Note the respiratory rate and rhythm (see Chapter 1, Vital Signs, for more information). If hypoxia is a concern, pulse oximetry is recommended. If oxygen saturation through a pulse oximeter is less than 90%, supplemental oxygen is recommended. If upon exercise oxygen saturation levels fall below 90%, supplemental oxygen during exercise is recommended.

Evaluate the resident's exercise capacity by progressing through the following sets of exercises as tolerance allows. Perform all exercises bilaterally, with 10 repetitions per limb. Perform them in the order given, but various physical disabilities may require some creative changes by the therapist. After each set of exercises, and within the set as indicated, monitor the resident's vital signs for changes indicative of cardiac decompensation.

- *Lower extremities (to be done seated):*
  - Dorsiflexion of the feet (feet on floor, lift toes only)
  - Ankle circles with the leg supported (place heels on the floor and make a circular motion with the toes)
  - Long-arc quadriceps sets (extend the knee by raising the foot; do not allow the thigh to lift off the seat)
  - Marching (hip flexion)
- *Upper extremities (to be done seated):*
  - Hand grasps with arms supported (make a fist, fully extend and flex the fingers, and keep the elbows on arm rests)
  - Elbow flexion and extension (place hands on knees, lift hands to the shoulders, bending arms at the elbows, and return hands to the knees)
  - Horizontal abduction and adduction (extend the arm straight out, keeping the hand at about hip level, and raise the hand to the opposite shoulder and back)
  - Do a vital sign check here.
  - Shoulder rotation forward (place a hand on the same shoulder and circle the elbow counterclockwise)
  - Shoulder rotation backward (place a hand on the same shoulder and circle the elbow clockwise)
  - Shoulder flexion (arms fully extended, raise hands to ceiling and then down)
- *Standing (using the back of a chair or parallel bars for support):*
  - Plantar flexion (raise up on toes)

- Marching (encourage the resident to lift the knees high)
- Semisquats (semi-deep knee bends)
- Lower extremity abduction/adduction (lift the foot and extend the leg out to the side, place a foot on the floor and shift the weight to that foot, shift the weight back to the other foot, and pick up the foot of the extended leg and bring it back to the center)
- Do a vital signs check here.
- Shoulder rotation forward (place a hand on the same shoulder and circle the elbow counterclockwise)
- Shoulder rotation backward (place a hand on the same shoulder and circle the elbow clockwise)
- Trunk rotation (place hands on the hips and twist the torso from right to left)
- Trunk lateral flexion (place hands on the hips and bend laterally at the waist from right to left)

The ability to complete all these steps indicates that the resident is ready to begin a more strenuous program. After completing all of the exercises, have the resident continue to move the legs slowly (with feet on the floor) in a semicircular motion for a 3-minute cool-down session. This prevents vasodilation and sudden drops in blood pressure.

Acceptable Vital Sign Changes

Check the resident's vital signs immediately after exercise, after a 3-minute cool-down, and after 2 minutes of complete rest. The following parameters apply:

- Heart rate. Heart rate can increase 20 beats or less per minute. The presence of new or increasing irregularity may represent cardiac ischemia and indicates a need to decrease exercise.
- Blood pressure. Blood pressure can increase safely by 30 mm Hg systolic and 10 mm Hg diastolic during exercise. A 10 mm Hg drop is acceptable after rest. Larger increases or

decreases in blood pressure may be indicative of cardiac ischemia or failure. Revise the program to an easier level.
- Respiratory rate. Respiratory rate can increase 8 to 12 breaths per minute. If the resident complains of dyspnea, immediately end the session.
- Oxygen saturation. An oxygen saturation higher than 90% is acceptable. If desaturation occurs with exercise (i.e., decreases to 90% or less), supplemental oxygen starting at 1 to 2 L/m is recommended.

When vital signs show no evidence of cardiac decompensation, the resident has demonstrated the ability to proceed in the rehabilitation program. The following are clinical symptoms of cardiopulmonary deconditioning:
- Dyspnea on exertion
- Decreased ability to perform ADLs
- Decreased ability to ambulate
- Tachycardia with minimal exertion
- Presence of an irregular heart rate
- Marked increase or decrease in blood pressure (greater than 20 mm Hg) with minimal exertion
- Refusal to participate in daily activities
- Increasing frequency of naps or bedrest
- Increased somatic complaints
- Fatigue

Any of these symptoms can indicate a variety of physical or emotional problems, so the resident should be evaluated by caregivers who are familiar with the his or her medical and emotional history.

The next step is to institute cycling, ergometry, or ambulation. Depending on individual capabilities, the program may consist of one modality at a time or a combination of modalities. The procedure to follow for cycling is as follows:
- Position the resident in the cycle seat so that his or her legs are comfortably flexed (about 20°) when the pedal is farthest from the body.
- Start with zero or very minimal tension on

the wheel.

- The first session should not exceed 3 minutes.
- Increase the sessions in 2 to 3 minute time intervals, as appropriate per vital signs.
- The maximum length of the cycling session should not exceed 20 minutes.

To further increase endurance once the 20-minute session limit is reached, slowly increase the wheel tension. Pay close attention to tolerance and vital signs.

- To build upper extremity endurance, add arm ergometry to the cycling program as follows:
- Seat the resident comfortably at a table, with the ergometer at elbow's length from the edge. The resident should not have to lean over the table or reach up to ergometer pedals. Adjust the seat height appropriately, using pillows if necessary.
- Start a 2-minute session. Increase in 1-minute intervals, as appropriate per vital signs indications.
- The maximum length of an ergometry session should not exceed 5 minutes. Five minutes of upper extremity exercise is equal to the maximal sustained upper extremity mobility used in ADLs.
- A total rehabilitation session should not exceed 20 minutes—e.g., 2 minutes on the ergometer, 18 minutes on the cycle; or 5 minutes on the ergometer, 15 minutes on the cycle, and so forth. Adjust the tension on both the cycle and ergometer to build further endurance.

If the resident is unable to cycle, use ambulation to build endurance. Ambulation is more physically stressful than cycling because of the associated weight bearing. The ambulation procedure is as follows:

- Ambulate 50 feet. Progress in 10-feet intervals.
- The size of the nursing unit or institution and the goals you and/or the resident set

will determine the maximum distance achievable. Use speed and arm swing to build further endurance.

NURSING CARE PLAN

The following sections describe the nursing care plan for pulmonary rehabilitation.

Activities of Daily Living

For a resident with respiratory problems, many ADLs will be affected. All the residents' ADLs will be made more difficult by the presence of respiratory disease. For a resident with a respiratory problem, successfully washing one's own face can be a triumphant experience. The nursing staff, especially the nurse assistants, need to monitor the resident's overall condition closely as the tasks of bathing, toileting, transferring, ambulating, grooming, and dressing are performed. These tasks should be broken down and done in an incremental fashion by the resident (*see* Chapter 29, ADL Rehabilitation, for more information). The resident may eat breakfast, rest in bed for 20 to 30 minutes, and then start to wash for the day. Use the principles of energy conservation. The nurse assistant needs to determine from the resident what ADLs the resident wants to do alone, and what leisure activities the resident wants to attend during the day.

Bathing and Dressing

For the resident to maintain independence in bathing, the nurse assistant may need to gather the equipment, fill the basin with water, and bring everything to the bedside, ready for the resident to use. The resident may need to rest before attempting the dressing tasks. Again, the nurse assistant may need to collect the clothes from the closet and drawers and bring them to the resident. If the resident becomes dyspneic while doing lower body dressing, then the staff may need to assist or perform this activity totally.

Perhaps the resident with a respiratory problem is a former concert pianist and lives for the music program held once a week. Unfortunately, if this same resident performs the morning care routine (bathing, dressing, and grooming), then he or she no longer has enough energy to sit up and enjoy the program. The nursing staff can discuss this with the resident, and if the resident identifies this as a priority activity, then the nurse assistants can follow through and on the music program day, perform total care on the resident, so that he or she may enjoy the program.

Toileting

Helping the resident with a cardiorespiratory problem with toileting can be very challenging. The physical act of transferring on and off the commode, toilet, or bedpan may be exhausting and overwhelming for the resident. Again, the nurse assistant needs to carefully time the ADLs to facilitate voiding and bowel evacuation. These residents may not have the energy for a complete bowel evacuation. Stool softeners and a high-fiber diet may be required. Nursing and dietary staff should warn the resident that it may take a few weeks to become accustomed to the high-fiber diet. Residents may need help with perineal hygiene due to decreased energy. Nursing staff must be aware of the resident's need for dignity and respect when being assisted with these very personal procedures.

Mobility

The nursing staff needs to consult and work very closely with the physical therapy staff on the resident's mobility plan. Whether the resident is working on wheelchair mobility or on ambulation, the physical therapist needs to be especially involved with the nurse assistants. Teach the nurse assistants how to assist the resident with ambulation or wheeling, and

how to help pace the resident during the activity.

Depression

Depression in residents with pulmonary disease can be a reaction to the decrease in function as the pulmonary disease progresses. The elderly may have atypical symptoms such as anxiety, restlessness, and irritability. They may focus on their physical health status (e.g., "I can't breathe"). The clinician needs to consider a depressive syndrome when these symptoms are present. Chapter 13, Depression, has more specific information about recognizing and treating depression.

Oxygen Therapy During ADLs

The nursing staff needs to be aware of any resident's oxygen therapy requirements. If the resident needs oxygen during specific activities, such as sleeping, the staff must be sure the oxygen is provided and used appropriately. Staff should also ensure that any respiratory equipment used is clean and properly stored when not in use.

Mouth Care

Meticulous oral hygiene is a necessity for residents with cardiorespiratory problems. Most are mouth-breathers and will have a dry mouth, often complaining of a bad taste in their mouths. Many of these residents are on various medications administered by inhalants and aerosols. These types of medications can dry the oral mucosa, predispose to the development of thrush, cause an unpleasant taste in the resident's mouth, and subsequently decrease the resident's appetite. The resident needs to do frequent oral hygiene, as often as every 1 to 2 hours. If the resident is independent, the nurse assistant can provide the equipment and reminders to perform the oral hygiene, as needed. The staff may need to perform the oral hygiene for the more dependent, or energy-compromised, resident. *See* Chapter 25, Oral Status, for more information.

Nutrition

Nursing and medical staff may need to consult with the dietitian about many nutritional concerns that arise in residents with cardiopulmonary problems. As previously mentioned, one of the primary concerns is oral hygiene. The taste of medications, as well as the nausea experienced by some elders on these medications, can produce a decrease or even a loss of appetite. The interdisciplinary team needs to review the medications. If possible, alter the dosages or substitute other drugs that have fewer side effects.

The drying of the oral mucosa can also make chewing, swallowing, and digestion of food difficult. Residents who are having problems with dry mouth should be served applesauce with meat meals, which will help moisten the meat and facilitate chewing, swallowing, and increased food intake. *See* Chapter 25, Nutritional Status, for more information.

Many of these residents need more attention to their nutrition due to an increased energy expenditure. For a resident with a compromised respiratory system, the physical act of breathing and conducting ADLs can produce a need for more calories. Some of the residents are unable to take in the needed nutrients, and can have a severe weight loss problem. These residents may have an uncomfortable sensation of bloating and fullness after eating. Some residents may need several small meals throughout the day and evening. Liquid supplements such as milkshakes and eggnogs can be offered to these residents to help increase their calories and prevent weight loss. The resident can be offered a small portion of a single food item at a time, and then rest in between food items. Food will need to be kept warm or reheated in a microwave during the meal. Some residents will have fears

of choking on food or liquids as they are trying to take in a breath.

The staff should acknowledge the resident's fears and encourage them to eat at a slow pace and take small bites. It may be necessary to have an oral suction apparatus at the bedside, and train the staff in how to perform the Heimlich maneuver.

Sleep

Sleep may be greatly disturbed in residents with respiratory problems. Residents may only be able to nap for an hour or so at a time during the day and night. Some may awaken frequently at night because of episodes of sleep apnea. Residents may also experience anxiety that can interfere with sleep as well as other activities throughout the day. Encourage the establishment of daily routines, exercise (as tolerated), and activities. Teach the residents relaxation techniques such as progressive muscle relaxation, guided imagery, and meditation, all of which may be very effective in relieving anxiety and enhancing sleep. The staff can talk with residents and their families and find out home bedtime routines that they can carry out in the facility. If there is loud snoring, frequent awakenings, and evidence of cardiopulmonary disease, refer the resident for evaluation of sleep apnea and possible therapy with continuous positive airway pressure overnight. *See* Chapter 6, Sleep Disorders, for more information.

Sleeping medications and antianxiety agents have deleterious effects on the elderly in general, and especially for those with respiratory symptoms. Use these agents cautiously and only on an episodic basis. The interdisciplinary team must carefully define the goals, frequency, and duration of such treatment and then carefully monitor the drug's desired and undesired effects on the resident's symptoms. *See* Chapters 6 and 14, Sleep Disorders and Psychotropic Drugs, respectively, for more information.

5
AIDS and HIV Infection

Linda Kilburn, MSSS
Liz Kass, MD
Steven Littlehale, MS, RNC, CS

The first case of Acquired Immunodeficiency Syndrome (AIDS) in the United States was recognized by the Centers for Disease Control (CDC) in January 1981. In the 15 subsequent years, more than 441,000 cases have been diagnosed. It is estimated that:

- *Between 1 and 1.5 million Americans are infected with the human immunodeficiency virus (HIV) that causes AIDS.*
- *Ten to 30% of the HIV-positive population will be diagnosed with AIDS within 5 years.*
- *The cost for caring for those currently diagnosed with AIDS exceeds $1 billion a year. Extensive research is under way, and major progress has been made in the development of drugs that inhibit disease progression. However, at present there is no known cure for AIDS.*

Home care-based and institution-based care providers—especially acute hospitals, hospices, home health agencies, and various community groups—are becoming increasingly involved in the care of persons with AIDS and HIV infection. Similarly, some nursing homes in large urban areas are rapidly gaining experience in caring for persons with AIDS and HIV infection, although most facilities throughout the country still have little or no experience with this type of resident. The physical, functional, and psychosocial needs of younger persons with AIDS in its later stages are, in some respects, similar to the needs of the typical elderly nursing home population. These similarities are especially pronounced in AIDS patients with dementia and in elderly persons with Alzheimer's disease and other dementias. It is important to note, however, that there are many aspects of caring for a person with AIDS that are profoundly different than caring for the elderly nursing home resident.

Our society assumes that the elderly are without risk for HIV infection, yet risk factors for acquiring HIV are the same for all age groups. As of June 1994, 10% of the documented cases of AIDS were in people over 50 years of age. The CDC reported that there were 5427 persons with AIDS 65 years or older by the end of June 1994. For many reasons the reported cases probably underrepresent the actual number of elderly with AIDS.

People over 65 years of age are the largest group of recipients of blood transfusions. In

1985, strict procedures for screening donated blood for HIV were implemented nationally. Some individuals who received contaminated blood transfusions prior to 1985 are just beginning to experience symptoms of HIV infection. Elders with HIV infection can present with symptoms similar to those of other chronic diseases seen in the elderly. In some cases, these symptoms may be attributed to disease processes other than HIV.

Persons with AIDS are competing for the same limited number of long-term care beds and supportive and subsidized housing services as are the elderly. With the increasing incidence of AIDS, more beds in nursing facilities will be needed to accommodate the long-term care needs of this population. Therefore, nursing home staff must become knowledgeable about AIDS, its clinical management, and the available community resources. Nursing home administrators must also consider the many issues that surround admitting persons with AIDS to their facilities.

In preparing for their first AIDS patients, nursing homes will need to do extensive preparation in terms of staff education and support, development of clinical procedures (including stricter enforcement of existing infection control protocols), and planning for the integration of the person with AIDS into the resident population. It is also essential to identify and establish links with persons and organizations within the community, or larger service delivery systems, which may have greater experience in the care of persons with AIDS. Hospices, AIDS organizations, and Departments of Public Health can provide both direct and/or referral services.

OVERVIEW

For the careplanning process to be comprehensive and humane, the differing perspectives of the people involved—that is, the person with AIDS or HIV infection, family members or significant others, and the individuals and institution providing care—must be considered.

Persons with AIDS or HIV experience the initial and ongoing trauma of knowing that they have contracted a disease for which there is no known cure. As the infection progresses, these individuals need an increasing amount of physical care. Common symptom management concerns include diarrhea, nausea, vomiting, edema, thrush, fevers, night sweats, open skin lesions, respiratory infections, and neuropathy. Late in HIV infection there may be significant neurologic impairment with associated cognitive and functional decline.

The emotional burden of AIDS is extremely high. Common reactions include panic, anger, guilt, blame, denial, shame, and feelings of desertion. Persons with AIDS may have lost their jobs or homes because of the stigma associated with the disease and the public's reaction to it. They may lack the support of friends or family. They may have inadequate financial or insurance resources.

For family members and significant others, there is often personal fear about contracting the disease, fear that other family members may have been exposed, anger or grief at learning that a loved one is homosexual or an intravenous drug user, or consternation about public or peer reactions. There may also be a wide range of emotions related to the impending loss of a loved one that is compounded over time by the increasing care and support needs of the person with AIDS. People with histories of illicit drug use have many complicated psychosocial issues that are rarely seen with elderly nursing home residents, and even in late stages of AIDS, drug addiction can continue to be an active issue.

Elderly parents, grandparents, and great-grandparents frequently assume primary caregiving roles for the younger family member with AIDS. When a person with AIDS dies, it is often the elderly parent who is left to raise grandchildren or great-grandchildren. If legal guardianship is not established in such cases, access to public support services can be very difficult.

AIDS and HIV in Nursing Homes

For nursing homes with relatively little experience in caring for persons with AIDS, the first admission can prove a challenge, both clinically and administratively.

First, there is the need for comprehensive staff education. The obligation of the nursing home administration is to:

- Learn more about AIDS, HIV, and related conditions.
- Identify the expected range of clinical care needs, and develop appropriate policies, procedures, and careplanning techniques (e.g., stringent compliance with universal precautions).
- Address the staff's personal fears about potential exposure and the uncertainty at dealing with a transmissible fatal disease. Such fears may be shared by their family members or significant others, which compounds the concern and creates more need for education and reassurance by nursing home administrators and health care providers.
- Address the staff's attitudes of people with different lifestyles, cultures, or sexual orientations than their own, as well as attitudes toward people with histories of addictions.
- Select nurses with particular knowledge and skills to serve as role models for the staff. For example, the nurse-trainer can accompany a fearful or resistant staff member during caregiving tasks, demonstrating, educating, and supporting the staff member until he or she feels more comfortable.
- Identify support services (e.g., social services) that the staff can call if they are needed by the person with AIDS, or his or her family or significant others. In some cases, family members may still be reeling from the news of the resident's diagnosis and its implications. They may need assis-

tance in becoming better informed and in dealing with their own reactions before they are able to aid in the support of the person with AIDS.

- Identify community resources that provide further AIDS education or linkage to specialized service and support networks operating in the immediate area or region.

Second, it is necessary to develop a plan for integrating the person with AIDS into the nursing home setting. Specific issues include:

- How to maintain confidentiality.
- How to meet the legitimate information or education needs of other residents (particularly any who may be roommates with a person with AIDS) and their families or significant others.
- How to address age-related issues since the majority of persons with AIDS are much younger than the average age of a resident of a long-term care facility. Address the need for special plans or assistance to integrate the person with AIDS into the life and activities of the nursing home. Address the need to develop more age-appropriate activities. Consider a special unit or separate facility if the number of persons with AIDS admitted warrant this.

ETIOLOGY OF AIDS OR HIV INFECTION

Human Immunodeficiency Virus causes AIDS primarily by attacking and destroying the immune system. HIV prefers attacking a type of white blood cell called the "helper" or CD4 lymphocyte. All white blood cells are essential for fighting infectious agents. In the late stages of HIV infection, as the number of CD4 cells diminishes, the infected person becomes increasingly susceptible to opportunistic infections and cancers that the immune system is no longer able to combat. These infections are termed opportunistic because they do not usually occur in people with normal immune systems, but take advantage of a damaged immune system and cause disease. The infections can be caused by viruses, bacteria, or fungi, often types that are in the environment, but do not cause disease in people with functional immune systems. Most of the infections are not contagious, except for tuberculosis, herpes viruses, and cryptosporidial infections. The HIV virus can attack various organs. When it attacks the brain, it can cause dementia.

People may be infected with HIV for over 10 years yet remain asymptomatic. The term AIDS refers to the late stage of HIV infection, when the immune system has become badly damaged. AIDS is currently defined by the CDC as the presence of a CD4 count of less than 200, or the presence of one of the conditions listed in Table 5-1, an AIDS surveillance definition.

Transmission and Persons at Risk

The HIV virus is transmitted through the exchange of body fluids, which occurs through sexual contact, shared needles and syringes, transfused blood products, and maternal/fetal blood exchange. HIV can be transmitted by any of these activities.

In the United States, specific groups are disproportionately infected by the HIV virus. These groups include men who have unprotected sex with other men and people who use injectable drugs and share needles and syringes ("works"). Outside of North America and Europe, HIV has been spread primarily through unprotected sex between heterosexual men and women. In the United States, the rate of heterosexual transmission is increasing rapidly.

Transmission of HIV may occur through oral, anal, or vaginal sexual contact. Because a carrier of the HIV virus can remain symptom-free for years, the potential to infect others unknowingly is greatly increased. While no cure for AIDS is yet known, there are an increasing number of treatments to manage the symptoms. The life expectancy of a person with AIDS has increased greatly as a re-

sult of these treatments. Consequently, AIDS should be considered a chronic disease.

The major contributing factors to the increased life expectancy of those contracting AIDS have been the development of a class of anti-AIDS drugs known as protease inhibitors. These drugs operate by blocking the protease enzyme, which the AIDS virus needs to reproduce. Three have been developed as of the date of this publication (ritonavir or Norvir, developed by Abbott Laboratories; saquinavir, developed by Hoffman-LaRoche; and indinavir, released by Merck and Company). The most effective of these drugs released to date is indinavir (trade name Crixivan) approved by the Food and Drug administration in March, 1996 just 42 days after Merck and Company submitted its application for approval. Indinavir, when combined with two more conventional AIDS drugs—AZT and 3TC—has been shown in initial trials to reduce the AIDS virus to undetectable levels in about 90% of patients after 6 months of treatment. Trials also indicate that the drug can prompt a marked increase in infection-fighting white blood cells, which are destroyed by the AIDS virus. Key concerns about these drugs include the high cost that acts as a major deterrent to access, as well as the fact that the AIDS virus has proven to have strong mutating capacity and it is unclear for how long the dramatic drops in virus can be sustained over time. Because of the rapidly evolving state of AIDS-related research, it is critical that persons and organizations involved in the care and treatment of persons with AIDS remain abreast of developments as they occur.

The elderly are at risk for contracting HIV infection in the same manner as younger people. According to the CDC end-of-the-year surveillance report for 1994, the two top exposure categories for people over age 65 years are men who have unprotected sex with other men and recipients of blood transfusions. A new blood test was approved by the United

Table 5-1. AIDS Surveillance Definition as Defined by the CDC in 1993

Candidiasis of bronchi, trachea, or lungs

Candidiasis, esophageal

CD 4 count below 200

Cervical cancer, invasive

Coccidioidomycosis, disseminated or extrapulmonary

Cryptococcosis, extrapulmonary

Cryptosporidiosis, chronic intestinal (lasting longer than 1 month)

Cytomegalovirus disease (other than liver, spleen, or nodes)

Cytomegalovirus retinitis

HIV encephalopathy

Herpes simplex: chronic ulcer(s) (lasting longer than 1 month) or bronchitis, pneumonitis, or esophagitis

Histoplasmosis, disseminated or extrapulmonary

Isosporiasis, chronic intestinal (lasting longer than 1 month)

Kaposi's sarcoma

Lymphoma, Burkitt's (or equivalent term)

Lymphoma, immunoblastic (or equivalent term)

Lymphoma, primary in brain

Mycobacterium avium complex or *M. kansasii,* disseminated or extrapulmonary

M. tuberculosis, disseminated or extrapulmonary tuberculosis, pulmonary

Pneumocystis carinii pneumonia

Pneumonia, recurrent bacterial (more than one episode)

Progressive multifocal leukoencephalopathy

Salmonella septicemia, recurrent

Toxoplasmosis of brain

Wasting syndrome due to HIV

Table 5-2. Summary of Classification System for HIV Infection

Group	Signs and Symptoms
Group 1: Acute HIV infection	Transient signs and symptoms at the time of, or shortly after, initial infection with HIV: a mononucleosis-like syndrome, with or without aseptic meningitis
Group 2: Asymptomatic HIV infection	No signs or symptoms of HIV infection; diagnosis based on positive HIV serology; hematologic and/or immunologic laboratory studies may or may not show abnormal findings consistent with HIV infection
Group 3: Persistent generalized lymphadenopathy	Palpable lymph nodes at two or more extra-inguinal sites persisting for more than 3 months in the absence of a concurrent illness or condition that might explain these findings
Group 4: Other HIV infection	*Constitutional disease* is defined as one or more of the following: fever lasting longer than 1 month, involuntary weight loss of greater than 10% of baseline, or diarrhea persisting longer than 1 month
	Neurologic disease is defined as one or more of the following: dementia, myelopathy, or peripheral neuropathy in the absence of a concurrent illness or condition that might explain these findings (myelopathy is damage to the spinal cord nerves causing extremity weakness, difficulty walking, loss of bowel and bladder control; peripheral neuropathy consists of burning, "pins and needles," numbness, or stabbing sensations in extremities, especially the feet, related only to neuropathy often difficult to treat with conventional analgesics)
	Secondary infectious disease is an infectious disease that is associated with HIV infection and/or at least moderately indicative of a defect in cell-mediated immunity (e.g., opportunistic infections)
	Secondary cancers are defined as one or more kinds of cancer that are associated with HIV infection and/or at least moderately indicative of a defect in cell-mediated immunity (e.g., Kaposi's sarcoma, non-Hodgkin's lymphoma)
	Other conditions in HIV infection are defined as the presence of other clinical findings or diseases that are not classified in the other groups and may be attributed to HIV infection or are at least moderately indicative of a defect in cell-mediated immunity

States Food and Drug Administration in March 1996, which should reduce HIV exposure rates of those receiving transfusions. However, there will continue to be cases stemming from periods in which blood testing and HIV screening were not as effective. The antigen test has the capacity to detect HIV in donated blood sooner than the formerly used test because it screens for the presence of antigens, or viral proteins, rather than antibodies.

It should be noted that many elderly people are still sexually active. The HIV virus that was initially transmitted to one partner may be transmitted sexually to another partner. A person infected through a contaminated blood product received during coronary bypass surgery, for example, can infect his or her partner through sexual intercourse and later die of heart disease before ever becoming symptomatic with HIV. Their partner is left with no suspicion about being infected with HIV.

Because AIDS may not be suspected in multiply-impaired elderly persons, it might be underdiagnosed in this population. Therefore, when presented with opportunistic infections in a resident, consider HIV infection before making the diagnoses of geriatric wasting syndrome, failure to thrive or dementia, particularly when the infection is accompanied by rapid physical deterioration.

Classification System for HIV Infection

Table 5-2 summarizes the classification system for HIV infections as developed by the CDC.

CAREPLANNING FOR THE PERSON WITH AIDS

Because of the extent of research currently under way, protocols and care interventions for persons with AIDS are constantly being reevaluated and updated. According to the CDC, 91% of all persons with AIDS or HIV infection presented with one or more opportunistic infections at the time of diagnosis.

Currently, the physiologic basis of providing care to a person with HIV infection requires a better understanding the nature of the opportunistic infections and malignancies associated with AIDS and HIV infection.

This section details the signs, symptoms, and recommended interventions for the opportunistic infections and cancers normally associated with AIDS or HIV infection. Many of the signs and symptoms of the indicated conditions are common to a variety of problems, so accuracy in diagnosis is critical. However, in all cases the appropriateness of the diagnostic work-up should be evaluated within the context of the following:

- The resident's overall condition
- The intrusiveness of the proposed diagnostic evaluation
- The resident's or significant other's desire for intervention
- The degree to which accurate diagnosis will have in impact on the resident's comfort
- Any public health considerations that may affect other residents or family (especially tuberculosis and skin conditions such as herpes)

Health Transitions Experienced by Persons with AIDS

Persons with AIDS may have periods of severe infection and debilitation followed by periods in which they are relatively symptom-free and quite functional. Therefore, failure by clinical staff to intervene and address symptoms aggressively, especially in the early stages of the disease, may result in a lost opportunity for the person with AIDS to realize another, relatively symptom-free period.

Hospitalizations may be frequent and interventions aggressive in the early stages of care, but as the overall condition of the person with AIDS deteriorates, aggressive and intrusive diagnostic and therapeutic interventions may become less appropriate. These issues deserve careful discussion with the ill person with AIDS and his or her relatives or significant others.

For nursing homes with relatively little experience in the care of persons with AIDS, educating staff and establishing links to community resources are strongly recommended. Resources commonly used include hospice team staff, AIDS support network personnel, AIDS advocacy groups, substance abuse treatment providers, test laboratories to assist in diagnostics, outpatient and inpatient resources of local hospitals, pharmacists, and state health department personnel. Physicians and other clinicians experienced in the care of persons with AIDS are invaluable as care needs are anticipated or identified.

In reviewing the following materials on AIDS and HIV-related opportunistic infections, it is important that nursing home staff consider the types of resources that are necessary for care, and differentiate between what the nursing home can provide internally and what it must secure externally. When nursing home staff arrange in advance for access to external resources, they can make necessary transitions more easily if the resident should need them.

The majority of persons with AIDS or HIV infection entering nursing homes are:

- In the late stages of their disease process
- In need of more intensive care and supervision and support than can be provided at home
- In need of skilled nursing care at the time of admission but may return to a higher level of functioning

In the first category, persons with AIDS are likely to remain in the nursing home until death. In the second and third categories, persons with AIDS who move into a temporary remission from symptoms may be discharged from the facility, although later they may be readmitted when their condition worsens.

Long-term care facilities discharge few residents; therefore, they have loosely structured

or informal discharge planning services. In caring for the person with AIDS, the facility must explore the concept of comprehensive discharge planning. Many persons with AIDS are homeless for a variety of reasons and will require assistance to find homes, supportive housing, and home health care services in the community when institutional long-term care services are no longer required.

MAJOR CONDITIONS ASSOCIATED WITH HIV INFECTION (IN ORDER OF EARLY TO LATER STAGES OF IMMUNE DEFICIENCY)

The following care planning information has been excerpted, revised, and adapted from Martin JP, et al. *AIDS Home Care and Hospice Manual,* ed 2; 1990, with permission of the authors. The Visiting Nurses and Hospice of San Francisco is one of the most experienced providers of care to persons with AIDS.

Because AIDS-related studies, findings, and recommendations continue to evolve at a rapid rate, it is strongly recommended that nursing homes caring for persons with AIDS develop and maintain close contacts with AIDS resource networks in their area, which ensures access to the latest information. Local and regional sources may also serve as conduits to additional, specialized information and services, such as the CDC, which publishes frequent updates to its findings and is an excellent resource on the complex of issues surrounding AIDS and HIV infection.

The recommendations presented here are primarily from a Western medical model. Alternative therapies such as acupuncture, massage, and reiki have been extremely helpful in the managing HIV- and AIDS-related symptoms.

Candidiasis (Yeast Infection)

Table 5-3 describes candidiasis types, signs and symptoms, and treatments.

Table 5-3. Candidiasis Types, Signs and Symptoms, and Treatments

Type	Signs and Symptoms	Treatment
Oral (thrush)	White patches on tongue and sides of mouth	Nystatin suspension swish and swallow four times a day, OR clotrimazole troches orally, OR fluconazole or ketoconazole (fluconazole is more effective and is more reliably absorbed but is very expensive)
Esophageal	Pain with swallowing; midchest pain	Fluconazole, to 100 to 400 mg once daily for 10 to 14 days; may require amphotericin intravenously if high dose fluconazole fails
Vaginal	White, odorless discharge; itching, burning	Nystatin or clotrimazole creamóoral treatment as above may be needed
Skin	Red, inflamed areas with distinct margins; seen particularly in moist skin folds	Topical nystatin or clotrimazole cream

Note: Candidiasis often becomes chronic and sometimes refractory with more advanced HIV infection.

Herpes Simplex

Herpes simplex presents the following signs and symptoms:

Signs and symptoms: Oral, esophageal, and/or genital lesions; which may appear as clusters of vesicles or large, painful areas of ulceration.

Diagnosis: Scrape lesions and stain or culture for the virus by immunofluorescent techniques. However, clinical inspection and presumptive diagnosis are often sufficient to begin therapy.

Treatment: Oral acyclovir five times a day for outbreaks. Intravenous acyclovir may be needed if oral therapy fails. Intravenous Foscarnet may be required for acyclovir-resistant lesions. Medication may need be administered indefinitely to control virus.

Comments: The lesions are contagious. Follow infection control precautions.

HERPES (VARICELLA) ZOSTER (SHINGLES)

Herpes zoster presents the following signs and symptoms:

Signs and symptoms: Clusters of erythematous, vesicular lesions, usually along a dermatome, that are often painful (burning), sometimes with itching.

Diagnosis: Clinical inspection is usually enough to diagnose the condition.

Treatment: Oral acyclovir, 800 mg five times per day for 10 to 14 days, or intravenous acyclovir (the dose is calculated by weight) every 8 hours for 7 to 10 days.

Comments: Postherpetic neuralgia may occur after the acute infection resolves, is very painful, and often responds poorly to usual analgesic medications.

People with no prior exposure to chickenpox can contract chickenpox from patients with herpes zoster.

Cryptosporidiosis/Isospora (Enteritis)

Cryptosporidiosis and isospora present the following signs and symptoms:

Signs and symptoms: Moderate to severe watery diarrhea; abdominal pain, cramping; volume depletion (dehydration); poor appetite; weight loss.

Diagnosis: Identification of *Cryptosporidium* organism in stool specimen (this must be requested specifically from the lab).

Identification of *Cryptosporidium* organism in gastrointestinal mucosa by biopsy.

Treatment: No effective treatment. Currently Paromomycin, 500 mg (or more) three to four times per day, is commonly tried.

Somatostatin subcutaneously is sometimes helpful.

Symptomatic control with antidiarrheal medications is often necessary (Lomotil, Imodium, or deodorized tincture of opium).

Symptoms tend to get more severe in late HIV infection.

Temporary intravenous fluid replacement or parenteral nutrition may be helpful in relieving dehydration and reducing malnutrition.

Comments: Crytosporidiosis is a common cause of refractory diarrhea. *Isospora belli*, another parasitic infection of the bowel, has a similar presentation and may respond to treatment with trimethoprim-sulfamethoxazole treatment.

Tuberculosis

There are two types of tuberculosis (TB) discussed here: pulmonary (the most common), and extrapulmonary (gastrointestinal tract, kidneys, central nervous system, disseminated). Tuberculosis presents the following signs and symptoms:

Signs and symptoms of pulmonary TB: Weight loss; fevers; cough, often with bloody sputum.

Diagnosis:
- Perform skin testing with purified protein derivative (PPD) antigen if the resident has no history of a prior positive PPD. Negative PPD results may well be inaccurate in later stages of HIV. Skin test controls (e.g., mumps, *Candida*) clarify whether or not the patient is anergic.
- Diagnosis requires finding acid-fast bacilli (AFB) in sputum (in the case of pulmonary TB) or other body fluid/tissue source, or granulomas on biopsy.
- *Mycobacterium avium* complex (MAC) also is an acid-fast bacilli. Currently, MAC cannot be distinguished from TB except on the basis of culture, which requires 4 to 8 weeks to be final. Start presumtive treatment for TB on the basis of AFB in the sputum pending identification of the organism.

Treatment:
- Drug-resistant TB strains are now complicating TB therapy and prevention. Initial treatment pending culture results and drug susceptibility testing (which takes 6 to 8 weeks) should include isoniazid (INH), rifampin, pyrazinamide, and Ethambutol unless INH-resistant infection is believed to be likely (in which case another anti-TB drug should be substituted for INH).
- Treat HIV-infected people who have positive PPD test (more than 5 mm) prophylactically with 1 year of INH.

Comments:

- TB can occur early or late in HIV infection.
- TB is contagious and can be transmitted to nonimmunodeficient people. TB spreads by aerosolization of the bacilli in respiratory secretions. Residents receiving appropriate medication, who no longer have bacilli found in their sputum, are no longer contagious. Residents suspected of having TB must be on respiratory precautions.
- Drug-resistant TB strains are now complicating TB therapy and prevention.

Pneumocystis Carinii (PCP) Pneumonia
Pneumocystis Carinii presents the following signs and symptoms:

Signs and symptoms: Fever; nonproductive cough; shortness of breath, especially with exertion; increased respiratory rate; often no sounds of chest congestion.

Diagnosis: Diagnosis is often made based on chest radiographic appearance of diffuse interstitial infiltrates in the appropriate clinical context. Induced sputum is often diagnostic but bronchoscopy is often required if sputum testing is unrevealing.

Treatment:
- Trimethoprim-sulfamethoxazole orally or intravenous therapy (the dose is calculated by weight) every 8 hours for 21 days.
- Intravenous pentamidine daily for 21 days.
- Atovaquone 750 mg orally three times a day for 21 days (for mild to moderate cases).
- Other: If toxicity or resistance to other agents develops, try clindamycin and/or primaquine.

Comments:
- PCP is an opportunistic respiratory infection that is a common cause of serious pneumonias in HIV-infected persons having a CD4 count less than 200, and is still the common major opportunistic infection diagnosed in association with HIV.
- Steroid treatment is recommended in moderate to severe cases of PCP with hypoxemia (PO_2 less than 70 mm Hg). Prophylactic treatment with trimethoprim-sulfamethoxazole DS once daily or aerosolized pentamidine is now used routinely in residents with CD4 counts of less than 200/mm^3, and has a decreased the frequency of PCP pneumonia. Dapsone is sometimes used in Bactrim-intolerant people.
- Drug intolerance is a problem. Residents may have severe allergic reactions or bone marrow suppression with trimethoprim-sulfamethoxazole; hypoglycemia, hypotension, or pancreatitis with pentamidine. Many persons with AIDS with a history of mild reaction to Bactrim may be safely desensitized.
- Bactrim is superior in preventing PCP, is much less expensive, and may have benefit in preventing toxoplasmosis active infection.

Central Nervous System Toxoplasmosis
Central nervous system (CNS) toxoplasmosis presents the following signs and symptoms:

Signs and symptoms: Fever; headache; lethargy; confusion; seizures; cognitive impairment; focal neurologic signs; depression; delirium.

Diagnosis: Diagnosis is often made based on lesions seen on computed tomography or magnetic resonance imaging of the head. Toxoplasmosis serology is usually (but not always) positive. Brain biopsy is a consideration in residents who fail to respond to empiric therapy.

Treatment: Continue drug therapy indefinitely to prevent recurrence. First-line therapy is sulfadiazine and pyrimethamine. Clindamycin with pyrimethamine currently seems to be the best alternative treatment regimen, with other newer approaches such as azithromycin. Residents intolerant to sulfa drugs may require treatment with Clindamycin, which can lead to chronic *Clostridium difficile* diarrhea. Folinic acid is always given with pyramethamine to prevent hematologic toxicity.

Cryptococcus

Cryptococcus is a fungal infection that is diagnosed most commonly as causing meningitis (although it is usually also detectable in the blood when meningitis is found). It presents the following signs and symptoms:

Signs and symptoms: Fever; mild-severe headache; nausea; vomiting; seizures; lethargy; stiff neck, double vision.

Diagnosis: Requires a spinal tap for diagnosis.

Treatment: Often initially treated intravenously with amphotericin, and long-term with oral fluconazole.

Requires maintenance therapy indefinitely or relapses occur.

Cytomegalovirus: Retinitis, GI, CNS

Cytomegalovirus (CMV) is a member of a group of large species-specific herpes-type viruses with a wide variety of disease effects. It presents the following signs and symptoms for the eyes, gastrointestinal (GI) tract, and central nervous system (CNS):

Signs and symptoms:
Eyes:
- Retinitis: blurry vision, floaters, blindness
GI tract:
- Esophagitis: pain with swallowing, chest pain
- Gastritis/duodenitis: abdominal pain, diarrhea
- Pancreatitis: epigastric and back pain, nausea, vomiting
- Colitis: abdominal pain, weight loss, fever, diarrhea
CNS:
- Encephalopathy/myelopathy: neurologic symptoms, sometimes focal

Diagnosis: Diagnosis is based on typical retinal findings in the case of retinitis, biopsy and culture in the case of GI disease, and cerebrospinal fluid culture in the case of CNS disease.

Treatment:
- Intravenous gancyclovir or foscarnet, requiring initial twice daily treatment for 2 to 3 weeks and often (particularly with retinitis) indefinite daily intravenous treatment.

Drug side effects:
- Gancyclovir causes bone marrow suppression (anemia, low white blood and platelet counts)
- Foscarnet can cause renal failure, rash, seizures, hypocalcemia, hypomagnesemia, hypokalemia

Comments:
- CMV infection occurs late in HIV infection, usually with CD4 count less than 50.
- CMV eventually often becomes resistant to treatment.

Mycobacterium Avium Complex

Mycobacterium avium complex presents the following signs and symptoms:

Signs and symptoms: Fever, weight loss, anorexia, weakness, abdominal pain, low blood counts (red blood cells, white blood cells, platelets), abnormal liver function tests (especially alkaline phosphatase).

Diagnosis: Identification of MAC in cultures of blood, or biopsy of tissues from bone marrow, lymph nodes, liver; subsequent cultures of these tissues demonstrate MAC; sometimes seen as AFB on initial screening; cannot currently be distinguished from TB until cultures grow out (which takes weeks).

Treatment: Treatment with multidrug regimens (no less than two of the following): rifampin, ethambutol, amikacin (intravenous), cycloserine, clarithromycin, clofazimine, ciprofloxacin.

Comments:
- Infection occurs late in HIV infection, usually with CD4 counts of less than 50.

- MAC has been found in approximately 50% of autopsies done on AIDS patients.
- Requires lifetime treatment, with multiple drug regimens; drugs are often not well tolerated and have variable symptom response rates.
- Prognosis is poor after diagnosis with MAC.
- Prophylactic regimens using Rifabutin or clarithromycin may prevent disseminated MAC infection in patients with CD4 counts of less than 50 (Rifabutin is recommended by the CDC but this is controversial).

Progressive Multifocal Leukoencephalopathy

Progressive multifocal leukoencephalopathy (PML) presents the following signs and symptoms:

Signs and symptoms: Neurologic deficits with variable onset and progression; motor and sensory deficits may include ataxia, clumsiness, muscle weakness, change in level of consciousness, tremor, paresis, decreased visual acuity, aphasia, incontinence, depression, dementia, delirium.

Diagnosis: Diagnosis is based on computed tomography or magnetic resonance imaging (multiple patchy defects), and ruling out other infections. Brain biopsy is definitive but rarely done.

Comments: PML is caused by a polyoma virus; no effective treatment is known.

HIV Encephalopathy (Dementia)

HIV encephalopathy (dementia) presents the following signs and symptoms:

Signs and symptoms:

Early stage:
- Cognitive: decreased attention span, decreased memory, slowing mental function
- Behavioral: social withdrawal, apathy, and personality change

Late stage (severe memory deficits):
- Global dementia, limited speech, multiple neurologic abnormalities, including bowel and bladder incontinence
- Consciousness usually intact

- Vacant stare
- Problem behaviors including agitation, paranoia, aggression
- Seizures

Treatment: There is no definitive treatment to reverse the condition. Refer to Chapters 10, 13, and 11, Cognitive Loss, Depression, and Delirium, respectively, for helpful management suggestions.

Comments: AZT in high doses sometimes improves cognitive function, but its toxicities must be considered. Psychotropics may reduce agitation. Psychostimulants (e.g., Ritalin) may improve psychomotor slowing and concurrent depression. Adapt the environment to promote consistency and continuity. Variable changes in levels of orientation may be observed. Progression is not well defined, but it may be rapid and debilitating.

Kaposi's Sarcoma

Kaposi's sarcoma presents the following signs and symptoms:

Signs and symptoms:

Characteristic early lesions:

Table 5-4. Antiviral Drugs and Their Side Effects

Drug	Side Effect
Zidovudine (AZT)	Anemia, leukopenia, myopathy, headache, nausea
Didanosine (ddI)	GI distress, nausea, diarrhea, pancreatitis, peripheral neuropathy (pain in extremities)
Zalcitabine (ddc)	Peripheral neuropathy, oral ulcers
Stavudine (d4t)	Peripheral neuropathy

- Faint beige-to-bluish, macular lesions
- Variable-sized red-to-purple, indurated plaques
- Often found on the face or in the oral cavity
- Do not blanch when pressed
- Painless
  Characteristic progressive lesions:
- Dark red-to-brown or blue tumor nodules
- Grow in size and coalesce
- Found on all body surfaces
- May be associated with pain and swelling
- Disseminated lesions, advanced Kaposi's syndrome:
- Widespread occurrence of lesions involving the skin, oral mucosa, lymph nodes, and visceral organs (particularly lungs and GI tract)
- Edema due to lymphatic blockage may occur in extremities and face
- Pain may be associated with edema and with oral lesions
- Respiratory distress and hemoptysis due to pulmonary lesions can occur
- Lesions in GI tract may be asymptomatic or may cause pain and bleeding

Treatment: Early asymptomatic lesions are often not treated. Symptomatic cutaneous, oral, or visceral involvement often initially responds well to chemotherapy.

Comments: Kaposi's syndrome is seen more frequently in gay men than other persons with AIDS.

Advanced disfiguring and malodorous lesions can lead to embarrassment and isolation.

Placing charcoal crystals in a bowl in the person's room may help control the odor.

Skin care management with advanced extremity lesions with edema can be extremely challenging.

Central Nervous System Lymphoma

Central nervous system lymphoma presents the following signs and symptoms:

Signs and symptoms: Neurologic changes: cognitive impairment, gait disturbance, behavior changes, stroke-like deficits.

Diagnosis: Diagnosis is made by computed tomography or magnetic resonance imaging, confirm with a brain biopsy.

Treatment: Steroids and radiation can slow progression by a few months but rapid progression is common. *See* Chapters 10 and 18, Cognitive Loss and Falls, respectively, for management suggestions.

Antiviral Therapy

Some persons with AIDS will be admitted to the nursing home on antiviral therapy with one of the drugs (alone or in combination) shown in Table 5-4, which also describes their side effects.

RESIDENT EDUCATION

Address the following issues with the person with AIDS residing in a nursing home:
  Infection control practices
- Resources available to them within and outside of the facility
- Addiction counseling and rehabilitation, if appropriate and desired.

By federal law, every resident has the right to privacy including disease diagnosis. The reality is that when a person with AIDS is admitted to a nursing home, especially for the first time, this information may become known by some residents. Resident education can alleviate some concern. It is best to educate residents and their families about HIV and AIDS before the initial admission of a person with AIDS.

UNIVERSAL INFECTION CONTROL PRECAUTIONS

These precautions must be followed by all caregivers when treating any resident. Gloves must be worn for contact with blood and body fluids. Hands must always be washed after gloves are removed before leaving room or caring for another resident. Gowns are only necessary if contamination of clothing is likely. Masks and protective eyewear are needed only if fluid splashes are likely, e.g., during suctioning and GI bleeding. Consider all used linen to be contaminated and place it in properly labeled receptacles. Sharps (e.g., needles, staples) must be promptly disposed of in sharps containers, which should be kept readily accessible.

Specific Infection Control Issues

The following subsections describe specific infection control issues.

Varicella (Chickenpox)–Herpes Zoster (Shingles)

Shingles is caused by the reactivation of the chickenpox virus. People who have never had chickenpox may be infected by people with chickenpox or shingles. Only people who have had chickenpox should care for patients with chickenpox or shingles. Specific infection control precautions include:

- Staying in a private room if a roommate has not had chickenpox
- Washing hands on entering and leaving room
- Wearing gloves for contact with skin
- Covering affected areas to limit contamination with drainage
- Continuing the precautions until all lesions have dried and crusted

Tuberculosis

Persons infected with HIV who have a past history of TB exposure have up to a 50% chance of developing active TB through reactivation. In people with HIV, PPDs are often negative because of immune system deficiency. Sputum smear and a culture for TB are often needed to make the diagnosis.

Nursing homes must have clear policies for respiratory isolation of patients with suspected TB. Facilities caring for populations with a high likelihood of having been exposed to TB should check staff PPDs every 6 months. Involve the local public health nurses in care and program planning.

CASE EXAMPLE

Mr. Y's admission to the nursing home presented the facility with two sets of issues: the clinical care issues and the administrative issues related to personnel involved in his care. The first portion of this case describes the clinical issues and care approaches. The second portion identifies personnel and organizational concerns, and reviews the steps taken by the home's administration to address these issues.

Clinical Issues

Mr. Y. was a 44-year-old divorced man diagnosed with AIDS. When his condition began to deteriorate, he moved from the major metropolitan area in which he had been living to a small city in a neighboring state where most of his family resided. At the time of the move, he was estranged from his father, who was unable to deal either with his son's diagnosis of AIDS or his homosexuality. Mr. Y.'s mother had been deceased for many years. There were two siblings, a brother and a sister, living in the area, who proved to be extremely supportive throughout his illness.

Lacking a primary caregiver, Mr. Y. made the decision to enter an area nursing home following his discharge from the local hospital. Upon admission, he was alert, wheelchairbound, and able to perform a portion of his self-care with assistance. He had toxoplasma encephalitis with a related seizure disorder, extreme perirectal irritation secondary to a herpes simplex infection of a prolapsed rectum, oral candidiasis, impaired vision due to CMV retinitis that had failed both Gancyclovir and Foscarnet intravenous therapy, urinary incontinence, and nutritional impairment.

Mr. Y. remained in the nursing home for 6 weeks until his death. Over the course of his stay, his condition deteriorated rapidly. He was on Dilantin to control the seizure activity and fluconazole for the candidiasis. He received multivitamins and nutritional supplements, as well as the antiviral drug AZT.

The goals of treatment were to maximize Mr. Y.'s comfort and maintain his independent functioning to the fullest extent possible. He was started on Percodan for pain, but soon required morphine, first orally and later subcutaneously. Oxazepam was added to relieve symptoms of anxiety and agitation. His decreasing respiratory function due to recurrent pneumocystis infection necessitated the use of oxygen and a bronchial inhaler. He was able to move from bed to chair with assistance, and required extensive padding when sitting upright. He was unable to use suppositories because of his prolapsed rectum. He interacted with other residents, making one close friend, an older man who was sympathetic to Mr. Y.'s impaired vision and assisted him at mealtimes.

Emotionally, Mr. Y. fared reasonably well for several weeks. The support of his siblings and their families, extensive staff reassurance, and interaction with other residents helped him deal with his deteriorating condition. At the physician's request, Mr. Y.'s estranged father made a visit but was unable to offer the acceptance his son desired. The unresolved issue was extremely difficult for Mr. Y., who required extensive staff support.

In the last 2 weeks of his life, Mr. Y.'s mental condition deteriorated significantly. He was increasingly unaware of care that was being given to him. This situation was not only difficult for him but also a source of frustration to nursing staff, with whom he enjoyed a good relationship and to whom he had repeatedly expressed appreciation for his physical care and the respectful way he was being treated.

Another psychologically difficult moment occurred after an eye examination, about 4 weeks into his 6-week stay. Mr. Y. had been hopeful that something could be done to improve his CMV retinitis and deteriorating vision, which was radically reducing his ability to maintain any independence. When he realized no useful intervention was possible, he experienced a significant sense of loss.

During his last few days, Mr. Y. became semicomatose and extremely agitated. His neurologic dysfunction made it virtually impossible for the staff to assess the effectiveness of their palliative techniques. His forgetfulness made it difficult for him to benefit from staff reassurances that he was being cared for and safe. It was important for the staff to understand that frequent, consistent reassurances on their part could enhance his sense of security. The introduction of Oxazepam reduced his agitation somewhat, but he still experienced periods of discomfort that the staff were unable to relieve entirely.

Administrative Issues

Mr. Y. was this nursing home's first resident with AIDS. Three years prior to this admission, the administration recognized it was only a matter of time before the increasing number of persons with AIDS would require that the facility assume some of the care responsibilities. The administration instituted periodic inservice education programs about AIDS and related care concerns, began exploring staff concerns about being involved in the care of persons with AIDS, and supported a stringent practice of universal precautions. Despite the level of education already received, the reality of a pending AIDS admission raised many concerns, and major efforts had to be made toward reeducation, reexploration of fears, and reaffirmation of plans and care approaches. The facility took the following actions:

1. Several more inservices were conducted, utilizing local expertise from the Visiting Nurses Association hospice team, which already had some experience in the care

of persons with AIDS. A representative from an AIDS advisory group was also invited to speak.

2. Mr. Y. visited the facility prior to his admission, so he and the staff had the opportunity to meet each other and break ground.

3. The local hospital's clinical care team (primary nurse, social worker) who were involved in Mr. Y.'s care visited the nursing home before his admission to review his current status, and recommended interventions and techniques to help meet his emotional and physical care needs.

4. Staff concerns about exposure and infection were extensively solicited. Both the medical director of the facility (who was also Mr. Y.'s personal physician) and the various inservice speakers offered additional support and clarification as staff issues and concerns were raised.

5. Staff voiced concern about Mr. Y.'s homosexuality. Some felt that their biases would interfere with providing good care. After diversity training and meeting Mr. Y., this concern was no longer raised.

6. Charge nurses and nursing home administration maintained a very strong presence on the floor, assisting and supporting the staff and bringing themselves into regular contact with Mr. Y. Both felt their own actions must show total commitment in order to provide a model for the staff's behavior.

7. Mr. Y.'s orientation to the nursing home was handled exactly the same as for any newly admitted resident. He was introduced to other residents, shown around the facility, and encouraged to participate actively in social and recreational activities.

8. Mr. Y. had a roommate. The availability of a bed was the driving factor in making the roommate choice. The roommate was not mentally alert and had few visitors. Staff would have preferred a private room because of the amount of time people spent in the room with Mr. Y.

9. Throughout Mr. Y.'s residency, the staff were provided with the latest information about AIDS.

10. A major effort was made to reduce staff anxiety by ensuring that appropriate protective garments and equipment were available. Gowns, aprons, gloves, and barrier shields were used and applicable items were sized to fit the staff.

11. After Mr. Y.'s death, a social worker came from the local hospice program to meet with the staff. This session offered them the opportunity to review the course of the case and their feelings about the resident's care. Three staff members subsequently attended Mr. Y.'s funeral.

6
Sleep Disorders

Sonia Ancoli-Israel, PhD[1]
Denise Williams Jones, MA
Patricia McGuinn, RN
Pauline Belleville-Taylor, RN, CS, MS

On any given night in a typical nursing home, a large number of residents are wide awake; and on any given day, a large number slouch in their chairs sleeping in common rooms or hallways. Conventional wisdom holds that daytime sleepiness and nighttime sleeplessness are a result of social isolation, lack of activities, or loneliness. These sleep patterns, however, may also be directly associated with various biologic causes, which can be controlled.

For example, sleep apnea, a disorder that disrupts normal sleep and promotes daytime sleepiness, is much more common in elderly nursing home residents than in people of comparable age living in the community. Chronic bed rest is defined as excessive time in bed, which is widespread in the nursing home setting. This excessive time in bed interferes with circadian rhythms, promoting insomnia and midsleep awakenings. Sedative-hypnotics, which are commonly prescribed in nursing homes, contribute to sleep problems and exacerbate symptoms of dementia.

[1]Supported by NIA AG02711, NIA AG08415 and the Research Service of the Veterans Affairs Medical Center

This chapter discusses the nature and incidence of the problems underlying the sleep disorders common to elderly residents of nursing homes, and also discusses current treatments and evidence for therapeutic interventions that might be available in the future.

OVERVIEW

The sleep/wake cycle is one of the circadian rhythms found in humans. The rhythm of wake and sleep is controlled by one or more internal biologic oscillators or clocks, by environmental stimuli, and by other processes that either promote or inhibit arousal. Sleep is divided into *rapid eye movement* (REM) *sleep* and *nonrapid eye movement* (NREM) *sleep*. NREM sleep is further subdivided into stages 1 through 4. Stage 1 sleep is transitional sleep; stages 2 through 4 get progressively deeper, with stage 4 being the deepest level of sleep. Most dreams occur during REM sleep. The first REM period in a normal, middle-aged adult begins approximately 90 to 100 minutes after sleep onset. The deeper levels of sleep (stages 3 and 4) occur primarily in the first third of the night and REM sleep occurs primarily in the last third of the night.

The amount of deep sleep begins to decrease at age 20 years, and by the sixth and seventh decades of life is almost nonexistent. Wakefulness may increase in the elderly since older people are more easily aroused by internal and external stimuli. In a normal older person, total sleep time should either stay the same or increase slightly beyond the amount the individual slept when younger. In addition, older people often experience advanced sleep phase syndrome (i.e., a disturbance in the sleep/wake circadian rhythm), which is an early-to-bed, early-to-rise pattern of sleep. Due to the sleep phase shift, these individuals are not aware that when they awaken in the early morning, they have already slept a full night. They then report early morning awakenings and difficulty returning to sleep.

The sleep of normal aging is not significantly different from the sleep of younger people. The need to sleep does not change with age, but the ability to sleep does. Daytime sleepiness and greatly disturbed sleep are usually signs of a sleep disorder.

Sleep disruption at night may be a result of environmental factors, circadian rhythm disturbances, specific sleep disorders (e.g., sleep apnea), chronic bed rest, medication side effects, depression, psychiatric disturbance, or dementia. It may also be secondary to other medical disorders. Whatever its genesis, the result is increased daytime sleepiness and napping, which further compounds the problem of disrupted sleep at night.

The following sections discuss these pathophysiologic categories of sleep disorders:

- Sleep fragmentation
- Sleep apnea
- Sleep apnea with dementia
- Sleeping pills and other medications
- Sundowning

Sleep Fragmentation

Elderly, infirm nursing home residents typically have very disturbed sleep. This *sleep fragmentation* may be secondary to underlying medical conditions (such as painful arthritis, nocturia, asthma, headache, gastrointestinal illness, chronic heart failure, and other causes), psychiatric conditions, or sleep disorders.

Some nursing home residents are never asleep for a full hour and never awake for a full hour throughout the 24-hour day. In one survey, residents on average had no more than 39.5 minutes of sleep per hour; 50% awoke three or more times per hour, with some awakening over 30 times per hour. The conclusion is that many elderly residents in nursing homes constantly fall asleep and wake up, both during the day and through the night.

Sleep fragmentation represents a major problem in the management of caring for elderly residents. While it is a normal consequence of aging to wake up more frequently at night, the amount of sleep one needs does not change. Well-meaning caregivers often encourage residents to spend more time in bed in order to catch up on their sleep. However, chronic bed rest interferes with the normal circadian sleep/wake cycle, rather than contributing to sleep improvement, so it actually contributes to the problem.

The circadian rhythm that controls wake/sleep behavior can also be weakened or desynchronized by environmental factors (e.g., lack of sunlight or inadequate interior lighting). The typical healthy, community-dwelling elderly person averages about 1 hour of bright light exposure (that is, 2500 lux) per day. A *lux* is a unit of illumination equal to the direct illumination on a surface that is everywhere 1 meter from a uniform point source of one candle. Patients with Alzheimer's disease who live at home generally average about 30 minutes of bright light exposure per day. The typical nursing home resident rarely experiences bright light exposure at levels of 2500 lux, and typically experiences only 19 minutes at levels of 1000 lux. There does appear to be a direct correlation between dim lighting in the nursing home environment and sleep fragmentation among the resident population.

Sleep Apnea

Sleep apnea is characterized by transient attacks of failure of the autonomic control of respiration during sleep, resulting in alveolar hypoventilation and hypoxia. It may also result in acidosis and in vasoconstriction of pulmonary arterioles, producing pulmonary arterial hypertension. Sleep apnea is a common condition in an elderly nursing home population. Its prevalence in community-dwelling elderly is 24%; in nursing home elderly, 42%. In one nursing home study of sleep apnea, 11% of the residents stopped breathing 20 or more times for every hour of sleep, an amount associated with an increased risk of mortality. Female nursing home residents with severe sleep apnea have been shown to be at significantly greater risk of death than those not having severe sleep apnea.

Sleep Apnea with Dementia

Some studies suggest that severe sleep apnea is closely associated with *dementia*. In nursing home residents, there are significant differences in dementia scores between those with no or mild sleep apnea and those with severe sleep apnea, with the latter group having significantly more severe dementia. The sleep disordered breathing leads to daytime fatigue and hypoxia, which can lead to decreased mental skills and cognitive impairment. This is especially pronounced in residents with dementia, and is likely to make the symptoms of dementia worse.

Sleeping Pills and Other Medications

In nursing homes, the use of *sleeping pills* is widespread and excessive. In a typical facility, 35 of the residents have a prescription for a sleeping pill; 5% have a prescription for two sedative-hypnotics; and 17% have a prescription for hypnotic and psychoactive drugs and antihistamines, which also have sedating effects. Chronic use of hypnotics can be deleterious for any age group, but the risks are especially grave for elderly residents. Because they metabolize and excrete sleeping pills more slowly than do young adults, they are subject to the cumulative sedative effects. Such "hangovers" may persist for weeks after the drug is withdrawn, making the effects (lethargy, confusion, impaired cognition, and personality changes) insidious and difficult to recognize. This symptomatology is similar to the symptoms of dementia. Therefore, the effects of sedative-hypnotics might mimic one or more dementia symptoms as well as exacerbate them.

Polypharmacy presents a wide range of potential problems. For example, since sedatives and hypnotics act as respiratory depressants, their action may make it more difficult for a resident to breathe at night. They are contraindicated in residents with sleep apnea. Using several medications to treat hypertension or cardiac, respiratory, gastrointestinal, and neurologic disorders may also have negative consequences for the sleep/wake cycle, since many of these medications have stimulating or sedating effects (*see* Chapter 2, Polypharmacy).

Every drug can affect the sleep/wake cycle. The resident can be stimulated by the drug (producing fragmented or decreased sleep), or the drug may cause a drowsiness or increase in sleep time (thus producing a disruption in the resident's sleep/wake cycle). Consider these factors in titrating resident medication. Changes in the time of day and the dose of medication administration may be needed.

For example, a resident is receiving phenytoin (Dilantin), 300 mg daily, in the morning and is experiencing daytime drowsiness. Switching to giving the medicine at bedtime may eliminate daytime drowsiness and enhance the resident's nighttime sleep.

Sundowning

Sundowning is a poorly understood phenomenon that may affect anywhere from 10% to 30% of the infirm elderly in nursing homes. In general, the term is used to describe confusion, disorientation, and agitation that occurs at night or near sunset. The mechanisms underlying the disruptive behaviors are unknown, but the problem seems to be more severe in the fall and winter than in spring and summer. Low illumination exposure during the daytime and frequent nighttime disruptions by caregivers may be a contributing cause.

Treating the Resident with a Sleep Disorder

The goal of all treatment is to improve sleep at night and to increase alertness during the day. Much of the intervention involves environmental or habit changes and improved sleep hygiene, and is discussed in the following sections.

Sleep Hygiene

Caregivers should encourage the following sleep hygiene practices:

Limit the time spent in bed. Residents should not go to bed until it is time for them to go to sleep. Twelve or 13 hours spent in bed to obtain only 8 or 9 hours sleep results in increased sleep fragmentation, since many of those hours are spent in frustrated wakefulness. Residents may request to go to bed constantly (usually due to boredom), but extensive bed rest is appropriate only when absolutely necessary for the resident's health.

Arise at the same time each day. Encourage residents to get out of bed every morning at the same time. Sleeping in on some mornings can disrupt circadian rhythms severely. Altering staffing patterns and shift times to better accommodate residents getting up in the mornings helps both the residents and staff. However, resident preferences should carry considerable weight so think about adjusting this practice to the wishes of the resident. In this situation, explain why it is important for the resident to rise at the same time every day, and that it is not only an issue of staff convenience.

Avoid caffeine. Most nursing homes serve only decaffeinated coffee to their residents. However, try to eliminate other sources of caffeine from the diet, such as caffeinated tea, chocolate (served in desserts, hot cocoa, snacks), and sodas. Be alert to the possibility that residents who are having trouble sleeping may be purchasing snacks such as chocolate bars in the nursing home gift shop. Talk to the residents and family about the benefits of caffeine restriction. Provide education to family, residents, and nursing assistants about sources of caffeine other than coffee. Specify caffeine restrictions on diet orders and notify volunteers and staff.

Diet. Certain foods (including milk, turkey, fish, and bananas) contain tryptophan, a natural amino acid with sleep-promoting qualities. A glass of milk at bedtime may help induce sleep.

Serve meals at a table in a social setting. Never serve meals in bed unless the resident is too ill to get out of bed. The bed should be reserved for sleep only. Eating at the same time each day will also help consolidate the circadian rhythms, and give the resident something to look forward to.

Avoid naps. Sleepiness naturally occurs in the early afternoon and the resident may benefit from one nap per day at this time. Try to discourage naps at other times of the day, since one needs only a certain number of hours of sleep per 24 hours, and any daytime sleep reduces nighttime requirements.

Keep nighttime noise level to a minimum. The night shift staff should avoid creating unnecessary noise. For example, converse in a low voice in communal areas, enter resident rooms as quietly as possible, and avoid conversations in the resident rooms to prevent disturbing a light sleeper. The staff can also help reduce environmental noise by quietly moving linen carts, medication carts, and other carts in the hall as needed. Be sure that medication carts are equipped with lights so nurses can see to distribute medications without turning corridor or room lights on. Encourage the use of penlights/flashlights when necessary to monitor residents while sleeping. If the resident requires personal care at night, deliver it when administering medication (if possible) to reduce the number of times the resident is disturbed. If the resident is on a prompted voiding program, arrange to give medications at the same time the resident is encouraged to void.

Keep the residents' rooms as dark as possible at night. Not all residents are so frail as to require open bedroom doors at night for nursing observation. Many are able to use a call bell when nursing assistance is needed, and a closed door provides privacy as well as a useful barrier against extraneous noise and light. Curtains near the door can be pulled to block out hallway light. For residents who get up at night to use the toileting facilities, a dim light or nightlight can be left on in the bathroom, providing a safe passage and an environment conducive to sleep.

Keep the residents' environment as bright as possible during the day. Light levels are important determinants of the quantity and quality of sleep. Most rooms have only 100 to 200 lux light; 1000 to 2500 lux are needed to synchronize circadian rhythms. Keep window curtains open during the day. Encourage residents to sit outdoors whenever possible to increase the amount of bright light exposure. If the weather does not permit being outdoors, sitting directly at a window is also beneficial.

Match roommates based on nighttime as well as daytime routines and behaviors. While the staff routinely considers factors such as level of function, level of nursing care, and daytime personality in matching roommates, they are usually unaware of residents' nighttime habits. Residents often attribute their poor sleep to roommate incompatibility. Ask the night shift staff for input about the resident's night time habits. Characteristics such as the level of nursing intervention needed at night (bedpan use, scheduled voiding, or regular turning in bed) or personal habits (e.g., wandering, snoring, dresser or closet rummaging, watching late night television, or reading), if well matched between roommates, can promote better sleep environments. Do not match incontinent residents who need to be changed or toileted frequently with continent residents.

Time cues. Everyone needs time cues to help synchronize their days and nights. Light is a very strong time cue. There are also others. Give meals at the same time each day so that the residents expect to go to the dining hall or common area to eat. Each day of the week (weekends included) should have appropriate activities planned, not only for purposes of stimulation but also as a mnemonic aid to residents in determining what time of day it is. For example, if music always appears on the schedule on Tuesdays at 10:30 AM, it becomes a time cue. Place clocks, calendars, and orientation boards throughout the facility and in large enough print for the residents to see. Bedtime routines should relax the residents and begin to prepare them for the idea of going to sleep. For example, one resident's bedtime routine consists of brushing her teeth and changing into her nightclothes around 9 PM. She then gets into bed and watches television until the news is over, usually falling asleep between 11:30 and 12 midnight. Consult the residents and families to determine prior bedtime habits and routines.

Regular exercise. Exercises appropriate to the resident's level of function should be done every day, but not right before bedtime. Keeping the body as active as possible has a beneficial effect on sleep. Demented residents tend to respond best when props such as musical instruments, beach balls, parachutes, and other props are used in conjunction with music to encourage participation in exercise programs. (*See* Chapter 29, ADL Rehabilitation, for more information.)

Circadian Rhythm Disturbances

There are two types of circadian rhythm disturbances: advanced sleep phase and delayed sleep phase.

Advanced sleep phase, which is characterized by the individual's biologic clock being phase-advanced in relation to the actual time, is a common condition in the elderly. Individuals with this disorder typically become sleepy late in the afternoon (around 6:00 PM), go to sleep, wake up about 8 hours later (around 2:00 AM), and complain of early morning insomnia. The current treatment for advanced sleep phase is 2 hours of evening bright light therapy (from approximately 7:00 to 9:00 PM, or for 2 hours before bedtime), which has the effect of delaying the rhythm. Such treatment is not currently available but it is being tested at several academic medical centers.

Delayed sleep phase, where the biologic clock is phase-delayed in relation to the actual time, is less common in the elderly. Nursing home residents with this disorder are wide awake at other residents' normal bedtime (i.e., at 11:00 PM). They do not become sleepy until 1:00 to 3:00 AM, go to sleep for 8 or 9 hours, and wake at 9:00 or 10:00 AM or later. They are difficult to arouse in the morning, and complain of sleep-onset insomnia. Treatment for delayed sleep phase is 2 hours of morning bright light (early in the morning), which has the effect of advancing the rhythm.

Sleep Apnea

Sleep apnea is a serious and potentially life-threatening problem. Residents are usually not aware of their recurring pattern of breathing cessation and consequent brief awakenings. Daytime sleepiness and snoring are indicators that a problem may exist. Night shift staff, alert to a resident's disturbed breathing while asleep, should always notify the staff on other shifts of the situation.

Evaluate the resident who is suspected to have sleep apnea to determine if this problem is actually present. This can be done by companies that go into nursing facilities to do sleep recordings. Noninvasive and well-tolerated portable equipment can be brought to the resident's bedside, and a sleep recording made. Oximetry can be also be used to determine the presence of sleep apnea. Oximetry is a noninvasive method of monitoring arterial blood oxygen saturation. A monitoring probe is clipped to the resident's ear or finger, and a computer printout is generated that will tell the physician when apneic episodes have occurred. The physician can decide whether to treat the apnea (if present) or to refer the resident to a sleep disorders specialist. A referral to a sleep disorders specialist is indicated in residents with severe apnea in whom therapeutic measures have been unsuccessful and cognition and daytime functioning have been affected.

When sleep apnea is confirmed, the available treatments include using a continuous positive airway pressure device, which is a hose with a nosepiece attached to a machine that produces positive pressure. The resident wears the nosepiece each night, with the positive pressure acting as a splint to keep the airway open. Another possible treatment for sleep apnea is uvulopaletopharyngeoplasty, but this surgery is not effective in many cases. For a resident with several medical complications, the surgical risk may not be warranted for a procedure that may prove to be ineffective. Other, more practical treatment approaches include:

Weight loss (for residents who are overweight, losing as few as 20 pounds can make a difference in the severity of sleep apnea)

Low doses of tricyclic antidepressants (e.g., nortriptyline, 5 to 20 mg)

In mild cases, keeping residents from sleeping on their backs, which is accomplished by sewing a tennis ball into the back of their pajamas or hospital gowns, or propping them up with pillows.

Not all of these treatments may be appropriate in any given instance; assess each case individually. Nevertheless, with timely identification, diagnosis, and treatment, sleep apnea can be improved, reducing some dementia-like symptoms, improving nighttime sleep, decreasing daytime sleepiness, and reducing the risk of mortality.

Medications

Most residents have multiple diagnoses with several medications prescribed, some of which dramatically affect the central nervous system. For example, bronchodilators stimulate the central nervous system and can cause nighttime awakenings. Evaluate residents to determine whether *all* of the medications they are taking are necessary, and consider it a goal to discontinue or reduce medications. A psychiatric consultation can determine the most appropriate medications as well as orders for titration to reduce drugs to the absolute minimum. Clinicians must be mindful of residents' sleeping problems when reviewing prescribed medications. For example, medications with a stimulating effect should be given in the early morning rather than at night. Careful observation by the nursing staff is extremely important, and the primary care physician must be informed about resident sleep complaints, behaviors, and previous interventions.

One of the most common types of drugs prescribed in the nursing home are sedative-hypnotics, which can create daytime sleepiness and promote insomnia rather than improve it. Since sedative-hypnotics are contraindicated for sleep apnea, and may exacerbate

the symptoms of dementia, use them with caution. In cases where sedative-hypnotics are considered necessary, prescribe them at half of the lowest possible dose and only on a short-term basis to help the resident who has difficulty falling asleep in a new environment or to sleep well for a few nights until a more permanent solution (e.g., improved sleep hygiene) is found. Never use sedative-hypnotics as long-term cures.

Almost all drugs have some effect on sleep, acting either as depressants or stimulants. By adjusting the dose and the time of day that medications are taken, clinicians can often ameliorate daytime sleepiness and nighttime insomnia while achieving the intended benefit of the drugs. (*See* Chapter 2, Polypharmacy, for more information.)

Dementia

Residents with dementia may have disturbed sleep at night, excessive sleepiness in the day, night wandering, disorientation and confusion, as well as problems with daytime behavior. Residents with dementia often have diffuse slowing of their brain waves, making it difficult to distinguish wake from sleep. Residents with dementia show more sleep disruption than elderly controls, including lower sleep efficiency, decreased total sleep time, more stage 1 sleep (and therefore less stage 2, 3, or 4 sleep), and more awakenings during the night.

Residents with dementia are difficult to treat. If none of the previous suggestions are effective, the staff might consider planning quiet nighttime activities for individuals who wander at night and cannot sleep. Such activities might help keep residents busy for a time and settle them down, which will enable them to sleep better later in the night. A full activity program during the day as well as volunteers to help maintain resident involvement during programs can increase wake time and may make residents sleepier at night. (*See*

Chapters 12 and 30, Behavioral Symptoms and Activities Programming, respectively, for more information.)

Depression and Sleep

Depression in the elderly is often associated with complaints of insomnia. Advanced age exacerbates sleep disturbances in depression. Sleep in depressed residents is characterized by early morning awakenings, shortened REM latency, decreased stage 4 sleep, sleep fragmentation, and decreased total sleep time.

Sedative-hypnotics are not the drug of choice for treating insomnia in the person who is depressed. Rather, the resident may benefit from treatment with an antidepressive drug that has sleep-promoting side effects. (*See* Chapter 13, Depression, for more information.)

Future Directions

Current research in sleep therapy is an outgrowth of the advances in scientific understanding of the mechanisms that regulate sleep. The importance of sunlight as a stimulant and regulator of the brain hormones that control sleep is increasingly recognized, and as such represents an exciting development that promises to change the recommendations for sleep interventions in the future.

New research examining the effects of light therapy on the consolidation and improvement of sleep have significant implications for nursing home residents, who typically receive minimal exposure to sunlight. Therapeutic intervention with bright light approximates the sunlight needed to stimulate the natural pacemaker located in the brain, which strengthens the daily rhythms of sleep. Researchers are continuing their efforts to determine the best dose of bright light for optimal therapeutic effects. Until then, increasing exposure to natural sunlight, with precautions against sunburn and ocular photosensitivity, can prove beneficial to nursing home residents.

Sunlight also regulates sleep by influencing melatonin production. Melatonin has natural sedating properties. If research into the potential use of melatonin as a sleeping aid proves fruitful, it may result in the availability of a sleeping pill that avoids the negative side effects common to many sedative-hypnotics.

CASE EXAMPLE

Mrs. S. is an 86-year-old woman who has been a nursing home resident for 2.5 years. On admission, her primary diagnoses were dementia, osteoarthritis, and hypertension. She is ambulatory with a walker and can assist with, although she does not initiate, her self-care. Since admission to the nursing home, her condition has deteriorated consistent with the progressive nature of her dementia and arthritis. Night shift nursing staff have noticed that she has developed the habit of getting out of bed at night, wandering the halls, and disturbing other residents. An observational evaluation of her day and nighttime sleep habits was recommended.

The charge nurse on each shift recorded Mrs. S.'s sleep habits for 1 week. Input was solicited from the nursing assistant responsible for her care during each shift. Time in and out of bed, sleep onset, awakenings, daytime napping patterns, medications, and dietary habits were recorded.

On the day shift, Mrs. S. was awakened around 7:00 AM. She arose with difficulty, dressed with assistance, and walked to the dining room for breakfast. After breakfast, she returned to her bedroom to watch her favorite game shows while lying on the bed. She would usually doze off in bed for about 45 minutes in the morning.

Mrs. S. claimed to be disinterested in activities with "all those old people." Due to her occasional irritability and reputation for being difficult, the staff allowed her to spend most of the day alone in her room. Because of her preference for watching television, her window curtains were drawn all day. Frequently, her nurse would awaken her for lunch. After lunch, she would return to her bedroom, lie on the bed again to watch more television, and once again doze off.

In the afternoons, she often received visits from family members who indulged her long-standing preference for chocolate treats. After asking Mrs. S.'s permission to check, the staff found a large amount of chocolate candy in her dresser drawers.

The day shift nurses were surprised to note how isolated and irritable Mrs. S. had become, but they did not suspect sleep problems. Rather, the day shift had requested an evaluation for a possible diagnosis of depression.

On the evening shift, Mrs. S. complained of fatigue early in the evening and would retire to bed soon after dinner, about 6:00 PM She would lie in bed watching television for 1 to 1.5 hours and fall asleep around 7:30 PM. She slept well for the early hours of the evening.

On the night shift, around 2:00 AM, Mrs. S.'s sleep problems were manifested. She would frequently awaken, get out of bed, and wander to the nursing station. On some nights, the nursing staff encouraged her to visit the activity room to watch television or look at magazines quietly. Mrs. S. would be in and out of bed, disrupting other residents until 4:00 or 4:30 AM.

The charge nurse noted that Mrs. S.'s roommate needed assistance with nighttime toileting. The roommate was very demented and became confused about how to operate the call bell at night. To accommodate the roommate's need for assistance with toileting, the bedroom door was left open so she could call for nursing assistance. This disrupted Mrs. S.'s sleep.

The interdisciplinary team reviewed the reports from all three shifts. Mrs. S.'s 24-hour patterns indicated circadian rhythm advanced sleep phase, poor sleep hygiene, and a poor choice of roommates. The following recommendations were made and discussed with Mrs. S. and her family:

- The day shift staff should open the bedroom curtains when arousing Mrs. S. in the morning. This will provide a cue to daytime wakefulness and improve the overall level of illumination while she is in her bedroom.

- Throughout the day, Mrs. S. should be encouraged to participate in group activities. Her favorite television programs are enjoyed by other residents in the home, and could be watched in the television lounge with other residents. If she goes on out-of-facility trips or participates in patio activities such as gardening, her level of stimulation and illumination exposure would both improve, providing dual benefits to day/night wake/sleep patterns.

- Within a typical 24-hour period, Mrs. S. is in bed approximately 15 hours and gets around 9.5 hours of sleep, with the main sleep period being between 7:30 PM and 2:00 AM. This sleep occurs throughout the 24-hour period, with the only periods of high physical activity coinciding with meals. Her high level of bedrest, self-imposed and not prescribed, increases the fragmented nature of her nighttime sleep. She should be encouraged to stay out of bed for as many hours of the day as she can tolerate. In addition, she should be discouraged from retiring for the night until later in the evening. Bright light exposure during the late afternoon would help delay her circadian rhythm so that she would not be as tired at 7:30 in the evening.

- An evaluation for physical therapy to improve muscle strength and range of motion has been ordered, and Mrs. S. will be encouraged to attend exercise classes. Improving her muscle and joint conditioning can reduce her need for bedrest and encourage her to attend activities.

- The staff will inform Mrs. S.'s family that the candy and snacks they bring her contain caffeine and probably contribute to her sleep problem. The dietitian will provide them with a list of alternative snacks.
- The team should review the appropriateness of the roommate situation, exploring alternatives (preferably a roommate who does not call out). This could eliminate the environmental stimulants of hallway noise and roommate interruptions that coincide with Mrs. S.'s arousal.
- A psychiatric evaluation for depression may be necessary. If sleep habits and daytime irritability do not improve following this specified treatment, a diagnosis of depression causing early morning awakenings should be considered by a psychiatric consultation. If Mrs. S. is found to be depressed, a low-dose antidepressant with sleep-promoting qualities (e.g., nortriptyline) can improve her nighttime sleep and daytime functioning.

7
Stroke

Claire Levesque, MD
Pauline Belleville-Taylor, RN, CS, MS
Germaine Odenheimer, MD

Cerebrovascular disease is the third leading cause of death in the elderly in the United States. It is a devastating, life-altering cause of significant, long-lasting, neurologic disability. Both the incidence and mortality rates for stroke have decreased this century, possibly due to better control of hypertension and changes in diet. Unfortunately, there is still no definitive therapy for acute stroke. The major advances have been in rehabilitation of stroke survivors, development of adaptive equipment, and stroke prevention.

Stroke is mainly a disease of the elderly, occurring in both men and women. Its prevalence is higher in African-Americans and Asians, with African-Americans having a worse prognosis than other population groups with regard to functional recovery.

Stroke is a common reason for placement in a nursing home. Because of age or intercurrent illness, nursing home residents are also at high risk for developing strokes or experiencing recurrence of cerebrovascular events.

This chapter describes the rehabilitation and care of the stroke survivor and techniques to identify new strokes.

OVERVIEW

Cerebrovascular disease encompasses both hemorrhagic and ischemic infarction of the brain. Hemorrhage accounts for about 10% of sudden cerebrovascular events. Ischemic infarctions, which are much more common, are characterized by a sudden alteration of neurologic function. The following sections describe hemorrhage and ischemic infarctions in more detail.

Ischemic Infarction

Table 7-1 describes the three mechanisms that are the probable cause for the majority of ischemic infarctions.

Ischemic infarctions are often categorized on the basis of size. Moderate or large lesions are caused by occlusion of a major intracerebral blood vessel, such as the middle cerebral artery, or occlusion of a major branch, such as the superior division of the middle cerebral artery. Small lesions, often called lacunes, are areas of ischemia measuring 1 cm or less on imaging or pathologic studies. Lacunes are seen commonly in residents with hypertension or diabetes and likely represent chronic damage to small blood vessels. Many syndromes have been associated with lacunar

Table 7-1. Possible Mechanisms that Cause Ischemic Infarction

Cause	Etiology
Thrombosis of a cerebral blood vessel	While difficult to prove, occlusion of a blood vessel through thrombosis is the likely etiology in about one third of ischemic events.
Embolization	This is the likely etiology in 30% to 40% of ischemic infarctions. Embolization can be from a cardiac source, including thrombus due to hypokinesis, arrhythmias, valvular problems, or rare atrial myxomas (intracardiac tumors). Embolization can also be artery-to-artery, with carotid artery plaques the most common source. Recent studies with transesophageal echocardiography implicate the aorta as a potential source in a subset of residents.
Unexplained causes	About 30% of ischemic infarcts are unexplained. History, physical examination, and laboratory evaluation reveal no obvious etiology.

infarctions in specific end arteries. An example is pure motor hemiplegia, a syndrome of hemiparesis without sensory disturbance that is caused by an infarct in the motor fibers in the internal capsule. The hemiparesis is often quite severe, demonstrating that small lesions in critical brain areas can produce marked functional impairment.

As with other ischemic events, the recurrence of lacunar infarction is common and can lead to multiinfarct dementia. In this syndrome, an accumulation of multiple small ischemic infarcts produces a stepwise deterioration of cognitive function. The resident's level of function may plateau, but the cognitive disturbance resulting from the succession of events can limit recovery from other motor deficits significantly. Multiinfarct dementia may be more

common than Alzheimer's disease as a cause of dementia in elderly African-Americans. The cognitive deficits make rehabilitation difficult in these residents. Nursing facilities may be able to provide rehabilitative and restorative nursing services.

Hemorrhagic Infarction

Hemorrhagic infarction is much less common than ischemic infarction. It occurs in two patterns, as described in Table 7-2.

COMMON STROKE SYNDROMES

Strokes are often described on the basis of the vascular territory involved. This can help predict the full range of deficits experienced by a resident. For example, a resident with a complete left middle cerebral artery infarction can be expected to have both language and motor disabilities. This section describes the most common vascular syndromes.

Internal Carotid Artery

A slow, gradual occlusion of the internal carotid artery can be asymptomatic. More sudden thrombosis produces a syndrome similar to middle cerebral artery territory strokes (*see* the next section). The ophthalmic artery, a branch of the internal carotid artery, supplies the optic nerve and retina. Occlusion of the ophthalmic artery produces transient monocular blindness, which is also known as amaurosis fugax. This occlusion is a transient ischemic attack (TIA), and usually lasts less than 30 minutes. It is described as a shade coming down over one eye. Transient monocular blindness is a frequent warning sign of impending stroke.

Dominant Hemisphere
Middle Cerebral Artery

The middle cerebral artery divides into two branches: the superior division and the inferior division. The deficit varies depending on the site and side of the occlusion. The dominant hemisphere of the brain is responsible for language. In most residents, even those who are left-handed, the left hemisphere is the dominant hemisphere for language function.

Proximal occlusions infarct the entire middle cerebral artery territory. In left (dominant) middle cerebral artery occlusion, the deficits include right hemiplegia, right gaze palsy (eyes deviated to the left), right hemisensory loss (loss of sensation on the right side of body and face), right hemianopia (right visual field cut), and global aphasia (the inability to understand or produce language).

Table 7-2. Types of Hemorrhagic Infarctions and Their Patterns

Type	Pattern
Subarachnoid hemorrhage	Usually caused by rupture of an aneurysm, this pattern typically presents as a severe headache, with alteration of consciousness and focal neurologic signs. Significant long-standing neurologic deficits encompassing a broad range of functional disabilities can occur as a consequence of the hemorrhage itself or subsequent vasospasm.
Intraparenchymal bleed	Often secondary to hypertension, this pattern is also seen in vascular malformations, coagulation defects (including anticoagulant and thrombolytic therapy), and congophilic amyloid angiopathy (a rare, often familial disorder of cerebral blood vessels leading to hemorrhages). Classically, residents with this disorder also present with headache, sudden change in consciousness, and neurologic deficits. However, some cerebellar hemorrhages and small bleeds in other areas of the brain mimic the clinical presentation of an ischemic event. These are identified by head computer tomography (CT) or magnetic resonance imaging (MRI). Surgical intervention for cerebellar hemorrhage can be life-saving and can maximize neurologic recovery. Neurologic deficits vary depending on the site and size of the hemorrhage.

If the superior division of the left (dominant) middle cerebral artery is infarcted, the resident will again have a right hemiplegia, right hemisensory loss, and gaze palsy. The language dysfunction is Broca's aphasia. In this syndrome, residents have marked difficulty producing language with some preservation of comprehension.

Infarction of the inferior division of the left middle cerebral artery produces a visual field cut, Wernicke's aphasia, and no disturbances of sensory or motor function. Wernicke's aphasia (fluent aphasia) is a severe disruption of language comprehension. Residents with this condition cannot comprehend their own language output so they speak freely but nonsensically.

Some left middle cerebral infarcts also cause apraxia. Residents with this deficit cannot perform skilled maneuvers, such as dressing or mimicking gestures, even though there is enough preservation of strength and sensation.

Small branch occlusions of the middle cerebral artery can occur. One such syndrome is transcortical motor aphasia, producing nonfluent language with difficulties in naming objects. Comprehension and repetition are intact. Transcortical sensory and mixed aphasias also occur and are thought to be due to watershed infarcts (*see* the section on watershed infarcts for more information).

Nondominant Middle Cerebral Artery

Infarction of the entire territory of the right middle cerebral artery produces left hemiplegia, left hemisensory loss, left gaze palsy, and left hemianopia. It also produces a neglect syndrome. *Neglect* means total lack of attention to half of the universe. These residents deny that their left arm belongs to them, dress and shave only the right side of their body, and ignore items in the left hemispace. They may also misinterpret nonverbal cues, especially the emotional content of language and facial expressions. They may have modest problems with naming objects but their overall language function is preserved.

Infarction of the superior division produces hemiplegia, hemisensory loss, gaze palsy and some neglect of the environment. The neglect syndrome is much less profound than in total occlusions of the nondominant middle cerebral artery.

Infarction of the inferior division causes a visual field disturbance and problems with some visuospatial tasks, such as copying complex drawings.

Anterior Cerebral Artery

Occlusions of the anterior cerebral artery usually produce a graded hemiparesis that is most marked in the foot. Urinary incontinence can occur. Abulia, a state in which residents lack spontaneity or motivation, and appear apathetic, is sometimes seen. These residents remain where caregivers put them and do not interact with other residents spontaneously.

Vertebrobasilar System

The posterior circulation, consisting of the basilar and vertebral arteries and their branches, supplies the brain stem, the cerebellum, and the occipital lobes. Multiple syndromes are caused by complete and partial occlusions of these vessels and branches. Common symptoms include dizziness, balance problems, visual disturbances, diplopia (double vision), swallowing problems, dysarthria (slurring of speech due to motor weakness with preserved language abilities), weakness, and sensory changes.

One common example of stroke in the brain stem is the lateral medullary syndrome, which is caused by occlusion of a branch of the vertebral artery. Residents with this condition have loss of sensation on one side of the face and on the opposite side of the body. They have dizziness, dysarthria, swallowing difficulty, and marked balance problems.

Lacunar Syndromes

Lacunar syndromes are occlusions of the small cerebral blood vessels. These strokes are small in size, but the deficits can be significant depending on the location of the lesion. Some examples include:

- *Pure sensory stroke.* Loss of sensation on one half of the body with preserved motor abilities.
- *Pure motor hemiplegia.* Loss of motor function without sensory loss.
- *Dysarthria-clumsy hand syndrome.* Slurred speech with clumsiness in one hand.

Watershed Infarcts

Watershed infarcts occur at the border zones between arterial supplies, and are usually caused by an episode of hypotension. As the blood pressure drops, blood flow in these small vessels drops, thereby causing ischemia.

One example of a watershed infarct occurs at the border zone between the anterior, middle, and posterior cerebral arteries in the left hemisphere. The result is transcortical sensory aphasia, a disturbance of language that causes difficulty in naming objects and in comprehension. Repetition and fluency are preserved.

Mixed transcortical aphasia is also usually due to a watershed infarct and causes nonfluent language with naming and comprehension problems, but with preservation of the ability to repeat. As noted in the section on the dominant hemisphere middle cerebral artery, transcortical motor aphasia is due to an occlusion of a small branch of the left middle cerebral artery.

Watershed infarctions can also cause other syndromes not related to language function.

COMMON DISABILITIES AFTER A STROKE

Thinking of strokes in broad terms, i.e., as vascular syndromes, helps the clinician identify other, less apparent deficits. However, in the nursing home setting, where a prime focus of caregiving is rehabilitation and restoration, it is also helpful to think of various stroke-related disabilities as isolated entities. This section describes five common problems after stroke that typically result in nursing home referrals.

Hemiplegia and Hemiparesis

Hemiplegia is total loss of strength (or paralysis) in half of the body. It is often accompanied acutely by flaccid muscle tone followed by development of spasticity.

Hemiparesis is the partial loss of strength, with strength quantified on the following scale:

- 5/5—Ability to oppose gravity and full resistance
- 4/5—Ability to oppose gravity and partial resistance
- 3/5—Ability only to oppose gravity
- 2/5—Ability to move only with gravity removed
- 1/5—Ability to contract the muscle without generating movement
- 0/5—No movement

Hemiparesis in stroke patients is often more prominent in the upper extremities. For example, a useful stable gait is possible in many residents who do not regain upper extremity strength and dexterity. The classic gait of a stroke survivor with hemiparesis is asymmetric, with circumduction (circular swing) and spasticity of the involved leg, and a rigid, flexed arm held close to the body.

Alteration of Sensory Modalities

Stroke patients can have disruption of both the primary and secondary sensory modalities. Primary modalities include light touch, pinprick, temperature, proprioception (position sense), and vibration. Loss of primary modalities can lead to injuries on the affected side. Some residents experience abnormal sensations, including dysesthesias (uncomfortable sensations such as burning) or hyperesthesias (increased sensitivity to sensory input such as discomfort from a sheet over the body area). In some thalamic strokes, these dysesthesias are debilitating (the thalamic pain syndrome).

In some residents with parietal lobe infarctions, the primary modalities may be preserved but secondary sensory modalities may be impaired. An example is sensory inattention. When stimulated simultaneously on both sides of the body, the resident perceives the input only on the unaffected side. This "extinction on double simultaneous stimulus" can lead to tactile misinterpretations.

After a parietal lobe infarct, residents may also have difficulty integrating more complex sensory stimuli on the affected side. Test for the following senses: graphesthesia (identification of letters or numbers written on the hand) and stereognosis (identification of small objects such as keys or coins placed in the hand). Residents with impairment of this type of sensory function often need to look at their affected side to augment tactile stimuli with visual cues.

Visual Disturbances

Strokes may produce visual field disturbances, the most common of which is a homonymous hemianopia (i.e., loss of vision in half of the visual field in both eyes). Residents with this type of deficit may run into things on the involved side and have a varying degree of ability to compensate. When combined with a neglect syndrome due to largely nondominant middle cerebral artery infarcts, a resident may never learn to pay attention to the affected hemispace, causing safety problems and difficulties with rehabilitation.

Language Disorders—Aphasia

This section discusses the language disorders associated with aphasia. Table 7-3 lists the language disorders that are commonly encountered in residents with stroke.

Global, Broca's, and Wernicke's aphasias are the most dramatic examples of language disturbance. Other, more subtle language dysfunctions can occur after both right and left hemisphere infarctions (see Chapter 16, Communication, for more information).

Evaluation of Aphasia

Aphasias are syndromes of disordered language that typically involve some degree of impairment of comprehension and/or fluid, grammatic expression of words. These syndromes are distinguished from speech disorders caused by problems with articulation or phonation in the context of preserved language. When speech is unintelligible, identify the language disorders by determining the proficiency of related aspects of language such as following commands, reading, or writing.

Identifying specific aphasias has diagnostic, prognostic, and therapeutic implications that can be approached in three general ways:
- Observational (informal)
- Task-specific (semiformal)
- Standardized (formal)

The typical clinical approach toward language assessment is informal. The resident, engaged in conversation with the examiner, is observed for the appropriateness of both spontaneous verbal output and behavioral responses, suggesting comprehension of the interchange. However, even moderately severe language deficits may go unnoticed with this technique because the resident may have well-preserved social skills. The resident may be adept at picking up nonverbal cues and may communicate effectively with gesture and a few common expressions.

The semiformal or task-oriented approach is useful to determine the general type and severity of language impairment and can direct management strategies. This approach has specific goals but can be done without special material or extensive training. The formal approach, using standardized tests, is usually

Table 7-3. Major Language Disorders Occurring in Residents with Stroke

Disorder	Symptoms
Global aphasia	This most profound language disturbance results from a large, dominant hemisphere, middle cerebral artery stroke. These residents initially have no language output and no comprehension of spoken or written language. As they recover they may regain a few phrases, but severe language dysfunction persists.
Broca's aphasia	Also known as *nonfluent* aphasia, this type of aphasia produces marked difficulty with production of language, but comprehension is preserved. The resident speaks in a halting, effortful style using short, telegraphic messages. This aphasia is caused by occlusion of the superior division of the middle cerebral artery.
Wernicke's (receptive) aphasia	Also known as *fluent* aphasia, it is characterized by an inability to comprehend language, with an ability to produce fluent language. The language output has little content, however, and ranges from paraphasic errors (incorrectly used words or minor word alterations, such as gamp for lamp) to completely unintelligible language-like sounds. Residents with Wernicke's aphasia can appear psychotic or delirious, since they become agitated and frustrated with staff's inability to comprehend them.

performed by trained speech therapists/pathologists or neuropsychologists. This approach is useful to detect subtle change in language function.

Language is organized predominantly on the left side of the brain in most individuals, so aphasias are often associated with deficits of motor and/or sensory function on the right side of the body. Some aphasia types suggest etiologies for which medical or surgical intervention may be indicated.

The most common causes of aphasia in adults are strokes, Alzheimer's disease, head trauma, and tumors. Aphasias can occur from lesions that affect cortical and/or subcortical structures. The subcortical aphasias have not been as well characterized as cortical aphasias.

The largest lobe of the brain is located behind the brow and is called the frontal lobe. It is responsible predominantly for action or preparation for action, such as the verbal production of words. When lesions occur in the frontal lobe on the left side, it is likely that difficulty producing chains of words will result and may yield telegraphic, agrammatic, and effortful verbal output. Language disorders associated with effortful output are sometimes referred to as anterior, expressive, or nonfluent aphasias.

The parietal, occipital, and temporal lobes of the brain are responsible primarily for reception and interpretation of incoming (sensory) information. A lesion on the left side of the brain involving one of the sensory lobes (especially the temporal or parietal) may be associated with problems interpreting words that are heard or read. Residents tend to produce words without effort but the words are often inappropriate. This type of language problem is often referred to as posterior, sensory, receptive, or fluent aphasia.

There are a few cautions to note when evaluating a resident with aphasia: the tests must be difficult enough to be sensitive to subtle changes but not so difficult that they are influenced heavily by educational factors. There must be language output in some domain (writing or speaking) to identify an aphasia. For example, a resident may be mute from severe depression with no language disorder. Many domains of language evaluation have been described but only four of them are discussed here: naming, repetition, fluency, and comprehension.

Naming

Anomia is the inability to name objects correctly, and suggests dysfunction of the left hemisphere of the brain and occurs in almost any language disorder (aphasia). Naming tasks can serve to screen for aphasia, but only if the tasks are difficult enough. For example, on the Mini Mental State Examination (MMSE) (Folstein, 1975), the resident is asked to name a pencil and a watch. This task is easy for many aphasics. To increase the sensitivity of the screen, ask residents less common words or parts of objects, such as watch band, clasp, and hands. Some names, such as winding stem, face, and crystal are educationally or culturally influenced, so interpret errors within this context.

Repetition

After establishing that the resident has an anomia, the task is to determine whether language deficits are evident from dysfunction in the primary language areas around the sylvian fissure (the peri-sylvian region). In the repetition task on the MMSE, "no ifs, ands, or buts," is very sensitive to repetition difficulties, but is culturally influenced in minor ways. For example, common but nonaphasic errors include omitting the plural "s" ("no if and or but") or changing the phrase to "no ifs ands and buts." Aphasic repetition errors are characterized by word order errors in this particular phrase, for which practice does not appear to benefit the patient. For example, residents may say, "no buts... no... no ifs... wait.... ands no."

Fluency

Fluent output does not mean correct language usage. It implies a quality of effortlessness with normal inflection and flow in word production. The part of the cortex largely responsible for activating and producing behavior, including language behavior, is the frontal lobe. Therefore, when language output is decreased, effortful, and agrammatic, there is likely dysfunction of the left frontal lobe. The so-called nonfluent language implies difficulty in producing strings of words with a grammatic organization. It is often referred to as telegraphic speech because the message may be comprised of meaningful words that are minimally connected, as in a telegram. There is also a tendency toward single-word responses. For example:

Examiner: "How did this happen?"
Resident: "Fell."
Examiner: "What kind of work did you do before?"
Resident: "Carpenter."

There is no specific bedside test to measure fluency. Consistently abbreviated responses, especially to open-ended questions in which the resident appears to be trying to express him- or herself, are likely to represent nonfluency.

Comprehension

Comprehension is vital to ensure that a resident can make competent decisions. Therefore, careful documentation of the level of comprehension has broad management implications.

Language comprehension is largely a task of the left temporal or parietal lobes. Sounds are heard first cortically in the primary auditory area in the temporal lobe. This information is transmitted to posterior regions that interpret the sounds. When residents have problems with comprehension, it is likely that they have dysfunction in the left temporal or parietal lobes. To have the resident perform the comprehension task on the MMSE, place a piece of paper in front of him or her and say, "Take the paper in your right hand, fold it in half, and put it on the floor," is a reasonable screen for comprehension. However, performance of the task can be influenced not only by aphasia but also by poor hearing or eyesight, inattention, poor memory, decreased motivation, or right/left confusion.

When errors are made, perform additional comprehension tasks to establish the basis for error. Do not assume that comprehension is normal based only on conversations with the resident. It is not unusual for the resident to appear to understand whatever you say and yet be unable to carry out simple commands, such as "Point to the ceiling." In the reading task on the MMSE, "Close your eyes," is another task that is easy for many aphasics. In general, comprehension for midline commands such as, "Close your eyes," "Open your mouth," "Stand up," "Turn around," and "Take off your glasses," may be preserved despite otherwise severe comprehension deficits.

Summary

The following list summarizes the domains of language function:
- Naming abnormal: **Left** hemisphere damage
- Repetition abnormal: **Peri-sylvian** damage
- Nonfluent: **Frontal** lobe damage
- Comprehension abnormal: **Parietal/temporal** lobe damage

Use of the word "normal" to describe the domains of language function is relative. For example, residents with isolated lesions of the left frontal lobe are typically nonfluent with relatively spared comprehension. However, given difficult enough tasks, residents with isolated frontal lesions often show subtle comprehension problems.

By examining four domains of language: naming, repetition, fluency, and comprehension, you can identify eight aphasic categories, which are shown in Table 7-4.

Neglect Syndrome

Residents with a neglect syndrome typically have sustained a nondominant hemisphere stroke. In the most profound cases, they do not recognize the affected side of their body as part of themselves, ignoring it while washing and dressing. They ignore the affected hemispace and run into obstacles in their affected visual field. They also deny their deficit by not believing that they have had a stroke. These residents benefit from bed placement and placement at meals and activities, which allow them to be with staff and other residents.

DISCHARGE PLANS FOR THE STROKE PATIENT

Admission of the stroke patient to a nursing home after hospitalization, rather than to alternative care settings, is generally determined by the functional disabilities present during the acute stage of the stroke and any intercurrent medical and psychiatric problems, as well as the ability of the nursing care facility to carry out a rehabilitation program. The following placement pattern typically applies:

- Patients with *minor* deficits are usually discharged to their homes after evaluation.
- Patients with *larger* deficits are considered for rehabilitation in a specialty hospital. Acceptance into a rehabilitation program depends on the type of deficit and its projected response to physiotherapy, as well as on the overall medical condition of the

Table 7-4. Eight Aphasic Categories

Naming	Repetition	Fluency	Comprehension	Site	Syndrome
ABN	ABN	ABN	N	Frontal	Broca's
ABN	ABN	N	ABN	Temporal	Wernicke's
ABN	ABN	ABN	ABN	Peri-sylvian Frontal Temporal Parietal	Global
ABN	ABN	N	N	Arcuate Fasciculus	Conduction
ABN	N	ABN	N	Frontal	Transcortical motor
ABN	N	N	ABN	Parietal	Transcortical Sensory
ABN	N	ABN	ABN	Watershed Frontal Temporal Parietal	Mixed Transcortical
ABN	N	N	N	Left brain	Anomic

ABN = abnormal; N = normal (relatively).

patient. Most rehabilitation centers require that the patient have a need for at least two therapy disciplines (physical, occupational, or speech), and that he or she possess the stamina to participate in the rehabilitative program for at least 3 hours a day.

- Patients with *larger deficits complicated by medical or psychiatric problems* are considered for rehabilitation in nursing facilities. Common coexisting disorders include depression and dementia, as well as medical problems such as chronic obstructive pulmonary disease, cardiac disease, and arthritis, which can complicate care.
- Patients with *very large deficits* may be placed in nursing facilities for total nursing care. These residents can still benefit from a restorative and rehabilitative care model.

IDENTIFYING RESIDENTS WITH ACUTE STROKE

Stroke is defined as an abrupt change in neurologic function. TIAs are episodes of alteration of neurologic function last less than 24 hours (by definition), but often last only minutes with complete recovery of function. However, these events can be warnings of impending stroke with permanent deficits. Strokes may also occur without warning, and frequently are present upon awakening.

Because of advanced age and problems such as heart disease, hypertension, smoking history, and diabetes, the typical nursing home population is at high risk for stroke. Early identification of the warning signs can sometimes result in preventing permanent deficits through prompt diagnosis and treatment. Table 7-5 summarizes these major warning signs.

While all of the symptoms shown in Table 7-5 can be seen in many other medical problems as well, health care providers must consider and evaluate them as precursors to a possible stroke. In residents with dementia or a previous stroke, new cerebrovascular events can be difficult to identify. Often, the major clue to a new event is an unexplained change in the resident's abilities to assist with activities of daily living (ADLs). Examples include the inability to manage finger foods, problems with transfers, or deterioration in interactive skills. Even confusion and a new onset of seizures in an elderly resident should prompt consideration of a stroke.

EVALUATING RESIDENTS WITH ACUTE STROKE

In a newly admitted resident with a history of stroke, or in a long-term resident with new symptoms suggestive of cerebrovascular disease, the first step in the evaluation process is to take a complete history of the event, review the risk factors, and conduct an examination with particular emphasis on cardiovas-

Table 7-5. Major Warning Signs of Possible Cerebrovascular Event

Sudden loss of vision or blurring in one or both eyes

Weakness on one or both sides of the body, sometimes including the face

Difficulty producing speech or language, or difficulty understanding language

Dizziness, loss of balance, or falling spells

Swallowing problems

Sudden onset of headache in a resident without chronic headaches

cular and neurologic involvement. Bruits or diminished pulses in the carotid arteries suggest stenosis and impairment of blood flow. Cardiac murmurs or rhythm abnormalities may predispose to thrombus formation and embolization. Blood pressure abnormalities, including hyper- or hypotension, may alter blood flow to the brain or cause chronic vascular damage. Since both endocarditis and a myocardial infarction may present as acute stroke, strongly consider these if there is fever, chest pain, or other cardiac symptoms. Obtain an electrocardiogram (ECG), and evaluate the cardiac enzymes if it is abnormal. Blood cultures are appropriate if the resident has a fever or new cardiac murmur.

Start the neurologic examination by observing the resident closely. Passive observation can yield important information about probable neurologic deficits and functional correlations. Does the resident use all of his or her extremities? Does he or she observe all surroundings? Can the resident provide a coherent history? Can he or she manipulate objects in the environment normally? Are the resident's posture and gait normal? Is there a new impairment in ADLs?

Staff members can perform additional evaluations, which are shown in Table 7-6.

DIAGNOSTIC AND THERAPEUTIC OPTIONS IN ACUTE STROKE

If stroke is suspected, place the resident on close observation, and monitor his or her pulse and blood pressure every 4 hours. In acute stroke, maintain the blood pressure at baseline or even slightly higher. Very tight control of blood pressure with the risk of hypotension can lead to cerebral hypoperfusion and cause extension of the infarction.

The nursing staff can conduct neurologic checks (i.e., a brief testing of language function and orientation, monitoring of pupil size, and hand grips) every 4 hours. Customize these checks to accommodate the resident's

Table 7-6. Resident Stroke Evaluation*

To evaluate	Procedure
Language function	Ask the resident to name objects, follow simple (one-step) commands, and repeat phrases.
Oral function	Note clarity of speech, ability to handle oral secretions, and swallowing function.
Orientation	Ask the resident to state his or her name, location, and the date.
Pupillary responses	Shine a light in one of the resident's eyes and observe the reaction in both. A normal response is a brisk constriction of both pupils. Repeat in the opposite eye.
Extraocular movements	Ask the resident to follow your finger or penlight with his or her eyes. Note any problems with extraocular movements and any forced deviation of the eyes.
Facial strength	Have the resident smile, show teeth, close eyes, puff out cheeks, noting any facial asymmetries.
Upper extremity strength	Test the hand grip for strength and symmetry. Test for drift by asking the resident to hold both arms out, palms up, straight in front with the eyes closed. When drift is present, the weak arm drifts downward and the palm turns in. Record any strength in the major muscle groups using the five-point scale. Note muscle tone by passive range of motion at the major joints.
Lower extremity strength	In an ambulatory resident, observe the gait. Observe other residents when transferring them. Record the ability to move the major muscle groups using the five-point scale. Note muscle tone by passive range of motion at major joints.
Sensory function	Test light touch with a cotton swab and pinprick with a safety pin, comparing the two sides of the body. Also test the face.
Reflexes	Test deep tendon reflexes by tapping with a reflexive hammer at the biceps, triceps, brachioradialis, knee, and ankle. Record the results on a 0-4 scale, with 0 being absent reflexes, 2+ being normal, and 4+ being increased reflexes with the presence of clonus (sustained rhythmic movement after the stimulus). Particularly note any asymmetries. Test for the Babinski sign by stroking the lateral aspect of the sole and observing the great toe. If the toe moves up, the Babinski sign is present (an abnormal response).

*This brief screening examination is useful in finding new deficits and following their progression. Physicians can perform further detailed examinations to elucidate other deficits.

abilities. For instance, a resident with dementia may not be able to answer typical orientation questions, but may be able to name objects or give a family member's name.

In some cases, transfer to an acute care facility will be warranted, but the decision must always be placed in the context of the resident's medical problems and any advanced directives or instructions from a health care proxy. Typical instances suggesting the need for acute care transfer include:

- New arrhythmias or heart murmurs, which may require observation in a cardiac care unit to rule out myocardial infarction, diagnose the new cardiac problem, and begin treatment.
- Alteration of consciousness or severe headache, which may indicate subarachnoid or intraparenchymal hemorrhage. Strongly consider an emergency head CT.
- Cerebellar findings such as dizziness or balance problems, or brain stem findings such as diplopia or crossed sensory or motor findings (e.g., right body and left face sensory changes), which raise the possibility of cerebellar hemorrhage. Since this is potentially a neurosurgical emergency, consider evaluation with an emergency head CT.
- Signs of increased intracranial pressure, such as sudden, significant depression of consciousness, asymmetric pupils, or an unresponsive pupil, requiring emergency imaging and potential neurosurgical intervention.

In other situations, decisions about the need for an imaging study depend on the overall medical condition and the potential for a therapeutic change. Small or moderate ischemic infarcts may not be apparent on imaging during the first day. However, with the passage of time, these infarcts will be seen on both CT and MRI. Computed tomography has clear advantages in demonstrating acute hemorrhage, and is better tolerated by residents. The high resolution of MRI will show lacunes, brain stem infarcts, and deep temporal lobe infarcts not seen on CT.

Computed tomography testing includes a limited exposure to x-rays, but a study without a contrast agent is very safe for persons who are not pregnant. An intravenous contrast agent is rarely used in studies on strokes and is contraindicated in renal insufficiency. Most individuals tolerate head CT well, but mild sedation is required occasionally. If needed, lorazepam, 0.5 to 1.0 mg by mouth, can be prescribed before the study. If the resident is taking an as needed sleeping medication, use this as an alternative choice. Low-dose, short-acting medications, such as oxazepam or lorazepam, are preferred. In general, it is best to avoid sedating medicines during the acute stage of the stroke since this complicates evaluation.

Magnetic resonance imaging is contraindicated in residents with pacemakers, magnetic clips from prior surgery, or intraocular metal (typical in welding injuries). The test requires the resident to lie still in a small tubelike structure with loud banging noises. It is not well tolerated by some individuals, especially those with claustrophobia or confusion. Use sedating medications to lessen anxiety, but consider this very carefully in the elderly and during the acute stroke. Cooperation with imaging studies is often increased if family or familiar staff accompany the resident to explain the testing procedure.

If hemorrhage is discovered, consider transferring the resident to an acute hospital for a neurosurgical evaluation. In ischemic infarctions, a search for the etiology of the event is warranted. An ECG may reveal arrhythmias and changes suggestive of cardiac ischemia. In residents with murmurs, new arrhythmias, or congestive heart failure, echocardiography is used to evaluate for possible valvular disease and thrombus formation. Holter monitoring is indicated in arrhythmias, in residents with pacemakers, and in strokes associated with syncope. An imaging procedure of the carotid arteries is indicated if endarterectomy is being considered, or to help delineate etiology.

The definitive imaging test for carotid stenosis is cerebral arteriography, an invasive procedure involving contrast. It carries an increased risk of morbidity and mortality in the elderly, including renal failure, cerebrovascular events, and injury to the peripheral vasculature. A new alternative is magnetic resonance angiography (MRA), a software technique that enhances visualization of major blood vessels on MRI without the use of contrast dyes. Since the technique is new, abnormalities seen on MRA may require confirmation by angiography or ultrasound. Carotid ultrasound provides information on stenosis and impaired flow in the internal and external carotids, but does not provide information about intracerebral vessels.

Therapy for acute stroke is limited. In residents with a new stroke who are not transferred to an acute hospital, maintain blood pressure at baseline or slightly higher. Place these residents on aspiration precautions; in some instances, these residents may need to take nothing by mouth during the initial stages. Start rehabilitation as early as possible by consulting with the appropriate therapies and develop a therapeutic plan. Initiate procedures that will prevent additional cerebral vascular events.

THERAPEUTIC MODALITIES IN STROKE REHABILITATION

After the acute phase of a stroke, the resident begins to have gradual recovery of neurologic function. Since neurons that have sustained ischemic damage do not regenerate, some functions return due to the development of alternative brain connections. These new brain programs can be facilitated by physical, occupational, and speech therapy.

Therapeutic Modalities

There are two approaches that are used to facilitate the return of abilities. The more traditional approach emphasizes training the unaffected side to take over all functions, such as one-handed dressing skills. The less traditional approach, known as the neuro-developmental or Bobath approach, aims to restore function to the affected side. Studies have shown no significant difference in return of function between the two approaches, but subsets of residents may respond more favorably to one approach than the other.

As soon as the resident is medically stable, involve the rehabilitation team. This interdisciplinary team consists of physicians, nurses, and ancillary therapeutic services. Nurses support and assist the resident with exercises, ADLs, and communication skills, and otherwise implement the individualized care plan developed by the team. Table 7-7 summarizes the specialized rehabilitation services. (See Chapters 29 and 16, ADL Rehabilitation and Communication, respectively, for further details.

Nurses and nurse assistants are responsible for maintaining continuity of therapy between sessions. Rehabilitation is modified to match the resident's needs. Often, this means scheduling short therapy times and frequent rest periods to accommodate decreased endurance. Cognitive or psychiatric disabilities are addressed through simplification of instructions. Even for residents with a large deficit or a remote history of stroke, a well-designed program of physiotherapy can result in continuing slow improvement, with the collateral benefit of an improved sense of psychological well-being.

Table 7-7. Specialized Stroke Rehabilitation Services

Rehabilitation Service	Description
Physical therapy	Deals mainly with the development of strength and return of mobility, and provides suggestions for the use of various walking aids and splints. Preventing contractures is also an important goal. The physical therapist can develop a program of passive and active range-of-motion and strengthening exercises tailored to the resident's needs. With proper instruction, this program can be carried out by the resident and nursing staff, particularly the nurse assistants.
Occupational therapy	Focuses mainly on return of function in ADLs (e.g., feeding and dressing). These complex activities require integration of a motor plan with visual and tactile cues. The occupational therapist also assists with finding adaptive equipment to maximize independence. Occupational therapy works with the nursing staff to help the resident perform ADLs.
Speech therapy	Useful to residents who, because of stroke, have difficulty either swallowing or communicating. For those with swallowing difficulties, the speech therapist evaluates the problem and recommends foods to avoid (e.g., thin liquids) in order to minimize choking. The speech therapist or staff member is present at meal times to retrain the resident in the act of swallowing. For residents with communication problems, the speech therapist works with them initially to develop a communication system for basic needs, then assists with the development of more complex language abilities. The resident practices these skills in conversations with staff, other residents, and visitors.
Recreation therapy	Allows residents to regain interpersonal skills and improve psychosocial well-being in a protected environment where the embarrassment about disabilities is minimized.
Cognitive therapy	Useful in residents with impairment of memory or other cognitive functions. The speech therapist or occupational therapist often incorporates this into sessions. Residents learn to use memory books and other techniques, and practice interactions with staff, other residents, and visitors.

Rehabilitation programs need to be used on an ongoing basis, according to the resident's physical condition and response to the program. Improvements in motor skills and strengthening can continue through the first year after a stroke, and significant changes in other modalities develop slowly over weeks and months. This places the nursing home staff in a key position

to carry out this more long-term type of rehabilitation program.

Assessment Scales

In addition to the care component, rehabilitation programs use various assessment tools and techniques, which may be useful in charting a resident's progress, determining areas for future emphasis, and assisting in evaluating the prognosis for recovery. However, note that all assessment scales oversimplify complex resident issues and are least helpful when applied to residents with multiple medical problems. Careful review of the resident's needs by all members of the care team remains the most accurate method for determining levels of care, prognosis and future plans. Table 7-8 describes some assessment scales that are commonly applied.

COMPLICATIONS OF STROKE AND THERAPEUTIC INTERVENTIONS

Stroke produces many complications, some of which are directly related to the neurologic process causing the stroke, while others are secondary to ensuing problems. Both types of complications are discussed in the following sections.

Preventing Recurrence of Stroke

A major issue in the management of stroke patients is the prevention of further cerebrovascular events. The recurrence rate for strokes is estimated at 25% in most studies. Prevention of stroke recurrence includes the reduction of risk factors and the chronic use of antiplatelet or anticoagulant medications. Anticoagulation with warfarin is indicated mainly in residents with chronic or intermittent atrial fibrillation, most heart valve replacements, and in residents with embolic sources such as a cardiac thrombus. Warfarin is contraindicated in individuals with bleeding disorders and recent hemorrhages. There are also multiple relative contraindications, including an unstable gait, which may lead to falls and possible injuries.

In other causes of ischemic infarction, aspirin has been shown to decrease the recurrence of stroke and cardiac disease. Most studies have included large numbers of white men, and clearly demonstrate significant decreases in relative risks in these patients. Smaller numbers of women and nonwhites have been studied, with less definitive results. An optimal dose and dosing intervals have not been determined; recommendations range from 90 mg every other day to 650 mg twice a day. The

Table 7-8. Assessment Scales

For assessment of	Scales
Self-care skills	Barthel's index assigns point values to the resident's level of independence in skills such as walking, transfers, dressing, and bowel and bladder continence. In the nursing home setting, the ADL items from the Health Care Financing Minimum Data Set should be well understood and provide information and resident involvement in these activities. Other self-care scales are Katz's scale and the Kenney self-care evaluation functional independence measure.
Cognitive difficulties	Folstein's Mini Mental State Exam is a brief multifaceted screening tool that is most helpful in care planning when the full results of each section are included in the chart, instead of the final score.
Depression	The Zung Self-Rating Depression Scale and the Hamilton Depression Rating Scale are useful to evaluate depression.

larger dose is used most often by neurologists. Enteric coated aspirin and lower doses are helpful in patients with a tendency toward gastrointestinal irritation.

A new agent, ticlopidine, has been shown to decrease the incidence of stroke in both men and women, but it has a higher risk of side effects and is contraindicated in residents with liver failure, a bleeding disorder, or neutropenia. Neutropenia occurs 3 weeks to 3 months after initiation of therapy, and is reversible on discontinuation of the drug. Liver function test abnormalities, diarrhea, and rash are also reported. Bleeding problems are similar in incidence to those for aspirin therapy. Monitor white blood cell counts every 2 weeks for the first 3 months, and check liver function tests during the first 4 months. The recommended dose is one 250-mg tablet twice a day taken with food. Ticlopidine is currently approved for use in patients who are aspirin-intolerant or in patients with stroke recurrence while taking aspirin (aspirin failures) who are not eligible for other therapeutic options, such as surgery or warfarin.

In addition to the previous approaches to reduce stroke recurrence, make attempts to reduce the risk factors in all residents, including those with no history of stroke. The major risk factors are smoking, hypertension, diabetes, and hypercholesterolemia. Smoking cessation programs for residents with appropriate cognitive skills, as well as good medical control of hypertension, diabetes, and hypercholesterolemia through diet and medication are key components in stroke prevention. With regard to treatment of hypertension, the goal of therapy is to slowly reduce systolic blood pressure to 135 to 150 mm Hg, and diastolic pressure to less than 90 mm Hg, while monitoring carefully to avoid postural and postprandial hypotension. Isolated systolic hypertension is also a risk factor for stroke, and its treatment is effective in reducing incidence of stroke.

Seizures

Residents with stroke can present with seizures as an acute manifestation of their cerebrovascular event, or they may develop seizures at a later date. Over 50% of new-onset seizures in the elderly are secondary to cerebrovascular disease. Some studies suggest that early seizures are a bad prognostic sign, but this has not been confirmed in more recent studies. However, early seizures do seem to predict recurrence of seizures, and are responsive to anticonvulsants. Seizures occurring later in the course should prompt a workup for other causes, including metabolic studies, review of medications and alcohol use, and imaging studies to exclude other mass lesions, such as tumors and hemorrhages. Imaging studies are essential if a new neurologic deficit persists after the seizure. Transient worsening of the old deficit can occur after a seizure.

Two types of seizures are most often associated with stroke. The first are generalized tonic-clonic seizures, which are characterized by loss of consciousness and jerking of the extremities lasting about 5 minutes, sometimes accompanied by incontinence or tongue biting, followed by drowsiness or confusion. The second are partial seizures, which are characterized by unilateral jerking or sensory symptoms such as numbness or dysesthesia without loss of consciousness. On rare occasions, status epilepticus occurs with convulsive seizure activity lasting for 20 minutes or more, or multiple seizures interspersed by poor responsiveness. This is a life-threatening emergency requiring transfer to an emergency room.

Anticonvulsants are not given prophylactically to residents with ischemic strokes. In some instances, a resident with a large hemorrhagic infarction may be placed on seizure prophylaxis. Residents who have one seizure after a stroke are at high risk of recurrence and an anticonvulsant should be started.

The choice of an anticonvulsant is determined by the clinical picture and the side effect profile. In most residents, the first choice for generalized and partial seizures is phenytoin. A loading dose of 1000 mg (10 to 20 mg/kg) over a 24-hour period is given in three to four divided doses by mouth after an acute seizure. The average maintenance dose is 300 mg in a single nighttime dose. Monitor the drug levels, complete blood cell count, and liver function tests (usually aspartate aminotransferase [AST]) in the early stages of treatment. The therapeutic range for phenytoin is 10 to 20 mg/mL in most laboratories. White blood cell counts less than 4000, an AST greater then twice normal, or a significant decrease in hematocrit or platelet count signal a need to consider discontinuation of the drug. In addition to bone marrow suppression and hepatotoxicity, phenytoin can cause rashes, including the potentially fatal Stevens-Johnson syndrome, which occurs early in treatment and is an absolute contraindication to restart the medicine. Cerebellar degeneration can occur after years of phenytoin use and causes ataxia. Phenytoin toxicity commonly produces confusion and ataxia.

Other anticonvulsants used in poststroke seizures are carbamazepine and valproate. Both require institution of therapy at low doses, with gradual increases and close monitoring of drug levels, white blood cell counts, and AST. Another anticonvulsant, phenobarbital, is rarely used in the elderly because of its sedating effects.

All seizure medications can produce some sedation and alteration of cognitive abilities, so their effects must be monitored closely. Common signs of anticonvulsant toxicity include ataxia and confusion. Monotherapy is preferred, but some patients require more than one medication to control their seizures, in which case drug levels must be monitored closely due to complex interactions. Close monitoring is also required for residents on a single anticonvulsant but with a long list of medications for other medical problems.

Depression

Another common finding in patients with stroke is depression, including major depression and dysthymic disorders. It is underdiagnosed and undertreated. The incidence of depression is 30% to 40% after stroke, and occurs after both right and left hemisphere lesions. Depression can present while the patient is hospitalized for stroke, during the recovery phase, or even years after the event.

Depression has a very significant role in functional recovery. Depressed patients are three times more likely to be discharged to nursing homes. Start treatment when the resident is medically stable. Antidepressant therapy decreases the depressive symptoms but may not improve functional outcome. Tricyclic antidepressants have been the drugs of choice but they have a long list of adverse side effects. In general, those with the least anticholinergic effects are preferred in the elderly. A new class of drugs, the serotonin reuptake inhibitors, are also efficacious in treating depression in the elderly. Further details about the evaluation and treatment of depression can be found in Chapter 13, Depression.

Muscle Tone Abnormalities

Hemiparesis, which is common in stroke, is often accompanied by spasticity (i.e., an increased resistance to passive stretch). Spasticity can be beneficial since it augments muscle strength, but it also produces contractures and discomfort due to unequal muscle forces, and may result in nonfunctional limb positions and difficulties with personal hygiene.

In stroke survivors, spasticity typically leads to flexion contractures in the upper extremity and extension contractures in the lower extremity, especially the ankle. Passive range of motion can decrease the probability of developing contractures but cannot eliminate the spasticity. Careful positioning and use of splinting techniques will reduce discomfort and minimize contracture formation.

Some medications that are helpful in reducing spasticity have significant side effects. Dantrolene produces weakness and can cause diarrhea and idiosyncratic hepatotoxicity, and is usually reserved for wheelchair-bound residents in whom the weakening effect on strength is less likely to influence function. The starting dose is 25 mg/day and can be titrated slowly to 100 mg four times a day. Liver function tests must be monitored. Baclofen is another antispasmotic that is usually not effective in spasticity caused by stroke, and stroke survivors appear to be more sensitive to its side effects. When the spasticity is most troublesome during sleep, low doses of short-acting benzodiazepines at bedtime can be helpful, but may cause excessive daytime sedation or confusion. A physiatrist may perform a local block with phenol or other agents for painful spasticity or when contractures impair local hygiene.

Flaccid muscle tone is present in some stroke survivors, particularly during the acute phase of recovery, and may persist in those with large infarctions with minimal functional return. Flaccid extremities require careful attention to positioning and the use of positioning devices. A common complication of decreased muscle tone is shoulder dislocation due to stretching of shoulder ligaments in a hemiplegic arm. Edema is frequent in the flaccid arm and hand and can be minimized through compressive gloves and elevation of the limb.

Both spastic and flaccid extremities can develop compression neuropathies, especially when the resident remains in one position for prolonged periods of time. Occupational and physical therapists can assess the resident and construct suitable splints to prevent and treat compression neuropathies. Nursing staff, especially nursing assistants, need to receive education about the proper application and timing of splints. Antidepressants, phenytoin, and carbamazepine have all been used with some success to ameliorate the pain and dysesthesias of neuropathies.

Pain Syndromes in Stroke

Identification of pain in a resident with dementia or a communication disorder can be difficult and requires careful attention to facial expressions and nonverbal cues.

In addition to the pain resulting from stresses on joints and compression neuropathies, a small percentage of stroke patients (including those with lacunes) develop a thalamic pain syndrome. The pain is usually not present initially, but develops weeks after an ischemic or hemorrhagic stroke located in the thalamus. Dysesthesia may be present at baseline, with debilitating pain when the involved areas are touched. Washing, the touch of a bedsheet, changing of position in bed, and other stimuli can elicit pain.

Use some simple means to minimize painful stimuli, such as a bed cradle at the end of the bed. If these measures are not successful, medications should be tried but they are often ineffective. Various antidepressants, carbamazepine, phenytoin, valproate and baclofen are all used in this syndrome. It is best to start with one medication and increase the dose to the maximum or until limited by side effects. If there is no beneficial effect, stop the first medication and try another. As with all chronic pain syndromes, avoid using narcotics.

Incontinence

A frequent complication of stroke is urinary incontinence. It resolves in many residents, but persists in those with large strokes, especially of the frontal lobe. Persistent incontinence should prompt an evaluation for possible urinary tract dysfunction and a review of medications. Residents with cognitive difficulties may also have incontinence because they cannot find the bathroom.

Incontinence is a common reason for transfer to a nursing home and may be a poor prognostic sign for functional outcome. Treatment modalities are described in depth in Chapter 27, Urinary Incontinence.

Fecal incontinence is less common after stroke, but can be seen in frontal lobe infarctions. Constipation related to immobility is a more common complaint, and can be managed by dietary changes, stool softeners and other bowel regimens. *See* Chapter 28, Bowel Disorders, for more information.

Effects of Immobility

Many problems are related to the reduced mobility of residents with a stroke. Problematic situations can be self-generating—immobility promoting further immobility through muscle deconditioning and decreased tolerance for physical and occupational therapy.

In residents who cannot reposition themselves in good alignment and who also have swallowing difficulties, there is a high risk of aspiration and subsequent pneumonia. Speech therapists can evaluate swallowing and develop a feeding program for nursing staff to carry out with the resident to minimize the risk of aspiration. If pneumonia does occur, respiratory therapy can help mobilize secretions, since residents with a stroke often have a weak cough. Pneumonia continues to be a frequent cause of death in residents with stroke.

Immobility also places residents with a stroke at risk for deep venous thrombosis and pulmonary embolism. To minimize these possibilities, low-dose subcutaneous heparin is recommended until the resident's mobility is increased. Elastic stockings alone are not ad-

equate. Space boots, which intermittently constrict the lower extremities, are also useful in reducing the risk of deep venous thrombosis in bedridden residents.

In residents with stroke, pressure ulcers can occur due to immobility compounded by areas of decreased sensation. Avoid pressure ulcers by repositioning the resident at least every 2 hours, and increase padding between the bony prominence and firm surfaces with pressure-relieving mattresses and seat cushions. Elbow and heel protectors may also offer benefit. Managing incontinence reduces the risk of pressure ulcers (*see* Chapter 22, Pressure Ulcers, for more information).

When erythema occurs, consider using a water mattress. Monitor any areas of erythema, especially areas of skin breakdown, with daily measurements of size and depth. Observe the affected areas for signs of cellulitis and culture them as indicated. (For full details of assessment and treatment, *see* Chapter 22, Pressure Ulcers).

Immobility can also cause osteoporosis, especially in white women. Hip fractures after minimal trauma are common in this population, and are a devastating blow to the person's chances for returning to a functional gait. Hip replacement after stroke poses additional rehabilitative needs, and these combined disabilities often result in wheelchair reliance. Therefore, consider all elderly white women for prophylactic treatment of osteoporosis. Also consider this therapy for other residents with stroke (*see* Chapter 18, Falls, more information). Further rehabilitation for hip fractures and techniques for their prevention are discussed in Chapter 19, Hip Fractures.

PROGNOSTIC INDICATORS IN STROKE

A large infarction and impaired consciousness in the first few days following an acute stroke are key predictors of poor outcome. The presence of a neglect syndrome, significant visuospatial problems, or dementia also implies a poor prognosis and suggests that the resident will have difficulty following rehabilitation instructions.

The persistence of urinary incontinence is likewise associated with an unfavorable outcome. If a resident has minimal motor function return after 1 month, the chance of significant motor recovery drops precipitously. Depression and coexisting cardiac disease imply poor prognosis. Advanced age may also presage an unfavorable outcome, but it is difficult to isolate the age variable from confounding features such as coexisting medical diseases.

However, all prognostic factors are relative. Every resident is an individual and every situation is, in many respects, unique. Some residents far exceed caregivers' expectations and others continue to find great pleasure in life despite significant disabilities. The goal of the caregivers is to optimize the resident's level of function, and to maximize opportunities for social interaction and involvement in meaningful activities.

CASE EXAMPLES

The following case examples describe two stroke scenarios.

Case 1

Mr. B. is a 75-year-old, right-handed African-American with hypertension and coronary artery disease. Retired after 40 years of trial law, he presented to an acute hospital with right hemiplegia and global aphasia. His hospital course was complicated by obtundation on day 3 due to midline shift, and edema surrounding a large, left middle cerebral artery ischemic infarction. He also developed aspiration pneumonia and a urinary tract infection. He had essentially no functional recovery of motor function, and occasionally made sounds and used hand signals to communicate needs. During the hospitalization, he was able to participate in physical therapy and speech therapy for a total of 1 hour a day. An initial swallowing study was abnormal, but with speech therapy training he was able to handle thick liquids and pureed foods.

He was transferred to a nearby nursing home for further rehabilitation and skilled nursing care. His only medications were an antihypertensive agent and aspirin for prophylaxis against myocardial infarction and stroke. He required assistance with all ADLs and needed repositioning every 2 hours. On admission, his right arm was flaccid and a built-up arm support on the right side of his wheelchair was used. A sling was used to maintain arm positioning while he was in bed. A gradual increase in muscle tone was noted in the nursing home and the sling was replaced with a band splint to prevent contractures.

He participated in physical, occupational, and speech therapy for about 2 hours each day. He loved family visits and enjoyed sing-alongs, participating by humming. He began to use a custom-designed communication board for some basic needs. Two months after his admission he began to stay in his room during sing-alongs and seldom smiled when his grandchildren visited. Depression was suspected and nortriptyline was started. Three weeks later he had clear-cut improvement and again began to participate actively in activities. He improved his transfers and did not develop contractures. He periodically developed areas of redness over bony prominence, but due to careful positioning, he did not experience skin breakdown.

After 2 years in the nursing home, he had several episodes of left-sided weakness that were suggestive of TIAs. On physical examination, he was globally aphasic with right spastic hemiparesis and no new neurologic deficits. His ECG revealed normal sinus rhythm, and a head CT showed the old left middle cerebral artery infarct and no new event. His dose of antihypertensive medications was decreased due to occasional episodes of relative hypotension (systolic blood pressure less than 110 mm Hg). Aspirin was discontinued and ticlopidine was started. No further TIAs occurred in the next few months.

This case shows an example of a large, dominant hemisphere, middle cerebral artery infarction and its effects. The loss of language function can be particularly devastating to residents such as Mr. B., who depend on verbal skills and take pleasure in reading and debating. Visuospatial cues can assist them in continuing interpersonal interactions, and they may enjoy other activities such as music. However, depression can occur and may manifest in subtle ways, such as withdrawal from activities. Treatment can relieve depressive symptoms. Residents with large middle cerebral artery infarcts are often admitted to nursing homes and can have very slow, gradual improvement with continuing rehabilitation. Immobility can lead to multiple problems, such as skin breakdown and deep venous thrombosis. The recurrence of stroke is frequent, but the risk can be decreased with aspirin or ticlopidine and treatment of other risk factors.

Case 2

Mrs. E. is a 70-year-old white woman with hypertension and diabetes treated with oral agents. She was brought to the hospital by her nephew about 1 month ago because she was confused and dragging her left leg. She was found to have a right temporoparietal ischemic infarction with left hemiparesis, intact language, left homonymous hemianopsia, and a neglect syndrome. She did very well medically and was transferred to the rehabilitation service.

However, the physical and occupational therapists found her to be very difficult. She totally neglected the left side of her body and denied her deficit. With much encouragement she was able to attend to her left leg, but still denied that her left arm belonged to her. Several times when getting out of bed she fell, sustaining bruises. Since she had reached the maximum rehabilitation benefit according to acute hospital criteria and was unable to care for herself and had an unsafe gait, she was transferred to a nursing home for further rehabilitation.

At the nursing home her deficits were stable, and physiotherapists continued to work with her. One night she was found on the floor next to her bed, moaning in pain. Radiography revealed a left hip fracture and diffuse osteoporosis. After surgical repair of her hip, calcium supplementation was begun. She returned to the nursing home where her room was rearranged to accommodate her left-sided neglect. A lower bed with a half bedrail on the right side was placed near the doorway, with her right side to the door. She then fell only occasionally, sustaining some bruising but no further fractures.

This resident has a neglect syndrome. She does not see left hemispace and tends to bump into and trip on objects on her left side. She does not recognize the left side of her body as belonging to herself, and cannot relearn to use it. Since her arm is weaker than her leg, she can ambulate but is susceptible to falling episodes because of the left-sided weakness, her inability to perceive obstacles on the left, and some left sensory abnormalities. She cannot learn from therapy instructions. She is best approached from her right side, and can appear paranoid when staff members stand on her left because she cannot see that side.

With her bed close to the floor, she has less risk of suffering injury in a fall. Also, more strength is required to rise from the low bed, so she is more likely to request assistance. Placing a half bedrail on her right side provides her with an assistive device for turning in bed and transferring out of bed. Eliminating full bedrails prevents her from falling over the rail or becoming caught in the rail and injuring herself. Positioning the bed so she can see the hallway allows her to view staff activity and enhance orientation during nighttime awakenings.

Residents who sustain strokes such as Mrs. E.'s have good language skills but often lose the ability to perceive emotional cues. They enjoy reminiscing groups and similar activities in which their verbal skills are used. Reading is usually impaired significantly due to the visual field disturbance, but residents who used to like reading may enjoy books on tape. Their neglect syndrome leads to problems with ADLs, such as dressing and eating, which may be quite resistant to rehabilitation attempts. These residents do best in an atmosphere where the staff value their strengths, such as their language skills.

8
Arthritis

Simon Helfgott, MD
Joanne Sandberg Cook, RN, C, MS
Pauline Belleville-Taylor, RN, CS, MS

There are over 100 diseases associated with the development of arthritis, but the vast majority of arthritic complaints in the elderly involve osteoarthritis. Less commonly found in a nursing home population are rheumatoid arthritis and crystal induced arthritis.

Many residents complaining of musculoskeletal aches and pains actually suffer from soft tissue disorders (e.g., bursitis, tendinitis, or nerve entrapment syndromes such as carpal tunnel syndrome). Although these conditions resemble arthritis, their treatment and prognosis differ.

This chapter describes the clinical features of various types of arthritis and the appropriate interventions and therapies for residents of long-term care facilities.

OVERVIEW

A joint is able to move freely because the bone ends are covered with cartilage—a tough, slippery, fibrous connective tissue that acts as a protective cushion between the bone ends. Cartilage is composed of two major substances:

- Proteoglycan, which functions as a highly viscous lubricant
- Type II collagen, an extremely large molecular weight protein that constitutes the fibrous substance.

As the body ages, cartilage begins to change, losing its thickness and resiliency. These changes are characterized by a progressive loss of water content from the proteoglycan and a breakdown of type II collagen into smaller components.

Osteoarthritis

Osteoarthritis is a form of arthritis in which one or many joints suffer from degenerative changes, including the breakdown of cartilage. The tendency of cartilage to break down with age is not yet fully explained, but contributing factors may include genetic predisposition, metabolic changes, and joint injury or trauma. Whatever the cause(s) in the individual instance, the effect of these changes is a progressive thinning of the cushion in the joint and less shock absorbency, so that the forces related to physical activity are passed through the joint and impact the articulating bony surfaces. For example, the progressive loss of cartilage in the medial aspect of the knee—a common site for osteoarthritis—results in greater forces being absorbed by the articulating surfaces of the femur and tibia.

The body's response to this jarring impact is to initiate a gradual, bony remodeling. This reaction is an attempt by the surrounding bone to transmit the received forces across a wider surface area, which produces the characteristic *osteophytes*, or bony pathologic protuberances, at the margins of the joint. Over time there may be complete loss of cartilage, large osteophyte formation (e.g., bone spurs), and bone rubbing against bone, resulting in progressive pain, stiffness, and loss of function in the affected joint.

Rheumatoid Arthritis

In *rheumatoid arthritis*, an inflammatory disease, the immune system cannot recognize the body's joint tissue as part of its normal self, so it attacks the joint tissue. Joints may become swollen, warm, and painful, but, unlike osteoarthritis, bony proliferation and osteophyte formation are not observed. As in osteoarthritis, however, joint damage can be extensive, often resulting in the need for joint replacement surgery.

Crystal-Induced Arthritis

Crystal-induced arthritis involves a metabolic disorder, specifically the inappropriate deposition of sodium urate (gout) or calcium pyrophosphate (pseudogout/chondrocalcinosis) crystals in the joint. It is characterized by intense pain and rapid swelling in the joint. Unlike rheumatoid arthritis, where symmetric, polyarticular joint involvement, especially in the hands and wrists, is the rule, crystal-induced arthritis is *oligoarticular* (involving only a few joints), asymmetric, and relatively short-lasting (i.e., a few days to a few weeks), even if untreated.

CLINICAL FEATURES OF ARTHRITIS

All arthritis sufferers will complain of pain, and many will experience considerable stiffness when they awaken. Generalized stiffness lasting longer than 30 minutes is often seen in rheumatoid arthritis. Arthritis patients typically feel worse in the morning hours, so they may be unable to perform independently activities of daily living (ADLs), such as dressing and hygiene. However, they may report a gradual loosening up as the day progresses and consequently become more functionally capable.

Joint swelling or bony enlargements (i.e., nodes) may also be observed around joints. *Heberden's nodes* (enlargements of the distal interphalangeal joints) or *Bouchard's nodes* (enlargements of the proximal interphalangeal joints) confirm the presence of osteoarthritis. Bony enlargements around large joints are harder to discern, so instead one may observe the development of an angular deformity such as varus (inward bowing) or valgus (outward bowing) at the knee or ankle.

Table 8-1 summarizes the clinical features of arthritis. The following subsections describe the effects of arthritis in various anatomic sites. Table 8-2 summarizes the possible causes of pain in these sites.

Arthritis of the Hip

Arthritis of the hip causes pain in the groin area, which is exacerbated by walking and often produces an unusual lurch to the gait. Since flexing the hip becomes progressively more difficult, activities such as putting on socks may be difficult or impossible without an assistive device. A simple bedside test to assess the extent of hip arthritis is to rotate the entire extended lower extremity (log-rolling) back and forth. Any pain experienced, especially with inward rotation of the leg, indicates arthritic damage to the hip. A radiograph will help assess the extent of the joint destruction.

Pain over the lateral aspect of the hip may be due to a trochanteric bursitis. The pain is made worse by applying pressure to the area, e.g., laying on the affected side may cause

Table 8-1. Clinical Features of Arthritis

Type of Arthritis	Typical Clinical Features	Commonly Affected Joints
Osteoarthritis	Progressive pain Bony enlargement Minimal swelling or warmth	Hips and knees; hands (DIPS: Heberden's nodes, PIPs: Bouchard's nodes)
Rheumatoid arthritis	Symmetric polyarthritis Joint swelling and increased warmth Prolonged morning stiffness, fatigue, malaise	Wrists; hands (MCPs, PIPs); shoulders; knees; feet
Crystal-induced arthritis (gout and pseudogout)	Acute asymmetric onset Severe pain, erythema Occasional low grade fever	Gout: first MTP, foot, ankle, knee Pseudogout: knee, wrist

DIPs = distal interphalangeal joints; MCPs = metacarpal-phalangeal joints; MTPs = metatarsal-phalangeal joints; PIPs = proximal interphalangeal joints.

nighttime pain to be noticed more.

Arthritis of the Knee

Arthritis of the knee may involve any of three compartments of the knee: patella-femoral, medial, or lateral. To confirm patella-femoral arthritis, flex the resident's knee fully and, with the other hand, feel for a bony crepitation (a noisy grating) over the knee joint. Crepitation may also be felt and heard over the medial or lateral compartments of the knee with flexion, and when present generally indicates more substantial arthritic damage to the knee. A radiograph (always taken with the knee in the weight-bearing position) can help to determine the extent of damage.

Shoulder Pain

Shoulder pain is generally attributed to *supraspinatus tendinitis*. Residents experience shoulder pain with abduction (drawing the arm away from the body) or external rotation (lifting the arm behind the head). This pain is often felt in the upper arm muscles just below the shoulder and tends to worsen with repeated pressure on the area, hence the characteristic nighttime symptoms. With repeated episodes, the supraspinatus tendon (the major component of the rotator cuff apparatus of the shoulder) begins to tear and cannot keep the humeral head in the shoulder socket. The result is the development of arthritis of the shoulder (glenohumeral) joint, which is uncommon. A frozen shoulder or adhesive capsulitis may occur if the resident avoids using the arm due to pain and if the condition is untreated. Loss of range of motion in the shoulder can occur rapidly, often within weeks. If untreated, an adhesive capsulitis or frozen shoulder may ensue.

Arthritis of the Spine

The most common form of arthritis affecting the spine is osteoarthritis. Narrowing of the space between the discs is an age-related condition. Combined with osteoporosis,

Table 8-2. Musculoskeletal Causes of Regional Pain

Anatomic Site	Possible Causes
Shoulder (and proximal upper arm)	Supraspinatus tendinitis Bicipital tendinitis Acromioclavicular osteoarthritis
Elbow	Arthritis (pain with pronation and supination) Epicondylitis (medial or lateral pain on palpation)
Hand	Carpal tunnel syndrome (numbness at rest) Rheumatoid arthritis Osteoarthritis Crystal-induced arthritis
Hip (groin)	True hip joint arthritis
Hip (lateral)	Trochanteric bursitis
Low back/ buttocks	Back pain with radicular symptoms (most commonly osteoarthritis)
Base of neck	Osteoarthritis
Knee (medial)	Consider osteroarthritis, osteonecrosis, anserine bursitis, meniscal tear
Knee (lateral)	Osteoarthritis
Knee (patella-femoral)	Osteoarthritis

scoliosis, and obesity, osteoarthritis typically results in adverse changes involving the facet joints at various levels, primarily the lumbosacral and lower cervical spine.

The most prominent complaint is pain, which may be localized to the portion of the spine that is most involved (e.g., low back, base of the neck). Radicular pain (sciatica) results in leg pain because the sciatic nerve innervates the lumbar and sacral (L4-S1) dermatomes. It is usually, although not always, associated with pain in the low back. Progressive osteoarthritic damage causes further bony overgrowth, which may severely limit the space available for nerve roots to exit through the spinal neural foramina (opening). Clinical features of this condition, called *spinal stenosis*, include cramplike pain in the buttocks and thighs, which is worsened by walking or prolonged standing. Some residents develop a forward flexion of the lumbosacral spine (stooped over posture), representing an attempt by the skeletal architecture to enlarge the neural foraminal space and to try to release pressure on the impinged nerve roots.

Spinal involvement in rheumatoid arthritis is limited to the cervical spine region, where synovial thickening of the atlantoaxial joint (C-C2) can result in myelopathic changes. With the new onset of low back pain in a resident with rheumatoid arthritis, evaluate for a vertebral compression fracture as a complication of corticosteroid use.

In any resident complaining of back pain, the severity and timing of the pain provide important diagnostic clues. Pain that worsens with activity and is relieved by rest suggests osteoarthritis. Pain that is experienced at rest, such as nighttime pain, and the new onset of back pain in an individual without a prior history of spine problems are suggestive of an infiltrative process such as a tumor (metastatic or myeloma) or infection.

Soft Tissue Disorders

Pain emanating from the tissues adjacent to joints (tendons, bursae, and nerve roots) may resemble arthritis. This pain is generally worse during rest periods or in the evening. This is due to the resident lying down, which puts pressure on the affected joints, thereby exacerbating the pain. The resident often presents with pain upon awakening. For example, bursitis, tendinitis, and epicondylitis are associated with more pain at rest or during the night. This may help to distinguish soft tissue pain from arthritis, which generally worsens with physical activity. Physical examination generally reveals tenderness on palpation of the affected tissue, which is adjacent to but not directly over the particular joint margin.

EVALUATING THE RESIDENT FOR ARTHRITIS INVOLVEMENT

To evaluate the resident for the presence or extent of arthritis involvement, perform the assessments described in the following subsections.

Range of Motion

To best assess the range of motion of joints, observe the resident performing normal ADLs (e.g., bathing, dressing, grooming). Determining how much assistance is needed during a bath or while dressing can indicate specific mobility deficits in areas of reaching, hand function, and lower extremity mobility. An inability to pull clothing over one's head can indicate decreased shoulder mobility. Buttoning requires fine finger mobility, which can be impaired by both pain and decreased finger movement. Difficulty in putting on shoes and socks can indicate decreased hip and knee mobility.

Pain

Determine the time or activity associated with maximal pain, and then quantify the pain using a visual analog scale, with 0 being "no pain" and 10 being "worst pain." Note that the resident makes a subjective assessment of pain at some point between these two extremes. This is useful in later assessing the effect of the intervention. Note the location,

intensity, radiation, and any accompanying redness or swelling.

Gait

Observe the resident's gait and note any leg discrepancies, pain, or use of assistive devices to aid in walking. (See Chapter 18, Falls, for more information.)

Muscle Strength

Examine muscle strength by asking residents to flex and extend each extremity against resistance by the examiner. Pay close attention to proximal and distal extremity strength and hand grip.

RECOMMENDED INTERVENTIONS

In an infirm, elderly nursing home population, interventions for arthritis focus on improving comfort, preventing concomitant deformities (e.g., contractures), and enhancing maximal resident function in self-care and leisure pursuits. Interventions typically involve medications for pain along with various hot or cold treatment modalities. Pain may be acute or chronic, resulting in disturbances in sleep, energy, mobility, posture, nutrition, and general health. There is no significant difference in pain management for osteoarthritis and rheumatoid arthritis. Residents who cannot verbally express pain (e.g., residents with dementia, aphasia) may communicate that they are in pain through agitated behaviors such as crying, calling out, moaning or rocking, or guarding the painful body areas.

Medications

Table 8-3 describes medications that are commonly used to treat arthritis.

The Role of Corticosteroids (Regularly and as Needed By Injection)

Oral corticosteroids are potent antiinflammatory agents. They are the preferred drug to treat *polymyalgia rheumatica*, a common in-

Table 8-3. Common Medications Used to Treat Arthritis

Type of Medication	Comments

NSAIDs
  Ibuprofen (Motrin, Advil)
  Naproxen (Naprosyn, Aleve)
  Aspirin (Ecotrin)
	Adverse side effects include gastrointestinal bleeding, renal impairment, hypertension, and fluid retention. Take with food. Gastrointestinal intolerance, including nausea, heartburn, abdominal pain, is often seen (20%). Adverse side effects of aspirin include gastrointestinal discomfort, anorexia, and bleeding. Signs of toxicity include tinnitus (ringing in the ears). Take with food or use enteric coated preparations.

Nonnarcotic analgesics: Acetaminophen (Tylenol)	Nonnarcotic drugs may help to relieve minor pain, so they are useful adjuncts to NSAIDs. However, they are not effective in alleviating stiffness.
Narcotics	As a rule, avoid narcotics. Use in residents with end-stage disease who are poor surgical candidates. In appropriate situations, they are most effective when given on a regular schedule, not "as needed."

Antidepressants
  Stabilizing sleep patterns may decrease musculoskeletal pain
  Examples are amitriptyline, nortriptyline, and trazodone
	In low doses, these drugs are used to alleviate nighttime pain and stabilize sleep patterns. Frequently observed side effects include cognitive impairment, daytime drowsiness, constipation, urinary retention, orthostatic hypotension, and dry mouth.

NSAIDs = nonsteroidal antiinflammatory drugs

flammatory musculoskeletal disorder in the elderly. They may be useful adjuncts in the treatment of rheumatoid arthritis. Fortunately, the doses required to treat these conditions are low, usually 10 mg/day or less. Give careful consideration to the risks versus benefits when using these agents in the elderly population. They have no role in managing osteoarthritis or back pain.

Using intraarticular joint injections as a treatment modality is highly effective in selected situations—for example, acute monoarthritis (noninfectious) at an easily injectable joint, such as the knee, wrist, ankle, shoulder, carpal-metacarpal, or hip (which requires fluoroscopic guidance). Avoid repeated injections to prevent complications such as tendon rupture, osteonecrosis, or sepsis.

Medical Treatment for Crystal-Induced Arthritis (Gout and Pseudogout)

The treatments of choice for crystal-induced arthritis (gout and pseudogout) include:
- Nonsteroidal antiinflammatory drugs (NSAIDs).
- Oral colchicine (maximum dose 1.2 mg/day). Adjust this dose downwards if renal dysfunction is present.
- Intravenous colchicine is extremely effective in managing polyarticular arthritis. Use low doses (1.0 mg/day or less) for a maximum of 2 to 3 days.

- Joint aspiration/injection with corticosteroids. This is the preferred treatment for monoarticular disease involving an easily accessible joint.
- Intramuscular adrenocorticotropic hormone gel is of questionable benefit; very short-term effects are noted.

The most common error in treating crystal-induced synovitis is the initiation of allopurinol therapy. Avoid this treatment until:

- A crystal-induced synovitis diagnosis is established by polarizing microscopy.
- The acute episode has completely resolved for at least 3 weeks
- The frequency of attacks has increased to at least three or four episodes per year
- There is clinical evidence of tophaceous gout
- There is no contraindication to the use of allopurinol, e.g., hypersensitivity or liver disease

Thermal Modalities

Apply thermal modalities, cold or hot treatments, depending on the indications or the resident's preference. Table 8-4 describes some thermal modalities.

Precautions for Thermal Modalities

Since thermal sensitivity may be reduced in elderly nursing home residents, and residents with cognitive impairment or language difficulty may be unable to report discomfort, observe the following precautions regarding thermal modalities:

- Check the resident often during treatment and do a careful skin assessment.
- Never use mentholated rubs in conjunction with externally applied heat.
- Warm water compresses are safer than heating pads (there is a risk of burns and electrocution). If used, wrap the heating pads in several layers of towels to avoid burning.

RECOMMENDED CHRONIC THERAPIES

The following sections discuss the recommended therapies for treating arthritis.

Exercise

A balanced program of exercise should focus on maintaining and improving motion, mobility, and muscle strength, and alleviating pain. Do not exercise acutely inflamed joints but put these joints through their entire range of motion each day. This may be done actively by the resident or passively by the nurse or therapist. Short periods of ambulation are beneficial in maintaining strength and building resident confidence.

The resident can perform simple range-of-motion exercises either in bed or while sitting or standing. Nursing assistants can be very helpful in carrying out range-of-motion exercises while doing bathing and dressing activities with residents. Try to maintain strength in the lower extremities by performing knee extension or straight leg raising exercises. A physical or recreational therapist should address specific problems with individual joints or atrophic muscles. Exercise groups led by a physical therapist, recreational therapist, nurse, or a specially educated nurse assistant or family member can be both therapeutic and enjoyable to the nursing home resident.

Rest

Rest is important during periods of increased disease activity (inflammation, swelling, severe pain). To aid in resting arthritic joints, use bed rests, chair rests, splinting of inflamed joints, or use canes, walkers, or platform walkers to minimize pressure on weight-bearing joints.

Distraction and Relaxation

Any activity that the resident enjoys (e.g., social activities, music, reading, or relaxation techniques) may divert the focus from pain, providing temporary pain reduction. Teach

Table 8-4. Thermal Modalities and Their Delivery Methods

Modality	Indications	Method of Delivery
Cold	Acutely inflamed joints with associated swelling New onset of back pain Soft tissue-related pain (e.g., tendinitis, bursitis) Resident preference	Chemical cold packs; crushed ice; ice collars/bags; or frozen gel packs 10 to 20 minutes every 2 to 4 hours, as tolerated.
Heat	Chronic pain Morning stiffness Resident preference	Warm showers/baths; hydroculator packs; microwave gel packs or mitts; warm moist towels; liquid paraffin soaks (for hands and feet). Usually applied daily or as needed for pain, for 20 to 30 minutes, as tolerated.

relaxation techniques to residents and staff so that the nurse assistants can reinforce these techniques. The following four-step process is recommended:

1. Find a quiet, relaxing environment.
2. Consciously relax the body's muscles one group at a time (e.g., relax the muscles in the right foot and then relax the muscles in the left foot).
3. Focus for 10 to 20 minutes on a mental image (e.g., word, prayer).
4. Assume a passive attitude toward intrusive thoughts.

Self-Care and Assistive Devices

The ability to perform self-care activities is directly influenced by rheumatic disease. However, the degree of deformity does not predict a resident's ability to perform self-care. Many other factors, including energy levels, endurance, and the resident's or staff's perception of how much help is needed, determine self-care ability. The resident's previous accommodation to a disability is also a major factor.

Assistive devices including reachers, dressing sticks, button hooks, long-handled grooming aids, raised toilet seats, grab bars, and other aids may enhance self-care abilities. Physical and occupational therapy can be very helpful in instructing both residents and staff in the use of these devices. Teach nurse assistants how to use these devices so that they can assist the residents. The nurse assistant needs to help the resident follow through on the teaching. Many residents react negatively to this adaptive equipment. If the staff does encounter resistance explore the reasons why and suggest alternatives. Family involvement in using assistive devices to perform ADLs may help the resident adjust to using the equipment. The key is to provide continuous education, positive reinforcement and limited introduction of change.

CASE EXAMPLES

The following case examples describe an osteoarthritis case and a pseudogout case.

Osteoarthritis Case Example

Mrs. L., an 81-year-old resident, noted the recurrence of low back and leg pain. There was no antecedent trauma. She complained that the pain was located primarily in the left thigh posteriorly, with radiation to the ankle. Sitting, standing, and walking more than 50 feet intensified the pain and bed rest alleviated it. She denied any neurologic symptoms. There was a long-standing history of osteoporosis and prior compression fractures involving the lumbosacral spine.

Physical examination revealed limited mobility of the spine, with pain intensified by attempts to extend (straighten) her forward-flexed lumbosacral spine. Motor strength was equal in both lower extremities. The deep tendon reflexes were 3+ at the knees, 1+ at the right ankle, and unobtainable at the left ankle. The toes were downgoing bilaterally. Sensory examinations to pinprick and vibration were normal.

The presumptive diagnosis, given the absent ankle jerk and presence of radicular pain, was osteoarthritis of the lumbosacral spine, with maximal features at the left L4-5 and L5-S1 vertebral segments resulting in spinal stenosis. The lack of resting or nighttime pain argued against a metastatic tumor or a new compression fracture as a cause of pain. While these diagnoses could be established by plain radiographs, one would normally expect to see some degree of osteoarthritic change associated with aging, so radiographs were not taken. Instead, the resident was treated with a course of physical therapy consisting initially of ice massage then deep heat and ultrasound applied to the lumbosacral spine. Stretching exercises were started.

An NSAID regimen was also started, but after 4 weeks of treatment there was only marginal improvement. The physical examination was unchanged. On the premise that Mrs. L. could benefit from an epidural corticosteroid injection, a magnetic resonance imaging study of the lumbosacral spine was obtained, which confirmed the presence of severe spinal stenosis at the left L4-5 neural foramina. A substantial reduction in pain followed her epidural injection.

Pseudogout Case Example

Mr. W., a 79-year-old resident, developed a sudden onset of pain and swelling of the right wrist. There was no prior trauma. The resident was in excellent health except for hypertension, which was being treated with a diuretic. Physical examination revealed intense erythema and swelling over the right wrist. There was limited right-hand function because of the pain. A temperature of 99.6° F was recorded. The remainder of the examination was unremarkable.

Mr. W. was told to rest the hand, and he was given acetaminophen with codeine for pain. After a restless night he was noted to have more extensive swelling of the wrist, which extended to the dorsum of the hand and some of the digits. A presumptive diagnosis of cellulitis was made, so he was started on a course of an intravenous cephalosporin. However, the pain and swelling persisted, and the following day he was transferred to an acute care facility. A hand and wrist film was notable for a few calcific specks in the wrist joint cartilage space. Wrist joint aspiration obtained slightly cloudy synovial fluid, which under polarizing microscopy revealed numerous calcium pyrophosphate crystals, establishing the diagnosis of pseudogout. The wrist was injected with a corticosteroid preparation and splinted. Because of the history of hypertension, NSAIDs were avoided, and instead Mr. W. was started on oral colchicine. The signs and symptoms of the wrist pseudogout resolved after 2 weeks of therapy.

9
Parkinson's Disease

Adam Burrows, MD
Susan Mitchell, MD
David Pilgrim, MD

Parkinson's disease is a degenerative disorder that reduces the availability of dopamine, a central nervous system neurotransmitter, in the basal ganglia. The basal ganglia are subcortical structures that coordinate complex motor activity to permit smooth, rapid movements and stable posture.

The prevalence of Parkinson's disease increases with age. One in every 100 persons over 60 years of age and one in every 40 over 80 years of age suffers from the disorder. The natural history of Parkinson's disease is characterized by progressive disability. Disabling symptoms include tremor, rigidity, slowness of movements, and postural instability. The goal of treatment in Parkinson's disease is to maximize functional independence.

Pharmacologic interventions attempt to restore the balance between dopamine and acetylcholine in the basal ganglia. The interventions of nursing, nutrition services, and various therapies (physical, occupational, and speech) seek to maintain and preserve the residents' physical and functional well-being. Careful observation and creative interdisciplinary interventions are the keys to successful management.

This chapter reviews the care of nursing home residents with advanced Parkinson's disease. It discusses the disease manifestations causing disability and reviews their recognition and management. Medications and adverse drug reactions are also discussed.

OVERVIEW

Idiopathic Parkinson's disease accounts for the majority of residents with parkinsonism. However, parkinsonism can also be due to other causes, and it is often difficult to determine the exact etiology without autopsy confirmation. In the nursing home setting, where the use of antipsychotic medications may be common, the prevalence of drug-induced parkinsonism is likely to be higher than in the general population. Similarly, because the prevalence of cerebrovascular disease is higher in nursing homes than in the community, there will be proportionally more cases of parkinsonism caused by stroke (basal ganglia infarcts). There are also several less common neurodegenerative syndromes that can produce parkinsonism. The clinician who observes signs and symptoms of parkinsonism should consider these other diagnoses, especially the possibility of medication effects (*see* Table 9-1).

Table 9-1. Medications Causing Parkinsonism

Class	Type
Antipsychotic neuroleptics	Phenothiazines Haloperidol (Haldol)
Antihypertensives	Methyldopa (Aldomet) Reserpine
Antinausea/GI medication	Metoclopramide (Reglan)

The average age of onset for idiopathic Parkinson's disease is in the sixth decade. A five-stage classification system developed by Hoehn and Yahr summarizes the symptomatic and functional progression of the disease. (Table 9-2).

Before the availability of levodopa therapy, the average time from onset of Parkinson's disease to stage IV disease was 8 to 10 years, and to stage V disease, 10 to 15 years. Levodopa has allowed a period of improved function early in the disease course, but it has not significantly delayed progression to advanced stages of disability (stages IV and V). Residents who are admitted to a nursing home with functional limitations related to Parkinson's disease tend to be younger than the overall nursing home population and, typically, have already enjoyed their period of benefit from levodopa therapy.

The life expectancy of patients with Parkinson's disease is only marginally shorter than that of comparison groups of the same age. Thus it is likely that parkinsonian nursing home residents will have relatively long lengths of stay. The leading causes of death are the same as for the general population, and include heart disease, cancer, stroke, and pneumonia. However, parkinsonian residents are more likely to develop problems that contribute to mortality, such as pressure ulcers, urinary tract infections, pneumonia, accidents, and surgical complications. These complications are primarily due to impaired mobility.

Table 9-2. Symptoms and Functional Progression of Parkinson's Disease

Stage	Manifestations	Functional Significance
I	Unilateral symptoms (tremor, rigidity, slowness)	Minimal functional impairment
II	Bilateral symptoms (tremor, rigidity, slowness)	Minimal functional impairment
III	Gait and balance impaired	Independent living possible
IV	Postural instability	Assistance with activities of daily living (ADLs) required
V	Severe disease	Restriction to wheelchair or bed

CLINICAL FEATURES

The classic triad of parkinsonian symptoms consists of:

- Resting tremor (involuntary rhythmic shaking movements)
- Rigidity (muscular resistance to smooth movements)
- Bradykinesia (slowness of movement)

The tremor of Parkinson's disease is present at rest and is characterized by fine pill-rolling movements of the thumb and hand. Postural instability, rigidity, and bradykinesia are major contributors to functional disability, especially in the advanced stages. They render the activities of daily living (ADLs) difficult, impair communication and mobility, and contributes to social isolation.

In the nursing home setting, a unique group of late symptoms contributes to functional disability and a reduced quality of life. In addition to the classic triad (tremor, rigidity, and bradykinesia), these late symptoms include:

- Falls and gait disturbance
- Dysphagia and malnutrition
- Dementia
- Depression
- Pain
- Communication problems
- Sleep disturbance
- Visual problems

These late manifestations demand a vigilant approach to recognition and often require creative approaches to intervention.

Table 9-3 summarizes the features of Parkinson's disease found in residents of long-term care facilities.

Falls and Gait Disturbances

Parkinsonian residents develop a characteristic gait and are at high risk for falls. The gait is easily recognized by the stooped posture, shuffling steps, absent armswing, and difficulty negotiating starts, turns, and stops. There is often a festinating quality (accelera-

Table 9-3. Features of Parkinson's Disease in the Nursing Home

I. Disease Symptoms
Classic triad
Tremor
Rigidity
Bradykinesia
Falls and gait disturbace
Malnutrition
Dementia
Depression
Pain
Communication problems
Sleep disturbance
Visual problems
Constipation
Urinary incontinence

II. Adverse Drug Reactions
Levodopa
Involuntary movements, freezing
Hallucinations
Orthostatic hypotension
Nausea
Nightmares
Anticholinergic medications
Urinary retention
Dry mouth
Constipation
Visual blurring
Confusion

tions and decelerations) as well. Falling is one of the most serious problems in advanced Parkinson's disease. Forty to 50% of parkinsonian residents fall, many of them frequently. Falls may result in serious injury, especially hip fracture, and also compound disability and isolation through the resident's fear of recurrence.

There are several causes of falls in Parkinson's disease, and multiple causes usually contribute to any falling incident. The primary contributing factors are:

- Unstable propulsion and retropulsion
- Delayed response to falling
- Muscle weakness
- Orthostatic hypotension
- Misinterpretation of visuospatial information
- Freezing secondary to Levodopa
- Stooped posture

Propulsion and *retropulsion* is the tendency of the parkinsonian resident to accelerate forward or backward, respectively, in a poorly controlled rush after the initial step or steps. If the resident is unable to recover before encountering an obstacle or losing balance, the result is a fall. A related problem is the absence of normal righting or stabilizing reflexes when balance is threatened. When the resident's center of gravity is extended beyond a comfortable radius, there will be an absence of the musculoskeletal postural adjustments and stepping reflexes necessary to prevent falling.

Various degrees of autonomic dysfunction often accompany late Parkinson's disease. Orthostatic hypotension (reduction of systolic blood pressure of 20 mm Hg or more upon standing upright) is noted in 10% to 15% of parkinsonian residents, and levodopa treatment may account for up to half of this prevalence. Staff should routinely evaluate postural symptoms (dizziness, lightheadedness) and blood pressure, especially after starting the resident on new medications or changing doses or timing.

Due to inactivity and difficulty eating and swallowing, parkinsonian residents are at risk for weight loss, malnutrition, loss of muscle mass, and muscle weakness. Weakness develops most notably in the large quadriceps and hip muscles needed for erect posture. Lastly, there is some evidence of impaired visuospatial reasoning, usually in the setting of Parkinson's-related dementia (*see* the discussion on dementia that follows). Residents with Parkinson's disease often have difficulty in determining the relative position of objects in their environment and in orienting their movements in specific directions. (*See* Chapter 18, Falls, for more information about treating residents who are at risk of falling.)

Recognition

The goal of recognition is to identify complications that place a nursing home resident at an increased risk of falling. Specific interventions may not always be possible, but identifying risk factors will optimize staff awareness and facilitate precautionary measures. Observe the parkinsonian resident while he or she is sitting, rising from a chair, standing, and walking. Time the resident while performing basic activities (e.g., rising from a chair, walking 20 feet) to establish a functional baseline and to evaluate functional declines or improvements. Challenge the standing balance by softly nudging the back and sternum to identify propulsion, retropulsion, and the absence of righting reflexes. Observe residents to assess balance and dynamic postural stability while they reach toward objects on a shelf. Obtain blood pressures as follows:

- Supine
- Standing
- Before meals
- A half hour after meals

Assess and document any reported symptoms. Quadriceps strength is best evaluated by watching the resident rise from a chair to a standing position. Rocking, multiple attempts, and the use of the upper extremities to push off the chair are all signs that suggest quadriceps muscle weakness. Table 9-4 summarizes the tests for balance and gait.

Interventions

Severe postural instability will necessitate staff assistance with transfers and ambulation. Symptomatic orthostatic hypotension can be managed by medication adjustments, (e.g., a

Table 9-4. Tests of Balance and Gait

Timed Observations
    Chair stand
    Twenty foot walk

Balance Challenges
    Nudge to back and sternum
    Reach for object

reduction in levodopa dosage) and simple nonpharmacologic measures (e.g., support hose, increased fluid intake). Refractory cases may require fludrocortisone (Florinef), starting at 0.1 mg/day. Muscle weakness should trigger a complete nutritional assessment and physical therapy consultation for muscle-strengthening exercises, as well as a search for other causes of weakness. All parkinsonian residents should perform regular range of motion exercises to retard the effects of rigidity and bradykinesia.

Nutrition

Despite apparent reductions in activity, parkinsonian residents may have increased energy expenditures and requirements. The cause is unknown, but it may relate to the energy requirements needed to sustain a tremor and rigid posture. Residents with Parkinson's disease may also suffer from diminished caloric intake. There are several possible reasons for reduced intake, including swallowing difficulties, gastrointestinal dysmotility, drug-induced nausea, and depression. Parkinsonian residents are also prone to constipation, which may lead to discomfort, anorexia, and confusion. An important consequence of malnutrition is loss of muscle mass and strength. In nonambulatory residents in the late stages of disease, malnutrition may also increase the risk of developing pressure ulcers.

Recognition and Intervention

All parkinsonian residents should have a thorough nutritional assessment, including observation at meals to ensure adequate intake and prevent aspiration. Encourage the resident to eat slowly and in small bites. An upright, seated posture is essential to facilitate swallowing. Prescribe multivitamins to prevent micronutrient deficiencies. Obtain weights weekly, and pursue any weight loss diagnostically and therapeutically. The clinician should be prepared to discuss the benefits and risks of tube feeding with the resident and family before swallowing difficulties become so severe that aspiration develops and nutrition is compromised. (*See* Chapter 23, Nutritional Status, for more information.)

Dementia

Up to 40% of parkinsonian patients develop cognitive impairment. In some cases, Alzheimer's disease and Parkinson's disease coexist. Other patients develop a characteristic parkinsonian dementia with features that are different from those of Alzheimer's disease. Its features are those of frontal/subcortical dementia, i.e., a generalized slowing of the thought processes as well as problems with initiating, organizing, and sustaining mental and physical activities. There may be problems with short-term memory, language, and praxis (ability to organize the steps of an activity into a logical sequence), but these are less pronounced in Parkinson's disease than in Alzheimer's. On formal neuropsychological testing, visuospatial construction is usually preserved, but there are often subtle problems with the interpretation of visuospatial information. The clinician should educate the direct care staff to recognize changes in cognitive function. It should also be stressed to the staff that reduced facial and verbal expression and slow responsiveness should not be misinterpreted to signify dementia.

Recognition

Parkinsonian dementia is often suspected by staff who observe the resident having difficulty organizing and conducting daily activities. Formal dementia screening methods, such as the Folstein MiniMental Status Examination (MMSE), may be insensitive to impairment because they emphasize orientation, memory, and language. However, testing of specific cognitive tasks, such as word list generation (the number of objects in a supermarket named in 1 minute) and visual pattern recognition, usually permit appropriate diagnosis (*see* Chapter 10, Cognitive Loss, for more information). Always consider depression in the differential diagnosis of subcortical dementia and treat when identified.

Intervention

As with other degenerative dementias, there is no cure for Parkinson's disease. Levodopa may help to accelerate thought processes that have become retarded, but the most useful interventions are often nursing measures designed to assist the resident with organizing, planning, and sustaining focus. Because of the associated rigidity and generalized slowness, nursing care of the demented, disabled Parkinson's resident requires considerable patience (*see* Chapter 10, Cognitive Loss, for more information).

Depression

Depression is a very common complication of Parkinson's disease. It is estimated that 40% of persons with parkinsonism are depressed, and this prevalence is even higher in nursing homes. Often, depressive symptoms in a disabled resident will be dismissed as an appropriate response to chronic illness and disability. Such an attitude is inappropriate. If depression is sustained, causes suffering, and compromises function, it requires appropriate

diagnosis and intervention. In actuality, depressive symptomatology in parkinsonian residents does not correlate with either age or the severity of the disability. Evidence suggests that depression in Parkinson's disease may be due to neurotransmitter abnormalities, particularly serotonin deficiency.

Recognition

The approach to diagnosing depression in parkinsonian residents is similar to that taken in the general nursing home population (*see* Chapter 13, Depression, for more information). However, there are potential hazards, since several typical parkinsonian characteristics (slowness of thought and movement, fatigue and loss of energy, lack of expressivity suggestive of apathy, and reduced food intake with weight loss) are also signs of depression. Too readily attributing features of depression to parkinsonism can result in a missed diagnosis.

The evaluation of possible depression in a Parkinson's resident should include careful assessment for each diagnostic sign and symptom of depression. These include:

- Depressed mood
- Disturbed appetite and sleep
- Anhedonia (loss of interest in pleasurable activities)
- Mood-congruent delusions (guilty, nihilistic, or somatic delusions)
- Suicidal thoughts
- The vegetative signs previously mentioned (anergy, retardation, and weight loss)
- If the diagnosis remains problematic, an antidepressant trial of adequate dose and duration may help to clarify the picture.

Intervention

Both pharmacologic and nonpharmacologic interventions are valuable in managing parkinsonian depression. Among antidepressant medications, there is good theoretic support for using serotonin reuptake inhibitors such as fluoxetine (Prozac), sertraline (Zoloft), and paroxetine (Paxil). Tricyclic antidepressants, especially nortriptyline (Pamelor), have been successful in treating depression in frail elders. However, tricyclic antidepressants may compound orthostatic hypotension and the anticholinergic effects of some anti-Parkinson drugs. Antidepressant MAO inhibitors are contraindicated in residents receiving levodopa because they inhibit the degradation of levodopa and its byproducts.

As a nonpharmacologic approach, group therapy may help residents not only through exercise but also by providing needed emotional support. Individual supportive psychotherapy may be a useful adjunct, especially in helping the resident confront progressive disability. Family members may also need education and support.

Pain

Assorted muscular aches and cramps are common in parkinsonism and may compromise the quality of life significantly. Residents often report painful cramps in the feet and calves, which may be dystonias secondary to long-term levodopa use. Back pain may be related to stooped posture. The most effective remedies are exercises designed to improve flexibility and range of motion. Physical therapy and daily exercises may alleviate painful rigidity, as well as prevent joint contractures, pressure ulcers, and other complications of deconditioning. Provide the residents with a set of stretching exercises to perform as a daily routine or when pain develops. Proper positioning in bed and chairs can also reduce pain. Oversized soft shoes are also helpful.

Drugs can be used in troubling situations that are not responsive to nonpharmacologic therapies. For foot dystonias, which occur in the morning, a nighttime dose of long-acting Sinemet can be helpful. Muscle relaxants, such as orphenadrine (Norflex), are more effective

but may be sedating. Antispasmodic agents, such as baclofen (Lioresal), may also be effective but have significant anticholinergic side effects.

Communication Problems

Parkinsonian speech is typically soft and monotonous. Residents may also encounter difficulties with enunciation and hoarseness. Palilalia, a repetitive stammering as if the speaker is stuck on a certain syllable, may be a particularly troubling problem. When compounded by reduced facial expression and difficulty with hand gestures, speech problems may severely compromise the resident's ability to communicate. In addition, the resident's handwriting will usually be micrographic (small letters) and difficult to read. As a consequence of communication difficulties, social withdrawal and depression may result, and a consultation by a speech-language therapist can be helpful.

Sleep Disturbance

Residents report frequent nocturnal awakening and often complain that sleep is not restorative. Painful myoclonus may be most troubling at night. Similarly, because the effects of levodopa usually wear off at night, the resident may become severely bradykinetic and complain of being unable to turn in bed. Long-acting Sinemet preparations prior to sleeping may be helpful. Other helpful measures include a later bedtime; smooth, silk sheets; pajamas that facilitate movement; and even a rope or grab bar on the bedside to facilitate self-turning.

Visual Problems

Parkinsonian residents blink less frequently and are prone to dry eyes. Artificial tears are administered frequently, and vigilance for complications such as conjunctivitis and corneal abrasion are recommended. As a preventive measure, remind residents to blink. Additionally, parkinsonian effects on the ocular muscles may impair extraocular motion and cause problems with tracking. As a consequence, residents often complain of the inability to read. Unfortunately, there is no helpful medical treatment, but staff can provide talking books and access to volunteer readers.

MEDICATIONS AND ADVERSE DRUG REACTIONS

The pharmacologic treatment of Parkinson's disease is directed at reducing symptoms. The mainstay of treatment is dopamine replacement, which is most often achieved by providing the resident with the dopamine precursor, levodopa. Levodopa is usually given in fixed combinations with carbidopa with the dose expressed as the proportion of carbidopa to levodopa (e.g., 25/100). The brand name of this combined preparation is Sinemet. In elderly facility residents, at least 50 mg of carbidopa must be administered daily to inhibit the conversion of levodopa outside the brain and thus prevent systemic side effects.

Levodopa treatment can be very effective in controlling rigidity and bradykinesia, which are the most disabling parkinsonian features. Unfortunately, effectiveness wanes over time, typically providing only a 4- to 8-year window of benefit. Although therapy usually continues beyond this period, the benefit is limited by disabling side effects (*see* the next section). In many advanced-stage Parkinson's residents, the effect of a treatment wears off after only 2 to 3 hours (on-off phenomenon). In some, it may end abruptly, resulting in sudden freezing episodes in which the resident is unable to move. In such cases, the resident may benefit from more frequent dosing or from long-acting levodopa preparations (e.g., Sinemet-CR).

Some neurologists recommend adding dopamine agonists to levodopa when response fluctuations are difficult to manage.

Two frequently recommended dopamine agonists are bromocriptine (Parlodel) and pergolide (Permax). These agents may also be used as initial therapy in the early stages of disability because of concerns that levodopa may actually accelerate progression of the disease.

Anticholinergic agents, such as benztropine (Cogentin) and trihexyphenidyl (Artane), may be helpful early in the disease, particularly before levodopa is started and when tremor is disabling. However, late in the course, the risks of anticholinergic medications invariably outweigh any potential benefits. Deprenyl (Eldepryl), or selegiline, is an MAO-B inhibitor that has been shown to delay the onset of disability requiring levodopa in early Parkinson's disease. It may also have some symptomatic benefits, but its role in late-stage disease is not yet well defined.

LEVODOPA SIDE EFFECTS

In the nursing home setting, the staff is often in the situation of managing the treatment of Parkinson's disease in its late stages, when the benefit from dopaminergic therapy is limited. Also, a resident's disabilities may actually be due as much to dopaminergic side effects as to the underlying disease itself. Watch the resident carefully and use creative pharmacologic manipulation to maximize the resident's function.

Involuntary Movements

After years of levodopa therapy, residents may develop various involuntary, or dyskinetic, movements. Commonly, these are twisting or writhing movements of the head, trunk, and extremities (chorea). Other dyskinetic symptoms include twitching and restlessness. Dyskinesia must be distinguished from tremor because of the very different treatment implications involved. Prolonged muscle spasms in awkward positions (dystonias) may develop in the hands and feet.

Recognition of dyskinesia is important because the condition responds to reducing the dose of levodopa. Major functional and symptomatic improvement can be seen, but levodopa doses may need to be substantially reduced or eliminated before improvement is noted. However, some residents cannot tolerate drastic dose reductions, and instead may require smaller reductions plus the addition of a dopamine agonist or a switch to long-acting preparations of levodopa. In others, fine-tuning with frequent dose adjustments will accomplish an optimal balance between control of dyskinesias and treatment of rigidity and bradykinesia.

Nausea

High peak levels of dopamine may provoke nausea and vomiting through its stimulating effect on the midbrain vomiting center. This can be avoided by delaying absorption of the drug, usually by administering it with a protein meal, which results in a slow, gradual rise in brain levodopa levels. Another alternative is to use long-acting levodopa preparations, which take longer to reach peak levels. However, many nursing home residents reveal their most urgent need for levodopa in the morning hours when they perform their ADLs. Thus, levodopa is often given when awakening so that function is maximized over the next 1 to 2 hours, when the resident is dressing, washing, and eating breakfast. Some patients with nausea may improve with 50 mg of pure carbidops.

However, the resident may become nauseated when taking levodopa on an empty stomach. The reaction usually resolves over 3 to 6 months, but the delay may be intolerable to some. Alternatives to waiting include giving the early dose with a small snack containing some protein or using antinausea medications. Metoclopramide (Reglan) is contraindicated because it can cause or worsen parkinsonism, but older antinausea agents, such as trimethobenzamide (Tigan), are better tolerated.

Hypotension

Levodopa usually causes a drop in blood pressure, which may be most pronounced on standing. A hypertensive resident started on levodopa, therefore, will often need a reduction of antihypertensive medication. Orthostatic hypotension may not be symptomatic, but should be documented. If illness, new medications, or hypovolemia supervene, asymptomatic orthostatic hypotension may become symptomatic (dizziness, lightheadedness), resulting in syncope or a fall. Symptomatic hypotension may also develop after meals.

SUMMARY

Clinicians in long-term care facilities usually encounter parkinsonian patients at the advanced stages of disability. Parkinson's disease accounts for the large majority of parkinsonism, but drug effects should be excluded. Rigidity and bradykinesia are two of the most disabling parkinsonian features, but there exists an array of late complications that impair function and compromise the quality of life. Falls, malnutrition, dementia, and depression are prominent among the late manifestations seen in the nursing home setting. Although levodopa is the mainstay of pharmacologic treatment early in the disease course, its effectiveness wanes over time while the burden of side effects increases. Careful observation and creative interdisciplinary interventions are the keys to successful management.

CASE EXAMPLE

Mrs. S. is a 78-year-old woman who was admitted to the facility from a rehabilitation hospital where she was recovering from surgical repair of a hip fracture.

She first noticed a tremor 14 years ago. When it began to interfere with her knitting 2 years later, she was referred to a neurologist who diagnosed Parkinson's disease and pre-scribed an anticholinergic medication, benztropine (Cogentin). Benztropine reduced the tremor but produced intolerable dry mouth and constipation. Two years later, she devel-oped stiffness and difficulty when getting in and out of a car. Her neurologist prescribed Sinemet, which allowed her to continue most of her activities for the next 6 years.

About 4 years ago, her posture became stooped and her steps became short and shuf-fling. Increasing doses of Sinemet were nec-essary to allow her to conduct her usual ac-tivities. She became increasingly fatigued. More recently, she has felt unsteady on her feet and has fallen while reaching for objects on shelves or cleaning in her home. Her last fall resulted in a hip fracture.

When the staff first met Mrs. S., she was attentive and complained of fatigue and of having little energy. She was sitting in a wheel-chair, speaking little, and exhibiting little fa-cial expression. She appeared thin and her clothes were loose fitting. On rising from a lying to a standing position, her blood pres-sure fell from 140/80 to 110/70 mm Hg, and she appeared unsteady. There were slow, coarse swaying movements of her head and trunk. There was mild upper extremity rigid-ity with a cogwheeling quality and minimal tremor. She ambulated with a walker in short, shuffling steps and could not stand upright without the walker or assistance. Cognitive testing demonstrated slow responses and dif-ficulty in generating a word list but no other significant abnormalities.

The physician suspected that the abnormal movements and orthostatic hypotension were due to dopamine sensitivity, and reduced her Sinemet dose from 25/250 four times daily to 25/100 three times daily. The staff was also

concerned that she was depressed, but chose to observe her through a period of adjustment to the nursing home. The staff was also wor-ried about weight loss and requested that the nutritionist evaluate her. The physical thera-pist was consulted to evaluate her gait and balance and to recommend an activity and rehabilitation program to be executed by the nursing staff.

One month later, the dyskinesias and ortho-static hypotension had resolved. With nutri-tional supplements, change to a soft solid diet, and instruction in swallowing technique, she has regained 5 pounds. She is working with the staff to improve her ambulation, but she remains fearful and unmotivated. She has fallen twice without injury while reaching to remove clothes from drawers. She expresses feelings of worthlessness and despair about her disabilities.

The staff next refered her to a weekly Parkinson's group for exercise and social sup-port. Following psychiatric consultation, an antidepressant trial of fluoxitene has begun, starting at 5 mg daily. Two months later she is in better spirits and is more active. However, she now complains that several hours after her Sinemet dose, she often gets suddenly stiff and cannot continue her activity. The physi-cian suspects an on-off phenomenon and adds pergolide (Permax) to her medical regimen, increasing the dose every few days until the on-off phenomena abate.

Mrs. S. has not regained her prior level of functioning and continues to fall periodically, but she is able, through an interdisciplinary approach and creative pharmacologic manipu-lation, to maintain some degree of indepen-dence and to continue personally satisfying activities.

10
Cognitive Loss

Nancy Mace, MA
John N. Morris, PhD
Nancy E. Lombardo, PhD
Thomas Perls, MD, MPH

Cognitive decline can be the result of many factors—dementia, delirium, the harmful effects of institutionalization, or a failure to treat medical or mood problems. More than one factor is often present. Approximately 60% of residents in long-term care facilities show signs and symptoms of intellectual decline. Fewer than 1 in 10 will have a full recovery, but many will improve. Achieving a partial recovery from cognitive decline requires judicious modification of medical regimens, caregiver vigilance, and maintenance of a residential environment that is both supportive and appropriately challenging.

Dementia is defined as the decline in multiple areas of cognition in a person who is awake and alert. More than 60 diseases can cause dementia, the most common of which is Alzheimer's disease. Progressing gradually over an average of 7 years from diagnosis to death, the duration of Alzheimer's disease is highly variable—a person can live with it for 15 years or more. It is currently incurable and results in total disability and death.

Multiinfarct dementia (MID), the second most common cause of dementia, results from multiple strokes—many so small as to be individually unnoticed. The progression of MID is potentially preventable by treating the risk factors for subsequent strokes.

Cognitive disability may lead to falls and injury, self-neglect, incontinence, malnutrition, isolation, depression, agitation, anger, inactivity, sleep disturbance, aggression, and wandering. Residents with dementia often lack insight into their disability and try to function normally, unwittingly exposing themselves to risk. This lack of insight also leads to resistance to care.

OVERVIEW

Once thought of as a normal aspect of aging, it is now known that dementias result from various disease processes (Table 10-1).

The American Psychiatric Association (APA) diagnostic criteria for dementia are shown in Table 10-2.

A decline in mental function distinguishes dementia from a lifetime pattern of limited mental function. The presence of a decline in more than one area of mental function distinguishes dementia from pure amnesic disorders. Chronicity and irreversibility are no longer part of the definition of dementia. The specific mental functions that show impairment vary depending on the disease process in-

Table 10-1. Conditions Causing Dementia

Degenerative Disorders of the Central Nervous System
Alzheimer's disease
Pick's disease
Huntington's disease
Parkinson's disease
Progressive supranuclear palsy
Hallervorden-Spatz syndrome
Spinocerebellar degenerations
Progressive myoclonic epilepsy
Progressive subcortical gliosis
Amyotrophic lateral sclerosis (ALS)
ALS-parkinsonism-dementia complex
Frontal lobe degeneration (non-Alzheimer type)

Metabolic Endocrine Disorders
Hypothyroidism
Wilson's disease
Hepatic encephalopathy
Prolonged hypoglycemia
Hypoxia
Cushing's syndrome
Hypopituitarism
Uremia

Cerebrovascular Disease
Multiple cortical strokes
Multiple subcortical strokes (lacunar state)
Cortical and subcortical strokes
Binswanger's multifocal leukoencephalopathy
Multiple etiologies

Deficiency Disorders
Alcohol-related syndromes
Pellagra
Marchiafava-Bignami disease
Combined systems disease or B12 deficiency

Toxins/Drugs
Heavy metals
Carbon monoxide
Medication

Brain Tumors
Direct effect
Paraneoplastic effects

Trauma
Sequelae of both open- and closed-head injury

Infections
Brain abscess
Bacterial, fungal, tubercular, and other forms of meningitis
Postviral encephalitic syndromes
Progressive multifocal leukoencephalopathy
Behçet's syndrome
Syphilis
HIV

Prion Diseases
Creutzfeldt-Jakob disease
Gerstmann-Sträussler syndrome
Kuru

Psychiatric Syndromes
Affective disorders
Schizophrenic disorders
Hysterical disorders

Other Conditions
Multiple sclerosis
Muscular dystrophy
Whipple's disease
Storage diseases, such as Kufs' disease
Obstructive hydrocephalus
Normal-pressure hydrocephalus
Sequelae of subarachnoid, intracerebral, or intracranial hemorrhage
Electrical injury
Hereditary dysphasic dementia

From: Mayeaux R, Foster NL, Rossor M, and Whitehouse PJ: The clinical evaluation of patients with dementia, *Dementia*, page 93, 1993.

Table 10-2. Diagnostic Criteria for Dementia and its Severity

Criteria for Diagnosis

1. Evidence of impairment in short- and long-term memory. Impairment in short-term memory (inability to learn new information) may be indicated by the inability to remember three objects after 5 minutes. Long-term memory impairment (inability to remember information that was known in the past) may be indicated by the inability to remember past personal information (e.g., what happened yesterday, birthplace, occupation) or facts of common knowledge (e.g., presidents, well-known dates).

2. At least one of the following:
   - Impairment in abstract thinking, as indicated by the inability to find similarities and differences between related words, difficulty in defining words and concepts and other similar tasks.
   - Impaired judgment, as indicated by the inability to make reasonable plans to deal with interpersonal, family, and job-related problems and issues.
   - Other disturbances of higher cortical function, such as aphasia (disorder of language), apraxia (inability to carry out motor activities despite intact comprehension and motor function), agnosia (failure to recognize or identify objects despite intact sensory function), and "constructional difficulty" (e.g., inability to copy three-dimensional figures, assemble blocks, or arrange sticks in specific designs).

   - Personality change, i.e., alteration or accentuation of premorbid traits.

3. The disturbance in 1 and 2 significantly interferes with work, usual social activities, or relationships with others.

4. Symptoms and signs not occurring exclusively during the course of delirium.

5. Either of the following:
   - Evidence from the history, physical examination, or laboratory tests of a specific organic factor(s) judged to be related etiologically to the disturbance.
   - In the absence of such evidence, an etiologic factor can be presumed if the disturbance cannot be accounted for by any nonorganic mental disorder, e.g., major depression accounting for cognitive impairment.

Criteria for Severity

Mild: Although work or social activities are impaired significantly, the capacity for independent living remains, with adequate personal hygiene and relatively intact judgment.

Moderate: Independent living is hazardous, and some degree of supervision is necessary.

Severe: Activities of daily living (ADLs) are so impaired that continual supervision is required, e.g., the inability to maintain minimal personal hygiene; the individual is largely incoherent or mute.

Reprinted with permission from: Diagnostic and Statistical Manual of Mental Disorders, ed 4, Washington DC, 1994, The American Psychiatric Association.

volved. A diagnosis of dementia cannot be made in the presence of delirium.

The two most commonly seen causes of dementia are Alzheimer's disease and MID. Although studies vary, Alzheimer's disease accounts for approximately 70% of dementia cases and MID for about 20%. There is some overlap of residents with both conditions. Five percent to 10% have potentially reversible causes. For residents with primary Alzheimer's disease or MID, the symptoms can sometimes be alleviated by treating the concurrent illness, depression, or delirium.

Identifying the Resident with a Cognitive Deficit

A clinical problem may exist when one or more of the following deficits are present:

1. A problem in long-term memory: difficulty recalling things from the distant past (e.g., name of spouse(s), children, date and place of birth, home address)
2. A problem in short-term memory: difficulty remembering recent events (e.g., breakfast foods eaten, whether medications were taken, whether a child visited in the morning)
3. Two or more problems in memory recall (e.g., problems identifying the season, staff names and faces, location of room)
4. Impaired decision-making ability about ADLs (e.g., choosing clothes, determining mealtimes, making correct decisions on how to get to the lunchroom)
5. Impaired ability to understand or communicate with others
6. Diagnosis of Alzheimer's disease or other dementia, mental retardation, or aphasia

Diagnostic Evaluation for Dementia

The goals of the diagnostic workup for dementia are as follow:

- Establish a diagnosis.
- Identify potentially or partially reversible factors for interventions.

- Identify other conditions that may exacerbate cognitive dysfunction or have an impact on resident care.

Diagnosing Dementia

Follow this procedure to diagnose a resident for dementia:

1. Obtain a careful history from both the resident and, most importantly, another informant (usually a family member). Notable points to obtain include
   - The particular changes in cognitive performance
   - The time period over which these changes have been seen
   - The rate and pattern of progression of these deficits
   - The identification of unique events (such as new medications or diseases)
   - The appearance of new or temporary physical findings such as a change in gait, urinary incontinence, and asymmetric neurologic phenomena
   - A list of prescribed and over-the-counter medications and a history of alcohol use (including current use)
   - History of trauma and falls
   - Family history of dementias, Parkinson's disease, Down syndrome, and malignancies
   - Determination of the risk factors for vascular disease
   - Explore with the resident the possibility of depression, looking in particular for changes in sleep pattern and appetite, a decline in interests, level of energy, and concentration ability, preoccupation with guilt, and the presence of psychomotor slowing or suicidal ideation. (*See* Chapter 13, Depression, for more information.)
2. Perform a mental status examination. Many residents are able, either consciously or subconsciously, to cover up cognitive deficits that can be exposed only after careful systematic examination of different facets of

cognitive performance. Screens for picking up particular deficits include the Mini-Mental-State Examination (MMSE) and asking the resident to draw the face of a clock depicting the current time (e.g., 11:10). A formal neuropsychological evaluation is very helpful in the workup of dementia.

3. Use laboratory and radiologic studies to rule out the following:
   - Infection (urinalysis, syphilis serology test—rapid plasma reagin [RPR] or Venereal Disease Research Laboratory [VDRL]—and complete blood count [CBC])
   - Electrolyte and metabolic abnormalities (full chemistry panel), thyroid dysfunction (thyroid function tests)
   - Head trauma, malignancy, and normal-pressure hydrocephalus (head computed tomography [CT] or magnetic resonance imaging [MRI])

When clinical suspicion warrants, other illnesses (and tests) to consider include pernicious anemia (vitamin B_{12} and folate levels); pulmonary disease (chest radiography and hemoglobin oxygen saturation); temporal lobe seizures (electroencephalography [EEG]); and toxic exposures (heavy metal screen). Residents with psychiatric illnesses, primarily depression, can also present with dementia, so a psychiatric evaluation is often warranted in the diagnostic workup.

Treating Dementia

Care for the resident with dementia consists of identifying and treating any potentially treatable causes, such as metabolic disturbances, toxic conditions (including medication use), hydrocephalus, psychiatric disorders, neoplasms, and head trauma syndromes. Any other illnesses or chronic pain should also be treated.

Many residents in long-term care facilities exhibit problematic behaviors, and often respond best to environmental interventions.

Helpful in some cases are low doses of neuroleptics, which also aid in treating hallucinations and delusions. Residents with dementia are vulnerable to side effects, so use the neuroleptics carefully for specific targeted symptoms. Problem behaviors often signal concurrent illness, pain, or drug reactions/interactions that, if treatable, may reduce the behavior. A successful model involves the close coordination of pharmacologic and environmental interventions. (If many residents in one facility are receiving fairly high doses of medication to treat problem behavior, this may signal that nondrug interventions have been overlooked.)

Sleep disturbances are common and may be treated with hypnotics. In a nursing home setting where supervision is available, prescribe these medications judiciously. Antianxiolytics may be used to treat anxiety, but even low doses of benzodiazepines can further impair cognition and increase falls. Antidepressants are useful for some residents (*see* Chapter 13, Depression), but should be selected with consideration for their side effects, including constipation, sedation, and falls.

Elderly people will metabolize and excrete drugs differently than younger adults, often increasing the drug effect. People with dementia often take multiple medications, thereby increasing the risk of interactions. The damaged brain itself is more vulnerable to interactions and side effects.

Practice the general geropharmacologic principles of treating residents with dementia: start low, go slow, and use as few medications as possible. Because acetylcholine is reduced in people with Alzheimer's disease, administer drugs with anticholinergic side effects carefully. Among these, phenothiazines, haloperidol, tricyclic antidepressants, and nondopaminergic antiparkinsonian drugs can cause a reversible dementia. The appearance of side effects may be delayed in this population, making it less likely that staff will associate them with medication changes.

Residents with cognitive impairment cannot be depended on to self-medicate or to use prescribed adaptive devices. As the residents' conditions progress, their need for and response to drugs will change, requiring regular monitoring.

ALZHEIMER'S DISEASE

Alzheimer's disease is the most common cause of dementia. It is characterized by the presence of two lesions on microscopic examination of the brain—neuritic plaques and neurofibrillary tangles—as well as a degeneration of neurons. Research has identified areas of the brain in which neuron degeneration is much more profound than in others. This partially explains the neurologic findings associated with Alzheimer's disease. People with this disease demonstrate decreased amounts or activity of acetylcholine, choline acetyltransferase, and acetylcholine esterase. Immunohistochemical studies reveal the reduction in choline acetyltransferase to be especially apparent in regions of the brain noted for their involvement in Alzheimer's disease: the hippocampus, midtemporal gyrus, and frontal and parietal cortices. Plaque counts also correlate with the decrease in choline acetyltransferase.

Meynert's nucleus, a cholinergic group located in the sublenticular region, receives afferent input principally from the limbic system and projects to most of the cerebral cortex. The nucleus is atrophic an Alzheimer's disease, which explains why many Alzheimer's patients display neurologic symptoms consistent with cholinergic deficiency, such as disturbances in sleep and slowed reaction times.

Severe nerve cell loss and atrophy, with or without extensive neurofibrillary degeneration or Lewy body formation, has been noted in the nucleus locus ceruleus along with changes in the hypothalamus and mesial termporal cortex. Neurofibrillary tangles are noted to occur preferentially in the hippocampal formation and the substantia innominata as well as in the temporal neocortex (Brodmann area 22). The hippocampus and parahippocampal gyrus have been of greatest interest given their crucial roles in memory and their unique susceptibility to Alzheimer's disease.

Correlates of Alzheimer's Disease

The incidence of Alzheimer's disease increases with age. It is extremely rare in people 40 to 50 years of age but its prevalence rises to 47% in people age 85 or older. Studies have consistently identified a genetic pattern in the disease. Fetal activity determination (FAD), an autosomal dominant form, occurs in less than 1% of cases.

Studies show that the cumulative risk to persons with one or more first-degree relatives with Alzheimer's disease increases significantly. However, there has been incomplete concordance in monozygotic twins. Together, these findings indicate that the gene may have age-dependent penetrance and that an environmental factor is involved.

Family members may be extremely concerned about their risk of inheriting Alzheimer's disease. Knowledge of the genetics of this disease is advancing rapidly, so refer concerned families to an Alzheimer's Research Center for the latest information. Families will need support and reassurance. Many family members remain at greater risk of developing other chronic or fatal conditions (e.g., heart disease or cancer) before they might develop a dementia. Reassure families that even when there is more than one afflicted family member, there is strong evidence that these family members were exposed to something in the environment that triggered the illness.

DIAGNOSIS OF ALZHEIMER'S DISEASE AS DEVELOPED BY THE NINCDS-ADRDA

The diagnosis of Alzheimer's disease can be difficult, and standards have been established relative to the diagnosis. Alzheimer's disease diagnoses are divided into three categories.

The diagnosis of *possible* Alzheimer's disease is made when no other disease or disorder appears to be responsible for the dementia, but the onset or symptoms are not typical of the disease. This diagnosis is also made when the resident has another illness that might be responsible for the dementia but the physician suspects the disease.

Probable Alzheimer's disease meets the following criteria:

1. Presence of a dementia (as determined by the APA) with deficits in two or more areas of mental function
2. Progressive worsening of memory and other cognitive deficits over time
3. Relatively intact level of consciousness
4. Onset between 40 and 90 years of age
5. Absence of any other process that can account for the cognitive deficit

Autopsies indicate that diagnoses are accurate about 88% of the time using these criteria.

The diagnosis of *definite* Alzheimer's disease is made when histologic evidence is found in the brain tissue of residents meeting the criteria for probable Alzheimer's disease.

Much of the diagnosis of Alzheimer's disease involves ruling out other conditions including MID. CT and MRI are primarily useful in ruling out the presence of MID and other etiologic factors such as hydrocephalus, hematomas, tumors, and other possible factors. Positron emission tomography (PET) and single-photon emission CT (SPECT) may have future potential as diagnostic tools.

Neurologic testing is useful, and certain findings (memory and language deficits) point to the presence of Alzheimer's disease. Some investigators report that scores on certain neuropsychological tests have a high predictive value and may be valuable in identifying who will later develop Alzheimer's disease. Research for a biologic marker is ongoing. Genetic testing is not yet sufficiently refined for clinical diagnostic use.

The clinical presentation of Alzheimer's disease may vary. The pattern of decline is gradual and insidious. Its course can range from less than 5 years to more than 20 years. Increasing memory loss and difficulties in using language are usually seen in the early stages. Apraxia, temporal orientation, visual discrimination, and constructional praxis usually arise early. Agnosias often appear as the disease progresses. For much of the disease, residents will be able to express emotions, communicate somewhat, participate in activities that sustain relationships, and respond to the qualitative aspects of life. These abilities gradually decline until the resident requires total care. Depression, tearfulness, suspiciousness, paranoia, hallucinations, delusions, wandering, purposeless or inappropriate activity, anxiety, fearfulness, irritability, verbal or physical aggression, physical threats, violence, agitation, day/night disturbances, and other psychiatric symptoms are common.

TREATING ALZHEIMER'S DISEASE

There have been exciting research breakthroughs, but the treatment of Alzheimer's disease is currently palliative. Treating the concurrent conditions can relieve distress as reflected in behavior problems. Management of symptoms is described in the section on treating dementia.

Many drugs have been proposed for the treatment of Alzheimer's disease, and more are developing as our understanding of the disease develops. At present, one drug, Cognex (Tacrine; tetrahydroacridine; THA), has been licensed to treat the disease, although its use is controversial. Tacrine, a centrally active cholinesterase inhibitor, increases the activity of cholinergic neurons. Tacrine is not a cure for Alzheimer's disease nor does it appear to stop disease progression. From what is currently known, Tacrine will elicit improvement in a minority of people with Alzheimer's disease in otherwise good health whose condition is mild or moderate. However, because of its potential toxicities, treatment with Tacrine is not for everyone. The most frequent side effects are an increase in alanine aminotransferase, nausea and vomiting, abdominal pain, diarrhea, indigestion, and skin rash. Weekly liver function tests and close follow-up by a physician are required.

At any given time multiple drugs are being tested for the treatment of this disease. The Alzheimer's Association provides a toll-free information line to physicians or others seeking the status of research drugs and drugs in clinical use: 1-800-272-3900. The association also provides fact sheets and lists of centers conducting drug tests.

Chelation has long been promoted as a treatment for Alzheimer's disease. No well-controlled large-scale studies have been conducted, however, perhaps because of the risks involved in chelation: nausea, hypotension, vomiting, arrhythmias, congestive heart failure, and kidney failure.

The Alzheimer's Association publishes numerous reports and newsletters that facilitate staying current in this rapidly changing field.

MULTIINFARCT DEMENTIA

The second most common cause of dementia, MID, results from a series of small infarctions. Information about its epidemiology is limited, but MID clearly contributes to disability in a significant number of nursing home residents. Table 10-3 lists the diagnostic criteria for MID according to the APA.

MID is most common in people 60 to 75 years of age. The risk factors are the same as for cerebrovascular disease. Hypertension—a

preventable factor—is present in most residents with MID.

The Hachinski ischemic scale is used widely to distinguish MID. The presence of hypertension, older age, a step-wise course, abrupt onset often with neurologic incident, frequent impairment of emotional control, relative preservation of personality, and mild but definite neuropsychological and neurologic abnormalities are hallmarks of the disease. Its time course is highly variable and symptom pattern will vary with the location of the lesions.

Neuropsychological testing plays an important role in revealing deficits characteristic of MID and in identifying areas of spared and impaired function, which are helpful in planning management strategies. CT and MRI are useful to rule out space-occupying lesion and

Table 10-3. Diagnostic Criteria for Multiinfarct Dementia

Dementia.

Stepwise deteriorating course with a "patchy" distribution of deficits (i.e., affecting some functions, but not others) early in the course.

Focal neurologic signs and symptoms (e.g., exaggeration of deep tendon reflexes, extensor plantar response, pseudobulbar palsy, gait abnormalities, weakness of an extremity).

Evidence from history, physical examination, or laboratory tests of significant cerebrovascular disease (recorded on axis III) that is judged to be etiologically related to the disturbance.

Reprinted with permission from: Diagnostic and Statistical Manual of Mental Disorders, 4th ed., Washington DC, 1994, The American Psychiatric Association.

normal- pressure hydrocephalus, and to identify lacunae indicative of vascular disease.

Treating MID includes the slow and gradual
lowering of blood pressure. Aspirin is reported
to reduce the incidence of stroke in residents
who have transient ischemic attacks (TIAs); it
may prevent the development of further lacunae in MID.

Binswanger's dementia is an uncommon
vascular disease that is also usually associated
with hypertension.

DEPRESSION

Depression is common in residents presenting with cognitive deficits and may be confused with symptoms of irreversible dementias.
Depression impairs function and causes significant suffering. Residents are at risk of suicide and severe anorexia. In the nursing home,
depressed residents are often apathetic, sometimes resisting care and suffering from incontinence. Their symptoms may go unnoticed
or their apathy may be mistaken for a symptom of Alzheimer's disease. Others may present
serious behavior problems including agitation,
paranoia, restlessness, or combativeness.
These symptoms may also be blamed on a
primary dementia, but will be more likely to
respond to treatment with antidepressants than
with antipsychotics. *See* Chapter 13, Depression, for a discussion of the diagnostic criteria
for a major depressive episode.

When psychosocial losses are contributing
factors, perform a careful workup to determine
the appropriate treatment. Never dismiss depression on the assumption that it is a normal
response to the losses of old age. The elderly
and those with cognitive deficits may deny
feeling depressed or their families may report
that "she was always like that." Neither should
be grounds for dismissing depression as a
working diagnosis.

Depression alone may cause significant
cognitive impairment, or it may deepen the
confusion of those with a primary dementia.

Studies show that in some residents presenting with both depression and dementia, the
dementia resolves when the depression is
treated.

The literature disagrees over whether the
cognitive impairments of depression (which
occur in adults of all ages with a major depression) are a pseudodementia or a true dementia. In either case, treating the depression
may improve cognition or behavior.

Depression is highly responsive to treatment. There are many antidepressant medications from which to select. Choose those that
will have the fewest side effects and greatest
response in a given resident. The brain-dam-
aged elderly may require very low doses. Trial
and error is required to identify the most successful drug and dosage. When treating depression it is usually necessary to address immediate psychosocial or environmental issues
as well as pharmacologic treatment. (*See* Chapter 13, Depression, for more information.)

Case Study Relative to Depression

A 79-year-old woman was transferred to a
special care unit. She had an MMSE score of
15 and denied feelings of depression. She was
diagnosed as having probable Alzheimer's disease. She was highly suspicious and insisted
that her husband had a new girlfriend and no
longer loved her. She paced for long periods
and would strike other residents and staff
without warning. She was treated with
neuroleptics and benzodiazepine without any
change, except for increased falls. Watchful
staff observed her husband in the garden with
his new friend. The social worker was able to
persuade him that his wife was still "with it,"
and although he chose to act as a loving husband around her, his wife's suspiciousness and
combativeness continued. Based on the negative content of her remarks and her affect, a
trial of Zoloft was begun, and the resident
relaxed considerably. She dropped her delusions, stopped striking people, and was able

to resume independent ADLs, but she remained arrogant and difficult.

DELIRIUM

Delirium is common in nursing home residents. The cognitive confusion of delirium is sometimes mistaken for a primary degenerative dementia. In such cases, the underlying cause of the delirium may go undetected. Delirium is often seen as an overlay in addition to a dementia, compounding the resident's cognitive and functional disability. The treatment of delirium cannot be overemphasized. People with dementia may present with mild symptoms in which worsened behavior is the most noticeable. When staff or family are not observant, delirium may persist and remain untreated for long periods. *See* Chapter 11, Delirium, for a description of the diagnostic criteria for delirium.

The minimum data set (MDS) defines a straightforward set of indicators for delirium that can be used by the nursing staff. Table 10-4 lists these indicators as shown on the MDS form (version 2.0). Residents triggering these indicators should be seen promptly by a physician.

The adverse effects of medications are the most common cause of delirium in the nursing home setting. Other important causes include infection, metabolic and electrolyte derangement(s), head trauma, pain, sleep deprivation, and intercurrent illness (e.g., congestive heart failure, acute stroke, pulmonary embolus). The aging brain is also vulnerable to a wide range of psychological stressors that compromise cognitive function (e.g., depression, grief, the stress of moving to a new setting, isolation, reaction to physical restraints, not being mentally involved to the extent possible). In addition, perceptual and other cognitive problems can be induced by bombarding the senses with noise, poor or disturbing lighting, and other environmental features such as crowding.

Because of their already impaired brain function, people with chronic dementia are more susceptible to developing a concurrent delirium. The diagnostic workup for dementia often identifies coexisting treatable environmental, psychiatric, or medical conditions for which appropriate treatment can improve intellectual function. These exacerbating factors, in the presence of a nonreversible dementia, are considered excess disabilities. Among residents with dementia, delirium often presents in subtle ways, such as a change in personality or behavior, level of alertness, activity level, or appetite. Appropriate treatment of the delirium can often improve cognitive function, even among people with dementia. For more information *see* Chapter 11, Delirium.

HYDROCEPHALUS

Hydrocephalus can be divided pathologically into nonobstructive and obstructive types. Nonobstructive hydrocephalus refers to ventricular enlargement, usually secondary to cerebral atrophy. Obstructive hydrocephalus is generally divided into communicating and noncommunicating types. Noncommunicating obstructive hydrocephalus occurs secondary

TABLE 10-4. INDICATORS OF DELIRIUM—PERIODIC DISORDERED THINKING/AWARENESS

Check if the resident's condition over the last 7 days appears different from usual functioning:
Easily distracted
Periods of altered perception or awareness of surroundings
Episodes of disorganized speech
Periods of restlessness
Periods of lethargy
Motor function varies over course of day

to a lesion such as a tumor, blood clot, or cyst that obstructs the ventricular outflow of cerebrospinal fluid (CSF).

Communicating obstructive hydrocephalus (also called normal-pressure hydrocephalus [NPH]) indicates a free flow of CSF from the ventricles, but obstruction at the subarachnoid channels leading to the sagittal sinus. Obstruction at this level can be due to a tumor, complications of bleeding (e.g., blood clot, fibrosis), postinfectious scarring, and other unknown causes. The hydrocephalic dementias are typified by a triad of signs: intellectual impairment, gait disturbance, and urinary incontinence.

The gait disturbance is often the most prominent finding but can vary greatly in its character. Usually there is lower extremity spasticity and the resident has difficulty starting movement, as if his or her feet were glued to the floor. There is often hyperreflexia, and with progression, extrapyramidal signs may emerge. Cognitive impairment is typically subtle at presentation and common complaints are similar to those with a subcortical type of dementia, i.e., mental slowing, memory impairment, and apathy. Urinary incontinence generally does not appear until late in the course. Imaging studies, including CT, MRI, and PET, are typically the most useful diagnostic aids for the hydrocephalic dementias.

AIDS

AIDS causes dementia in roughly half the residents with the disease, either primary to the virus itself or secondary to AIDS-related diseases. (For more information, *see* Chapter 5, AIDS.)

PARKINSON'S DISEASE

A epidemiologic study found that about 40% of the people with Parkinson's disease also have a dementia. Researchers are seeking to define the relationship, if any, between the two diseases. Managing symptoms in a resident with Parkinson's' disease and dementia is challenging because many drugs that treat hallucinations and behavior problems worsen parkinsonian symptoms, and antiparkinsonian drugs may aggravate other symptoms of dementia. Environmental supports have proven highly successful.

DIAGNOSTIC EVALUATION FOR DEMENTIA

Much of the diagnostic workup for dementia involves ruling out the possibility of a treatable cause for the decline in intellectual function. Furthermore, the workup often identifies coexisting environmental, psychiatric, or medical conditions for which appropriate treatment can effect improvement in cognitive function even if the main disorder is irreversible.

Start the workup with a careful history obtained from the resident as well as, importantly, from family and caregiver(s). Notable points to obtain include:

• The particular changes in cognitive performance
• The time period over which these changes have been seen
• Behavior and personality changes that have been observed
• The rate and pattern of progression of these deficits
• The identification of unique events (e.g., new medications or diseases) that may have been seen during the most recent period of decline

The appearance of new or transient physical findings such as a change in gait, urinary incontinence, and asymmetric neurologic phenomena are important. Include a list of prescribed and over-the-counter medications; history of alcohol use, trauma, and falls; family history of dementias and malignancies; and a determination of risk factors for atherosclerosis. Explore with the resident the possibility of depression, looking in particular for changes in sleep pattern and appetite; a decline in interests, level of energy, and concentration ability; preoccupation with guilt; and the presence of psychomotor slowing or suicidality (*see* Chapter 13, Depression, for more information).

Perform a careful mental status examination (*see* the section on diagnosing dementia for details), and use laboratory and radiologic studies to rule out the following:

- Infection (urinalysis, syphilis serology test—RPR or VDRL tests—and CBC)
- Electrolyte and metabolic abnormalities (full chemistry panel)
- Thyroid dysfunction (TSH)
- Head trauma, malignancy, and normal-pressure hydrocephalus (head CT or MRI)

When clinical suspicion warrants, other illnesses (and tests) to consider include pernicious anemia (vitamin B_{12} and folate levels); pulmonary disease (chest radiography and hemoglobin oxygen saturation) temporal lobe seizures (EEG); and toxic exposures (heavy metal screen). Psychiatric illnesses, primarily depression, can also present with dementia, so a psychiatric evaluation is often warranted in the diagnostic workup.

Assessment of cognition is not based entirely on formal tools, many of which have a high floor effect, that is, they are not useful in differentiating residual cognitive capacity beyond a certain point in the illness; residents with differing cognitive abilities will have the same low score. Observe the resident closely. In the severely ill, observe eye tracking, facial expression, and body language. Also observe the resident in a quiet place, and look for very simple skills such as walking, grasping, eating with fingers, or petting a dog. Even very impaired residents will be able to do some things in a relaxed and supportive environment.

ASSESSMENT OF RELEVANT CAUSAL FACTORS AND TREATMENT STRATEGIES

A focused, ongoing assessment of cognitive status and daily function, psychosocial needs, and remaining abilities is the guide to intervention. Start with a medical workup and a complete history at intake followed by a 1-month course of focused, daily assessment by licensed nursing and other professional personnel. Rather than a perfunctory overview, this review must be an extensive hands-on assessment. Professional expertise and careful attention is necessary to identify those areas in which intervention will be most therapeutic.

The assessment must be detailed enough to guide care planning directly. For example, a statement such as "resident incontinent of urine" is of limited use in care planning. Assessment must also question, for example, is the resident aware of the need to urinate? Can the resident find the toilet and manipulate his or her clothing? Is the staff recognizing the resident's cues and responding quickly enough? A statement such as "resident refuses activities" must go on to query the following: Is the resident overwhelmed by the size of the group? Does the activity make sense to the resident? Is the resident depressed?

Base the assessment on input from medical, nursing, and activities and social work staff as follows:

- Observe the resident at different times of the day and in different situations.
- Talk with the resident.
- Get input from the caregivers.
- Observe the behavior of the caregivers on all shifts.
- Get information from and (if possible) observe the family.
- Observe the resident interacting with other residents.
- A search of the hospital and facility records

(there is often information or patterns here that have been forgotten).

Emphasize positive information, such as one caregiver who does not have trouble with a resident and another who has found that if she starts a resident eating, the resident can continue independently.

Assessment also includes intense information exchange to and from caregivers, among professionals, and with the family. For example, only the family may know that a female resident is lactose-intolerant (which explains the diarrhea); only the assessing nurse may know that the resident has arthritic pain in her shoulder (which is why she fights the caregivers when they dress her); and only the day shift may know how to calm her when she gets upset. The weekend shift may know none of this, which explains why the resident needs more medication at that time.

An intensive 1-month assessment is generally done on admission, but successful care does not end there. Successful care is a process of ongoing reconsideration. Partial assessments are done when there is change and at periodic intervals.

A thorough medical workup is the basis for all resident care. Include input from this workup from the nursing staff, complete with a history, a systems review, and a drug review, taking into consideration that people with dementia are vulnerable to drug reactions and interactions. Disease may be occult or overlooked. Symptoms such as fever are muted in the elderly, and confused residents often deny symptoms or report confusing information. In considering disease status, consider what impact, if any, the disease has on function. When assessing falls, consider medication, rushing, the physical plant, the noise levels, and resident characteristics. Adequate hydration and good nutrition are critical to good care. It can be difficult to see into some

resident's mouths, but infection or pain can contribute to nutrition problems, behavior problems, and poor general health. The medical review provides evidence of excess disability, delirium, and depression.

Confirming Cognitive Assessment

Assessment includes the resident's interpersonal history and customary routine. Use the psychosocial assessment to obtain useful information for the caregiving staff by asking these questions:
• Is the resident shy?
• Who does the resident call out for?
• What things might embarrass the resident?
• What things has the family done to manage the resident's behavior?
• What signs does the resident use to signal the need to use the bathroom?

The social worker should ask caregivers about the practical information that is important to *them*. Practical information saves time and confusion in the first few days of an admission.

An assessment consists of communication and hearing patterns and should go into some detail. For example:
• Does the resident hear better on one side?
• Does he or she communicate better when rested?
• Does he or she communicate better in a quiet space?

Often, the first two or three words a resident with dementia says are relevant but the meaning diminishes as speaking continues. Observation by both caregivers and professionals in a quiet, well-lighted place will help determine visual patterns and hearing deficits.

Observe the resident's ADLs and continence over time and on different shifts. As well as assessing performance, look for reasons for poor ADL performance other than cognition. For example:

- The caregiver's behavior
- Light
- Confusion
- Life-long patterns
- The physical environment
- Facility routine

Identify those ADLs or parts of ADLs that the resident can do him- or herself. Determine the circumstances needed to ease performance (e.g., a one-step command or a two-step command). Determine how quickly the resident fatigues and assess whether time-out periods will help. There is a tendency to both overestimate (she should be able to understand that she has to have a bath) and underestimate (he cannot help at all getting dressed) resident function.

Assessment of mood and behavior problems includes assessing times that problems arise; the staff, family, or other residents involved; and data from the medical workup. Consider the quality of resident behaviors (e.g., afraid, angry, response to a put down, always negative). Assess for apathy as it is often evidence of a treatable condition.

Assessment also identifies the triggers for a resident's angry outbursts. Keep a log of the events, the times they occur, who was with the resident, and what happened just before the outburst. A pattern will emerge that will enable the observer to identify ways to avoid outbursts.

Important factors of the activity assessment include:

1. How long is the resident engaged in an activity versus the amount of down time in the entire day?
2. Does the resident enjoy the activity and appear to know what is going on?
3. Is the resident involved or tuned out?
4. Is the group size appropriate?
5. Does the activity reinforce the resident's abilities or disabilities?

A month-long assessment allows an opportunity to assess the efficacy of current treatments for acute and reversible mental health problems. Feedback and immediate teaching about daily care approaches can be offered. Observe how successful interventions are used by caregivers.

Problems often have multiple causes that assessment will identify. For example, if a resident is not eating, there may be many related explanations:

- Depression
- Gastrointestinal or swallowing problems
- Physical illness
- Problems using utensils, paranoia (which may lead the resident to fear that he or she is being poisoned)
- An overreaction to the noise and confusion in the dining room
- Frightening hallucinations (which may cause the resident to scream, become agitated, or withdrawn).

It is not unusual for two or more of these factors to be at work simultaneously. Symptoms may not obviously match cause; depression may manifest as agitation or causes of stress may be hard to see. For example, one woman would sit peacefully in the dayroom for a long time as staff brought other residents back from lunch before suddenly becoming agitated. The staff finally realized that it was the number of people in the day room that overstressed her. The assessor must cast a broad net to determine the problem.

INTERVENTIONS

The completed assessment should provide a list of the required interventions; the care plan follows directly from a good assessment. Intervention is then followed by documentation of its success, identifying techniques that have worked and areas that need a new strategy. There are nine broad areas of intervention to consider. Small changes in multiple areas will result in reductions in behavior problems, some improvements in function, better social interactions, and family satisfaction.

1. Consider the brain damage itself

Data from multiple mental status tests, neuropsychological testing (if available), and observation provide information about what the resident can or cannot do. Brain damage is often exacerbated by untrained caregivers who fail to recognize what the resident can and cannot do (e.g., a resident cannot remember that he or she needs to urinate in the time it takes to walk to the toilet).

2. Treat concurrent illness, pain, and medication reaction or interaction (excess disability)

People with dementia are vulnerable to even mild concurrent illness or pain. Many medications worsen cognitive function or contribute to falls and constipation. It is important to treat these conditions directly and to ask whether there is an insidious relationship between these conditions and cognitive function (see the section on diagnostic evaluation). Symptoms may be only affective or may manifest only as a change in behavior. Do not assume a worsening of function or behavior to be a necessary consequence of dementia. When this attitude occurs, treatment of the condition may not be appropriately aggressive. It is more successful to treat problems early than to try to reverse an established condition. Therefore, train caregivers to report even minor changes.

For example, bladder incontinence is often treatable. Residents with Alzheimer's disease usually do not become incontinent from the dementia alone until the end stage of the disease. Most incontinence in residents with early-, middle-, or even late-stage dementia has the same etiology as in other people. Consequently, in many residents, incontinence can be prevented or treated. Unnecessary incontinence can cause residents to refuse to participate in activities, resist help in changing, or become depressed. It is also an unnecessary added workload (and cost) for the caregivers. Interventions for incontinence are multifaceted:

- Eliminate the factors that may aggravate the problem, such as medications or a urinary tract infection
- Ease elimination (e.g., dress the resident in easily removed clothing, easy availability of toilets, and regular patterns of toileting)
- Prevent conditions that can lead to incontinence, including fecal impaction and recurrent strokes (see Chapter 27, Urinary Incontinence, for more information).

Addressing problems often requires the efforts of several disciplines. For example, a resident dozed through activities even though the staff felt sure she needed the stimulation. The staff reviewed her treatment protocols, preferences, and expanded list of problems. Ultimately, a change in her medications made her more alert so that she could participate and begin to regain her self-esteem.

Even residents who seem reasonably articulate may deny pain or report it to be in the wrong place. It is easy to overlook pain from dental problems, mild arthritis, or the discomfort from sitting in one position for a long period.

Residents with dementia are more sensitive to medications and commonly require lower doses than younger adults. Anticholinergic medications may cause worsening of function. Drug interactions are common. A careful adjustment of the resident's total medication load may improve function. Changes in staff behavior may also make it unnecessary to increase medications that have increased side effects. When staff are alert to resident functioning, early intervention can often prevent problems.

3. Support sensory function

Residents with dementia cannot compensate for vision and hearing loss and often forget to wear their glasses or hearing aids. This excess disability can lead to immobility (fear of not seeing where one is going), suspiciousness (someone is talking about me), and combativeness (not hearing or seeing someone who approaches). Keeping up with glasses and hearing aids may seem a nuisance to staff, so devise a system to manage and find them (e.g., use eyeglass straps, find a set place for housekeeping to put found items).

Facilities that plan remodeling need to consider plant designs that increase light levels, reduce glare, and absorb noise.

4. Treat psychiatric disorders

Memory, communication, and other skills may be severely damaged, but most residents with dementia appear to retain and show emotions. Fear, anxiety, anger, and depression make function worse. Moreover, psychiatric disorders may respond well to treatment. Mood disorders in this population are often undiagnosed. Because these residents have a limited ability to express themselves accurately, recognizing and interpreting nonverbal cues of either mood distress or contentment are essential. The steps described in Chapter 13, Depression, will result in greater resident involvement and fewer behavior problems.

The resident with dementia is often surrounded by psychological stressors but usually has lost the coping strategies he or she used in the past. Among factors to be considered are sadness, grief, fatigue, the stress of moving to a new setting, isolation, and physical disability. Many have experienced a loss of self-esteem, a loss of dignity, the loss of the ability to control even simple things in one's life, and limited opportunities for simple successes (getting one's clothes on, finding the way to the dining room). These disabilities leave residents unable to find anything

meaningful to do or the ability to initiate doing it. In addition, many residents must cope with insensitive staff and a nonsupportive environment. It is not surprising that this negative emotional burden results in problem behavior. It is usually possible to modify some of these burdens for people through the combined expertise of the physician, social worker, nurse and caregivers.

5. Facilitate communication

Residents often have difficulties expressing themselves and understanding others, which can lead to frustration (often expressed as agitated behavior) and isolation. The same difficulties are highly frustrating to staff and contribute to stress. For example, Mr. S. had difficulty making himself understood, and often became angry and tearful during encounters with staff and visits with family. In addition, because of impaired hearing he had difficulty understanding others. To address the problem, Mr. S. was provided with primary nursing assistants on each shift who became adept at both verbal and nonverbal communication with Mr. S. This continuity provided a chance to develop relationships. The staff made efforts to address him as an equal, speaking slowly but treating him with respect.

A primary goal is to ensure that caregivers, family members, and residents communicate clearly and effectively with each other. Identify in the care plan the best way to encourage (using verbal and nonverbal cuing) or involve the resident. Describe how tasks must be broken into steps, how to best approach as well as not approach resident (avoiding factors that may lead to an explosive or catastrophic resident response), and how the resident expresses needs and preferences. Identify those problems that call for a review by a licensed professional (e.g., speech therapist).

Residents with dementia retain nonverbal language longer than verbal language. Close observation of behavior and facial expression will help the staff learn what the resident wants and how he or she is feeling. The staff should help each other examine their own facial expression and body language, because these can comfort or anger those they care for. For example, a caregiver may speak slowly and calmly but her body may say "rush."

Residents who are no longer able to use spoken language often remain alert to patronizing behavior and may react with anger. It is difficult not to be patronizing when caring for impaired people. Discuss patronizing behavior in staff meetings. The staff can learn by listening to their own voices and body language. Supervisors should consider carefully the behaviors they model.

Many seemingly incomprehensible behaviors such as screaming or striking out can be treated when they are seen as an effort to communicate. When a restrained or immobile resident screams, he or she may be expressing a need to urinate, pain, discomfort from the need to reposition (this problem is not limited to those who are restrained), fear from not understanding the restraint or the care he or she is being given, or sadness and humiliation.

Use touch to communicate affection, sympathy, and friendship. Meet people's eyes. Be aware that touch that communicates restraint, control, or is patronizing will be understood by even very impaired people. Do not push those who dislike touch from strangers or they will shy away from any touch at all.

6. Create a supportive environment

Residents with dementia are highly reactive to stressors and conversely will often have fewer behavior problems in a supportive environment. For example, not seeing well, not understanding what is going on, excessive noise, feeling an urgent need to "go home," or feeling put down all cause stress in residents and can trigger behavior problems. Modifying the physical environment and

changing the behavior of the staff usually have a significant impact on behavior.

The physical environment Noise, large groups of people (more than 8 to 10), people rushing about, caregivers from other units cutting through a resident's unit, poor lighting, and things the resident cannot explain or understand (e.g., the public address or paging system) are all considered as likely stressors that can be modified. Review and modify the physical environment and interior design features as resources that support the functioning of cognitively impaired residents, accommodate behaviors and maximize functional abilities, promote safety, and encourage independence in residents. These features should also facilitate the caregiver's work. Many design changes are not costly, especially when the caregiver's time is saved by reducing problem behaviors. Fabric banners in the dining room can reduce noise. Repainting doors in bright colors that contrast with walls help residents find their way. Curtains or blinds can reduce glare. The most important aspect of the physical environment is to make it feel like a nice place to live. The Alzheimer's Association lists the design guidelines in Table 10-5 to address environmental issues.

The Alzheimer's Association emphasizes the need for adequate space in nursing homes, including small, intimate spaces, outdoor spaces, and space for residents' personal belongings. It also encourages positive sensory cues, pleasurable smells, reduced background noise, and adequate lighting. Facilities must control resident departures, control the security of medications, and ensure safety.

The goal of the physical environment in a nursing home is to compensate for disabilities by supporting function and by placing the resident in an environment that is tolerant of his or her behavior. For example, transferring a resident to a dementia unit that is secure will allow for wandering to continue. Small units are far less stressful and allow residents

Table 10-5. Guidelines for Action

Residents' Needs	Physical Design
Identity and self-esteem	Personal items for meaningful activities: desk, typewriter, photo album
Communication/human interaction	Furniture groupings, private dining area
Appropriate exercise	Exercycle, outdoor and indoor wandering paths
Minimized hazards and risks of falls	Sturdy and comfortable chairs (recliners and those that provide assistance to get up), ramps, noncluttered space
Nurture, comfort, and security	Soft music by pillow, familiar bedspread or afghan
Cues and way finding assistance	Signs and arrows, handrails along pathways, visible destinations (i.e., not hiding activity areas behind closed doors)
Minimized agitation	Bird feeder, pets, activity areas for art projects, games or gardening
Independence	Identified and accessible bathrooms

Reprinted with permission from: Guidelines for Dignity; Goals of Specialized Alzheimer/Dementia Care in Residential Settings, Chicago, 1992, Alzheimer's Association.

to form bonds with other members of a homogeneous group. It is much easier to manage a resident who removes things from others' rooms, walks uninvited into rooms, makes strange noises, or acts somewhat bizarre on a small, intimate unit of residents with similar strengths and weaknesses. It is not necessary to limit such a unit to Alzheimer's disease; residents with dementia from various causes will usually mix well.

The interpersonal environment Residents with dementia may be unable to use words effectively, but they remain sensitive to the people around them, including staff, family, and other residents. The people around them can have a significant impact on their restlessness, angry outbursts, feelings of self-worth, and behavior. The nursing home can change staff behavior, but must consider the impact of other residents and family members in problem-solving. Helpful staff behavior includes the following:

- Little things can help the resident feel like he or she is being treated as a person. Smile and look directly at the resident when speaking; do not ignore efforts to communicate. This can be very difficult for caregivers who are busy or when the resident says the same thing over and over. Remember that from the memory-impaired resident's point of view, it is being said only once. Speak as one adult to another instead of sounding patronizing.

- Since people with dementia think slowly, let the resident take the time instead of rushing him or her. Give only one bit of information at a time, allowing the resident time to think about what is being said. Instead of saying, "After lunch we're going to take a walk; now don't you think you ought to take a shower before that?" try, "Come with me"—pause—"Are you hungry?"—pause—"Lunch is ready." If you need to get the resident showered, talk about just that.

- Ask the resident to do things one step at a time rather than asking for more than he or she can manage. Mistakes can make the resident with dementia angry or ashamed, so try to fix things so he or she will not make many errors.

- Always be pleasant; residents with dementia cannot cope with rudeness.

- Find ways to make residents feel that their privacy is being respected. Close their doors when you dress them; talk *to* them, not at them.

- Residents with dementia often have difficulty following directions. Eventually they will become so impaired that they cannot follow instructions at all, but many can be assisted to participate in tasks. Use only one-step instructions; simplify what you say; show as well as tell; try a calmer environment or a different time of day; and let your behavior be shaped by the resident's responses.

- Let a resident do as much as he or she can.

For example, can the resident hold his or her shoe while you put the sock on? Can she get her dress over her head if you guide her arms? Let a resident do things that might seem odd but are not dangerous (e.g., rolling up her skirt or carrying things around). Often people with dementia get angry because they feel you are trying to control them.

- Find out who among staff and family is most successful with the resident and do what that person does that is successful.

- Good leadership, training, and adequate staffing are necessary to implement these approaches.

7. Reduce stress for the resident with dementia

The damaged brain makes many things difficult for the resident with dementia. One can sympathize with the resident who finds him- or herself in the shower, with no idea how he or she got there and strangers caring for his or her body. Further, the damaged brain cannot process as much information, even when the information can still be understood. A resident may be unable to cope with the noise, confusion, and activity in the dining room and be unable to eat even when he or she can manage well in a calmer setting. Knowing which things are overwhelmingly stressful to a resident allows the staff to avoid combativeness and agitation.

People need stimulation, involvement, relationships, and activity as well as a low-stress life. The challenge is to determine what is desirable stimulation and what is likely to overstress a person and trigger an angry outburst.

The following factors that contribute to stress have been discussed:
- Health status
- Pain
- Drugs that dull thinking
- The struggle to communicate

- Sensory deficits
- An inability to make one's needs known or to understand others
- A facility that is noisy or hard to understand
- Staff whose behavior is thoughtless

The impact of these stressors is cumulative. For example, the resident who is not feeling well may be more upset by the shower than he or she would be when feeling well. The resident who was rushed and insulted by the day shift may be harder for the second shift to manage. Considering the sum of the day's stresses will help staff predict how much stimulation a person can tolerate.

Many types of stimulation or stress situations are subjective. For example, a visit from five family members may be a pleasure for one resident and seriously upset another, who needs to see his or her family members one at a time.

Boredom itself can be a stressor. Staff often observe a resident who begins wandering aimlessly and soon is going faster and faster, shaking the doors and headed for an outburst. Residents need to be engaged at their own levels. Avoid long periods when the resident has nothing to do (e.g., waiting for meals or activities). A slow, laid-back pace, periods of rest, or flexibility that allows spontaneous singing if lunch is delayed will help a resident stay involved but not overwhelmed. You may have to walk alongside the resident who paces all day or sit a while with the depressed resident who stays in his or her room.

Avoiding stress and providing stimulation at an acceptable level is one of the most effective ways to manage problem behaviors. Consider explosive resident behavior as communication that the resident is overstressed. Good detective work to identify the trouble spots can reduce or even eliminate these outbursts. An observant staff can learn to anticipate and avoid problems, rechannel energies into other areas, defuse anger, and increase communication. When the resident is less stressed, he or she may also be more cooperative in carrying out ADLs. Most solutions are individual and there are few fixed rules for what residents can tolerate. Many factors that may stress residents cannot be changed. However, because stress is cumulative, problem behaviors can be reduced when even some changes are made.

8. Maximize the meaning and involvement in daily life

The resident with dementia faces a diminishing ability to initiate, participate in, and complete many tasks. The resident may not remember when to come to the dining area for meals or how to do something as simple as getting dressed. He or she is often unable to find or initiate any positive activity. For these residents the days may be long and empty. They may become passive or seek stimulation by wandering, pounding, or shouting.

In the rush to provide care, ADLs become something that is done *to* the resident without his or her involvement, and activities are often secondary to resident care—underfunded and overcrowded.

However, the things residents do all day shape who they are and how they behave even when they have a severe dementia. When tasks are done in a patronizing, demeaning way or when residents are idle for long periods, they are more likely to be uncooperative or angry. Make activities part of the total care plan and base them on the assessment findings. Regard the ADLs as an opportunity for therapeutic interventions, not simply a task to be done.

Many residents with dementia are severely impaired, i.e., completely dependent in ADLs and with limited mobility. It can seem as if getting them to participate in meaningful activities is unrealistic. Look for simple, brief ways to involve them. Increase the number of times staff speak to them and touch them, if only for a minute each time. Minimize crafts and verbal activities that require skills this group has lost. Try household tasks for both men and women (anybody can knead biscuit dough with their fingers). Repeat activities that are successful; familiarity is comforting. Arrange for residents to do things you know they can do (holding the napkins while you set the table), and protect them from doing things at which they would fail (laying out the napkins). Residents who do not know how to do something may still know that they failed.

Be creative. Sometimes a staff member will stumble onto an activity that will help a resident feel more in control and that is low in cost as well. For example, one resident spent time shaking the locked door knob, saying he needed to go home; he was angry because he was locked in. The director gave him her keys. There were several keys and the lock was stiff, so he was never able to unlock the door. He returned after a while to report that the lock was broken. He subsequently borrowed the keys whenever he felt restless. He was unable to get out, but he no longer felt locked up. Obviously, this will not work with everyone; trial and error and individualization are tools to improve communication and self-esteem successfully.

As residents become more impaired, try to become involved in brief activities with them, e.g., pausing to admire a family picture, smiling or speaking briefly with a resident, or asking a resident to sand a block of wood. Sanding wood is a role for men and takes advantage of the tendency to repeat a motor activity. It is not possible to fail.

9. Behavior management strategies

Chapter 12, Behavioral Symptoms, discusses problem behavior. However, as a part of the care of residents with dementia, it will be discussed briefly here. If these nine strategies are followed, resident units will be easier to manage and the risk of accident will be reduced. *Problem behavior is not caused solely by the dementia.* Brain damage is a contributing fac-

tor, but other reversible causes intensify symptoms. For example, in a specific resident:
Dementia + Pain + Isolation = Screaming and Hitting
or
Dementia + Treated Pain + Mild Engagement = Confusion + Mild Anxiety
Consider another example:
Dementia + Being Rushed + Rude Care = Biting and Hitting
or
Dementia + Slow Pace + Kindness = Confusion + Grumbling
The complete resident assessment is essential to behavior management because it identifies causal factors.

It is much easier and more successful to prevent behavior problems than it is to cope with them when they arise. Assessment and monitoring will identify potential problems before they become serious or permanent. This means considerable cost savings in nursing time. *Behavior management is individual.* It is successful when the resident is understood and when considerable work is done to identify the causes of stress in a given resident. However, this is not a one-time fix: problem behaviors will recur if interventions are pulled back.

Consider ignoring behaviors that pose no threat to safety, health, or the well-being of others. Unnecessary control of the resident can be harmful and counterproductive. Behaviors such as making faces, pacing, taking one's clothes off, or chewing on nonpoisonous but inedible objects may distress staff but are harmless. If these behaviors distress residents in a heterogeneous unit, consider a unit change. Staff who are well supported by management will be able to tolerate rude treatment, accusations of theft, and even racial slurs, but management is the essential component. Make vigorous efforts (usually by identifying and avoiding resident triggers) to protect staff from being pinched, bruised, or otherwise physically assaulted.

It is much easier and often more effective to change the staff's behavior than it is to get the residents to change. For example, a resident who responds to personal care with anger may be more cooperative when the caregiver changes his or her approach. Flexibility in facility routines helps avoid confrontations with residents. Learn to recognize the cues each resident gives that he or she is becoming upset and try to stop the resident before he or she explodes.

Behavior that seems to be uncooperative, manipulative, or spiteful may not be so. Consider angry outbursts, screaming, and aggression as communications that the resident has been pushed beyond endurance. The resident may be frightened, may not understand, or may be overwhelmed by the negatives in the environment. Residents with dementia usually have difficulty controlling their impulses. If a caregiver responds harshly, the resident may become more belligerent or angry. The caregiver should back off and try a new, low-key approach. A different caregiver may be more successful.

Take the resident aside and help him or her calm down in quiet environment. The best approach with a very angry resident is to back off and do nothing—let him or her calm down. Consider an angry resident who was pounding on the wall with a stapler, leaving marks. This resident was at risk of injuring himself and other residents. When a management person entered the room and tried to gain control of the stapler, the resident hit him, leaving serious bruises. A second management person entered, and the first manager left, taking the remaining residents with him. Removing the residents is a much safer procedure than removing the angry resident. Alone in the room with the angry resident, the second manager sat down at some distance and made sure that the resident would not hurt himself. After a while the resident wore out and they had a quiet cup of tea together. After the wall was scrubbed, the small dents did not show and no one else had been hurt. The next staff meeting was devoted to a discussion of what instigated this episode and how to better manage the resident. There were no further incidents and no medication was used.

Caregivers who support each other, with adequate staffing to allow a caregiver to take time out to control his or her own anger, can be productive. Without these opportunities, caregiver frustration is communicated through body language and adds to the continuing conflict.

The way staff view problem behavior in residents is important in planning appropriate interventions. As staff learn that behavior is not manipulative or deliberately nasty and begin to see it as communication, a signal that something is wrong, a misunderstanding, or a response to an overwhelmingly confusing world, they will find responses that reduce problems. Table 10-6 lists ways to manage angry outbursts and combativeness.

Staff Training

Even more important than a special unit for residents with dementia are the highly specialized skills required of the staff. Registered nurses need the ability to recognize concurrent illness and pain in a nonverbal population, and physicians need skills to treat multiple problems without overmedicating this fragile group. Physical and occupational therapists need special skills to accomplish rehabilitation (where possible) in residents who do not understand directions or do not cooperate. In addition, all professionals are role models and teach caregivers informally. A wise, caring physician with a professional demeanor will have a profound impact on caregiver attitude.

Nonprofessional caregivers can become experts with highly impressive skills in managing residents with dementia and are role

Table 10-6. Managing Angry Outbursts and Combativeness

1. Cause: Overreaction to a minor stressor; when the crisis is over, identify the stressor
2. Early warnings: Restlessness, stubbornness, fidgeting
3. Precipitants: Not understanding what he or she was asked
   - Too many things happening at once
   - Noise, confusion, poor lighting
   - Being stopped or restrained
   - Inability to communicate
   - Fatigue
   - Frustration
   - Response to patronizing or demoralizing treatment
   - Long periods of idleness
   - Being rushed
   - Not feeling well
4. Intervention: Do not restrain, argue, explain, hold, or force the resident. This forces the resident to strike out or hit.
   - Remove the cause
   - Back off, be quiet, and watch the resident
   - Be calm and reassuring
   - Stop everything as soon as you see any indication of a warning signal

5. Prevention strategies:
   - Prevention is the only approach that is safe and successful
   - Keep the resident healthy
   - Know the resident's limits; never rush the resident
   - Keep things simple
   - Plan environmental cues that say "this is home"
   - Fill in when the resident seems to be groping for a word or skill
   - Plan difficult tasks, like showering, at the resident's best time of day
   - Give positive reinforcement only
   - Avoid rushing the resident
   - Check that you are not misunderstanding the resident
   - Keep a log to help you identify warning cues and triggers
   - Remember that the cause of behavior is usually concrete; it is not psychodynamic or rooted in the past
   - Individualize your interventions
   - Be flexible: try things in a different way; accept some odd behavior

Modified from: Mace NL, Whitehouse PJ, Smith KA: Management of Patients with Dementia, Dementia, Philadelphia, 1993, F.A. Davis.

models to others. Acknowledge these skills. Four components are required:
- Recruiting people who have the proper temperament and interest in this kind of work
- Good management, which provides support and leadership
- Training
- The flexibility to allow caregivers to try out their ideas

Caregivers must understand that the behavior and disabilities of the resident with dementia are not within that resident's control.

Equally important, the staff must know what to do when jobs have to be done, residents get upset, and activities do not work out. Without being taught the special skills of caring for this challenging group, caregivers will continue to create difficulty.

Because people with dementia are sensitive to nonverbal interpersonal communication, caregivers need to be taught to be attuned to their own and the residents communication. Caring for people with dementia is stressful for hands-on caregivers, and training must include strategies to reduce that stress or it will be reflected in resident care.

People with dementia are more responsive to staff behavior than they appear to be at first. Staff behavior toward the resident helps to shape the resident's behavior. Caregivers need to know correct behaviors that they can use instead of harsh words, avoidance, ridicule, punishments, and taking control of resident's everyday activities.

A formal training course is followed by ongoing informal training and problem-solving. Schedule regular case conferences in which a resident is presented and care is discussed by members of the disciplines and the nurses' aides. Elicit a caregiver's natural knowledge. Plan these case conferences to highlight a resident who is causing problems, or to discretely focus on staff problems (e.g., when staff raises the overall noise level by calling out to one another, or everyone tends to ignore or rush a specific resident who is not very likable). This avoids pointing a finger at one or two people.

Supervisors need to observe the interactions between staff and residents. When they observe that the caregiver is having problems, supervisors need to teach by doing (role modeling) and give immediate explanation and feedback. Positive feedback is much more effective than correcting the caregiver. For example, the supervisor might say, "I've noticed that Mrs. T. tries to hit you when you dress her. She doesn't see well and doesn't recognize our voices. Try introducing yourself before you touch her, and ask her if it's OK if you help her dress."

The Alzheimer's Association recommendations for staff training are shown in Table 10-7.

Caregiver recruitment considerations

Not everyone has the capabilities to care for this challenging population. Look for staff (both leadership and caregivers) who are interested in taking responsibility, are flexible, can work as a team, are patient, are willing to learn new skills, who have a natural capacity to see the resident and the resident's strengths beyond the often overwhelming impairments, and who have a sense of humor. Residents with dementia need caregivers who can communicate affection and sympathy as well as respect and courtesy. For many facilities, recruiting desirable candidates may be a challenge.

Staffing patterns A major cause of poor care and caregiver stress is inadequate staffing. It is almost impossible not to rush residents or treat them as objects, to hurry through the ADLs, and to avoid long periods of resident idleness when the staff have too many people to care for. Employ enough caregivers and other staff to implement the full day and evening program. There should also be enough staff for caregivers to have time to assist residents in small group activities. The night shift must be adequate to meet resident's needs without relying on sleeping medications.

A primary nursing model is preferred. Residents will gradually be reassured by the familiarity of the same person even though they may not "recognize" the person. Equally important, the caregiver will become familiar with the resident's needs, what triggers outbursts, and what form of reassurance works.

Adequate staffing is so important that consideration should be given to limiting costs in other areas, such as elaborate plant modifications.

Management

A key to the success of any program is its leadership. Good staff, ample funding, and an excellent facility cannot overcome the devastation wrought by poor leadership. Management ensures a solvent program, maintains standards, locates and trains good staff, responds to families, negotiates essential resources, is concerned about caregiver stress, ensures interdepartmental cooperation, sets the attitude and values by which the caregivers carry out their daily tasks, and performs many other tasks essential to good care. Unfortunately, the importance of good management is often overlooked.

TIPS TO HANDLE CAREGIVER STRESS

Caring for people with dementia is stressful. Even caregivers who say they love their jobs and who remain by choice in caregiving

Table 10-7. Staff Training Recommendations for Alzheimer's Disease and Dementia

1. Explanation of Alzheimer's disease and related disorders
   - Diagnosis (dementia, delirium, and other coexisting conditions)
   - Symptoms/behaviors characteristic of dementing illness
   - Reversible symptoms (depression)
   - Excess disability
   - Progression, stages, variability and individual differences
   - Awareness of lost or diminished abilities and the role of former personality
2. The specialized Alzheimer's dementia care program
   - Knowledge of philosophy and Mission Statement
   - Goals and guidelines
   - Program policies
   - The careplanning and implementation process
3. Communication with Alzheimer's dementia residents
   - Verbal and nonverbal communication
   - How residents communicate with staff
   - How staff communicate with residents
   - Communication techniques (including nonverbal communication)
   - Spiritual support (the grieving process and support methods)
4. Family issues
   - Communication with family
   - Assisting family to interact in the program
   - Assisting family with techniques for coping
   - Identifying roles and responsibilities
5. The supportive program environment
   - The influence of the environment (both human and physical)
   - The facility itself and safety issues
   - Use of the physical environment as a therapeutic resource
   - Intentional programming to reduce and eliminate the use of restraints (physical and pharmacologic)
   - Orienting to the program, to roommates, other residents, staff
6. Therapeutic techniques and strategies
   - Approach, reassurance, and distraction
   - Therapeutic activities, ADLs, and instrumental activities of daily living (e.g., making bed, setting table)
   - Interventions (i.e., for ambulation, dining, and so on)
   - Therapeutic recreation (daily calendar, techniques, and goals)
7. Protocols for specific needs/behaviors
   - Anticipating and preventing behaviors
   - Understanding behavior as communication
   - Ambulation, wandering, pacing
   - Appropriate staff responses
   - Tracking antecedent behaviors
   - Meeting nutritional needs (menu modifications, devices, and techniques)
8. Staff support
   - Stress management techniques
   - Team building approaches

From: Guidelines for Dignity, Goals of Specialized Alzheimer/Dementia Care in Residential Settings. Chicago, 1992.

positions for many years report high levels of stress. If caregivers are to respond gently to anger, respond kindly to abuse, respond supportively to fear, and respond without being patronizing to gross disability, then the high stress level of the job must be recognized and caregivers must be supported.

The most important intervention for treating caregiver stress is management. Caregivers who have no voice, whose work environment is unpredictable, and who receive no praise and no recognition of their work will burn out or take their frustrations out on their charges. People treat those they care for as they themselves are treated. Dignity cannot be mandated: it can only be passed down.

Troubleshooting

When staff problems or staff/resident problems arise, begin by identifying the source of the disturbance. Ask the following questions:

- Has the resident "gotten" to the staff member?
- Does the staff member lack the basic knowledge of the resident being cared for?
- Is the facility understaffed and the staff member overburdened?
- Was the staff member placed on the unit without a full training program?
- Are daily instructions for care sufficiently specific? Is the staff member aware of the amount of care and staff time the resident requires?
- Is the staff member able to come to grips with working with demented residents? Not all staff members can manage such residents.
- Does the staff member's behavior or communication style lead to inappropriate and aggressive behavior with others?
- Is there any possibility of reallocating available resources to increase direct care coverage or expand the number of hours of activity programming each day?
- How strong a case can be made with the administration of the need for more staff support?

- Is the staff member experiencing stress in other aspects of his or her life (e.g., family, finances, illness, school)?
- Can the staff member whose job performance is in question be replaced or reassigned?
- Is there any possibility of reallocating available resources to increase direct care coverage or expand the number of hours of activity programming each day?
- How strong a case can be made with administration of the need for more staff support?
- Does the staff feel in conflict with the facility (resentment, rumor)?
- Do conflicts among staff members create tension in the environment?
- Do staff members work well together, sharing their expertise and time to help each other?
- Are management strategies supportive of the staff?
- Is the supervisor's style supportive and enabling?
- Are staff encouraged to seek solutions to their own and the resident's problems?
- If a staff member is overstressed, but likes the work on a particular unit, is it possible for that staff member to take time out by working on another unit and returning to this unit when his or her stress level is lowered?
- Do staff rotations add to resident stress? Has a primary nursing model been considered?
- Is role modeling used regularly as a training method?

Begin a plan to correct staff-related problems by addressing possible deficiencies in the training or care planning processes at the facility. These problems warrant immediate action. It is costly to expect direct care staff to respond appropriately when the facility has thrown them into the lion's den.

If the facility has had a problem maintaining its full staff complement, base an appropriate response on whether the situation is temporary or chronic. If it is temporary, talk with the troubled staff member, bring on additional staff, and closely monitor the situation. If it appears to be permanent, ask the following questions and take corrective action based on the insights gained in this review:

- Can the staff be better prepared to work within the bounds of available resources?
- Can orientation and ongoing educational programs be improved?
- Can residents be better placed within the facility, i.e., bringing demented residents together in smaller-care, homogeneous groups, providing an environment in which staff can gain experience in dealing with residents with specific problems?
- Can the direct care staff member whose job performance is in question be replaced or reassigned?

OVERCOMING THE MYTH

For many years, the cognitive decline that is common in late life was believed to be a normal part of the aging process. This false assumption about cognitive decline led to a pervasive assumption that nothing could be done to help these residents. This assumption still governs many care decisions from the attitude of the nursing assistant to the reluctance of some physicians to search aggressively for concurrent illness. Funding for resident care clearly reflects the public opinion that nothing can be done. Even research was influenced by this negativism: virtually no research was funded until the mid-1980s.

It was not until the 1960s that Blessed, Tomlinson, and Roth's epidemiologic studies showed that many very old people had normal mentation and that those who had cognitive decline had the same pathologic changes as younger people with Alzheimer's disease. During the same period, research showed that vascular dementia was not caused by hardening of the arteries but by infarcts.

The knowledge of care has changed dramatically in the past 15 years. Many ideas for care that claim to improve the resident's quality of life or reduce disruptive behaviors have been advanced. However, time, costs, regulation, and the availability of skilled staff make some interventions seem impossible. Facilities also try interventions only to have them fail. All of these factors contribute to sustain the common assumption that nothing can be done for these residents. Overcoming this attitude and creating an optimistic team may be the biggest challenge of caring for residents with dementia.

The reality is that a creative approach to individualized care with judicious tinkering with health and mental health status, interpersonal life, and the environment will result in gains. These gains will usually be small but their cumulative effect will be significant. Change may be seen in self-care; maintenance of safe ambulation; decreased fear, anxiety, and agitation; moments of genuine pleasure; improved social interactions; and a reduction in combative and aggressive behaviors. Improvements often benefit the caregiver and other residents as well as the confused resident.

Staff at all levels may express the opinion that residents are "not there," "gone," "mean," "manipulative," or "disgusting." Primary nursing helps staff to discern the subtle distinctions of character that shine through the disability. Ongoing training teaches staff the techniques that will bring out a smile "just for them," and the unexpected sense of humor that is so often retained. It also teaches staff that negative behavior is the result of the disease process and is not deliberate and personal.

Consider the following case. Mr. E. had known a staff member for 2 years and had come to expect the silly, shared finger game they enjoyed. At the end of his life, Mr. E.

moved to a new facility, but when the staff person visited him a month later, even though he could no longer walk or speak, his face lit up and he raised his fingers for the faintly remembered game. Mr. E. died a few days later. The person beneath the profound dementia must be unmasked by removing excess disability and unnecessary stress and by offering friendship.

It is no myth that regulations, building design, costs, limited hiring pools, inadequately trained professional personnel, and limited medical resources, among other things, limit a facility's options. A facility's capacity to carry out the suggestions listed in this chapter may be restricted. The answer is to understand the principles and concepts of good dementia care. With flexibility and good leadership, interventions can be invented that will work for any facility.

People with dementia are highly responsive to even minor positive changes—a strong motivation for doing what one can now.

CASE EXAMPLE

Mrs. W. was recently admitted to the facility from a hospital. She had been living alone until she was hospitalized with herpes simplex afflicting the trigeminal nerve. However, she had apparently gotten lost in her own neighborhood and had trouble making change before she fell ill. Her daughter reported that she had declined dramatically during her 3 weeks in the hospital.

Facility staff reported that she was anxious and thought that she was grieving over coming into the facility. She had made several attempts to leave the facility, saying that she wanted to "take the bus home."

The intake evaluation, using the items in The Health Care Financing Administration's MDS revealed that Mrs. W. was experiencing problems with short- and long-term memory. She was moderately impaired in decision-making, knew the location of her room, and was

able to make herself understood (by constantly saying, "I want to go home"). However, she had some difficulty understanding others, she did not really understand that she is in a long-term care facility, and did not recognize her caregivers.

Her current diagnosis is severe confusion (ICD 9-CM code 298.9) in conjunction with Alzheimer's disease. However, it is premature to assume that her confusion is due to an untreatable dementia. A recent acute illness, multiple medications, and relocation are enough to trigger suspicion that some of her difficulties may be due to a treatable delirium. The MDS indicated that Mrs. W. has the following conditions that have generally been found to be associated with delirium (acute confusional state):

- She has had a recent acute illness from which she is still recovering.
- She has periods of motor restlessness.
- Her cognitive state has declined in the last 90 days (since her hospitalization).
- She is losing weight. Her total protein and serum albumin are down and during the MDS review her refusal to eat was noted.
- During her hospitalization she was placed on medications with anticholinergic effects (confusion, constipation, urinary incontinence), including the antipsychotic Haldol and the antidepressant Elavil. She was also taking Dalmane to control sleep and Monogesic for pain control. These medications continued to be given daily.
- She only recently entered the facility and appears to be experiencing a major grief reaction secondary to the move. These steps were followed to care for Mrs. W.:

1. The first step was to manage Mrs. W.'s function and mental status by identifying and treating all potentially treatable conditions. This included a review of the need for medications and their reduction, elimination, or replacement with other drugs less inclined to cause delirium, and monitoring of her

recovery. Physical therapy to reduce the permanent paralysis from her illness was started and a dietary plan was designed to stabilize her weight. A plan was established with her daughter to let Mrs. W. make some decisions about the disposition of her most treasured possessions. Several things were brought to the facility and secured to her dresser so they would not be lost. Mrs. W.'s delirium gradually cleared, the Haldol and Dalmane were discontinued, she was better able to plan for her relocation, and she gradually became involved in more activities. This first step confirmed for the staff that Mrs. W.'s situation was not hopeless. Resolution of the complicating factors led to considerable improvement. The value of staff monitoring of medications and illness, especially in residents who cannot express themselves, is reaffirmed.

• While it is difficult to distinguish a primary dementia from complicating problems such as delirium, treatment of the conditions known to be treatable will usually result in gains. These symptoms, such as anxiety, depression, irritability, stubbornness, and apathy, are just symptoms—they may indicate an underlying primary dementia, reversible conditions, or both.

• An underlying impairment such as Alzheimer's disease increases the resident's vulnerability to other stressors such as illness, medications, relocation. While Mrs. W. made considerable gains as her delirium resolved, she retained some disability from her shingles, some cognitive impairment, and considerable sadness. Her aggressive treatment did not end with the treatment of her delirium.

The next step was to treat the reversible conditions. The following interventions were put in place gradually as Mrs. W. improved.

2. The next step was to confirm the diagnosis of Alzheimer's disease. In Mrs. W.'s case, this diagnosis had not been made properly, but had been given during her hospitalization when she was very confused from illness and drugs. Her daughter was referred to a physician for Mrs. W. to obtain a dementia workup. A few dementias are treatable or reversible.

3. A regimen was then established to assist Mrs. W. with the effects of her residual disability. Mrs. W.'s eye drops fogged her vision, making it worse than necessary. She became anxious and withdrawn. Other forms of eye care were essential to help her continue to function well.

4. The cause of Mrs. W.'s evident sadness and grief was determined. While the staff assumed that her grief was a reaction to relocation, they did not know this for sure. When this assumption is made, an underlying depression may be overlooked. Like the treatment of delirium, the treatment of depression can improve both life quality and function.

5. Staff began a plan to help Mrs. W. build a new life in her new setting. Grief, restlessness, anxiety, and sleep disturbances can result when there is no way for a resident to put down roots or find meaning in her new home. This does not happen automatically when people are impaired. A 6-month plan of reengagement and socialization was planned by the activity director and carried out by the caregivers, activity staff, and Mrs. W.'s daughter.

11
Delirium

Katharine Murphy, RN, MS
Sue Levkoff, ScD
Lewis A. Lipsitz, MD

Delirium is an acute, reversible organic mental disorder that is characterized by the reduced ability to maintain attention to external stimuli and disorganized thinking as manifested by rambling, irrelevant, or incoherent speech. There is also a reduced level of consciousness, sensory misperceptions, disturbance of the sleep-wakefulness cycle and level of psychomotor activity, disorientation to time, place, or person, and memory impairment. Delirium may be caused by a number of conditions that result in derangement of cerebral metabolism, including systemic infection, poisoning, drug intoxication or withdrawal, seizures or head trauma, metabolic disturbances such as hypoxia, hypoglycemia, fluid, electrolyte, or acid-base imbalance, or hepatic or renal failure. Risk factors include age greater than 80 years, prior cognitive impairment, symptomatic infection, fever, uncontrolled pain, fractures, and use of narcotic or neuroleptic drugs.

OVERVIEW

Delirium is a transient and complex acute brain syndrome that is characterized by concurrent disorders of attention, perception, thinking, memory, psychomotor behavior, and the sleep-wake cycle. Although geriatricians often refer to delirium as an acute confusional state, in nursing home records a variety of other terms may also be found to denote the condition, including acute brain failure, acute organic reaction, agitated confusional state, altered mental status, metabolic encephalopathy, pseudodementia, reversible dementia, and toxic encephalopathy. These variations in terminology can be a source of unnecessary confusion to caregivers, who may fail to identify a presenting condition or to recognize more complex manifestations as a distinct indication of delirium. Rather than being overly concerned with diagnostic labels, caregivers should concentrate on recognizing the signs of delirium so that they may promptly identify potentially reversible causes and initiate treatment.

It is widely recognized that delirium is a common phenomenon among hospitalized elderly. Less well known is that delirium presents an array of symptoms that can be caused by almost any disease or drug regardless of setting. The precipitating causes of delirium are usually external to the brain. Delirium may be a result of a physical illness (e.g., myocardial infarction) or challenge (e.g., surgery), environmental stress (e.g., sensory deprivation or overload), or toxicity or withdrawal from therapeutic doses of common prescription and over-the-counter drugs as well as alcohol.

Drugs with anticholinergic properties, such as antipsychotic, antiparkinsonian, antihistamine, analgesic, or antidepressant drugs, are particularly problematic. In the nursing home setting, infections, congestive heart failure (CHF), dehydration, drugs, and fecal impactions are major contributors. Delirium is often the first sign that a resident is experiencing a new illness or an exacerbation of a chronic one, or is having a reaction to treatment.

IDENTIFYING THE RESIDENT IN NEED OF CARE

The following sections describe how to identify residents with delirium who are in need of care.

Predisposing Factors

Anticipate delirium in elderly residents with any of the following predisposing factors, especially as new, troubling symptoms emerge.

New Admission to the Nursing Home

In one study, investigators found that 9.6% of newly admitted residents have delirium. Frail elderly residents admitted from home or from another largely unsupervised setting may not have been managing their health, medications, or nutrition appropriately. Therefore, evaluate for delirium in any new resident who appears confused, lethargic, or agitated, recognizing that such symptoms may also be reflective of the grief that is often associated with relocation (e.g., loss of one's home, independence, lifestyle, and friendships).

Admission to the Nursing Home from an Acute Care Hospital

Ninety-six percent of patients who developed delirium in the hospital are discharged with at least one sign of delirium remaining. Many are discharged to nursing homes. Delirium may last as long as 6 months, even if the underlying cause has been treated successfully. Provided that the underlying causes of delirium were addressed, careplanning should focus on helping the resident adjust to the new environment, resolve any residual physical or emotional problems, and restore function in self-care and leisure activities.

Multiple Medications

Drug toxicity, especially due to neuroleptic medications or other drugs with anticholinergic properties, as well as toxicity associated with some other commonly used prescription drugs, is one of the most frequent causes of delirium. Where multiple medications are involved, the chance of an adverse drug reaction increases significantly.

Alzheimer's Disease or Other Dementia

Delirium commonly occurs in residents who have dementia. When delirium is superimposed on dementia, cognitive function may worsen acutely. Therefore, it is important to recognize that treatment of the delirium may enable a resident to return to baseline cognitive function—perhaps making the difference between severe functional dependence and participation in self-care activities. When delirium is misdiagnosed as dementia, or mistaken for the natural deteriorating progression of dementia, treatment of the underlying illness may be delayed, often with serious consequences.

For the resident currently in a long-term care setting, the key to detecting subtle but important mental and behavioral changes is the staff's familiarity with the person's usual cognitive, sleep, and communication patterns, and his or her general response to the world at large. For the new admission, it is important that staff promptly gather information from someone who knows the resident well (i.e., family/significant others), so that any potentially reversible decline can be identified. Nursing staff should always monitor and document symptoms, even if they feel uncertain about the diagnosis.

Sensory Impairment

Approximately 30% of residents who are identified by the Health Care Financing Administration's Resident Assessment Instrument (HCFA RAI) to have signs of delirium also have severe vision impairment. Confusion also appears to be worse if the resident is hearing impaired. Sensory problems often contribute to misinterpretation of the environmental stimuli necessary for making sense of one's surroundings.

Withdrawal from Medication or Alcohol

Withdrawal from benzodiazepines, particularly Valium, or alcohol, may lead to delirium. This situation can occur inadvertently when either of these substances is taken at home or in the hospital but is not received in the nursing home.

Signs and Symptoms of Delirium

Delirium is suspected if any of the following behavioral or cognitive symptoms represent a change from the resident's usual functioning (new onset or worsening of symptom):

- **Easily distracted.** The resident may have impaired ability to focus, sustain, and shift attention; the resident gets sidetracked.
- **Periods of altered perception or awareness of the environment.** The resident may misperceive the environment; illusions and misinterpretations of environmental stimuli are common. There may be evidence of disorientation, such as the resident thinking he or she is somewhere other than in the facility, or confusing the time of day (e.g., getting dressed in the middle of the night to "catch a bus"), or of being more confused and agitated at night.
- **Episodes of disorganized, incoherent speech.** Speech patterns may be rambling or content is irrelevant.
- **Periods of motor restlessness** (e.g., grasping/picking motions; agitation; increased speed of response) **or lethargy** (e.g., sluggishness, staring into space, difficult to arouse, slow motor response).
- **Cognitive function varies over the course of the day.** The resident may have periods of lucidity as well as periods of confusion.

Most of the residents who are identified by these features will also manifest functional decline, aberrant behavioral symptoms, and other symptoms such as falls, all of which are often associated with acute confusion. The Minimum Data Set (MDS) data reveal that approximately 70% of residents suspected of having delirium will also have a physical symptom or condition associated with a potentially reversible problem that may be causing the delirium.

Recognizing Delirium

To facilitate the detection of delirium, perform the following steps during assessments:

- Determine if the resident's presenting level of function and behavior is the usual status, or whether it represents a change (i.e., new onset or worsening)?
- o To distinguish between dementia and delirium, especially if delirium is superimposed on dementia, it is necessary to determine the resident's baseline or usual function. Since the confused resident is often unable to provide accurate information, solicit input from someone who knows the resident and the situation well.
- o For the new admission, ask the family or significant others, or contact other professionals who have recently worked closely with the resident (e.g., Visiting Nurses Association nurse or primary acute hospital nurse).
- o For the long-term resident, discuss the

situation with caregivers who have had regular close contact with the resident, particularly nurse assistants who are in the best position to detect subtle but important changes. Because signs of delirium can be highly variable throughout the day (i.e., sometimes present, sometimes not; sometimes better, sometimes worse), communicate with caregivers who regularly provide care to the resident on multiple shifts. Using a behavioral symptom flow sheet for documentation (*see* the case example at the end of the chapter) across shifts can facilitate this monitoring process. Information exchange is most productive and accurate when there are permanent staff assignments for resident care. This type of nursing model enhances continuity of care, which enables the caregiver to recognize cognitive, functional and behavioral changes associated with delirium.

- Consider delirium as a possibility if the resident has been medically unstable at home or has transferred from an acute hospital setting, where delirium is often iatrogenic (i.e., caused by drugs, treatments, tests, surgery, anesthesia, sensory overload). Despite its prevalence do not assume that confusion is merely a manifestation of the stress and grief that accompany relocation to a nursing home.
- Check whether the resident has ever been delirious in the past and if so, under what circumstances and predisposing factors. Ask the family and review the record. Having a history of delirium is often a marker of risk for developing delirium again.
- Consider delirium as a possibility if the resident exhibits an alteration in perception (e.g., a hallucination or illusion) or thought disorder (e.g., delusion). A *hallucination* is a false perception that occurs in the absence of any real external stimuli. It may be audi-

tory, visual, tactile, olfactory, or gustatory. An *illusion* is a misinterpreted perception of actual external stimuli, such as mistaking a moving curtain for a person climbing through the window or a television show for something real. In schizophrenia, hallucinations are primarily auditory. In delirium related to drug toxicity and acute illness, hallucinations and illusions are usually visual. A *delusion* is a false idea (e.g., belief that one has cancer or that the food is poisoned).

o Residents experiencing an alteration in perception may appear easily distracted, have difficulty paying attention to a conversation, pause for a long time before responding to your voice, or be seen moving their lips as if talking to someone who is not present. In the delirious resident, aberrant behavioral symptoms such as noisiness, unsafe climbing, wandering, disrobing, and picking at bedclothes or tubing often occur in response to mental confusion, and sometimes represent the resident's attempt to flee or fight scary hallucinations.

o Few residents will report their altered perceptions. Therefore, the caregiver should make the resident feel comfortable talking about what is being perceived by phrasing questions in a helpful, straightforward manner. For example, say, "It is common for unusual things to happen to people when they are sick. Have you heard or seen anything unusual recently?" or "I noticed you were moving your lips. Were you speaking with someone you believe is present?" or "I noticed you picking at something. Is there something bothering you?" Listen carefully and probe regarding the nature of the misperception. Do not validate its presence or argue with the resident about it.

- If a previously socially engaged or noisy resident has become quiet or withdrawn consider delirium:

o Some delirious residents who are hypoactive and apathetic are often overlooked or misdiagnosed because they may be easy for caregivers to care for and do not bother anyone. Look for an adverse reaction to a drug, a physical illness (e.g., hypothyroidism, CHF, dehydration, infection), a family or past history of depression, a recent significant loss (e.g., death of a family member or roommate, termination of a favorite nursing assistant, loss of function secondary to stroke), or a change in environment (e.g., move to a new unit).

Diagnosing the Underlying Cause of Delirium

Perform the diagnostic steps described in the following sections if delirium is suspected.

Review of Health Status

To review the resident's health status:

- Check vital signs and compare them with baseline. Include blood pressure, temperature, pulse, respiration, and weight. If a change from baseline is found, look for the underlying cause (see Chapter 1, Vital Signs). Check also for the following conditions:

  o *Fever:* Fevers are usually associated with infection. Rectal temperatures above 100°F (38°C) are considered significant. Remember that many frail elderly persons have normally low basal temperatures (96°F to 97°F) and respond to infection with temperature increases that merely reach the usual normal range (98°F to 99°F).

  o *Hypothermia:* The resident is considered hypothermic if his or her temperature is lower than 95°F. This may occur in a nursing home particularly if the facility's temperature is low from air conditioning or

drafts. Check for hypothermia using a rectal thermometer that has readings from 84°F to 108°F. In addition to confusion, other signs of hypothermia include pale, cool skin and the absence of shivering.

  o *Alteration in blood pressure, pulse, and respiration:* Alterations in these vital signs may be indicative of systemic problems related to adverse drug reactions, internal bleeding, cardiac or respiratory disease, dehydration, stroke, or infection.

  o *Weight changes:* A weight increase may indicate the presence of CHF, which in the elderly may not present classically with shortness of breath or other symptoms. Unexpected weight loss may be a sign of dehydration from inadequate intake or diuretic effects.

- Does the resident suffer from, or have a history of, recurrent infections?

  o Infections—usually pneumonias or infections of the gastrointestinal tract, urinary tract, and skin—commonly cause acute confusion. Infections often present with fever, elevated heart rate, and malaise. When the infection is local, there may be signs of inflammation and pain.

  o In the elderly, it is also common for infection to present atypically with confusion, anorexia, restlessness, and weakness. In debilitated residents, fever, tachycardia, and an elevated white count may be absent. Multiple chronic conditions may mask signs of infection.

  o Recurrent lung aspirations, which often occur in persons with dysphagia or in those receiving tube feedings, may predispose a resident to pneumonia. The decreased level of alertness associated with delirium may itself result in aspiration pneumonia. An indwelling catheter is a risk factor for urinary tract infections (UTIs).

- Does the resident suffer from, or have a history of, CHF?

o Although many frail residents present with typical signs and symptoms, such as shortness of breath (dyspnea), peripheral edema, and increased urine output, it is more common in this population to find CHF marked by confusion, anorexia, restlessness, fatigue, and falls.

o Dyspnea may be absent, and peripheral edema is not a reliable indicator of CHF, since many elderly residents who sit for long periods may have peripheral edema without CHF. Better indicators include distended neck veins, pulmonary bibasilar rales, an S_3 gallop, and weight gain.

• Check urinary output and compare with baseline.

o Decreased urinary output may be a sign of dehydration or urinary retention. Acute urinary retention is usually accompanied by pain and tenderness in the suprapubic area and a distended bladder. However, in some cases pain may be absent. In a diabetic, increased output may be a sign of hyperglycemia.

• Does the resident have a history of constipation or fecal impactions? Check the resident's bowel pattern and compare with baseline.

o A review of the bowel record may provide clues yet yield inadequate information for this purpose. If so, solicit information from nurse assistants who know the resident well. Are stools infrequent, small, hard, or liquid? Liquid stool may be indicative of stool leaking around a high fecal impaction. This is often accompanied by fecal incontinence without adequate bowel evacuation.

o Anorexia, nausea, vomiting, and abdominal and/or rectal discomfort may be present. Confused residents who are unable to communicate their discomfort may be found disimpacting themselves.

On examination, look for abdominal distension and the presence of hard or pasty feces in the rectum. An empty ballooned rectum may suggest impaction higher up. Also, note any painful hemorrhoids or fissures that may be prohibiting bowel evacuation.

• Has the resident been receiving any new medications?

o Any change in medication may precipitate delirium. Review to determine whether there is a temporal relationship between onset or worsening of delirium and the start of new medication.

o In addition to new medications, consider whether the resident has been experiencing physical decline that may affect how long-term drugs, such as digoxin, are being metabolized. For example, if the resident has worsening renal failure or liver function and is unable to excrete the drug properly, he or she may become confused. This is commonly seen when digoxin is given during an acute illness and oral intake is compromised. The development of dehydration and decreased renal perfusion may reduce digoxin excretion and lead to toxic accumulation of the drug. If the drug is necessary, lowering the dose or reducing the frequency of administration may alleviate the problem.

• Review the type and number of medications the resident receives.

o The greater the number, the greater the possibility of adverse drug reaction or toxicity. Review medications to determine the need and benefit of each. Check to see whether the resident is receiving more than one class of drug to treat a given condition.

• Review the drug regimen for those that cause delirium. Eliminate any of the following drugs that are unnecessary:

o *Psychotropics:* antipsychotics, antianxi-

ety/hypnotics, antidepressants
- o *Cardiac:* digitalis glycosides (Digoxin); antiarrythmics—e.g., quinidine, procainamide (Pronestyl), disopyramide (Norpace); calcium channel blockers—e.g., verapamil (Isoptin), nifedipine (Procardia), diltiazem (Cardizem); antihypertensives—e.g., methyldopa (Aldomet), propranolol (Inderal)
- o *Gastrointestinal:* histamine H_2 receptor antagonists—e.g., cimetidine (Tagamet), ranitidine (Zantac)
- o *Analgesics*: Darvon; narcotics—e.g., morphine, Dilaudid
- o *Antiinflammatory:* corticosteroids—e.g., prednisone; nonsteroidal antiinflammatory agents—e.g., ibuprofen (Motrin)
- o *Over-the-counter drugs* (especially those with anticholinergic properties): sedatives, antihistamines—e.g., Benadryl; caffeine; antinauseants; alcohol
- Is the resident in pain? Postoperative pain or pain associated with fractures, malignancy, acute abdomen, or local lesions can present as delirium.

Physical Examination

The goal of the physical examination is to detect physical illness that may be causing delirium. Give special attention to the neurologic, respiratory, and cardiovascular systems. Look also for the presence of infection, keeping in mind that infections of the respiratory and urinary tracts are most common in this population. Focus the examination on any problem that may have precipitated delirium in the resident in the past.

Laboratory Studies

Laboratory studies are targeted by findings from the resident's history, drug intake, and physical examination. Typically, the studies include:
- Complete blood count (CBC) with differential, electrolytes, blood urea nitrogen (BUN),

creatinine, glucose, and liver enzymes
- Urinalysis with culture
- Serum drug levels
- Chest radiography, electrocardiography, thyroid function tests, and other tests as indicated

Be alert to the possibility of hyper- or hypoglycemia in the diabetic resident, azotemia in the resident taking diuretics, or acute myocardial ischemia.

CARE PLANNING FOR THE RESIDENT WITH DELIRIUM

The goals of care planning are to restore cognitive, behavioral, and self-care functioning to baseline status, to promote safety, and to prevent complications. A care planning strategy for symptoms of delirium must be:
- Sensitive to the resident's usual daily patterns as well as health and functional status
- Tolerant of the acute confusion and agitation the resident is experiencing
- Responsive to the underlying causes of the condition

Whether the approach is nonpharmacologic or pharmacologic, the resident's need for security, order, and environmental predictability must be recognized and accommodated.

In the resident who is not presently delirious, but is at high risk for its development, take all efforts to minimize the risk and potential complications. Risk factors include male gender, surgery, prior cognitive impairment, pain, neuroleptic or narcotic use, and a past history of delirium. By identifying residents at risk, caregivers can attempt to minimize risk factors and monitor regularly for early detection of delirium to decrease the associated morbidity.

Treat the Underlying Cause

The first step in the management of delirium is to treat the underlying cause. Sometimes this requires active medical intervention, e.g., antibiotic therapy for infection or diuretics for

CHF. At other times it may require a period of careful observation in the absence of new interventions, e.g., when the resident is recovering from surgery.

Successful detection and treatment of the condition causing the delirium will lead to a return to baseline cognitive function within a few months in the majority of cases (*see* Chapter 3, Infection, and Chapter 28, Bowel Disorders). Note, however, that sometimes treatments for the underlying cause (e.g., diuretics for CHF, intravenous fluid for dehydration) as well as for signs and symptoms of delirium (e.g., haloperidol for hallucinations) may prompt a secondary delirium. In addition, if recovery from delirium is prolonged, progression of an underlying disease process, such as Alzheimer's disease, may leave the resident more impaired than at baseline by the time the delirium resolves. In cases in which treatment for delirium is delayed or never initiated, delirium may have adverse consequences, including irreversible dementia, prolonged institutionalization, functional dependency, or death.

If the causes of delirium cannot be identified or treated in the nursing home setting, consider transfer to an acute care hospital. If transferred, for the sake of continuity of care, be sure to send any of the resident's belongings that will enhance orientation and communication, and provide a sense of security. Send eyeglasses, hearing aids, family pictures, religious articles, and other belongings. It is also important to send a copy of the care plan and an outline of resident's daily routine.

Nonpharmacologic Approaches

The following subsections discuss nonpharmacologic approaches to managing delirium.

Milieu

The environment should minimize stress and facilitate mental and behavioral reorganization. For example:

- Reduce stimuli that may be confusing to the resident. Minimize unnecessary distractions such as a loud television or radio or caregiver conversations in the resident's room. Limit the number of unfamiliar contacts (i.e., multiple direct caregivers).
- Provide quiet, well-lit, calm surroundings with orienting stimuli such as clocks, calendars, and familiar objects and people.
- If the resident appears more comfortable among other people, do not isolate the resident in his or her own room.
- Avoid abrupt relocation, such as to another unit or to a room closer to the nurses' station for better supervision, unless absolutely necessary.
- Be sure the resident is wearing eyeglasses, hearing aids, or prosthetic devices if he or she ordinarily uses them.

Emotional Support

A calm, quiet, gentle but firm approach by familiar caregivers is important. For example:

- Reintroduce yourself with each contact. State the purpose of your interaction and keep explanations simple and brief. Reorient as necessary.
- Reassure the resident (and family) that he or she is safe, the situation is temporary, and that the resident will start to feel better soon and is not going crazy but is sick from (name of illness or medications).
- Listen to and acknowledge concerns and fears.
- Neither agree nor argue with the resident about his or her misperceptions, such as hallucinations, delusions, or illusions, since argument may aggravate the agitation. Focus instead on validating the resident's feelings. For example, say "I don't see any bugs, but it must be frightening to you."
- Be alert to nonverbal cues. For example, touching the resident may increase or decrease anxiety.

- Arrange contact with familiar people by engaging family or significant others in care routines and by staying with the resident.

Daily Routines

Maintain familiar routines to the extent possible given functional deficits or medical restrictions. For example:

- If the resident is used to walking around the unit each afternoon but currently has mild shortness of breath, take the resident for a short walk at the usual time if medical status permits.
- For the new admission, review customary routines for ideas, such as a daily afternoon nap or daily contact with relatives. Try to ensure that baseline sleep routine is maintained (e.g., milk and snack at bedtime).

ADL Performance and Support

The resident's continued participation in activities of daily living (ADLs), even at a minimal level, will add structure and order to a confusing situation and provide the resident with a sense of control. For example:

- Temporarily compensate for the resident's functional deficits while maintaining the resident's participation to the fullest extent possible (*see* Chapter 29, ADL Rehabilitation).
- Throughout each day, reassess functional needs until the resident is stabilized. During the acute phase of delirium, these needs will likely fluctuate with changing cognitive status. Maintain a flexible approach to care.

Mobility

Allow the resident as much mobility as possible. Do not restrict movement arbitrarily with physical restraints, since they have been shown to aggravate delirium and cause greater harm in the form of injurious falls, strangulation, and depression. Likewise, be cautious in deciding to use bed rails if the resident does

not use them ordinarily. Also, note the following points:

- If possible, provide one-on-one supervision. Walk, pace, or wander along with the resident. Encourage family participation to avoid using restraints. Exercise is often useful for treating agitation.
- If, after all other options have been explored, it is determined that a physical restraint is absolutely necessary in order to administer treatment (e.g., parenteral hydration, intravenous antibiotics, bladder decompression), use the least restrictive alternative.
- Inform the family about the burdens and benefits of restraint use as they affect the resident. Engage them in the decision-making process. Solicit their input in care planning and involvement in carrying out the plan (e.g., providing companionship, taking walks) (*see* Chapter 31, Restraint Reduction).

Comfort

Maximize nonpharmacologic measures to promote comfort and decrease agitation. Specifically: provide proper positioning, massage, soothing sensory input (e.g., soft music), constant temperature, nutrition and hydration, and anticipation of toileting needs.

Preventing Complications

Anticipate complications such as pressure ulcers, aspiration, dehydration, accidents, and falls in any resident who has delirium and abnormal psychomotor activity. Institute the appropriate measures to prevent such problems from occurring. (*See* the appropriate chapters for tips on preventive approaches to care.)

Continuity of Care

Document the resident's response to interventions using a behavioral symptom flow chart to depict the approaches that are working and identify those that are not. Orient caregivers on all shifts to the most effective approaches.

Pharmacologic Approaches

The following subsections discuss the pharmacologic careplanning approaches to delirium.

Criteria

If the resident's thinking is severely disorganized, agitation is severe, safety is impaired, and hallucinations and/or delusions are present, psychoactive drugs may be necessary. There is no ideal drug that yields the intended benefit without possible adverse side effects, so before considering psychoactive medications consider the following:

- Is the resident currently receiving a psychoactive drug that may be causing the delirium?
  - o Even therapeutic doses may cause or aggravate mental and behavioral disturbances. Akathesia is a common side affect of neuroleptics that mimics the psychomotor restlessness of delirium. One of the most common mistakes in treating the delirious resident is to increase the dose of neuroleptic medication when increased restlessness and agitation are observed. It is important to recognize that such restlessness may be a side effect of the neuroleptic, and that the proper treatment is a *reduction* in dose or discontinuation of the medication (*see* Chapter 14, Psychotropic Drugs).
- Has the resident had an adverse response to any psychoactive drug in the past (e.g., delirium, agitation, lethargy, depression)? Were the problems related to drug type or dose?
  - o Review the record to identify the drug, dosage, frequency, circumstances of administration, and adverse effects. If a particular drug has caused problems in the past, try a different drug or a lower dose.
- Is the resident hypoactive, lethargic, drowsy, or difficult to arouse?
  - o If so, psychoactive drugs are contraindicated, even in the presence of confusion, agitation, or altered sleep patterns.

Principles of Psychoactive Drug Therapy

When choosing a psychoactive drug to treat delirium, the following principles apply:

- Antipsychotics (neuroleptics) are the drugs of choice. They help to organize thinking and diminish hallucinations and delusions. Benzodiazepines are used less often because they cause drowsiness and paradoxic agitation. Short-term benzodiazepines such as lorazepam (Ativan) can cause delirium.
- Use these drugs on a short-term basis only. Begin to taper the drug as signs of delirium diminish. Stop the drug as soon as cognition approaches baseline.
- Always start with the *lowest possible dose*. Tailor the dosage to the individual and adjust according to the drug's effect.
- Give the antipsychotic on a *regular* basis two to three times a day initially to minimize the possibility of hypotension. It is best given 1 to 2 hours before expected agitation if possible.
  - o "As needed" (PRN) doses alone are usually contraindicated because the variability of delirious symptoms can prompt erratic drug administration.
- Increase the dosage slowly as necessary. Provide guidelines (orders on medication sheets) for reviewing the resident's response and postural vital signs before each increment in dose.
- Anticipate that the effective dose will lead to adverse side effects if administered regularly for several days.
  - o The neuroleptics are fat soluble and may accumulate after several days of use. Therefore, monitor closely and taper the dose after a therapeutic effect is achieved.

Specific Psychotropic Drug Options

There are many psychotropic drugs that can be used to help reduce the agitation and anxiety of a person with delirium, but it is best to become familiar with two antipsychotics that represent different extremes of anticholinergic versus dyskinetic side effects. Drugs like haloperidol (Haldol) have more extrapyramidal (dyskinetic) effects, while thioridazine (Mellaril) is more anticholinergic with associated sedating and hypotensive side effects.

If agitation is present and it is important not to overly sedate the resident:

- Give haloperidol (Haldol), 0.25 mg orally, as an initial dose. Monitor behavioral and physical effects. Repeat the dose in 30 to 60 minutes if agitation continues.
- Thereafter, 0.25 to 1.0 mg may be given orally two or three times a day, with careful monitoring and titration.
- If unable to administer an oral dose because of resident combativeness, agitation, or inability to follow directions to take a pill, haloperidol may be given intramuscularly.
- Monitor closely for adverse side effects such as, akathisia, parkinsonism, tardive dyskinesia:
  o Haloperidol (Haldol) has relatively low anticholinergic properties and may be used in cases of delirium when a sedative effect is not desired or potential anticholinergic side effects (e.g., orthostatic hypotension, urinary retention) would be too risky for the resident. Nevertheless, it still can cause sedation and hypotension. Do not use this drug in residents with parkinsonism. Haldol is manufactured in scored form and the lowest dose (0.5 mg) can be cut in half easily. A liquid concentrate is also available.

If severe agitation is present, particularly at night when sedation is desirable:

- Give thioridazine (Mellaril), 10 mg orally, as an initial dose. Monitor behavioral and physical effects. If there is no effect, give thioridazine, 10 mg orally, within 30 to 60 minutes.
- Thereafter, thioridazine, 20 to 25 mg, may be given orally two or three times a day

with careful monitoring and titration until severe agitation subsides with treatment of the underlying cause of delirium.

- If unable to administer an oral dose because of severe agitation or combativeness, chlorpromazine (Thorazine) in 5 to 10-mg increments may be given intramuscularly two or three times a day until the resident is able to take thioridazine orally.
- Monitor closely for adverse side effects such as excessive drowsiness, hypotension, worsening delirium, urinary retention, and constipation.
  o Mellaril is appropriate for severe agitation since its anticholinergic properties have sedative effects. However, do not use this medication in residents with glaucoma, urinary retention, or orthostatic hypotension. The pill form is enteric-coated and not scored. To achieve accuracy in administering doses lower than 10 mg (the manufacturer's lowest dose), use the liquid concentrate. Mellaril is not available for injection, so use Thorazine intramuscularly if sedation is necessary.

There are many other neuroleptics available with varying anticholinergic and dyskinetic effects. Newer agents, such as Respiradone, may have fewer adverse side effects, and with further clinical experience may prove useful in the treatment of delirium.

CASE EXAMPLE

Mrs. K. is an 88-year-old woman with dementia. She has been a resident of the nursing home for 3 years. Over time she has slowly become more forgetful, but still performs her ADLs when provided with simple cues. She needs supervision and redirection for daytime wandering behavior. She is oriented to person and knows she lives in the nursing home, but cannot find her room. Although she has difficulty finding the right words to express herself, she is usually understood by staff and family. Despite her impairments, she is an energetic woman who is a regular and eager participant in group sing-a-longs, dances, outdoor walks, and reminiscing. Her course has been relatively stable except for recurrent UTIs.

Recently, the night nurse reported that Mrs. K. had a restless night, awakening more confused than usual, very frightened, and newly incontinent of urine. With much nursing effort and reassurance, Mrs. K. finally returned to bed and eventually fell asleep for the rest of the night.

The following day, Mrs. K.'s nurse assistant reported that the resident was "acting differently and just didn't look good." She had difficulty paying attention for more than a few seconds. She could not follow directions during her usual self-care routines and therefore required extensive assistance, even with eating. She picked at her food and took in very little fluid. In the afternoon, Mrs. K. refused to go to a unit social and was later found sleeping in another resident's bed. Upon being awakened, she did not recognize Anna, her long-term nurse assistant. She spoke gibberish and was anxious and combative when Anna tried to help her get up. Anna said that when she touched her to calm her down and walk her back to her own room, her skin felt warm. She readily fell asleep once helped into bed.

Mrs. K.'s nurse recognized a familiar pattern emerging, and wondered if the cognitive and behavioral decline were indicative of a recurrent UTI. She examined the resident and found her to be lethargic and unable to participate in a mental status examination. Her tongue was dry and furrowed. Her temperature was 101°F rectally. Vital signs were as follows: blood pressure 140/90 mm Hg; pulse, 88 beats per minute; respirations, 26 per minute. Her lungs were clear. Because she was drowsy and had worsening cognitive functioning, incontinence, fever, and possible dehydration, the nurse suspected she had acute delirium caused by a UTI. She notified the physician of the resident's condition, telling him, "In the past, whenever Mrs. K. has been more confused she has had a UTI."

A urine culture and sensitivity, antibiotics, and increased oral fluids were ordered. Mrs. K. was monitored closely, and after a couple of days of drug and fluid therapy, assistance with self-care, and gentle reorientation and reassurance, she began to act like her old self.

This case describes the classic presentation of delirium in a nursing home resident who also has baseline dementia. Delirium is often overlooked as a reversible cause of functional decline in frail, chronically ill residents, especially residents having subtle signs of a mild, chronic delirium or those with dementia who are at high risk for developing delirium.

The key to recognizing the syndrome in this case example was the deterioration in Mrs. K.'s cognition, behavior, communication abilities, self-care function, and activity level. Nursing staff were quick to notice and report significant changes. Moreover, instead of dismissing these symptoms as a progression of her dementing illness, the caretakers questioned whether these changes were manifestations of a reversible condition. Through prompt recognition and treatment of both the delirium and its underlying cause, the staff not only prevented further decline but also saved Mrs. K. an unnecessary trip to the hospital. Suspect delirium in any resident who suddenly becomes more confused or has an abrupt change (worsening) of cognition, communication, mood, behavior, and sleep pattern.

12
Behavioral Symptoms

Barry Fogel, MD

Behavior patterns of nursing home residents become problematic when they:
- *Put the resident or others at risk for injury*
- *Interfere with the resident's care or his or her performance of activities of daily living (ADLs)*
- *Are socially inappropriate or unacceptable*

Determining when a specific behavior pattern is disruptive enough to be considered a "problem in need of intervention" depends on its frequency or severity. Some clinicians have a higher threshold of tolerance than others. However, vague definitions of appropriateness or acceptability aside, most clinicians agree that any physically assaultive behavior warrants immediate assessment and probably intervention. Likewise, so does any behavior that may lead to injury to self or others, or that may evoke violent responses from other residents.

When the clinician's response to problem behaviors is poorly planned, there may be harmful consequences. Social isolation and ostracism of the resident may result, adversely affecting the well-being and mood of the resident or others on the unit. In addition, there may be serious physical and mental compli- *cations, especially when the intervention involves using psychotropic medications or restraints. An inappropriate response by staff may worsen or prolong problem behaviors, further disturbing interactions with the staff and leading to a downward spiral of staff burnout, mutual staff and resident distrust, and counterproductive behavior on both parts.*

Problem behaviors reflect an interaction of the resident's personality traits, current physical and mental status, and the facility environment. In addition, specific interpersonal conflicts with staff, family, or other residents can contribute to problem behaviors.

OVERVIEW

By habit and convention, clinicians commonly use certain terms to describe problem behavior, e.g., agitation and self-injurious behavior. These terms can be rigorously defined and reliably applied, but in practical terms they are usually too general to be useful as a guide to planning care. A better approach is to construct a concise statement of the specific behavior that is causing or threatening to cause adverse consequences for the resident or others. For example, *wandering* is a better term

157

than *agitated* to describe the resident who is continually on his or her feet and becomes upset if prevented from walking around. If appropriate, replace wandering with a more accurate term, such as exit seeking, pacing, or akathisia, which refers to the continual purposeless motion of residents experiencing an adverse neurologic side effect of neuroleptics.

The five generally recognized categories of problem behaviors are:

- Wandering
- Verbally abusive behavior
- Physically abusive behavior
- Socially inappropriate/disruptive behavior
- Resistance to care

These behaviors represent problems for the facility regardless of the resident's intent.

Wandering

Wandering refers to seemingly purposeless walking, particularly when the walking interferes with care or risks injury (e.g., on a stairway), and the resident resists being redirected. It is usually described as "seemingly" purposeless because the resident may have a purpose (e.g., trying to leave the facility or relieve muscular discomfort). By discerning the agenda underlying the resident's wandering behavior, the clinician may be able to develop a more effective therapeutic plan.

Verbally Abusive Behavior

Verbally abusive behavior includes threats, curses, screaming, and other highly emotional verbal behaviors directed at specific individuals. For careplanning purposes, clinicians must distinguish between verbal abuse directed against a particular individual, an identifiable group (e.g., people in uniform), or everyone in general.

Physically Abusive Behavior

Physically abusive behavior includes hitting, pushing, shoving, biting, grabbing, kicking, and throwing objects at other people. As with verbally abusive behavior, the descriptive statement should identify the persons or group being targeted.

Socially Inappropriate/ Disruptive Behavior

Socially inappropriate/disruptive behavior refers to behavior that is not hostile but still has the effect of evoking annoyance, upset, or other unpleasant feelings in witnesses (in the caregiving staff, for example, because the resident's behavior makes their job more difficult or unpleasant). In some cases, these behaviors may not have caused problems when the resident was living alone or with a tolerant family member, but they do cause difficulties in the more public situation of a nursing home. Such behavior may include screaming, making loud or unpleasant sounds or noises, disrobing or masturbating in public, making sexual overtures to other residents or staff, smearing feces, throwing food, rummaging through others' belongings, hoarding food, or wearing grossly soiled clothing. Markedly poor personal hygiene is also socially inappropriate in a group setting, even if it is tolerated in a reclusive person living in the community. This category describes a broad range of behaviors, each with multiple possible causes or motivations, so the clinician must be as specific as possible when describing the particular disruptive or socially inappropriate actions.

Resistance to Care

Resistance to care refers to focused resistance to taking medication, assistance with ADLs, or cooperating with necessary medical procedures (e.g., physical therapy or skin care). Residents who fail to care for themselves without cues, yet ignore or resent cueing by staff, are regarded as resisting care. Within this category of problem behavior, try to distinguish residents who specifically object to elements of care (e.g., those who do not wish certain medications or who complain that particular procedures are painful) from residents who are generally resistant to most or all care interventions by staff. To identify residents with specific objections to particular care practices, ask the caregiving staff and family to offer examples of cooperation with care. If several examples of cooperating are offered, resistance must be somewhat specific, and careplanners can try to infer the resident's objectives if the resident is unable to express them. If specific objections can be identified, these care elements can often be avoided, eliminating the problem behavior.

Observe Underlying Motivations

Observing the underlying motivations of most problem behaviors makes them more understandable. For example, the resident may not understand a situation, or may fail to consider alternatives or take into account the likely consequences of a particular action. Dementia or other cognitive impairments often compromise the resident's ability to generate a positive and socially appropriate response to feelings or needs. When thinking about the pathophysiology of problem behaviors, it is often useful for the clinician to consider the following factors:

- What is the resident's perception of the current situation?
- What is the resident's level of arousal? Is the resident hypervigilant, excited, or agitated?
- Is the resident aware of the social context and likely consequences of any action?
- Does the resident have any capacity for impulse control?
- Is the resident afraid?
- Does the resident have any alternative outlets for self-expression? In particular, can he or she communicate specific feelings in words or gestures?
- How does the environment influence the resident's behavior (e.g., an intrusive pub-

lic address system that causes a negative response in the resident)?

Such a conceptual framework eases the identification of possible medical and psychiatric diagnoses, and encourages clinicians to look systematically for remediable components to the problem behavior, regardless of cause. For example, a resident whose screaming was triggered by hallucinations in a darkened room might respond to a change in lighting. The resident may be comforted by the intervention regardless of the underlying diagnosis.

CAUSES OF PROBLEM BEHAVIORS

Problem behaviors arise as a result of the interaction between residents' personalities, their underlying medical and/or psychiatric illnesses, and their environment—including the medications they are given. Therefore, the causes of problem behavior have many interacting factors, and the solutions usually involve care plans with more than one component. The physician and nurses' primary goal is to identify the contributing causes that are most likely to respond to intervention.

To start this process, get a careful history at admission. Have the interdisciplinary team follow up on known behavioral problems. Health Care Financing Administrations's MDS contains a series of relevant items referencing either the pre-nursing home period or the resident's status at admission. Use these items, such as the "Customary Routine" questions, as a starting point in this assessment. As problems emerge after admission, review the intake social history and talk with both the resident and family to determine whether the resident's new behavior has historical roots.

The following sections describe frequently identified causes of problem behaviors.

Personality Disorders and Longstanding Behavior Patterns

A significant proportion of the general population, including those who reside in nursing homes, has maladaptive personality traits or habitual patterns of behavior that may be either self-defeating or offensive to others. Well known examples include:

- Paranoid personalities who are generally suspicious and mistrustful
- Narcissistic personalities who are frequently demanding and entitled
- Emotionally unstable personalities who may display intense anger and disappointment intermittently

When individuals with rigid and maladaptive personality traits are placed in nursing home facilities, they are forced to be intimate with people they did not choose, and they are in an environment they do not control. Moreover, cognitive deficits and physical limitations may limit their range of alternatives for dealing with negative emotion. Coping styles and behaviors that worked in the resident's prior life situation may be ineffective in the nursing home. The outcome often is physically or verbally abusive behavior, screaming or agitation, or focused resistance to care.

Underlying personality traits such as an entitled attitude, or a tendency toward passive-aggressive behavior, are best identified by history from the resident's family and primary care physician. While personality traits, as such, cannot be modified, knowledge of the resident's history can aid the clinician in identifying the specific aspects of the current situation that are most likely to evoke negative emotion. The history may also identify interventions that have helped the resident in the past.

One way to identify problematic personality traits is to ask family members whether there are some ways in which the resident has been hard to get along with, or has caused conflict in the family. Another way is to obtain a brief life story of the resident, inquiring in detail about life events that suggest interpersonal difficulties, such as being fired from a job, separation or divorce, estrangement from

family members, or legal troubles. If family members identify specific behavioral problems that preceded nursing home admission, ask them for details about what seemed to aggravate or help the behavior.

For example, a resident might make continual unreasonable demands for special treatment. A life history might reveal that the resident was estranged from a sibling because of feeling intolerably slighted when the sibling forgot a birthday. The family might go on to say that only profuse professions of love and gratitude would calm the resident down when agitated. With this information in mind, the clinician would infer narcissistic personality traits, and try to help the resident feel sufficiently special to deter unacceptable behavior.

PHYSICAL AND MENTAL DISORDERS

The following sections describe some physical and mental disorders that affect behavior in residents.

Conditions Causing Pain and Discomfort

Pain, shortness of breath, anxiety, or other unpleasant physical sensations may all produce inappropriate behaviors while simultaneously interfering with a resident's ability to concentrate or think logically about alternatives. Pain and discomfort can precipitate or aggravate problem behavior, so symptomatic relief may reduce or eliminate the behavior, even if the underlying cause of the pain cannot be corrected. For example, an agitated resident with osteoarthritis may be helped by treatment with acetaminophen (Tylenol).

Frontal Lobe Dysfunction

The frontal lobes of the brain have a crucial role in perceiving social context as a control on impulse, and in providing capacity for insight and judgment. In the latter stages of dementia, frontal lobe function is usually compromised. For example, a resident with impaired frontal lobe function might be disoriented and fail every item on a memory test, yet insist that there was nothing wrong with her memory. Likewise, a resident with impaired frontal lobe function might verbally state that a sign that read "Not an Exit" meant that one should not open a door, yet attempt to open the door a few minutes later. Nondemented people also can have dysfunction of the frontal lobe (e.g., head injury victims, chronic schizophrenics, and people with frontal lobe strokes). The nondemented resident with frontal lobe impairment typically shows poor planning, poor judgment, and poor impulse control with relatively preserved memory, orientation, and verbal abilities.

Some people with frontal lobe dysfunction have such impaired impulse control that they cannot refrain from impulsive behavior even with a policeman at their elbow, so they require environmental controls (e.g., dining at a particular table) and other measures to redirect their impulses to more appropriate behaviors (e.g., completing a meal without taking other's food). Others, by contrast, are able to behave appropriately if they are consistently and repeatedly reminded by suitable cues of what behavior is expected from them. For example, consider a resident who attempts to rearrange the furniture in another resident's room. Interventions can include putting a stop sign on the back of the chair that the resident tries to move. If the cue is enough to inhibit the resident's behavior, the problem is solved. However, if the resident understands the meaning of the stop sign but still cannot control the action, a better strategy might be an electronic warning device that sounds an alarm when the resident goes into areas that are off limits. At those times, a staff person would physically redirect the resident, perhaps by saying, "Let's go for a walk."

Dementia

Dementing illness contributes to problem

behaviors in various, predictable ways. Most people with dementia have, or eventually develop, frontal lobe dysfunction. Moreover, the general loss of intellectual function that characterizes dementia makes residents less able to articulate their problems, wishes, and needs, and to identify alternatives when they feel an impulse to act. Misperceptions of reality, including visual illusions and misunderstanding of others' comments, are often the motivating force behind agitated behavior. Memory loss causes residents to forget past negative consequences of a particular behavior, and to forget alternatives that may otherwise satisfy their needs.

In addition to the general problems associated with dementia, residents may also suffer from one of the frequent complications of dementia, i.e., depression or psychosis. When depression is present, there is an increase in negative thoughts and feelings, and often a decreased level of tolerance for minor annoyances. When psychosis is the complicating factor, there are often paranoid misconceptions of reality and threatening hallucinations, which produce a motive for disturbed behavior and agitation.

When dementia is identified as an underlying cause of disruptive behavior, the clinician must be satisfied that all the treatable causes of dementia have been addressed. Both depression and psychosis, when they complicate dementia, have specific pharmacologic treatments that should be tried (*see* Chapter 14, Psychotropic Drugs for more information).

Delirium

Problem behavior often accompanies delirium, but the behavior is typically overshadowed by disorientation and altered consciousness. However, delirious states may show a predominant behavior disturbance, with the change in orientation and awareness identifiable only after observation and assessment. Delirium usually represents a specific toxic or metabolic problem, so it must be identified promptly.

For example, when a resident with no prior history of delerium suddenly develops problem behavior, or if problem behavior escalates dramatically or begins to fluctuate uncharacteristically, assume it is delirium and start the appropriate assessment and monitoring (*see* Chapter 11, Delirium, for more information).

Medication Side Effects

While it is unusual for prescription drugs to produce gross and persistent problem behaviors in otherwise healthy young adults, it is common for them to cause or aggravate problem behaviors in elderly nursing home residents, particularly if they already suffer from several other potential causes of problem behavior. The prescription drugs most often associated with problem behaviors are those that alter mood, cognition or perception. For example, Sinemet and L-Dopa commonly cause hypersexuality which can result in inappropriate sexual advances or masturbation in public. Many medications can cause paranoid delusions, particularly those associated with delirium such as digoxin, phenytoin, lithium, cimetidine, and other psychoactive drugs.

Theophylline or beta-adrenergic agonists for chronic obstructive pulmonary disease can cause agitation by creating an excessive level of arousal. Alcohol is an important drug that may be used secretly by residents or may be administered inadvertently in cough suppressants. Its administration or withdrawal may result in problem behaviors. This also applies to caffeine, nicotine in cigarettes, and benzodiazepines.

Primary Psychiatric Illnesses

In otherwise healthy young adults, the behavioral disturbances produced by primary psychiatric illnesses occur along with the char-

acteristic combinations of mental symptoms. To diagnose psychiatric syndromes in older adults who are relatively intact cognitively, perform a careful history and mental status examination. In older adults with significant impairment of cognition and/or communication, some of the characteristic symptoms of mental illness may be missing or impossible to determine. When some major symptoms such as depressive mood or paranoid delusions are combined with information on past psychiatric history, a tentative diagnosis of a primary psychiatric illness (modified by dementia) can be made.

Anxiety disorders can produce problem behaviors. For example, residents with specific phobias (e.g., fear of needles, fear of enclosed spaces, fear of elevators) may show problem behavior in order to escape from the feared situation. Residents with compulsions (e.g., hand washing, checking or rearranging behaviors, hair pulling, and nail biting) may display problem behavior if they are prevented from carrying out their compulsive rituals.

Depression causes problem behavior by increasing negative thoughts and emotions, aggravating cognitive deficits, and limiting frustration tolerance. Problem behavior is particularly likely if the depression is accompanied by delusions or marked physical agitation.

Manic-depressive illness (bipolar disorder) can produce severe problem behavior in both the depressive and manic phases. In the manic phase, the resident shows an elevated rate of speech and movement, and a decreased need for sleep. The resident may display aggressive, irritable, or hypersexual behavior, and may become loud or violent if the staff try to interfere with the behavior. Loss of insight is always a problem in the manic resident.

Residents with psychotic illnesses such as schizophrenia may show problem behaviors throughout their course. The facility environment as well as changes in physical and cognitive function may modify the expression of these problem behaviors.

Bizarre behavior may increase if there is no social contact with mentally intact persons. The resident with both schizophrenia and dementia may be unable to talk about delusions, but may still act upon them.

ENVIRONMENTAL AND SITUATIONAL FACTORS

The following sections describe some environmental and situational factors that may affect behavior in residents.

Overstimulation and Understimulation

All individuals have a range of sensory and emotional stimuli that they find tolerable or pleasant. This range varies (sometimes greatly) according to personality. However, when cognitive and adaptive capacities are lost, the individual's range of response usually narrows, and discomfort is experienced if there is too much or too little stimulation. For example, residents left alone much of the day in a private room without any structured activity might develop problem behaviors. Other residents might manifest most of their problem behaviors when excessively stimulated, such as during a large group meal or visits with multiple family members. Some residents are overstimulated by some visitors and not by others.

Therefore, the clinician is obligated to determine the optimal level of stimulation by direct, systematic observation, incorporating input from family members, significant others, and direct care staff. Demented residents often get agitated if too many demands are placed on them, e.g., during encouragement to perform ADLs, physical or mental status examinations, or activities that interfere with the daily routine. A log of visitors, activity, and behavior over a few days may help identify situations that are overstimulating and might provoke problem behavior.

Changes in Environment or Relationships

Residents with diminished cognitive and adaptive capacities may be overwhelmed by environmental changes or changes in their interpersonal world. A move to a different room, a new roommate, or illness or death of a family member or roommate can precipitate agitation and problem behaviors.

Specific Environmental Problems

Just as people in general have pet peeves, nursing home residents may find particular environmental stimuli to be intolerable. Understandably, many residents are intolerant of other residents' screaming, particularly if the screaming is continual. However, when coping mechanisms are impaired, the resident who is annoyed by an environmental difficulty may develop problem behaviors. It is not unusual for one screaming resident to set off an entire nursing unit (sometimes including the staff) while residents are gathered for meals or other activities.

Specific Interpersonal Difficulties

Troubled relationships between a resident and other people, such as family, staff, or other residents, can manifest as problem behaviors. This is a likely explanation when the problem behavior is focused on a particular individual or appears only when that individual is present. Specific interpersonal problems often have a realistic provocation or a contribution from the resident's history and personality (i.e., transference).

For example, an aide who evokes agitated behavior might actually have handled the resident roughly on a previous occasion, or might physically resemble an abusive relative who injured the resident in the past. The loss of cognitive ability in a demented resident makes it difficult for the resident to interpret the intentions of others. Therefore, a particular act or gesture by a caregiver may be misinterpreted, which may lead to inappropriate behaviors.

PROBLEM IDENTIFICATION

The first step to evaluate a problem behavior involves identifying the triggering incident. The second step is to obtain a detailed description of the behavior, implicitly addressing the question, "Is the observed behavior severe enough to warrant identification as a "problem behavior?" Include in this description what happened, the context or situation in which the incident occurred, and, if the incident was interpersonal, who else was involved. In the severity assessment, include how frequently the behavior occurs, and how the behavior affects—or threatens to affect—the resident's or other people's safety, the resident's care, the resident's function, and the social environment of the facility. Also determine how the resident responds to staff, other resident, or family efforts (if any) to address the problem.

If the observed situation is severe enough to warrant intervention, obtain the following information to develop a specific treatment plan:

1. An estimate of the resident's baseline personality, with particular attention to the resident's strengths as well as longstanding maladaptive personality traits, characteristic ways of relating to other people, what "pushes the resident's buttons," and what the resident finds comfortable or agreeable.
2. A review of all active medical problems, including a comprehensive drug list and the most recent data from physical examination or laboratory tests. The workup for an acute onset problem behavior is the same as the delirium workup; the workup for the chronic problem behavior follows the lines of the medical evaluation for factors aggravating depression or anxiety.
3. A review of the current physical symptoms, particularly emphasizing pain and discom-

fort. In residents with impaired communication or severe dementia, symptoms might be inferred from behavior.
4. A past history of psychiatric illness and treatment, and past responses to psychotropic drugs and psychosocial therapies.
5. A description of the current status of mood and cognitive function.
6. A description of specific mental symptoms, such as hallucinations, delusions, or compulsions.
7. A history of recent environmental changes or changes in relationships.
8. A personal history of known or suspected abuse, neglect, or hostile relationships.
9. A description of current nursing practices in talking with the resident, restraining the resident, and encouraging the resident.

TREATMENT

Treating problem behaviors is typically subdivided into nonpharmacologic treatments (e.g., providing behavior therapy and instituting deliberate changes in the environment) and medical/pharmacologic interventions (e.g., giving neuroleptics). Nonpharmacologic interventions also work by affecting specific causes of problem behavior. For example, explanation and reassurance by a caregiver may alter the perception of the current situation by a cognitively intact resident, or a resident with severe cognitive impairment may not be able to understand the explanation, but the level of arousal might be reduced by positive human contact and a calm, soothing voice.

To evaluate the possible courses of treatment, it is also useful for the clinician to think in terms of the pathophysiologic mechanism being affected. For example, when a neuroleptic is used to treat paranoid delusions, the drug will influence the resident's perception of the current situation. When a neuroleptic is used in a nonpsychotic resident to provide sedation, it works by decreasing excitement, hypervigilance, agitation, or other manifestations of increased arousal. It may not have a specific effect on delusions or hallucinations. If doses of neuroleptics make the resident stiff or functionally impaired, then the problem of impulse control is being addressed inappropriately by chemically restraining the resident's capacity for action.

NONPHARMACOLOGIC INTERVENTIONS

The following sections describe some nonpharmacologic interventions that can affect behavior in residents.

Interventions to Alter the Resident's Perception of the Current Situation

These interventions are aimed at enabling residents to perceive their environment more accurately. These efforts include:

- Taking steps to improve the resident's vision or hearing
- Making improvements in ambient lighting
- Speaking more clearly to the resident
- Positioning signs so that they are more easily read
- Reducing unnecessary noise and other external stimuli

Carefully explaining to the residents how they may be misperceiving reality, and providing reassurance when frightening misperceptions occur, may also be helpful in dealing with problem behaviors triggered by altered perceptions. Make these explanations easy to understand when the resident is cognitively impaired.

When the resident's problem behavior is triggered by misperception of interpersonal situations, such as when actions by the staff are somehow regarded by the resident as threatening, make efforts to:

- Modify the staff's behavior to avoid triggering the predictable response
- Modify the resident's perception of the staff's behavior

In general, staff validates the resident's experience, i.e., even though the staff may disagree with the resident's interpretation of an experience, they should acknowledge that the resident is having it. For example, the resident may perceive insects that are not present. Staff should not argue that they are not present, but acknowledge how upset or frightened the resident might feel. Residents with more intact cognition may be helped by talking about their problem with a sympathetic staff member, or in some cases by receiving formal psychotherapy. Some residents with less intact cognition may be helped by touch, others may not. Use these observed responses to direct the staff's approach.

A one-on-one relationship is helpful. At times, an actual environmental or interpersonal situation may be perceived correctly by the resident, and it may be truly noxious. In such cases, identify the triggering relationship or behavior as precisely as possible and make efforts to remove the noxious stimulus. Examples include:

- Assigning a different aide to care for the resident
- Limiting visits of people who disturb the resident
- Consciously altering the approach to the resident when specific triggers are identified

The clinician should always look for a modifiable environmental factor that may be aggravating the problem behavior. Sometimes changing the environment will be enough to end the problem behavior; at other times, environmental interventions will supplement other treatments by giving a better result or reducing the need for psychotropic medication.

Interventions to Modify the Level of Arousal

These interventions are aimed at providing the resident with an optimal level of stimulation. For residents needing more stimulation, this may mean more visitors, more organized activities, more verbal interaction with caregivers, and so forth. For residents who are overstimulated, the opposite tactic may have the desired effect.

One form of these interventions is aimed at regulating arousal directly. Such efforts include:

- Teaching residents a formal means of relaxation by conducting guided relaxation exercises (e.g., having a staff person lead residents through a visualization of pleasant scenes, focusing on diaphragmatic breathing, or first tensing and then relaxing successive muscle groups)
- Having residents exercise vigorously on a regular basis (see Chapter 29, ADL Rehabilitation, for more information)
- Providing physical comfort by warm baths, massage, or touching

Increased arousal related to strong emotion may also be modified by sympathetic listening and offering the resident opportunities to complain and ventilate negative emotion, either on a one-to-one basis or in a group. Efforts to channel discontent into constructive activity, if successful, can also reduce arousal. Music is also helpful in channeling emotional energy or distracting an agitated resident.

Interventions to Improve Awareness of Context or Consequences of Action

These interventions are aimed at clarifying social context and expectations by providing cues to the residents in the form of visual signs or verbal reminders.

One form of these interventions is generally referred to as formal behavioral therapy. The intent is to improve the residents' perception of context and the consequences of their actions by responding in a consistent and predictable manner to particular behaviors. For example, the staff might reinforce positive behavior by providing tokens or tangible rewards and verbal praise. They might also institute a program of nonpunitive time-outs for

socially inappropriate behavior. Time-out training is also a useful response to problem behaviors related to excessive arousal.

Many cognitively intact residents may also be helped by clear, consistent, and repeated discussion of what is the expected behavior and its likely consequences. Residents who retain some insight can often participate in choosing cues or systems of reinforcement that they find helpful in controlling their behavior and that are not offensive to them.

Interventions to Improve Impulse Control

These interventions consist of simple strategies for residents to uncouple impulse from action. A simple example is asking the resident to count to 10 before acting on an impulse to strike out. Unfortunately, such strategies are of little use for most residents with severe organic impairment of impulse control, since the majority of these residents also have significant cognitive difficulties. In such cases, the goal of nonpharmacologic intervention is to disconnect impulsive behavior from harmful consequences. Examples include placing a screaming resident with a deaf roommate, and providing safe places for residents to wander freely without the risk of injury or escape.

One of the cornerstones of successful institutional behavior management is to place the resident in situations in which their behaviors are no longer disruptive. For example, a child's playful behavior may be inappropriate in a museum, but perfectly acceptable in a playground. Similarly, if a noisy resident is grouped with residents who are noisy, or a wandering resident is put in a safe environment where wandering is acceptable, the behavior is no longer a problem. Institutions can deal with problem behaviors more effectively if residents are grouped on units where the staff are skilled in behavior management, and the behaviors are more acceptable.

Interventions to Help Residents Find Alternative Behaviors

Individual or group sessions on how to resolve problems and cope with the stresses and difficulties of life in the nursing home may be useful for more cognitively intact residents. In individual counseling, it is particularly helpful to identify strategies that the resident has used effectively in the past to cope with stresses and conflicts.

Coping skills groups should have four to 10 residents and be led by a social worker, nurse, or psychologist. The group meeting should last from 45 to 90 minutes, and might address such themes as what makes life meaningful in old age, how current problems among residents or with the staff might be resolved, and how people feel about living in a different environment. The leader is responsible for allowing ventilation of complaints, but not permitting a purely negative "gripe" session. Allow reminiscences about prior experiences but limit them so that the group returns to a positive, current approach to coping. Residents who participate should be verbal, with at most mild cognitive impairment, and have a history of positive involvement in group activities.

Coping groups are inappropriate for residents who never liked group activities or who lack the cognitive capacity to participate actively.

For residents too cognitively impaired to think in terms of alternative behaviors, it may still be possible to rechannel behavior that is aggressive or inappropriate. A simple example is to give the resident who physically strikes out at objects or people an opportunity to hit a punching bag instead.

MEDICAL/PHARMACOLOGIC INTERVENTIONS

The following sections describe some medical/pharmacologic interventions that can affect behavior in residents.

Interventions to Modify Perception of the Current Situation

If a resident has hallucinations, illusions, or other sensory abnormalities, the clinician's intent should be to address specific causes, such as deafness or visual impairment. Review the resident's medication list, and wherever possible eliminate any drugs that are suspected of causing a disturbed mood or altered perception of the environment (*see* Chapter 14, Psychotropic Drugs, for more information).

If the resident has a specific mental disorder, such as depression, an anxiety disorder, or a psychotic condition that is leading to a frightening or negative perception of reality, the clinician can diagnose this and provide specific pharmacologic treatment for that mental disorder (*see* Chapter 14, Psychotropic Drugs, for more information). If it is not clear whether the resident has such a condition, obtain a psychiatric consultation.

Interventions to Modify the Resident's Level of Arousal

To modify a resident's level of arousal, begin with efforts to treat any medical symptoms, such as pain or shortness of breath, that are raising the level of arousal. The clinician can review prescribed medications and eliminate or change any medications likely to cause increased arousal. These medications include stimulants, bronchodilators, and neuroleptics if they are causing akathisia.

Short-term drug therapies for increased arousal include short-acting benzodiazepines and low doses of neuroleptics. If long-term treatment is needed for increased arousal, the clinician should find a nonneuroleptic, nonbenzodiazepine alternative. *See* Chapter 14, Psychotropic Drugs, for more information.

Interventions to Improve Awareness of Social Context

The interventions to improve awareness of social context include treatment of remedial causes of sensory impairment and treatment aimed at improving cognitive status. Discontinue or change any drugs that are causing reversible cognitive impairment, such as sedatives, centrally active antihypertensives, and some of the cardiac drugs (Digoxin, beta-blockers, antiarrhythmics). Reassess the resident's nutrition, and, where appropriate, provide supplemental nutrition. Also, when possible, correct minor metabolic abnormalities not severe enough to cause frank delirium.

There are no drugs that improve cognitive function reliably in residents with dementia. However, in residents in whom awareness or reasoning is impaired by depression, the appropriate treatment of depression may help. Likewise, residents with untreated or undertreated parkinsonism may show an improvement in awareness of their environment and reasoning ability if their parkinsonism is better treated. Residents whose awareness of context is linked to severe apathy may on occasion benefit from stimulants (e.g., Ritalin).

Interventions to Improve Impulse Control

The interventions to improve impulse control involve removing any drugs that impair impulse control, especially benzodiazepines, alcohol, and barbiturates (*see* Chapter 14, Psychotropic Drugs, for more information). These need to be tapered gradually before discontinuation. Medical interventions to improve cognition, as previously discussed, may also improve impulse control.

Giving tranquilizers to impulsive residents generally does not improve impulse control. Rather, they reduce the level of arousal so that the impulses with which the resident has to deal are less strong, or they chemically restrain action by causing rigidity or akinesia. Paradoxically, a worsening of behavior may result from sedative use if their negative effect on cognitive function or inhibitions outweighs their positive effect on the level of arousal.

Summary of Medical/Pharmacologic Interventions

Regardless of the type of problem behavior being evaluated for medical/pharmacologic intervention, a medical review, attention to sensory impairments, and careful reconsideration of the resident's drug list is always justified. Psychotropic drugs may have beneficial effects on some factors causing the behavior while having adverse effects on others. Typically, a neuroleptic or sedative decreases resident agitation, but impairs cognition or problem-solving ability. Reassess both the behavior and the resident's overall physical, cognitive, and social function after starting a new drug.

INTERVENTIONS FOR RESIDENTS CURRENTLY RECEIVING PSYCHOTROPIC DRUGS OR RESTRAINT WHO NO LONGER SHOW PROBLEM BEHAVIOR

Because restraints restrict a resident's freedom and autonomy, and because virtually all psychotropic drugs have some significant side effects and risks, consider reducing the restraints or psychotropic drugs in residents who are currently free from the precipitating problem behavior. To determine whether to decrease or discontinue restraints or drugs, several principles apply:

• If restraints or psychotropic medications were used for a very brief time, and the problem behavior appears to be due to a nonrecurring event (e.g., relocation) and has resolved, then medication or restraints can be discontinued rapidly. However, if benzodiazepines were used to control behavior for more than 1 week, gradually decrease the dosage to prevent benzodiazepine withdrawal symptoms.

• If more long-standing problem behaviors have come under control with restraints or psychotropic drugs, then the problems are likely to recur when restraints or medications are removed unless a contributory condition has changed. In some cases, changes in the resident's underlying physical or mental health may have altered the likelihood of the problem behaviors. However, in most cases, some other intervention by the facility or caregiving staff will be needed to substitute for the effects of restraints or medications. Therefore, before tapering medication or restraints, analyze the problem according to the guidelines presented in this chapter.

- In most cases, gradually remove restraints or medications. For restraints, this may mean reducing the amount of restraint or the times per day they are applied. For medications, this means reducing the dosage no more than 10% to 20% at a time, with intervals of several days after each dosage reduction to evaluate how the resident's behavior has changed. If problem behaviors re-emerge with tapering of medication or reduction of restraints, try other means to manage the problems unless the behavior is putting the resident or others at immediate risk.

- When problem behaviors are a direct consequence of a specific diagnosed mental disorder for which long-term drug therapy is appropriate, medications may need to be continued indefinitely. The classic example is the resident with disturbed behavior due to manic-depressive illness who responds well to lithium. In the absence of a specific medical problem caused by lithium, it is not necessary to reduce the medication. Residents with chronic psychotic illnesses, such as schizophrenia or organic delusional disorders, who have done well on neuroleptics should have periodic attempts at neuroleptic discontinuation. If several attempts have led to a recurrence of symptoms, consider long-term drug therapy.

- However, most nursing home residents have chronic progressive medical and/or neurologic problems. As a resident becomes more physically or cognitively impaired, neuro-

leptic use may become more risky, even though the drug is still effective for the resident's psychotic symptoms. Therefore, periodic reconsideration of the appropriateness of neuroleptic therapy is necessary.

- When restraints or psychotropic medications are to be tapered in a resident with chronic problem behaviors, inform in advance all relevant people in the caregiving system about what to expect in terms of potential benefits, possible injuries, and possible aggravation of problem behavior. Have the interdisciplinary team start and share a schedule of monitoring and charting both problem behaviors and functional status. In particular, explain the plan to families and aides who work with the resident every day and give them an opportunity to provide their input. Furthermore, if there are specific signs that a resident's behavior is likely to change for the worse, encourage family members to report them promptly. Families must understand that such efforts are not without risk but are motivated by the goal of securing the best possible well-being for the resident.

- Document in the resident's record any plans to taper or discontinue restraints or psychotropic drugs.

CASE EXAMPLE

Mrs. H., a 75-year-old woman with multiinfarct dementia and a history of severe traumatic brain injury from a fall, exhibited two problem behaviors. The first was loud screaming, which often continued for hours at a time. The second was resistance to physical care, particularly bathing and dressing, which was characterized at the worst by hitting, kicking, and biting her aide.

Mrs. H. was aphasic from multiple strokes and completely dependent in all ADLs. She was fed with a jejunostomy tube, and had an indwelling Foley catheter.

Her behavior was identified as a problem

because of the risk of injury to caregiving staff, and because her screaming was distressing to other residents of the facility.

Assessment began with a review of her prior history and personality. She had always been an anxious, irritable, demanding, high-strung, and controlling person who became angry and lashed out verbally if she did not have her way. Her husband, a somewhat meek man, invariably responded by catering to her and relinquishing control to her for most major family decisions.

The second step in the assessment process was a review of Mrs. H.'s medical and psychiatric issues. It was noted that she had a number of active problems currently under treatment. These included a seizure disorder treated with phenytoin and hypothyroidism treated with thyroid replacement. Retesting of her thyroid function showed that she was still mildly hypothyroid, and the dosage of thyroid hormone was increased. Her phenytoin level was checked and found to be within normal limits. However, suspicion that the mental side effects of phenytoin might be contributing to the problem led to a gradual substitution of carbamazepine, an antiepileptic drug with fewer behavioral side effects.

The review of her psychiatric history was positive for a definite episode of major depression following her first stroke 2 years earlier. Her husband noted that she was unusually negative and irritable during that depression. No specific treatment had been given at the time, and her husband suspected she had never completely recovered.

The third step in the assessment process was to review the environmental and situational factors. The charge nurse noted that Mrs. H.'s screaming was most likely to occur during her husband's daily afternoon visits, and typically would abate after he left. This led to the hypothesis that some kind of emotional interaction between the husband and wife was contributing to the agitation. Direct

observation showed that the husband responded to his wife in a highly solicitous manner while displaying a facial expression of anxiety. The staff suspected that Mrs. H's husband's attention was overstimulating, while at the same time his look of worry and concern might be provoking an emotional reaction in his wife. The husband was encouraged to join a support group for caregivers. He was counseled to adopt a less stimulating but more reassuring demeanor. As a result, the screaming associated with his visits decreased.

Because of the association of physically aggressive behavior with daily care, two episodes of morning care were carefully observed. In both instances, the resident appeared frightened by the aide, and despite her aphasia was heard to say, "Don't hurt me." There was no evidence she had ever been mistreated at this facility, but there was some history of rough treatment by an attendant during an episode of acute hospital care. The staff suspected that Mrs. H. feared physical harm during her care, and they tried to reassure her. Unfortunately, because of communication difficulties and the resident's extreme arousal when anticipating her care, reassurance and explanation were not helpful.

Therefore, she was treated with thioridazine, 10 mg every morning, the reasoning being that the combined antianxiety and antipsychotic effect of this very small dose of medication might enable Mrs. H. to tolerate physical care and accept explanation and reassurance from staff. Monitoring of her blood pressure showed no subsequent orthostatic hypotension. She had no complications of confusion, constipation, urinary retention, or visual change. The intervention was successful, and there were no further occasions of hitting, biting, or kicking during care. Because intervention with her husband had reduced but did not eliminate episodes of screaming, and because her history suggested an element of depression, an antidepressant dose of trazodone was given. The screaming stopped completely after 4 weeks of treatment.

In this case example, medical, psychopharmacologic, and environmental interventions were combined to address two problematic behaviors. Previous attempts to treat Mrs. H. with psychotropics alone were unsuccessful. These efforts included giving a full antipsychotic dose of haloperidol, and giving lorazepam when she screamed. Haloperidol caused muscle stiffness and aggravated the agitation; lorazepam made Mrs. H sleepy and confused. The "drugs only" approach did not address her depression, nor did it identify the medical issues of hypothyroidism and possible behavioral toxicity of phenytoin.

Before formal assessment and combined intervention, psychosocial interventions also had been tried without success. Trying to explain and to reassure Mrs. H to quell her fears of daily care were unsuccessful. Her husband did not respond to the nurses advising him to spend less time with his wife because he did not see how that would help her. His own anxiety about his wife's condition did not permit him to leave her bedside. The psychosocial intervention that succeeded was similar in spirit to the one that had failed, but was eased by the appropriate medical and psychopharmacologic treatment, as well as by placing it in an explanatory framework that made it acceptable to both family and staff.

13
Depression

Andrew Satlin, MD
Katharine Murphy, RN, MS

Among infirm, elderly nursing home residents, depression and anxiety are prevalent, closely associated with morbidity and mortality, and frequently reversible with proper treatment.

Major depression—defined as depressed mood and/or loss of interest and pleasure, combined with five or more additional neurovegetative symptoms—occurs in 10% to 15% of nursing home residents, with combinations of depressive symptoms that do not meet the criteria for major depression appearing in an additional 15% to 50%. These rates are considerably higher than those reported for elderly persons living at home or in congregate housing. A significant morbidity is associated with mood disorders. Among the correlative factors are:

- *Poor adjustment to the nursing home*
- *Loss of independence*
- *Uncooperativeness with daily care*
- *Inability to participate in social and recreational activities*
- *Isolation from loved ones*
- *Increased risk of medical illness*
- *Possible impaired immune response*
- *Decreased cognitive ability*
- *Increased sensitivity to physical pain*

Major depressive disorders present a significant risk factor for mortality. According to one study, nursing home residents with depression were 59% more likely to die over a 1-year period than those without depression. This increased risk may be accounted for by the increased rates of medical illness, particularly cardiovascular disease, found in residents; but it also may be due to other, unknown factors.

The risk of suicide also is higher in the elderly than in younger persons, with a rate of 26.5 per 100,000 persons 80 to 84 years of age, compared with 12.4 per 100,000 in the general population. Data are not available on the rates of suicide among the elderly in institutional settings.

However, despite the high rates of depressive illness and associated complications, mood disorders are very treatable. Elderly depressives are as likely to respond to conventional therapeutic modalities as younger patients. It is tragic when depression and other mood disorders go unrecognized and untreated among nursing home residents.

This chapter discusses the causes and pathophysiology of mood disorders, how to identify the resident in need of treatment, and how to develop appropriate treatment plans.

OVERVIEW

A disturbance of mood is present when the resident feels sadness that is out of proportion to or more prolonged than the circumstances warrant, or when the resident's mood has labile and apparently unprovoked fluctuations. Any of these changes may reflect a disorder of brain neurochemistry that is commonly referred to as *affective illness*.

Such a disorder typically is accompanied by a spectrum of abnormalities of neurovegetative function, including sleep, appetite, energy, arousal, concentration, curiosity, and interest. Generally, however, the first indication of a problematic situation will be the resident's depressed affect (i.e., the appearance of a sad face, listless body posture, motor retardation, or apathetic response to external stimulation). Collectively, these symptoms of disturbed mood and abnormal behaviors comprise the syndrome of *depression*. When a total of five neurovegetative symptoms are present, including depressed mood and/or loss of interest or pleasure, the depression is said to be major.

Although the syndrome of depression is very treatable once it is recognized, it often goes unrecognized in many elderly persons—especially nursing home residents—for two reasons. First, the elderly may have atypical symptom clusters, such as the absence of a subjective mood complaint; or they may report anxiety, irritability, or a sense of not feeling anything at all or of feeling numb. They may also focus on the sensation of physical pain or discomfort or physical health status rather than on their inner mood state. To the observer, the resident may appear to be restless, fidgety, aggressive, or overly concerned about minor aches and pains, rather than presenting a typically depressed affect.

Second, the resident or clinician may attribute symptoms to causes other than depression. For example, impaired sleep, loss of appetite, decreased energy, loss of interest, and the inability to sustain arousal or concentration may be ascribed to medical illness, medication use, dementia, or more generally to the aging process. Attributions to other medical causes may prove correct, but a depressive syndrome should always be considered when these symptoms are present. Depression is never a normal age-related change.

CAUSES AND PATHOPHYSIOLOGY

The following sections discuss the causes and pathophysiology of depression.

Neurochemical Abnormalities

The neurochemical abnormalities that underlie the pathophysiology of depression are not yet fully understood. The most likely hypotheses implicate disturbances of serotonergic and noradrenergic neurotransmission. These deficiencies account for the known antidepressant effect of medications that block serotonin and norepinephrine reuptake at nerve endings in the brain. However, the exact anatomic localization of these neurochemical alterations is uncertain.

Risk Factors

Whatever the root causes, the risk of developing major affective illnesses increases with a history of these disorders in first-degree relatives. For residents who develop their first depressive episodes late in life, the familial connection is less predictable. Other biologic risk factors may include cognitive impairment, cerebral atrophy, deep white matter changes on magnetic resonance imaging, and a variety of medical illnesses. Social and demographic risk factors include female sex, widowhood, forced retirement, and a low availability or quality of social supports such as close relatives and friends. Nursing home admission also may be associated with many of these risk factors, and is itself linked to higher rates of depression over the year following placement.

Medical Illness

Table 13-1 shows the medical illnesses associated with increased rates of depression. Many of these disorders are common in the elderly, particularly cardiovascular disease, cancer, renal failure, and endocrine abnormalities such as hypothyroidism and hypercortisolism (Cushing's disease).

Among neurologic diseases, stroke and dementia are the most common causes of depression in the elderly. There is increasing evidence that cortical strokes cause depression at rates far higher than those found in people with comparable disability due to other causes (e.g., orthopedic disease), which suggests a specific biochemical or anatomic etiology of poststroke depression.

Dementia

The relationship between depression and dementia is highly complex. Rates of depression appear highest in elders with early or mild dementia (roughly 25%), which suggests that their depression may represent a psychological reaction to the loss of cognitive ability, independence, and functionality. However, depression in the later stages of dementia may be more common than suspected. Residents with more severe dementia and concomitant language deficits are less able to recognize and report depressive symptoms. These factors also make it more difficult for the staff to recognize depression. Resident depression may be manifested in agitated behaviors such as pacing, wandering, or repetitively calling

Table 13-1. Medical Disorders Commonly Associated with Depression

Central nervous system diseases	Jakob-Creutzfeldt disease
Alzheimer's disease	Influenza
Cerebrovascular accidents	Acquired immune deficiency syndrome
Neoplasms	**Nutritional deficiencies**
Parkinson's disease	B_{12} deficiency
Multiple sclerosis	Folic acid deficiency
Amyotrophic lateral sclerosis	Thiamine deficiency
Huntington's disease	**Electrolyte imbalance**
Myasthenia gravis	Hyponatremia
Paraneoplastic syndromes	Hypokalemia
Endocrine disorders	Hyperkalemia
Hypothyroidism	Hypercalcemia
Hyperthyroidism	**Systemic diseases**
Autoimmune thyroiditis	Systemic lupus erythematosus
Hyperparathyroidism	Temporal arteritis
Diabetes mellitus	Uremia
Addison's disease	Disseminated carcinomas
Cushing's disease	Rheumatoid arthritis
Infectious diseases	**Cardiovascular diseases**
Tertiary syphilis	Myocardial infarction
Viral encephalitis	Angina pectoris
Infectious mononucleosis	

Table 13-2. Commonly Used Drugs that can Cause Depression

Alcohol	**Cardiovascular medications** Digitalis, lidocaine
Analgesics Nonnarcotic: indomethacin Narcotic: morphine, codeine, meperidine, pentazocine, propoxyphene	**Estrogens**
	Gastrointestinal medication Cimetidine
Antihypertensives Propranolol, methyldopa, reserpine, clonidine, hydralazine, guanethidine	**Hypoglycemic agents**
	Progestational agents
Antibacterials	**Sedatives** Barbiturates, benzodiazepines, mep- robamate, chloral hydrate
Antiparkinsonian drugs Levodopa	
Cancer chemotherapeutic agents Tamoxifen, vincristine, vinblastine, hexamethylamine	**Steroids**

for help, and may be mistaken for a progression of the dementing illness. There is also some evidence that degeneration of subcortical cholinergic neurons in severe Alzheimer's disease may reduce the clinical expression of depression.

Since many of the symptoms of depression and dementia overlap, diagnosis can be difficult. Depression may even cause a cognitive impairment that closely mimics dementia. This so-called pseudodementia is not aptly named, however, because the dementia of depression (a preferable term) is as real and disabling as that caused by a presumed neurodegenerative condition.

Drugs

Table 13-2 lists drugs generally believed to increase the risk of depression. Common medications such as beta-blockers and antihistamines may lead to depression. Chronic use of sedative medications, frequently inappropriately and overprescribed in nursing homes, may result in an apathetic depressed state with associated cognitive impairment, lack of coordination, falls, and injury.

Alcohol use (an option in the daily routine in many nursing homes), which is often overlooked by those who work with the elderly, may result in a chronic depression, or its use may be a marker for underlying depression.

**IDENTIFYING THE RESIDENT
IN NEED OF TREATMENT**

The following sections discuss how to identify residents who need treatment for depression.

Signs and Symptoms of Depression

The hallmark of depressive illness is a depressed mood state, which may be communicated by the verbal expression of sad mood or by behavior that is consistent with sad mood. For example, the resident may:

- Complain of feeling sad, low, down, blue, empty, hopeless, or worthless; or may have a sad facial expression, easily become tearful, remain in bed, not attend to personal appearance, move slowly, or withdraw from contact with others.
- Manifest related mood states, such as anxiety, tension, anger, irritability, or an apparent inability to feel anything at all; or may appear restless, agitated, and hyperactive; or may be withdrawn, hypoactive, and unresponsive to external stimulation.
- Complain of apparently unrelated conditions, such as aches and pains, an inability to walk or perform activities of daily living, or impaired vision, hearing, sensation, or taste. The resident may sit without moving and refuse to talk or to take medications. Frequently he or she may seek help, medical attention, medications, or other care (e.g., blankets, hot water bottles, enemas, or assistance with eating or going to the bathroom), or alternatively may resist care or attention.

In general, if the resident having these symptoms does not respond to the staff or family's encouragement, positive statements, or attempts to cheer the resident up, suspect a major depression. The clinician should ascertain the approximate time of onset of symptoms that are most obvious, distressing, or limiting to the resident's functioning.

Associated Symptoms

The clinician should try to determine whether there are other, related symptoms with the same time course as the depressed mood or affect that might suggest the presence of a mood disorder.

Such related symptoms include:

- Loss of interest or pleasure in previously enjoyed activities (e.g., visits from family, reading, group activities)

- Sleep disturbance, including difficulty falling asleep, restlessness, frequent awakenings during the night, or waking in the early morning and being unable to fall asleep again
- Fatigue or loss of energy
- Impaired concentration or memory, or a subjective sense that thinking is slowed down
- Loss of appetite or a feeling of having to force oneself to eat, often accompanied by weight loss and constipation
- Ideas of guilt, which may reach delusional proportions, other delusional ideas such as the incorrect belief that one is poor, or somatic delusions (e.g., has cancer)
- A diurnal variation of mood (e.g., many depressives experience more intense depressed mood or other symptoms in the morning, with a gradual lessening of the intensity of distress as the day progresses)
- Feelings of hopelessness and helplessness
- Wishes to die or suicidal ideation

Many clinicians find it difficult to inquire about suicide. Usually, it is easiest to approach the topic in stages, and then building on the resident's responses. Begin by asking the resident if the feelings ever get so bad that the he or she thinks that life is no longer worth living. Then ask whether the resident sometimes wishes that his or her life were over. Does the resident think about death frequently? Has the resident ever thought about doing something to end his or her life? What thoughts about this has the resident had? Has the resident had these thoughts today, this afternoon, in the last hour? Has the resident thought about any specific means that might be used? How much of a possible plan has the resident started to carry out? Does the resident think about actually carrying this plan out?

Residents who exhibit self-destructive behaviors, such as refusing to eat, refusing medications, resisting care, or sustaining frequent accidents, also may harbor the wish to die, but these behaviors are common in depressed residents and do not per se indicate suicidality. Explore other causes for these behaviors with the resident. Does the resident refuse food because he or she thinks it may be poisoned (i.e., is he or she delusional)? Does the resident refuse medications because of uncomfortable side effects or a belief that the drugs do not help? Does the resident resist care because he or she no longer cares about appearance, or feels guilty about receiving attention or help, or is in physical pain that is exacerbated by nursing care routines?

Significant Change

The next step in assessment is to determine whether the resident's depressive symptoms represent a clear change from baseline. For staff who are familiar with the resident over a long period of time, it may be relatively easy to recognize a new condition. Discussion among staff who work different shifts may be revealing. It is often more challenging to evaluate a newly admitted resident, particularly if he or she is unable to express verbally feelings of being depressed or sad. Ask family or friends to provide information about the resident's usual affective state before admission to the nursing home. Does the resident's current status represent a change in mood?

In order to warrant intervention, the change from baseline must be persistent. Observe the resident over at least 1–2 weeks. It is often helpful to maintain a written behavioral flow sheet to record the resident's symptoms and response to attempts to be cheered up over all three shifts for 1 to 2 weeks. Again, information from staff working different days and shifts should be shared. The altered affective state most often will not respond to external stimulation, including events or news that the resident ordinarily would find pleasurable.

FURTHER ASSESSMENT

When preliminary assessment indicates that a mood disorder is present, the next step in the care planning process is to identify any associated conditions that may contribute to the problem or suggest specific modes of treatment. Perform further history gathering, physical examination, and laboratory tests. Consult with the geriatric internist and psychiatrist to collaborate on the assessment and treatment planning if this has not already occurred. Obtain the information discussed in the following sections.

History

Obtain the following historical information about the resident:
- Cognitive decline. Determine whether there has been a progressive cognitive decline, which suggests a concomitant dementia. Careful history taking regarding the course of the disorder is essential, because clinically cognitive impairment due to depression may be indistinguishable from that due to a progressive dementia from other causes. Look for:
  o A course of cognitive decline with a well-defined onset (usually over a period of days to weeks) and a rapid escalation of depressive symptoms are suggestive of affective illness.
  o A more insidious onset and slowly progressive course is more typical of dementia. Family members often debate its true beginning and disagree by a year or more.
  o Try to pin down whether the depressive symptoms preceded or followed the onset of cognitive impairment, suggesting that one or the other may be causative. Remember that recent research indicates that significant cognitive impairment is rarely due to depression alone, and that when memory deficits coexist with depressive symptoms a combination of dementia and depression is most often present.
  o Many of the secondary symptoms of depression and dementia, such as apathy,

lack of interest, decreased concentration, insomnia, decreased appetite, and anxiety, are similar in both disorders. In residents with mild to moderate cognitive impairment, complaints of sad mood, tearfulness, guilty thoughts, and suicidal ideation are better indicators of the presence of depression than are secondary symptoms.

o In residents who are further along in the course of dementia, it is usually advisable to suspect depression in any resident who has an acute decline in function or an acute increase in agitation that cannot be explained by an intercurrent medical illness, medication side effect, or environmental stressor; the natural progression of dementia is slow and gradual, so any deviation from this pattern requires an evaluation.

o If depression is suspected, and other treatable conditions have been ruled out, antidepressant treatment is generally warranted even in questionable cases because the potential benefit is great.

- **Medical illnesses.** *See* Table 13-1.
- **Medication or alcohol use.** *See* Table 13-2.
- **Recent emotional stress** (e.g., death of or loss of contact with significant others or loss of physical abilities, cognitive abilities, or financial resources; or change in a primary caregiver).
- **Disruptive environmental change** (e.g., recent admission to the nursing home; change of room, roommate, or staff; or loss of treasured or familiar possessions).
- **Past history of depression.** A history of previous depressive episodes, with a cyclic pattern of remission between acute depressive illnesses, strongly suggests that a current change in affective state represents recurrence of a depressive disorder. Ask the resident and family about their perceptions

of the situation as well as what triggered depression in the past and what has helped. Were episodes accompanied by specific precipitants or associated conditions?

- **Past treatment history.** If the resident had a past history of depression what was the specific treatment regimen? For example:
  o Did previous depressions respond to a specific treatment regimen, including the use of antidepressant medication?
  o If medication treatment was not successful in the past, were all classes of antidepressant agents tried? Were doses adequate? Were medication trials of sufficient duration?
  o Did past antidepressant use result in intolerable side effects (i.e., side effects that outweigh the benefits of treatment)? If so, what adverse effects did the resident (or surrogate decision-maker) consider intolerable?

Physical and Mental Status Examinations

Perform physical and mental status examinations and look for the following symptoms:

- Delusions indicating the presence of psychotic depression. A *delusion* is a false idea or conclusion about an experience (e.g., the food is poisoned; a roommate is stealing; a daughter is withholding information; the resident is dying). Determine the content of the delusion from the resident without validating or challenging it.
- Fluctuating level of consciousness and impaired attention indicative of delirium. (*See* Chapter 11, Delirium, for more information.)
- Focal neurologic symptoms or signs consistent with stroke.
- Level of cognitive function. Determine whether there is an underlying dementia, and assess the resident's ability to understand and cooperate with a treatment plan.
- Physical examination for intercurrent medical illnesses.

Laboratory Studies

Conduct the following laboratory tests to obtain more information:

- Complete blood count to look for anemia, leukemia, or chronic infection
- Electrolytes, blood urea nitrogen, and liver enzymes to rule out metabolic disorders
- Thyroid function tests to exclude hyper- or hypothyroidism
- Drug levels to check for potential drug toxicity (e.g., digoxin, anticonvulsants, antiarrhythmics, bronchodilators)
- Nutritional indicators: vitamin B$_{12}$, folate, albumin

Resident Strengths and Resources

Ask the following questions to assess the resident's strengths and resources:

- Does the resident have a good support system? Are family and friends (or close staff members if the resident has no significant others) available and willing to be involved in supporting the treatment plan, including psychosocial interventions?
- Does the resident have enough physical ability, energy, and motivation to participate in recreational therapy or exercise?
- Does the resident have sufficient cognitive ability and verbal skill to benefit from psychotherapeutic modalities? Is the resident willing to talk with a trusted professional?
- Are the resident's hearing and vision adequate for participating in group therapy? (*Adequate* is defined as sufficient for receptive communication so that the resident does not become further frustrated or isolated by misinterpreting group interaction or feeling left out.)

FORMULATING THE TREATMENT PLAN

Base the resident's treatment plan on all of the information gathered about precipitants, associated conditions, symptoms, the resident's strengths and resources, and past response to drug and psychological therapy. The goals of treatment are to alleviate discomfort, ensure safety, increase function, promote understanding of the illness by the resident, family, and direct care staff, and prevent relapse. Treatment will generally require an interdisciplinary approach. Frequent interaction and cooperation among medical, psychiatric, social work, recreational therapy, and nursing staff is essential.

The major components of treatment for depressed mood in the nursing home setting are discussed in the following sections.

Involve the Resident and Family

To the fullest extent possible, inform the resident and close relatives about treatment options and encourage them to participate in the treatment decisions. It is especially important to discuss possible adverse reactions to medications or changes in medication regimens for other medical conditions. Family members may find visits with a depressed relative at the nursing home to be stressful especially if conversation is sparse, they feel they have to cheer the resident, or the resident is angry and abusive. This may lead to fewer visits and a greater sense of loneliness in the resident.

Visits may be less stressful when staff provide families with tips for visiting that do not involve verbal struggles (e.g., taking the resident for a walk, bringing a favorite food from home, giving the resident a manicure). Encourage families to share with the staff their feelings about dealing with a depressed relative. Families may find this easier to do when the staff openly acknowledge the stress this may cause. Referral of family members to individual or group counseling may be indicated. Many families have difficulty accepting the need for counseling. For reluctant families, facility staff may need to discuss this suggestion many times over a period of time.

Treat the Underlying Causes and Associated Conditions

To address the underlying causes and associated conditions of depression:

- Treat the medical or neurologic conditions that might be contributing to the depressive symptoms. Often, resolution of syndromes such as congestive heart failure, hypothyroidism, or vitamin B$_{12}$ deficiency will improve mood substantially.
- Minimize or eliminate the use of alcohol or medications that may be causing the depression.
- Address sources of discomfort and other health concerns that may be contributing to the depression (e.g., pain, constipation, or poor sleep). When possible, treat the condition without adding another medication, especially one that may cause distressing side effects (e.g., excessive daytime drowsiness) and interfere with ongoing assessment and management of depression.
- Address the environmental or psychosocial stress factors that are amenable to change (e.g., extremes of heat or noise; a wandering resident who may be rummaging through the depressed resident's belongings; lack of visitors; or conflicts with staff or roommates).

Protect the Resident from Self-Harm

If the resident has expressed suicidal ideation, determine whether he or she has any active intent to attempt suicide. If so, admission to a psychiatric unit or hospital is indicated even if the resident cannot describe any specific plan. If the resident denies any active intent, and can contract with nursing staff to inform them of any increased inclination toward suicide, then perform repeat assessments of suicidal intent each shift while treatment for the underlying depression is started. Continue these assessments until the resident no longer expresses any wish to end his or her life.

Ensure Adequate Nutrition and Hydration

If the resident is losing weight and has poor intake consult with a dietitian. (*See* Chapters 23 and 24, Nutrition and Dehydration, respectively for more information.) The resident may require nutritional supplements. Find out whether the resident has specific food or drink preferences that can be accommodated. Family members may be able to respond to the resident's requests. Additionally, some residents experience gastrointestinal side effects from antidepressants. If an antidepressant is given, monitor for side effects that interfere with intake such as nausea, anorexia, constipation, or diarrhea. Taking medication with meals can reduce these effects.

Encourage the Resident to Take Part in Daily Activities

Invite the resident to outings, recreational therapy, special unit activities, and exercise programs. Participating in such activities can serve to increase self-esteem, provide opportunities for social support, distract from worries and concerns, and channel anger and restlessness. However, do not coax the resident to participate when he or she is clearly too depressed, psychomotorically retarded or agitated, anergic, oppositional, or delusional to be able to participate or derive any benefit. Start with activities the resident found enjoyable in the past. Take the cue from the resident, but note that depression is an illness that prevents function in its acute stages. Any premature attempt to overcome this inability to function may lead to a greater sense of failure and frustration. (*See* Chapter 30, Activities Programming, for more information.)

Initiate Psychotherapy

A variety of modalities may be useful to treat the resident with depression. Contrary to common beliefs, older people can benefit from psychotherapy. Any of the following modalities may be provided alone or concurrent with antidepressant medication:

- **Cognitive behavior therapy** to help restructure the resident's thinking from more negative interpretations of life changes to more positive ones. This treatment is appropriate for residents with intact cognitive ability who have distorted (but not psychotic), negative self-perceptions as a prominent part of their depressive syndrome.

- **Behavior therapy** to help the resident change behavior by using alternative coping strategies, and to reduce anxiety by using relaxation and desensitization techniques. This treatment is indicated in residents who are cognitively intact but less comfortable with talking therapies, and especially for those with prominent anxiety and attention- or medication-seeking behavior.

- **Supportive interpersonal therapy** to help the resident strengthen positive self-esteem. This treatment may be beneficial even if some mild cognitive impairment is present, and is suited to residents who express hopelessness. Some education about the nature of depressive illness and its treatability is frequently useful and can be incorporated into this modality.

- **Supportive group therapy** to help the resident reduce loneliness and isolation and the sense that one's problems are unique and therefore insoluble. This treatment will be of the greatest benefit to residents who have experienced losses and who need help with socialization.

- **Short-term psychodynamic therapy** to help the resident explore the antecedents of feelings and behavior, with the goal of inducing a structural change of personality and altering ways of thinking that perpetuate the depressive symptoms. This treatment requires insight and may not be helpful in the acute stages of a major depressive episode. However, it may be very useful for residents who have recurrent episodes of illness and who appear to follow patterns of self-defeating behaviors that may precipitate or exacerbate depressive syndromes.

- **Other therapies** that straddle the boundary between traditional psychotherapies and activities programs. These include movement therapy, art therapy, and other forms of expressive therapy. They may provide a benefit through the opportunity to engage in behavior that is positively reinforcing, or through the chance to explore feelings that may be more difficult to express verbally. These therapies may be especially useful for residents with mild to moderate dementia or aphasia.

Initiate Biologic Therapies

The biologic therapies used to treat depression are antidepressant medication or electroconvulsive therapy (ECT). The following subsections discuss these therapies.

Antidepressants

Many studies indicate that antidepressants are effective in the treatment of acute depression, and most of the antidepressants are thought to be equally effective in the elderly. Decisions about which drug to use depend on the side-effect profile of the drug and considerations about individual residents to determine which side effects might be least tolerated.

In most cases, consult a psychiatrist before using antidepressant medication, and ongoing psychiatric follow-up is recommended during this form of treatment. The following guidelines discuss the rational use of antidepressants in the elderly. Consult a geriatric pharmacology text for more detailed information about drug side effects, interactions, blood levels, and so forth. (*See* the reference section for more information.)

- The initial drug should be a tricyclic antidepressant, one of the selective serotonin reuptake inhibitors, or one of the newer agents that inhibit the reuptake of both serotonin and norepinephrine. Residents in good medical health with no contra-indications to the use of a tricyclic may be started at night on nortriptyline, 10 to 25 mg, or desipramine, 10 to 25 mg. These drugs have the advantage of known thera-peutic blood levels that can be used to guide therapy. In general, the tricyclics with a sec-ondary amine structure (i.e., those previ-ously mentioned) have less severe anticho-linergic and hypotensive side effects than the tertiary amines such as amitriptyline, imipramine, or doxepin, which generally should be avoided. Among the selective serotonin reuptake inhibitors, fluoxetine, sertraline, or paroxetine may be used. The side effects of these drugs include gastro-intestinal symptoms, insomnia, agitation, and anxiety. Newer antidepressants such as venlafaxine and nefazodone also may be useful.

- Medication trials must be of adequate dos-age to be effective. Side effects often limit the achievement of an adequate dose and require careful monitoring. Start with low drug doses (one third to one half the usual young adult starting dose) and increase them slowly at intervals of at least 5 days.

- Medication trials must be of adequate dura-tion to be effective. In general, the elderly often require trials of 6 to 8 weeks for re-sponse, and may need up to 12 weeks.

- If the resident has a partial response to the first antidepressant trial, try the addition of an augmenting agent such as thyroid re-placement (triiodothyronine-T3) or lithium. A partial response may be defined as remis-sion of some symptoms, or a reduction in severity of some symptoms, without a com-plete remission. Continue the augmenting agent and the antidepressant for another 1 to 3 weeks.

- If the resident fails to respond to the first antidepressant (failure to respond is defined as minimal or no improvement in any symp-toms), reconsider a diagnostic review for the possibility of comorbid conditions (psy-chiatric, medical, social, environmental) that might be interfering with treatment response and that might require therapy. If none are identified, discontinue the antidepressant medication, and start a trial of an alterna-tive agent selected from a different class of medications. If a tricyclic was used first, try a serotonin reuptake inhibitor or one of the newer agents. Again, after an adequate trial, augmentation may be attempted if there has been a partial response. If there is no re-sponse, other alternatives may include the use of monoamine oxidase inhibitors (e.g., phenelzine, tranylcypromine), bupropion, stimulants such as methylphenidate, or ECT. Methylphenidate has the advantage of a rapid onset of action. Many of the antide-pressants cannot be given concurrently, and may require a period of discontinuation before starting another medication. Obtain a consultation if a change from one antide-pressant to another must be made.

- Concomitant delusions usually require a combination treatment with antipsychotic agents. Always treat delusions in the pres-ence of depression. Some residents with dementia who are not depressed may have misperceptions of their environment that are due to their cognitive impairment and are more accurately called *illusions* rather than delusions. Illusions per se do not always require pharmacologic treatment.

- Frequently assess for side effects, and stop the trials if the side effects are not tolerable or manageable with supportive measures. In practice, one would assess this risk-ben-efit ratio the same way one would assess the depressive syndrome itself. To the ex-tent that the resident can convey a discom-fort from side effects that significantly com-promise the benefit from the medication, that assessment should be relied upon. In cases in which the resident cannot make such a judgment, collateral information from other sources will be necessary. In particular, be alert to orthostatic hypotension, sedation, and anticholinergic side effects, including delirium. Peripheral anticholinergic symptoms include constipation, blurred vision, urinary retention, and tachycardia. A bulk laxative may relieve constipation.

- Once improvement has occurred, continuation of maintenance medication is required. The maintenance dose should be the same as that required to achieve remission. An attempt may be made to discontinue the medication after 6 months for a first episode of depression, and after 12 to 18 months for a second episode. Chronic treatment should be considered if the resident has had three or more depressive episodes in late life alone.

Electroconvulsive Therapy

For severe, life-threatening depression, or if medication trials cannot be tolerated because of side effects, consider ECT. *Life-threatening depression* is present if it results in the refusal to eat or drink or leads to active suicidal ideation. The decision to use ECT may be reached at any time during the course of medication treatment trials. ECT has the advantage of working more rapidly than antidepressants in many cases, and of avoiding the side effects caused by antidepressants. ECT places stress on the cardiovascular system and may be relatively contraindicated in residents with recent myocardial damage. The use of ECT requires thorough evaluation and clearance by an internist and anesthesiologist before this form of treatment is begun.

PREVENTION

Nursing home staff may minimize some of the psychosocial and environmental risk factors for depression by creating a milieu in which the resident can receive social support and maximize functional independence. The following are examples of strategies for reducing risk:

- Facilitate the new admission's adjustment to the nursing home by orienting the resident to surroundings and unit routines. Help the resident enhance the network of social support by introducing him or her to peers and inviting him or her to social and recreational activities. Involve the resident in setting up his or her room to make it as homelike and functionally accommodating as possible. Designate one staff member to help each resident through the transition process. (See Chapters 15 and 30, Psychosocial Well-Being and Activities Programming, respectively, for more information.)

- Assist the resident to be as independent as possible. Associated with independence is the opportunity to have a sense of control in one's daily life. Staff can enhance a resident's sense of control by helping him or her prepare for an anticipated change (e.g., discharge, new staff), involving him or her in health care decisions, and offering choices (e.g., dietary, selection of clothing, timing of routines). (*See* Chapter 29, ADL Rehabilitation, for more information.)

- Help the resident pursue and maintain involvement in activities that are meaningful to him or her. Look for ways to adapt the activity to the resident's cognitive and physical skills if necessary.

- Help the resident achieve a sense of continuity in life by facilitating connections with the past. Reminiscing, celebrating religious and cultural traditions, looking at and talking about family pictures, and family involvement in care are some ways to enhance continuity.

- Anticipate the resident's having a grief reaction to loss (e.g., death of another resident; transfer of a favorite nursing assistant) and provide support for the natural grief process.

CASE EXAMPLES

The following case examples describe two depression scenarios.

Case Example 1

Mr. S. has been a resident of the nursing home for 2 years. Five years ago he was diagnosed with Alzheimer's disease. He had a successful adjustment to his residential unit and made new friends easily. However, over the past few months staff have noticed him becoming more frustrated and anxious with slowly increasing cognitive impairment. His difficulty is primarily with word finding and learning new things in new situations. Although he is not always able to find the exact words he wants to say, he is generally able to advocate in his own behalf and ask his physician pertinent questions about his medical condition. His memory for old events is good, and he enjoys reminiscing with family and friends about old times. He maintains familiar daily routines, including twice daily walks outdoors in good weather. However, he becomes anxious with any change in routine (e.g., float nurses, clinic appointments).

On three occasions in the past month, Mr. S. expressed sadness that his mind is going. He becomes tearful at these times and ventures back to his room to nap for a while. However, he is easily cheered up and re-engaged in life at the facility. The primary care team discussed these changes and referred him to an expressive therapy men's group to help him deal with his cognitive losses.

This case describes an elderly man who is aware of increasing deficits and responds with anxiety and depressed mood. However, he does not have a major depression. Current care plans should focus on prevention of major depression.

Case Example 2

Mrs. F., a 70-year-old woman, has been a resident of the facility for 1 month. Staff no-

ticed a deterioration in her behavior during this time. Mrs. F. is alert and oriented in all spheres. She has no deficits in either short- or long-term memory. She organizes her daily routines, chooses to keep to herself, and remains in her room except for meals. She does not socialize with other residents who she complains are much too old and sick for her. Her appetite has been poor since admission and she has lost 5 pounds.

Mrs. F.'s speech is intact but because she has a tendency to be agitated she does not always communicate clearly with her caregivers and becomes frustrated. To understand her speech, staff must remind her to slow down and speak more clearly. Likewise, Mrs. F.'s anxiety prohibits her from fully understanding others. She has a tendency to misperceive the intent of messages, believes that she is disliked, and needs constant reassurance. When she is severely agitated, the staff provide her with only simple and direct messages until she is more relaxed and better able to comprehend.

Mrs. F. is angry and constantly complains to the staff that she was dumped in the home by her ungrateful daughter. Lately, during her daughter's visits, Mrs. F. berates her mercilessly to the point that she leaves in tears.

During the past week, Mrs. F. has been noisy, constantly calling out for someone to help her or get her something. She wakes up many times during the night and has difficulty getting back to sleep. She has several daily conflicts with caregivers in which she is verbally abusive. On one occasion during the last 7 days she threw a brush at her nurse assistant and told her to "get the hell out of here and leave me alone." The staff do not always understand what Mrs. F. wants when she gets frustrated. Then, after blowing off steam, she becomes very tearful and full of remorse and is not easily cheered up. She says that she is useless and would "rather be dead than stuck in this place."

A geropsychiatrist was consulted and made the diagnosis of depression. He met with Mrs. F. and her daughter to discuss treatment options. Mrs. F. was started on an antidepressant trial of nortriptyline, 10 mg every night. The dosage was gradually increased to 40 mg every night and her medication blood level stabilized at 75 ng/mL. She received weekly psychiatric visits for individual supportive therapy. As her symptoms lessened, individual therapy was discontinued and Mrs. F. began group therapy for increased socialization and support.

As Mrs. F. improved, she was better able to deal with her anger and grief over her admission to the nursing home. At dinner one night she met an old friend and accepted her invitation to attend a unit social. With the support of a recreation therapist Mrs. F. slowly became more involved in facility life.

14
Psychotropic Drugs

Barry Fogel, MD

A majority of nursing home residents receive at least one psychotropic drug during their stay. Until recently, these drugs were often prescribed to nursing home residents without the benefit of psychiatric diagnoses to justify their use, and without systematic monitoring to minimize their adverse effects. The passage of the Nursing Home Reform Act, implemented in October 1990, was influenced significantly by a mounting body of evidence suggesting widespread psychotropic drug misuse in nursing homes. The law now requires that in nursing homes receiving Medicare or Medicaid reimbursement, psychotropic agents must be used in accordance with a diagnosis and resident care plan determined by a comprehensive interdisciplinary assessment of the resident at the time of admission and at least every 3 months thereafter. It also empowers the Health Care Financing Administration (HCFA) to set minimum essential standards for nursing home operators and surveyors regarding the use of psychotropic drugs and to impose penalties on nursing homes found to be prescribing them inappropriately.

While it is relatively easy to identify cases of gross drug misuse, it is more difficult to specify generally applicable guidelines for the appropriate use of psychotropic drugs. Primarily, this is because of the vast individual differences in drug metabolism and drug response in an elderly nursing home population. Appropriate dosing requires that drug dosages be individualized in every case.

The difficulties associated with psychotropic drug use have both a clinical and an administrative dimension. Clinical challenges arise because no psychotropic drug is without risks. Thoughtful decisions must be made about whether to use psychotropic drugs at all, which drug or drugs to choose, the duration of treatment, and how to monitor the resident for both therapeutic benefit and potential side effects. Clear thinking about a strategy for monitoring can protect the resident not only against more severe adverse events, but also against undertreatment or needless continuation of ineffective treatment. The administrative challenge in psychotropic drug therapy is to ensure that proper procedures for consent, therapeutic decision making, and outcomes monitoring are carried out and documented properly. This provides the basis for both effective risk management and continuous quality improvement regarding psychotropic drug prescription practices.

OVERVIEW

Psychotropic drugs (i.e., antidepressants, antianxiety and hypnotic drugs, and neuroleptics) are among the most frequently prescribed agents in the nursing home setting. Studies of nursing home drug usage suggest that more than half of all residents receive psychotropic medications at some time during their stay.

The potential for drug side effects in frail, chronically debilitated residents with multiple disease conditions and physical disabilities is high. Side effects may impair physical, mental, and social function, and can be difficult to differentiate from primary disease states or worsening of the mental or behavioral problem for which the drug was prescribed. Adverse effects commonly include central nervous system (CNS) problems (e.g., drowsiness, confusion, unsteady gait, motor agitation) and involuntary movements, such as tardive dyskinesia, that can compromise eating and social interaction. The potential for side effects increases when the older person is sick or taking other medications that may interact adversely with the psychotropic drugs.

Despite the special problems and expertise that is required to prescribe and monitor these drugs appropriately, they are widely overused and misused in the nursing home setting. At the same time, they are underused in certain situations in which their benefit has been established. Overuse and misuse occur primarily among demented, agitated residents in connection with attempts by the staff to control behavior. Underuse typically occurs with quietly depressed or psychotic residents who may not have been evaluated adequately and could benefit from receiving an appropriate psychotropic drug.

The use of any psychotropic drug in elderly residents requires striking a careful balance. This class of medications has done much to relieve the suffering of elderly individuals who have incapacitating mental disorders such as depression, schizophrenia, and paranoid psychosis of later life. These disorders are not normal concomitants of aging, but rather are diagnosable and treatable illnesses. Therefore, psychotropic drugs can be a valuable component of the total treatment approach to the psychiatrically impaired older person.

However, like any treatment modality, psychotropic drugs can be misused. They are often used as a substitute for a therapeutic relationship between the health care professional and the resident. Sometimes they are used as the only treatment modality in situations in which other interventions should be tried first or in conjunction with drug treatment. They are often used before a comprehensive medical, psychological, and social assessment of the resident is made.

There is an inevitable trade-off between symptom control and side effects. The appropriate weighing of risks versus benefits must be resident-specific, and functional status—including performance in activities of daily living (ADLs), social interaction, and cognitive state–should be used as a criterion for assessing these trade-offs. Those drug therapies that enhance a resident's overall function are usually appropriate, even if some side effects are encountered.

IDENTIFYING THE RESIDENT IN NEED OF INTERVENTION

The following residents require an individualized treatment plan:

- Any resident already on a psychotropic drug regimen in which no treatment plan was initially provided
- Any resident on a medication who is showing functional decline, cognitive decline, or possible adverse side effects
- Any resident failing to improve over a time period appropriate to the drug and indication
- Any resident receiving long-term psycho-

tropic drug therapy; conduct reassessments no less than twice a year

In addition, reassess psychotropic drug use in any situation in which the resident shows symptoms that may be attributed to the well-known side effects of the drug being administered. To identify these side effects from specific items on the Minimum Data Set (MDS), see Table 14-1.

After determining that a resident needs a therapeutic plan of care for psychotropic drug use, but before constructing the plan, the clinician should collect and assess six data categories of information, which are discussed in the following sections.

History of Psychotropic Drug Use

To obtain a history of psychotropic drug use, review:

- The reason the drug was prescribed
- The sequence of dosage changes
- Other drugs given concomitantly
- The relationship of current symptoms to the timing of drug initiation or dosage changes

Response of Target Symptoms or Disorder to Treatment

Assess how the resident's mental or behavioral symptoms have changed since the beginning of treatment. For diagnosed mental disorders such as depression, disease-specific

Table 14-1. Possible Psychotropic Drug Side Effects and the MDS Indicators for Them

Possible Side Effect	Indicators That Adverse Side Effects May be Present
Orthostatic hypotension (decline >20 mm Hg in systolic blood pressure when changing position from supine to sitting or standing)	Resident is on a neuroleptic and/or antidepressant and also has hypotension, dizziness/vertigo, syncope, or falls
Movement disorder (antipsychotic-induced)	Resident is taking a neuroleptic and also has a loss of voluntary limb movement, unsteady gait, loss of ability to position, balance, or turn, repetitive movement (motor agitation), Parkinson's disease, tardive dyskinesia, or a chewing or swallowing problem
Gait disturbance (other than antipsychotic-induced)	Resident is taking an antianxiety or hypnotic drug and has poor balance, unsteady gait, difficulty in positioning or turning, dizziness or vertigo, or falls
Cognitive or behavioral impairment	Resident is taking any psychotropic drug and has (a) delirium or disordered thinking, depression, hallucinations, or a major change in ADLs or self-performance; and/or (b) deterioration in cognition, communication, mood, or behavior
Anticholinergic effects (dry mouth, constipation, hypotension, visual blurring, urinary retention)	Resident is taking any psychotropic drug and has constipation, fecal impaction, or urinary retention

rating scales such as the Hamilton Depression Rating Scale are available. For behavioral symptoms such as aggressive behavior, there are symptom-specific scales such as the Overt Aggression Scale. For mood and behavior in general, use the MDS scales for Mood, Behavior, and Psychosocial Well-Being. Table 14-2 lists some common, well-accepted scales for measuring symptoms of mental disorders.

Current Drug List

This drug list includes all drugs, both psychotropic and nonpsychotropic, whether given continually or intermittently. The list should be screened for potential drug interactions. There are two kinds of screening for interactions, one done most conveniently by nursing staff, the other by the physician or pharmacist. The nursing staff should consider the problem of multiple drugs with additive or more-than-additive side effects. The following examples show common situations of this type:

- **Sedation:** Temazepam (or another benzodiazepine) for sleep plus propranolol (or another centrally acting antihypertensive) for

high blood pressure plus cimetidine for esophageal reflux
- **Hypotension:** Hydrochlorothiazide (or another diuretic) for hypertension plus nortriptyline (or another tricyclic) for depression plus a nitrate for angina pectoris
- **Anticholinergic effects:** Imipramine (or another tricyclic) for depression plus diphenhydramine (or another antihistamine) for allergies
- **Dopamine blocking effects:** Haloperidol (or another neuroleptic) for hallucinations plus metoclopramide for esophageal reflux
- **Insomnia:** Fluoxetine (or another stimulating antidepressant) plus theophylline for chronic obstructive pulmonary disease plus prednisone for polymyalgia rheumatica

The other type of drug interaction screening consists of checking, either manually or by computer, the resident's drug list against a standard reference on drug interactions. The reference section describes a partial list of references on this topic. This check is for more specific interactions between particular drugs, based on their metabolism or chemical properties, rather than the more general screening

Table 14-2. Possible Psychotropic Drug Side Effects and the MDS Indicators for Them

Symptom/Syndrome	Rating Scale	Source
Depression	Hamilton Depression Rating Scale; Geriatric Depression Scale; Cornell	Hamilton M (1960) Yesavage et al (1983) Spitzer et al (1978)
Anxiety	Hamilton-Anxiety; Zung Anxiety Scale	Hamilton M (1959) Zung WWK (1971)
Psychosis	Brief Psychiatric Rating Scale; Columbia University Scale	Overall and Gorman (1962) Devanand et al (1992)
Aggression/behavior problem	Overt Aggression Scale; Nursing Home Problem Behavior Scale	Yudofsky et al (1986) Ray et al (1992)

for overlapping drug actions previously described.

Vital Signs

A check of vital signs includes an accurate temperature and orthostatic blood pressure and pulse. The temperature is particularly important for residents taking neuroleptics, since these drugs can affect temperature regulation, leading to hypothermia or high fever. Measure the pulse and blood pressure when the resident is lying down and remeasure after he or she has been standing for 1 and 3 minutes. Note whether the resident experiences dizziness, vertigo, or other discomfort after standing.

Gait Abnormalities and Involuntary Movements

Observe the resident's gait or determine what prevents the resident from walking without assistance if that is the case. Note involuntary movements of the hands, trunk, mouth, and face both at rest and when the resident is walking or doing a purposeful activity with the hands.

When observing gait and movements in a resident receiving neuroleptics, look for signs of parkinsonism (decreased arm swing, slow movement, difficulty with turning and stopping, rest tremor), as well as dyskinetic movements of the face or limbs that may represent tardive dyskinesia. Also, if the resident on neuroleptics continually fidgets and cannot keep still, the likely cause is akathisia, another movement disorder commonly caused by neuroleptics. The presence of any of these movement disorders is a reason to seriously consider reduction of neuroleptic dosage. Another option is to use a lower-potency neuroleptic or risperidone, which will have fewer extrapyramidal side effects. Thioridazine (Mellaril) has the fewest extrapyramidal side effects of the typical neuroleptics.

When dosage reduction or drug substitution is not feasible or when the movement disorder is so uncomfortable as to require immediate treatment, specific drug therapy is available for parkinsonism and akathisia (the latter may respond to beta blockers).

Rest tremors, muscular rigidity, abnormal posturing, shuffling gait, and other signs of drug-induced parkinsonism are best treated with antiparkinson drugs. The dopamine agonists amantadine (100 mg every day or twice a day) and bromocriptine (1.25 to 2.5 mg/day) are best for rigidity and akinesia, but may cause nausea or hypotension. The anticholinergic drugs benztropine (1 to 2 mg/day) or trihexyphenidyl (2 to 5 mg/day) are most effective for rest tremor, but can cause delirium and produce the full range of other anticholinergic effects. For akathisia, i.e., restlessness and the inability to sit still, the most effective treatments are beta blockers (e.g., propranolol, 20 mg three times a day) or benzodiazepines (e.g., lorazepam, 0.5 mg three times a day). The medical contraindications to these drugs are well known: bronchospasm or aggravation of heart failure are the most serious risks of beta blockers, and ataxia and falls are the major risk of benzodiazepines in this setting.

For residents on antidepressants, antianxiety drugs, or mood-stabilizing drugs (thymoleptics), the most frequent gait problem is ataxia, or unsteadiness of gait. In extreme cases the resident staggers or lurches; in mild cases the difficulty is noted on turns, on stopping and starting, on responding to a gentle push by the examiner, or on walking heel-to-toe. In all cases the appropriate response is to reduce the dosage or to taper and discontinue the responsible drug.

Antidepressants, thymoleptics, and stimulants can cause or aggravate action tremors shaking of the hands on purposeful activity such as writing or eating with a fork. Residents with preexisting familial essential tremor are at the highest risk for developing this side effect. Dosage reduction or drug substitution is the usual response, but if the resident is doing exceedingly well on the drug in other respects, suppress the tremor with a benzodiazepine or a beta blocker. (Note that using drugs to control drug side effects introduces new risks, so the decision to do it is best made with input from a psychiatric consultant who can assist in balancing the risks and benefits.)

Resident's Subjective Impressions and Observations by Family

If the resident is not profoundly demented or unable to communicate, ask for subjective impressions about the drug being taken and its positive and negative effects. This information can help to confirm the presence of side effects and to weigh the positive versus negative drug actions. For example, akathisia is most easily diagnosed when the resident describes a subjective sense of urgency to continually move the limbs in the absence of some other motive for moving, or a particularly great anxiety. Or, a resident recovering from a profound and frightening major depression may be willing to accept side effects such as constipation or dry mouth, rather than risk a relapse of a horrifying mood state. When residents are seriously cognitively impaired or have difficulty communicating, observations by family members or significant others may substitute for the resident's subjective impressions of positive and negative drug effects. Family members are particularly likely to notice changes in residents' mood, level of comfort, and spontaneous behavior. Family impressions supplement residents' subjective impressions when residents are mentally reliable, but the resident's judgment of benefit should take precedence if there is a disagreement.

Modifying Therapy to Reduce Side Effects or Improve Therapeutic Response

After reassessing the resident's current psychotropic drug treatment, there are several options available to the clinician:
- Make no change in the therapy.
- Increase or decrease the dose.
- Discontinue the drug.
- Switch to another psychotropic drug within the same therapeutic class.
- Switch to a different class of psychotropic drug.
- Add a second drug to augment the therapeutic response (e.g., adding lithium when a resident has partially responded to an antidepressant).
- Add a drug to mitigate a side effect.
- Modify therapy for an underlying medical condition.
- Start or change nonpharmacologic therapy for the mental disorder or problem behavior.

The choice among these therapeutic options depends on how much benefit the resident has obtained from the drug therapy, what potential drug-related problems have arisen, and how much the drug-related problems are specific to a particular drug, a particular chemical grouping, or a particular drug class.

Choosing, Monitoring, and Assessing Psychotropic Drug Therapy

When a new psychotropic drug is started, the clinicians should clearly identify:
- What disorder or symptoms are to be treated
- How the response to treatment is to be measured
- How long a trial is reasonable
- How the dosage will be adjusted
- What side effects must be anticipated
- How the resident will be monitored for those side effects

In addition, the clinicians, resident, and family should agree on the process for deciding whether a particular balance of benefits and side effects is acceptable, or whether alternative therapies should be tried. If a resident is already on a psychotropic drug, the same questions must be asked.

CLASSES OF PSYCHOTROPIC DRUGS

There are five classes of psychotropic drugs with which the clinician should be familiar:
- Neuroleptics
- Antidepressants
- Antianxiety drugs
- Mood-stabilizing drugs
- Stimulants

This section discusses these medications and their side effects.

Neuroleptics

Neuroleptics, also known as antipsychotic drugs or major tranquilizers, are a large class of drugs that share the property of blocking dopamine receptors in the CNS. Well-known neuroleptics include haloperidol and thioridazine. Several widely prescribed neuroleptics belong to the chemical class of phenothiazines. However, not all phenothiazines are neuroleptics, and many widely prescribed neuroleptics are not phenothiazines.

All neuroleptics have side effects on the motor system, which are usually referred to as *extrapyramidal side effects*. The extrapyramidal motor system has a major role in the control of gait, posture, and the coordination of movement. The motor side effects are due to the consequences of blocking dopamine receptors on the function of this system. Extrapyramidal side effects include:
- Parkinsonism
- Tremor
- Akathisia (the inability to remain still)
- Akinesia (a lack of voluntary movement)
- Dystonia (involuntary posturing--experi-

enced by the resident as muscle spasm)
- Dyskinesia (repetitive involuntary movements)

Some recently released neuroleptics have substantially less effect on the motor system than the conventional agents. The only ones currently available in the United States at this time are clozapine and risperidone.

Neuroleptics also have nonmotor side effects, including sedation, anticholinergic effects, and orthostatic hypotension. In general, the agents with relatively fewer motor side effects have relatively more nonmotor side effects, and vice versa. A specific agent should be selected that minimizes the side effects that are most problematic for a given resident. Table 14-3 displays the potencies and side effect profiles for commonly prescribed neuroleptics.

Choosing and Monitoring a Neuroleptic

Conventional neuroleptics usually cause detectable side effects on the motor system. Therefore, only prescribe them for psychosis or for dangerous or disabling levels of agitation, and then use the lowest effective dose. Low-potency neuroleptics, such as thioridazine and chlorpromazine, have the least motor side effects, but they have the most sedation, anticholinergic, and hypotensive effects. High-potency neuroleptics, such as haloperidol and fluphenazine, usually cause some detectable motor side effects, but are relatively free of anticholinergic and hypotensive effects. The high-potency agents are approximately 50 times as potent on a milligram basis as the low-potency agents. Therefore, one milligram of haloperidol is roughly equivalent to 50 milligrams of thioridazine.

Because of their lesser systemic toxicity, the high-potency agents are generally preferred for treating psychosis in frail elderly persons. Risperidone, with its low systemic toxicity, mild motor system effects, and high antipsy-

Table 14-3. Relative Incidence of Side Effects of Neuroleptic Drugs

Generic Name	Trade Name	Approximate Dosage Range (mg/day)	Sedation	Hypotension	Extrapryamidal Symptoms	Anticholinergic Symptoms
Chlorpromazine*	Thorazine Chlor PZ	10-300	Marked	Marked	Moderate	Marked**
Chlorprothixene*	Taractan	10-300	Marked	Marked	Moderate	Marked**
Thioridazine*	Mellaril	10-300	Marked	Marked	Mild-Mod.	Moderate
Acetophenazine	Tindal	10-60	Moderate	Moderate	Moderate	Moderate
Perphenazine	Trilafon	4-32	Moderate	Moderate	Moderate	Moderate
Loxapine	Loxitane	5-100	Moderate	Moderate	Moderate	Moderate
Molindone	Moban	5-100	Moderate	Moderate	Moderate	Moderate
Trifluperazine	Stelazine	4-20	Moderate	Moderate	Mod.-marked	Mod.-mild
Thiothixene	Navane	4-20	Moderate	Moderate	Mod.-marked	Mod.-mild
Fluphenazine	Prolixin	0.25-6	Mild	Mild	Marked***	Mild
Haloperidol	Haldol	0.25-6	Mild	Mild	Marked***	Mild
Risperidone	Risperdol	0.25-6	Moderate	Moderate	None-Mild	Mild

* Has quinidine-like cardiac effects; contraindicated if resident has heart block of greater than first degree.

** Contraindicated in residents with narrow-angle glaucoma or lower urinary tract obstruction.

*** Contraindicated if there is a history of parkinsonism or severe rigidity with neuroleptics.

chotic potency, may soon emerge as the drug of choice. However, when the primary indication for neuroleptics is agitation rather than psychosis, thioridazine occasionally may work better because of its sedative and antianxiety actions. If the resident had no significant prior history of heart disease, hypotension, or intolerance of anticholinergic drugs, first try thioridazine. If the thioridazine works at a dose lower than 100 mg per day, continue it. If a higher dose appears necessary, use a high-potency agent.

Begin a neuroleptic at the lower end of the recommended ranges for elderly persons, and do not increase it more frequently than weekly for elective therapy. If an acute dosage of a neuroleptic is needed for a behavioral emergency, start a lower and more deliberate dosage when the emergency is over.

Since neuroleptic side effects may develop over weeks, check the resident on neuroleptics at least weekly for involuntary movements, gait problems, cognitive changes, and diminished ADL performance. Monitor residents receiving low-potency agents for anticholinergic effects (constipation, urinary retention, blurred vision, and other symptoms) and for orthostatic hypotension (see Chapters 18 and 1, Falls and Vital Signs, respectively, for more information).

If tremor, muscular rigidity, and a fever develop in a resident on antipsychotic drugs, the resident may have the neuroleptic malignant syndrome. This is a life-threatening condition that also includes skeletal muscle breakdown, elevated creatinine phosphokinase, unstable vital signs, and the risk of renal failure or shock. Immediately refer the resident for acute medical care.

Modifying Therapy to Reduce Side Effects or to Improve Therapeutic Response

The following sections discuss the common side effects of neuroleptics and how to improve the therapeutic response to these drugs.

NEUROLEPTIC-INDUCED HYPOTENSION

Neuroleptic-induced hypotension is usually caused by a low-potency phenothiazine neuroleptic such as thioridazine or chlorpromazine. If the resident's symptoms are well controlled by one of these drugs, the first step is dosage reduction. If the symptoms are not well controlled, switch to a higher-potency drug such as fluphenazine or haloperidol, or risperidone at an equivalent dose (i.e., about one fiftieth the milligram daily dose of the low-potency agent).

If an excellent clinical response to a low-potency neuroleptic justifies an attempt to continue it despite hypotension at the minimum effective dose, other steps to manage hypotension may be taken, as described for antidepressant-associated hypotension. If these are unsuccessful, switch the resident to a high-potency drug. If the clinical response to the higher-potency drug is less satisfactory, obtain a psychiatric consultation about other drug treatments.

NEUROLEPTIC-INDUCED MOVEMENT DISORDER

Neuroleptics cause a wide range of movement disorders, which can emerge during treatment and persist or become worse after treatment is discontinued. The disorders that develop late and persist are called *tardive movement disorders*, and include tardive dyskinesia, tardive akathisia, and tardive dystonia.

For all neuroleptic-induced movement disorders, the best approach is to reduce the dose of the drug or discontinue it altogether. If the resident is on a conventional neuroleptic, try substituting risperidone. When the drug is of substantial benefit but causes a distressing or functionally significant movement disorder at the minimum effective dose, try adding a second drug to control the movement disorder.

NEUROLEPTIC-INDUCED GAIT DISTURBANCE

Neuroleptic-induced gait disturbance usually is due either to parkinsonism or to orthostatic hypotension. Manage these problems according to the guidelines for movement disorders.

Antidepressants

Antidepressant drugs are most often used to treat major depression, but they are increasingly being used for a number of other psychiatric and nonpsychiatric indications, including:

- Dysthymia (minor depression)
- Anxiety disorders
- Obsessive-compulsive disorder
- Eating disorders
- Chronic pain syndromes
- Migraine
- Irritable bowel syndrome

There are several classes of antidepressants, including:
- Tricyclic antidepressants
- Serotonin reuptake inhibitors
- Monoamine oxidase inhibitors

All antidepressants have approximately the same efficacy in the treatment of major depression, but may have different efficacy for other indications. Also, a resident with major depression may respond well to one drug but not to another. Each class of antidepressant drug has a distinctive set of side effects, and within classes there are more subtle but clinically relevant differences among drugs. For example, the tricyclic antidepressants, but not the other classes, have substantial quinidine-like effects on the heart, and are not safe for residents with higher degrees of heart block. Within the tricyclics, the secondary amine tricyclics nortriptyline and desipramine cause less sedation, orthostatic hypotension, and anticholinergic effects than the tertiary amines amitriptyline and imipramine. Table 14-4 lists antidepressants with their usual dosages and side effect profiles.

Choosing and Monitoring an Antidepressant

The choice of an antidepressant begins by ruling out drugs that are strongly contraindicated for the resident, such as a tricyclic antidepressant in a resident with second-degree heart block and no pacemaker, or bupropion in a resident with epilepsy. (These strong contraindications are highlighted in Table 14-4.) Next, consider the symptoms of depression that cause the resident the most distress or disability, and identify the drugs most likely to relieve those symptoms early in treatment. Finally, choose a drug that is least likely to cause side effects that the resident will tolerate poorly. In the event that this process leaves no options, a psychiatric consultation is advisable to balance the risks and benefits of treatments expected to have both therapeutic and adverse effects.

When the major symptoms of depression are weight loss, anorexia, and insomnia, first consider the tricyclic antidepressants. A second choice is trazodone if the resident is very intolerant of anticholinergic effects. When the major symptoms are irritability, moodiness, and negative ruminations, consider a serotonin reuptake inhibitor. Venlafaxine appears to be suitable for both symptom profiles. When the major symptom is apathy or lethargy, consider a stimulating antidepressant such as bupropion or fluoxetine.

The following side effects are common:

- Anticholinergic and hypotensive effects with the tricyclics
- Hypotension and sedation with trazodone
- Agitation and gastrointestinal symptoms with the serotonin reuptake inhibitors
- Agitation and insomnia with bupropion
- Nervousness or sedation with venlafaxine

Monitor residents on a regular basis for the common side effects of the class of drug they

Table 14-4. Relative Side Effects of Antidepressants

Drug	Approximate geriatric dosage range mg/day	Sedation	Hypotension	Anticholinergic Side Effects	Altered Cardiac Rate and Rhythm
Tertiary Amines					
Imipramine	10-150	Mild	Moderate	Mod-strong**	Moderate*
Doxepin	10-150	Mod.-strong	Moderate	Strong**	Moderate*
Amitriptyline	10-150	Strong	Moderate	Very strong**	Strong*
Trimipramine	10-150	Strong	Moderate	Strong**	Strong*
Clomipramine	10-150	Strong	Strong	Strong**	Strong*
Secondary Amines					
Desipramine	10-150	Mild	Mild-moderate	Mild	Mild*
Nortriptyline	10-150	Mild	Mild	Moderate**	Mild*
Amoxapine	10-150	Mild	Moderate	Moderate**	Moderate*
Protriptyline	5- 15	Mild	Moderate	Strong**	Moderate*
Maprotiline	10-150	Mod.-strong	Moderate	Moderate**	Mild
Atypical					
Trazodone	25-300	Moderate	Moderate	Mild (except dry mouth)	Mild-moderate
Bupropion	75-225	Unusual	None	Mild	None
Venlafaxine	25-150	Variable	Occasional	Mild	None
Selective Serotonin Reuptake Inhibitors					
Fluoxetine	5- 20	Unusual	None	None	None
Paroxetine	5- 20	Variable	None	None	None
Sertraline	12.5-100	Variable	None	None	None

* Contraindicated if the resident has heart block more severe than first degree.

** Contraindicated in residents with narrow angle glaucoma or lower urinary tract obstruction are given. For example, for residents on tricyclics, monitor for bowel and bladder dysfunction and orthostatic hypotension. In addition, frequently ask the resident and family about any new symptoms or any problems they attribute to the drug. Pose this as a question about any effects, positive or negative. If therapy is not urgent, start with a low dose, and make sure that there are no troublesome side effects before increasing to the next higher dose. In the severely depressed resident, general somatic distress may make it impossible to separate side effects from symptoms of depressive illness. In this case, dosage titration should follow a gradual, predetermined schedule, and a combination of physical and functional assessment should be the main indicator of drug safety.

Obtain an electrocardiogram (ECG) before initiating tricyclic antidepressant therapy, and obtain a follow-up ECG after the resident has been established on a therapeutic dose to identify prolongation of QT interval.

Modifying Therapy to Reduce the Side Effects or Improve Therapeutic Response

The following sections discuss the common side effects of antidepressants and how to improve the therapeutic response to these drugs.

ANTIDEPRESSANT-ASSOCIATED HYPOTENSION

Antidepressant-associated hypotension is seen with tricyclics, with trazodone, and occasionally with venlafaxine. Among the tricyclics, imipramine and amitriptyline have the most hypotensive effect, and nortriptyline has the least. While switching to a less hypotensive agent should be considered first, it is not always the best choice. Some residents have a better antidepressant response to tricyclics than to newer antidepressants, and others may be intolerant of alternatives for

other reasons. In particular, residents with marked anorexia, insomnia, and agitation may do worse on bupropion or a serotonin reuptake inhibitor. These drugs depress appetite and can cause difficulty falling asleep.

If a tricyclic appears to be the drug of choice for a particular resident, but hypotension is a problem, reasonable options include:

- Switching to nortriptyline if the resident is not already taking it
- Reducing the dose gradually, especially if the resident's depression has already remitted
- Reducing or discontinuing other drugs, such as diuretics or antihypertensives, that also cause orthostatic hypotension

Salt intake may be liberalized, and blocks may be placed under the head of the resident's bed to reduce nocturnal diuresis and minimize hypotension on arising from bed.

ANTIDEPRESSANT-INDUCED MOVEMENT DISORDER

The most common movement disorder that can be induced by antidepressants is tremor. The typical antidepressant tremor is an action tremor indistinguishable from familial essential (senile) tremor. The resident shows shaking of the hands or head that is brought out by purposeful action or by stress. There is often a personal or family history of tremor that precedes exposure to the drug. Appropriate management is dosage reduction when feasible. Switching to a different class of antidepressant is not necessarily helpful; it works best when a drug of a different class can be given at a substantially lower dose. If necessary and if not contraindicated, antidepressant-induced action tremors can be controlled by the same drugs that work for essential tremor: beta blockers, benzodiazepines, and primidone. However, due to its sedative effects, primidone is the least well tolerated of the three.

The serotonin reuptake inhibitor drugs, especially fluoxetine (Prozac), can cause severe restlessness and the inability to sit still, which are regarded by many psychiatrists as indistinguishable from neuroleptic-induced akathisia. When this occurs, use a different antidepressant. All antidepressants can provoke a state of physical agitation, especially soon after initiation or dosage increases. These states will aggravate any preexisting movement disorder the resident may have. They are prevented by conservative dosage titration and treated by dosage reduction. If movement disorder absolutely prevents adequate treatment of a serious depression, the psychiatric consultant may be able to suggest a combination of an antidepressant with an antianxiety drug, thymoleptic, or neuroleptic that will permit adequate antidepressant treatment. In view of the general risks of polypharmacy, such combinations should be carried out with ongoing consultant follow-up.

Two commonly prescribed drugs, amoxapine (Asendin) and amitriptyline-perphenazine (Triavil), are marketed as antidepressants but actually are neuroleptics as well, with the full range of neuroleptic side effects. Never use them as first-line treatment for depression.

ANTIDEPRESSANT-INDUCED GAIT DISTURBANCE

Gait disturbance associated with a tricyclic antidepressant or trazodone should immediately raise the suspicion of orthostatic hypotension. If unsteady gait develops despite normal blood pressure on any antidepressant, drug-induced ataxia is a possibility. The presence of ataxia of gait is demonstrated by showing that the resident cannot walk on a narrow base, or stand securely with feet together or pointing heel-to-toe. (In the case of residents with preexisting gait problems, look for an aggravation over baseline.) The response to

antidepressant-induced ataxia is dosage reduction or switching to a different antidepressant.

In addition, gait disturbance in residents taking antidepressants can develop as a feature of drug-induced delirium. Residents with delirium often are less able to walk, since their ability to compensate cognitively for sensory, motor, and orthopedic impairments is reduced. The condition is diagnosed by mental status examination; drug discontinuation is mandatory if the drug is implicated in causing delirium.

Antianxiety Drugs

Antianxiety drugs are used to treat anxiety symptoms, anxiety disorders such as panic disorder (recurrent panic attacks), insomnia, and memory impairment. The most prescribed antianxiety drugs are the benzodiazepines, a chemical class that includes diazepam (Valium) and alprazolam (Xanax), as well as the three most-prescribed sleeping pills: triazolam (Halcion), temazepam (Restoril), and flurazepam (Dalmane). All benzodiazepines have a common set of side effects that comprises sedation, impaired motor coordination, and respiratory depression.

A clinically important distinction among benzodiazepines is in their half-life and whether they have active metabolites. Drugs with long half-lives and active metabolites, such as diazepam, accumulate progressively with continued use, potentially leading to excessive sedation and falls. Drugs with short half-lives and without active metabolites lack the problem of accumulation, but may be more likely to cause amnesia or confusion after a single dose. They may also cause intense withdrawal symptoms of anxiety and insomnia if they are discontinued abruptly.

The nonbenzodiazepine antianxiety drug buspirone (BuSpar) is much less likely than the benzodiazepines to cause ataxia, sedation, or memory impairment. However, not all residents whose symptoms respond to benzodiazepines will respond to buspirone. Dosage of buspirone must be individualized. Individuals' metabolism of the drug varies greatly, so that some residents will get a therapeutic response to as little as 10 mg/day; others will need 60 mg. Further, full therapeutic benefits may take

as long as 4 weeks.

A number of other medications are often used to treat anxiety, including the antihistamines diphenhydramine (Benadryl) and hydroxyzine (Vistaril), barbiturates, and meprobamate. These drugs are not currently recommended for this purpose, because they are

Table 14-5. Antianxiety and Hypnotic Drugs

Generic Name	Brand Name	Usual Geriatric Dose Range(mg/day)	Elimination Half-Life
Benzodiazepines (short half-life)*			
Triazolam	Halcion	0.125-1	Very short
Oxazepam	Serax	10-60	Short
Temazepam	Restoril	15-60	Short
Lorazepam	Ativan	0.5-4	Short
Alprazolam	Xanax	0.25-2	Medium
Estazolam	Prosom	0.5-1	Medium
Benzodiazepines (long half-life)*			
Chlordiazepoxide	Librium	10-100	Long
Diazepam	Valium	2-30	Long
Clorazepate	Tranxene	3.75-15	Long
Halazepam	Paxipam	10-40	Long
Quazepam	Doral	7.5-15	Long
Flurazepam	Dalmane	15-60	Very long
Clonazepam	Klonopin	0.125-0.5	Very long
Non-Benzodiazepine			
Buspirone	BuSpar	7.5-60	Short
Zolpidem	Ambien	5-10	Short

*Relatively contraindicated in residents with chronic lung disease with carbon dioxide retention.

regarded as more toxic and no more effective than the benzodiazepines. Administering diphenhydramine as a hypnotic for use at bedtime remains controversial. Critics of its use as a hypnotic point to its anticholinergic effects, including the potential for confusion, as a major drawback. Table 14-5 summarizes the features of the different antianxiety drugs.

Choosing and Monitoring an Antianxiety Drug

There is only one relatively strong medical contraindication to the use of benzodiazepine antianxiety drugs: lung disease with carbon dioxide retention. In this situation, the depression of hypoxic respiratory drive by benzodiazepines creates a risk of respiratory failure (*see* Chapter 4, Pulmonary Disorders, for more information). Lung disease without carbon dioxide retention is not a contraindication; benzodiazepines can reduce dyspnea in some residents with emphysema without impairing respiration. Buspirone, the other drug approved specifically for symptoms of anxiety, does not have any major medical contraindications.

A relative contraindication to the use of benzodiazepines is gait impairment since benzodiazepines can aggravate gait disturbance of any cause, and invariably can cause ataxia if the dose is high enough. Confusion or memory loss is another contraindication. Benzodiazepines cause measurable impairments in cognition that are especially relevant in people with preexisting dementia. However, if anxiety or agitation has a large effect on the person's ability to concentrate, cognitive abilities for everyday function may actually improve on a benzodiazepine dose just sufficient to reduce anxiety.

After noting contraindications, and assuming that medical problems causing pain, discomfort, or insomnia are addressed adequately, choose an antianxiety drug based on the most likely cause of the anxiety, the probable duration of treatment, and the prior history of drug treatment.

Benzodiazepines are the first choice in the following situations:

- The cause of the anxiety is mainly situational, and the expected duration of treatment is short
- Panic attacks
- The resident has a long-term problem with generalized anxiety, and a long history of good responses to modest doses of benzodiazepines

If panic attacks are prominent, alprazolam or clonazepam may give better results than other benzodiazepines.

When initiating benzodiazepine therapy, use shorter-acting benzodiazepines without active metabolites. The dosage can be adjusted easily and the problem of gradual accumulation of active metabolites is avoided. Typical dosages are oxazepam, 10 mg, lorazepam, 0.5 mg, and alprazolam, 0.25 mg. Doses are given on a once to twice a day schedule depending on the resident's response. Decrease these doses by half if the resident develops ataxia, excessive sedation, or confusion following a dose; in cases of more severe intolerance, discontinue the drug. If anxiety or agitation persist, increase the dosage every 2 to 3 days.

While longer-acting benzodiazepines are not viewed as drugs of first choice in the elderly, there are four situations in which their use may be appropriate:

- Very occasional use in a resident known to respond well to them
- Continuation at a low, stable dose in a resident who has responded well to them and does not have problems with cognition or gait
- Use as a substitute for a short-acting drug to facilitate the tapering and discontinuation of benzodiazepines, since withdrawal

symptoms are milder with longer-acting agents
- Use as a substitute for a shorter-acting agent when the short-acting drug produces uncomfortable anxiety when it wears off between doses (in this situation, first try more frequent dosages of the shorter-acting drug)

Monitoring of benzodiazepine therapy should consist of the following:

- A measure of the therapeutic benefits for anxiety or agitation
- Frequent checking of cognitive function and stability of gait–daily during dose increases and weekly for at least a month after stabilizing the dose
- A weekly overall functional assessment as the dosage is adjusted to establish whether the relief of anxiety symptoms has led to improved function

If cognitive function or gait become impaired in the resident on a benzodiazepine, reducing or discontinuing the dosage may be necessary. Discontinuation should be gradual to avoid precipitating a benzodiazepine withdrawal delirium.

If the resident has a long history of nervousness, anxiety, irritability, and tension, but does not have panic attacks, an obvious situational precipitant, or a long history of benzodiazepine use, try buspirone. This drug does not have the cognitive and gait effects of benzodiazepines, so it is safer. However, it can cause the nuisance side effects of dizziness, tinnitus, headache, and gastrointestinal upset, as well as insomnia or increased anxiety at the start of therapy. Start the drug at a low dose (e.g., 2.5 mg three times a day) to minimize these problems, but increase the dose every 3 or 4 days as tolerated until symptoms are relieved, side effects develop, or a maximum dose of 20 mg three times a day is reached. The full therapeutic effects may take

4 weeks or more to develop.

Treat residents with anxiety due to agitated depression with antidepressant drugs. However, many such residents become intolerably anxious when antidepressants are first started. Under these circumstances, start with a very low dosage and raise it slowly. On occasion, the short-term use of a benzodiazepine along with the antidepressant is appropriate. The decision to use this therapy should be made by a consulting psychiatrist.

Treat residents with anxiety due to paranoid fears, as well as residents with long histories of severe personality disturbance whose anxiety is accompanied by dangerous behavior, with neuroleptics. In this situation, low- to medium-potency neuroleptics such as thioridazine or perphenazine are preferable to high-potency neuroleptics such as haloperidol, because they have more intrinsic antianxiety effect and are less likely to cause akathisia. Risperidone, although a high-potency agent, may have some antianxiety effects.

Modifying Therapy to Reduce Side Effects or Improve Therapeutic Response

The following section discusses the common effects of antianxiety drugs on gait disturbance, and how to improve the therapeutic response to these drugs.

Antianxiety Drug-Induced Gait Disturbance

Gait disturbance developing in a resident taking benzodiazepines usually is due to drug-induced ataxia, which is a predictable consequence of benzodiazepines if the drug level is sufficiently high. It is particularly likely to occur in residents given long-acting benzodiazepines because the blood level of those drugs can rise steadily over several weeks on a fixed dose. Depending on the severity of the problem, the appropriate response is dosage reduction or drug discontinuation. Try to use an alternative treatment for anxiety, such as buspirone or an antidepressant. If the benzodiazepine is given for insomnia and nondrug treatments have been tried and found wanting, alternative hypnotics deserving consideration are zolpidem (a nonbenzodiazepine with lesser ataxic effects) and trazodone.

When antihistamines, which are used in some facilities to treat anxiety, cause gait disturbance, they usually also cause confusion or sedation. Since these drugs are of doubtful value, the development of gait problems while taking one of them would warrant discontinuation.

Mood-Stabilizing Drugs

Mood-stabilizing drugs, or thymoleptics, are primarily used in the treatment of bipolar disorder (manic-depressive illness) and related conditions. They are also used to treat the instability of mood that may accompany other mental disorders, including schizophrenia and dementia. Lithium is the best known; the antiepileptic drugs carbamazepine (Tegretol) and valproate (Depakote) are of equal efficacy, and can be used as alternatives or as adjuncts to lithium. Residents with bipolar disorder may respond better to one thymoleptic than another, and some only respond to combinations.

The major common side effects of lithium include tremor, weight gain, and a partial loss of the kidney's ability to concentrate the urine. This side effect can provoke or aggravate incontinence and dehydration in nursing home residents. Lithium has an antithyroid effect, and can precipitate clinically significant hypothyroidism. Its therapeutic index is low, and life-threatening toxicity can occur if it is given without proper monitoring of blood levels, or if it is continued in the face of dehydration. The common side effects of carbamazepine include sedation, ataxia, and anticholinergic effects. To minimize the side effects of carbamazepine, slowly increase the dosage.

Carbamazepine can cause neutropenia or hyponatremia, but neither effect usually is severe enough to require drug discontinuation. The common side effects of valproate include sedation, tremor, and weight gain. Both carbamazepine and valproate can cause abnormalities of liver function but clinically significant hepatitis is rare in older persons. Monitoring blood levels is necessary for most residents taking thymoleptics, at least during the initiation of therapy, and upon any change in clinical condition. The therapeutic and toxic levels are well established. Table 14-6 summarizes the features of the mood-stabilizing drugs.

Choosing and Monitoring a Mood-Stabilizing Drug (Thymoleptic)

Choosing a drug to treat manic-depressive illness or a related mood disorder is usually the task of a consulting psychiatrist. However, nursing home staff have a major role to play in identifying residents who need psychiatric assessment for mood disorder, and for monitoring the effects of the prescribed drug therapy.

Any resident with marked ups and downs, particularly if these symptoms last weeks to months, may have a mood disorder that will respond to treatment. Lithium is most helpful for residents with distinct highs and with relatively long mood cycles. The antiepileptic drugs carbamazepine and valproate are especially helpful in people with shorter cycles (i.e., lasting weeks rather than months and more than two per year). However, a resident with a mood disorder who has not done well on one drug should try the other if there is no contraindication.

Monitor residents on thymoleptic drugs for mood stability as well as cognitive and behavioral function. As with all other psychotropics, the goal is both to relieve symptoms and improve overall function. In addition, each of the three main thymoleptics is associated

Table 14-6. Mood-Stabilizing (Thymoleptic) Drugs

Drug	Indications	Relative Contraindications	Usual Side Effects	More Serious Side Effects
Lithium	Bipolar disorder Antidepressant adjunct	Impaired kidney function Tremor Atrial arrhythmia Hypothyroidism	Polyuria Tremor Weight gain Hypercalcemia Atrial arrhythmia	Impaired kidney function Hypothyroidism
Carbamazepine	Rapid-cycling or lithium-unresponsive bipolar disorder Epilepsy Neuropathic pain	Neutropenia Impaired liver function Greater than first-degree heart block	Sedation Ataxia Diplopia Anticholinergic effects	Neutropenia Hepatitis Hyponatremia Heart block
Valproate	Rapid-cycling or lithium-unresponsive bipolar disorder Epilepsy Neuropathic pain	Impaired liver function Bleeding diathesis	Sedation Weight gain Nausea	Increased bleeding time Hepatitis

with specific medical concerns and side effects. The following subsections discuss these concerns.

Lithium

Lithium always impairs renal concentrating capacity, sometimes impairs general renal function, and occasionally causes hypothyroidism or hypercalcemia. Therefore, residents on lithium should have baseline kidney and thyroid function tests and a baseline calcium. Repeat these tests every 3 months. A thyroid-stimulating hormone (TSH) level usually is sufficient to monitor thyroid function after completing baseline studies. Because lithium can aggravate atrial arrhythmias, most clinicians also obtain an ECG before starting lithium. If the baseline is normal, no follow-up ECGs are necessary if the resident is asymptomatic.

Lithium increases urine volume, so it can aggravate incontinence. It also causes tremor and aggravates tremor in residents with preexisting essential tremor. For this reason, both urinary incontinence and essential tremor are relative contraindications to lithium. However, if lithium has marked benefit for a resident, both of these problems can be managed with appropriate dosing strategies, with adjunctive medications, or in the case of urinary incontinence, with a toileting program.

Monitor blood levels on a routine basis in residents on lithium. Therapeutic levels for lithium are generally given as 0.6 to 1.5 mEq/L. However, many older people, particularly those with cognitive impairment or parkinsonism, cannot tolerate levels above 1.0, and some will respond well to levels as low as 0.3. Furthermore, very low levels of lithium can be effective as an adjunct to an antidepressant drug in the treatment of depression. Therefore, the target range for lithium levels often needs modification to a lower level, in consultation with the psychiatrist. However, a lithium level above 1.5 mEq/L is never acceptable in an elderly resident.

A suitable schedule to monitor lithium blood levels depends on two factors--the stability of the resident's hydration and renal function, and how close to the upper end of the range the resident's level usually lies. Quarterly levels may be adequate for a resident with stable renal function and hydration and a usual level of 0.6; weekly or even more frequent levels may be more appropriate for a resident with a creatinine of 2.0, recent weight loss, and a usual level of 1.0.

Early signs of lithium toxicity include nausea, vomiting, and coarse tremor. When these symptoms appear acutely in a resident on lithium, immediately obtain a level and withhold the drug until results are available. Residents on lithium should have blood urea nitrogen, creatinine, and TSH levels obtained quarterly to screen for renal insufficiency and the development of lithium-induced hypothyroidism.

Carbamazepine

Carbamazepine resembles tricyclic antidepressants chemically, and can cause virtually all of the side effects of tricyclics, including anticholinergic effects, sedation, ataxia, and quinidine-like effects on the heart that can aggravate heart block. However, it usually does not cause orthostatic hypotension. Second- or third-degree heart block is a relatively strong contraindication to this drug.

Carbamazepine commonly lowers serum sodium and lowers the white blood cell (WBC) count. Because of the effect on the WBC count, a baseline WBC count of less than 4000 cells/μl is a contraindication, and a WBC count should be obtained on any resident on carbamazepine who develops an infection or fever. However, persistent neutropenia or agranulocytosis is rare, so routine monitoring

of the WBC count is not necessary or helpful. Carbamazepine's effect on lowering serum sodium makes it relatively contraindicated in residents who are already hyponatremic, and requires that electrolytes be checked if a resident on carbamazepine shows new cognitive impairment.

Carbamazepine frequently causes mild abnormalities in liver enzymes, but rarely causes true hepatitis; therefore:

- Pre-existing liver disease is a relative contraindication
- Routine monitoring of liver enzymes is not necessary or helpful
- Development of anorexia, nausea, or other signs of hepatitis warrants an immediate checking of the liver enzymes

Because carbamazepine induces hepatic metabolic enzymes, it is involved in many drug interactions, generally in the direction of lowering the level of the other drug. However, two common drugs—erythromycin and verapamil—can interact with carbamazepine and raise its level dangerously. Since carbamazepine induces its own metabolism, gradually increase the drug dosage over the first few weeks of therapy in order to safely reach and maintain a therapeutic blood level. In the frail elderly resident, a starting dose of 100 mg at bedtime is reasonable; increase the dosage every 2 or 3 days as tolerated until therapeutic effects are obtained, side effects develop, or a blood level of 12 μg/dL is reached. Start measuring blood levels when the resident reaches a dosage of 200 mg three times a day. Repeat as necessary to titrate dosage or to evaluate for potential toxicity or nonresponse.

Valproate

Valproate has a similar therapeutic spectrum to carbamazepine in bipolar disorder, but slightly different side effects and greatly different metabolism. Its principal side effects are sedation, tremor, ataxia, and nausea. The major serious, but rare, side effects are drug-induced hepatitis and bleeding due either to thrombocytopenia or to decreased synthesis of clotting factors. The approach to monitoring is similar to that used in carbamazepine; check the liver enzymes as indicated by the symptoms. Check a coagulation panel if the resident develops bleeding or bruises, or if the resident is scheduled for surgery. Start the dosage in elderly residents at 125 mg twice a day; gradual increases should aim for a blood level of 50 to 100 μg/dL unless the symptoms are well controlled at a lower level. Valproate inhibits the metabolism of many other drugs, raising their blood level.

Monitoring the Mood-Stabilizing Drugs

Since the maximum therapeutic effects of all three mood-stabilizing drugs occurs 2 to 4 weeks after reaching a therapeutic dose, weekly monitoring of disease-specific symptoms and general function is reasonable when a resident is beginning therapy or a dosage has been changed. For the resident stabilized on therapy with a thymoleptic, a monthly assessment of general function, cognition, mood, and behavior is appropriate. Residents on lithium require routine monitoring of kidney and thyroid function. If there are any changes in health status, obtain lithium blood levels, calcium, and electrolytes. Residents on carbamazepine require a complete blood count and differential, liver enzymes, electrolytes, and carbamazepine blood level in the event of worsening health status. In this situation, residents on valproate require monitoring of liver enzymes and a blood level.

Modifying Therapy to Reduce Side Effects or Improve Therapeutic Response

The following sections discuss the common side effects of the mood-stabilizing drugs and

how to improve the therapeutic response to these drugs.

Mood-Stabilizing Drug-Induced Movement Disorders

All of the mood-stabilizing (thymoleptic) drugs can cause action tremors similar to those caused by antidepressants. At toxic blood levels, lithium can cause coarse, flapping tremors of the shoulders and arms. The occurrence of such movements in a resident taking lithium warrants immediate discontinuation of the drug, a lithium blood level, and medical consultation. At toxic blood levels, or when given to residents with pre-existing parkinsonism, lithium can cause parkinsonian tremor and rigidity. The occurrence of parkinsonian tremor at the lowest lithium level that will control the resident's mood symptoms is an indication to switch to a different thymoleptic. Adding an antiparkinson drug is a distant second choice in view of the risks of additive systemic toxicity.

All of the mood-stabilizing drugs can aggravate neuroleptic-induced movement disorders. Neuroleptic-thymoleptic combinations, while occasionally necessary for the control of severe chronic mental illness, require close monitoring, with both the neuroleptic dose and the thymoleptic blood level kept as low as possible while still controlling major mental symptoms.

Mood-Stabilizing Drug-Induced Gait Disturbance

All of the mood-stabilizing drugs can cause ataxia. The effect is dose-related, and the management is to decrease the dose. If the drug is ineffective at the highest dose that does not cause ataxia, use an alternative drug.

Stimulants

Direct stimulant drugs, including methylphenidate (Ritalin), dextroamphetamine (Dexedrine), and pemoline (Cylert) are indicated primarily for the treatment of attention deficit hyperactivity disorder in children, but are frequently used to treat fatigue, sluggishness, apathy, and some forms of transient depression in residents. While the stimulant drugs have been tested and found ineffective for treating major depression, extensive case reports, case series, and published informed opinion support their utility for treating apathy and impaired motivation, particularly in the context of chronic medical illness. The most compelling evidence is for patients with apathy and lethargy following major surgery, and for patients with AIDS. However, these drugs have been used in a wide range of medical and neurologic conditions in which apathy, sleepiness, or lack of motivation are prominent symptoms. The stimulants are also recognized as a useful adjunct to antidepressant drugs in situations in which the antidepressants improve mood symptoms but leave the patient apathetic and unmotivated.

Among the stimulant drugs, methylphenidate and dextroamphetamine have very similar effects; pemoline is less potent, substantially longer acting, and may not work as well. The typical dosage of stimulants in a resident is dextroamphetamine, 5 mg once or twice a day, methylphenidate, 5 mg once or twice a day, or pemoline, 18.75 to 37.5 mg daily.

Both the therapeutic and side effects of stimulants tend to occur immediately. The common side effects include increased pulse rate, increased blood pressure, tremor, insomnia, and nervousness. Anorexia may also occur, but patients whose apathy is helped substantially by the stimulant may actually eat more when taking the drug.

Choosing and Monitoring a Stimulant

Consider stimulant therapy in residents in whom apathy, lethargy, or lack of motivation are causing significant emotional distress or functional impairment, in those who are not significantly nervous or agitated, and in those who do not have an unstable cardiac condition that would be aggravated by a possible mild increase in heart rate or blood pressure. Residents with a partial response to antidepressants but with persistent motivational impairment might also be suitable candidates for stimulant treatment. Either methylphenidate or dextroamphetamine is a good initial choice because these drugs have a relatively short duration of action. Pemoline has a long duration of action and is only appropriate for the occasional stimulant responder needing long-term treatment. Watch for insomnia on this longer-acting agent. The starting dosage for methylphenidate or dextroamphetamine is 5 mg morning and noon, or 2.5 mg morning and noon if the resident is particularly frail or has a low body weight. If there is no obvious response to that dosage, double the dosage on the following day.

Therapeutic response should appear immediately. After a resident has had a therapeutic response for 2 to 4 weeks, make an effort to taper and discontinue the drug. If the resident has become more active, continued stimulant therapy may be unnecessary. However, chronic therapy is appropriate if the drug is helpful, has no significant side effects, and efforts to taper the drug resulted in recurrent symptoms.

During the initial trial of treatment, check the blood pressure and pulse 1 to 2 hours after each dose. An ECG is unnecessary unless the resident develops an irregular heart rate or complains of cardiac symptoms. No routine blood monitoring is necessary.

Note the resident's sleep and eating patterns on stimulant therapy for the first few weeks. Significant insomnia or weight loss are reasons to reduce or discontinue stimulant therapy.

If stimulants are given together with tricyclic antidepressants, the tricyclic blood level can be raised by a pharmacokinetic interaction. In this situation, carefully monitor the resident for signs of tricyclic side effects such as anticholinergic symptoms or hypotension. Reduce the tricyclic dose if such side effects develop.

Stimulant-Induced Movement Disorder

The most common movement disorder that can be induced by stimulants is tremor. The typical stimulant tremor is an action tremor indistinguishable from familial essential (senile) tremor. The resident shows shaking of the hands or head that is brought out by purposeful action or by stress. There is often a personal or family history of tremor that precedes exposure to the drug. Appropriate management is dosage reduction when feasible. Switching to a different class of stimulant is not necessarily helpful; it works best when a drug of a different class works at a substantially lower dose. If necessary and if not contraindicated, stimulant-induced action tremors can be controlled by the same drugs that work for essential tremor: beta blockers, benzodiazepines, and primidone. However, primidone is the least well tolerated of the three due to its sedative effects.

All stimulants can provoke a state of physical agitation, especially soon after initiation or dosage increases. These states will aggravate any preexisting movement disorder the resident may have. They are prevented by conservative dosage titration and treated by dosage reduction.

If movement disorder absolutely prevents adequate treatment of a serious depression, the psychiatric consultant may be able to suggest a combination of a stimulant with an antianxiety drug, thymoleptic, or neuroleptic that will permit adequate stimulant treatment. In view of the general risks of polypharmacy, such combinations should be carried out with ongoing consultant follow-up.

Two commonly prescribed drugs, amoxapine (Asendin) and amitriptyline-perphenazine (Triavil), are marketed as stimulants but actually are neuroleptics as well, with the full range of neuroleptic side effects. Never use them be used as first-line treatment for depression.

DELAYED PHARMACOLOGIC EFFECTS

Both the therapeutic and the adverse effects of psychotropic drugs can be delayed, and may not appear until the resident has been taking the drug for several weeks. Neuroleptics can relieve agitation within hours, but their full effect on hallucinations and delusions may take weeks. The neuroleptic side effect of dystonia occurs within hours if it occurs at all, but parkinsonism can develop gradually over days to weeks, and tardive dyskinesia can develop over months to years of neuroleptic exposure. The delayed appearance of neuroleptic effects has several causes:

- The gradual accumulation of the neuroleptic in the brain, as the drug, which is highly fat-soluble, saturates brain membranes
- The gradual exhaustion of the brain's compensatory increase in dopamine release in response to dopamine blockade by the drug
- Changes in the function of other neurotransmitter systems as a secondary consequence of persistent dopamine receptor blockade

In addition, some common neuroleptics, such as chlorpromazine (Thorazine), have active metabolites that accumulate in the blood.

Antidepressants, thymoleptics, and the antianxiety drug buspirone are known to take 1 month or more to achieve peak therapeutic effect. Therapeutic effects are related to secondary changes in the brain that result from the immediate drug effect, so that improvement in symptoms can continue for weeks after the blood level of the drug has reached a steady state.

Benzodiazepine antianxiety drugs have their therapeutic and toxic effects immediately, given a specific level of the drug in the blood and the brain. However, benzodiazepines with long half-lives and active metabolites may not reach a steady state level for weeks, so that both benefits and side effects can build up over time. Benzodiazepine effects are also influenced by tolerance. A resident who has taken benzodiazepines for a long time may show fewer side effects and less benefit at a given dose than someone who has just been started on the drug.

Because of the delayed effects of psychotropics, dosage adjustment often is needed after several weeks of treatment. For neuroleptics and for benzodiazepines, the usual dosage adjustment is to reduce the dose after the symptoms are under control, or in response to the delayed emergence of side effects.

DRUG-INDUCED MENTAL STATUS OR BEHAVIOR CHANGES

If a resident develops delirium or impaired cognition shortly after initiating or increasing the dose of a psychotropic drug, discontinue the drug and watch the resident carefully to see if the cognitive change resolves. If the situation is not urgent, tapering is generally better tolerated than abrupt discontinuation of the drug, particularly if the resident has been taking it for a long time (see Chapter 11, Delirium, for more information).

If a resident taking a psychotropic drug for a condition other than depression develops depression, perform a full diagnostic reassessment. The sedative effects of psychotropic drugs can mimic or aggravate depression. If clinically significant depression is present, start an antidepressant drug therapy and other measures to treat depression. If the resident has depressive symptoms of recent onset and does not have a major depressive syndrome, try tapering and discontinuing the offending drug with a reassessment of the mental status while the resident is off the drug.

If a resident develops visual hallucinations

while taking a psychotropic drug, drug toxicity is the most likely cause. Drugs with potent anticholinergic effects are most likely to cause visual hallucinations, but virtually all psychotropic drugs can produce hallucinations, particularly in people with prior brain impairment or unusually high psychotropic drug blood levels. If the hallucinations are of acute onset, discontinue the drug. Obtain drug levels if the drug is a tricyclic antidepressant or a thymoleptic. If the hallucinations are more chronic and not troublesome to the resident, slow dosage reduction is likely to be better tolerated.

Visual hallucinations should trigger investigation for inadvertent drug withdrawal. Sudden reduction or elimination of sedating drugs, especially benzodiazepines, can produce a withdrawal state similar to delirium tremens, with visual hallucinations as a feature.

To treat the side effects of psychotropic drugs, follow these guidelines:

- If a resident taking a psychotropic drug has dramatic fluctuations in functions according to the time of day, chart the cognitive and behavioral symptoms against the time of psychotropic drug administration to see if there is a pattern. If a linkage is established, interventions are the same as if the drug were causing a persistent decline in cognition or function.

- If a resident taking a psychotropic drug shows a significant decline in cognition, communication, or any ADL function linked to the initiation or increase of the drug, reduce, discontinue, or change the drug. The decision will depend on whether the drug trial has been adequate in duration, and the extent to which the resident has shown a positive therapeutic response to the drug. When a therapeutically useful drug causes unacceptable side effects despite efforts at dosage reduction, the usual next move is to substitute another drug in the same therapeutic class that is less likely to cause the troublesome side effect. For example, if a resident had good anxiety relief from a benzodiazepine but developed memory loss, try buspirone. Or, if a resident got relief of hallucinations from haloperidol but showed a large drop in initiative, consider substituting risperidone, a new neuroleptic much less likely to cause akinesia.

ANTICHOLINERGIC EFFECTS

Anticholinergic side effects may result from using psychotropic drugs. To treat these side effects, follow these guidelines:

- If a resident maintained on an antipsychotic or antidepressant drug develops anticholinergic side effects (e.g., constipation, fecal impaction, urinary retention, or dry mouth), management depends on how effective the drug has been therapeutically. If the resident has had a good therapeutic effect, the first step is to reduce the dosage gradually to the minimum effective dose, then offer symptomatic treatment for the anticholinergic effects. Treat constipation with stool softeners, bulk-forming agents, a higher-bulk diet, increased fluids, and increased exercise. Treat dry mouth with artificial saliva or other wetting agents. Try hard candy if it is appropriate.
- If therapeutic response is not satisfactory, or if the anticholinergic side effects remain troublesome despite symptomatic treatments, or if significant side effects develop before a trial of therapeutically adequate dosage and direction can be given, switch the resident to a less anticholinergic agent within the same therapeutic class. Among the antidepressants, trazodone, venlafaxine, and the serotonin reuptake inhibitors are least anticholinergic. Among the neuroleptics, the high-potency agents haloperidol and fluphenazine are relatively low in anticholinergic effects, as is the medium-potency agent molindone and the new risperidone.

INADEQUATE TREATMENT RESPONSE

Follow these guidelines to treat an inadequate response to psychotropic drug therapy:
- If a resident's mental disorder or symptoms fail to respond to a psychotropic drug, ask the following questions
  o Is the diagnosis correct?
  o Is the dosage appropriate?
  o Has the drug been given for an adequate duration?
- The most common diagnostic error leading to drug nonresponse is the misdiagnosis of depression as an anxiety disorder or nonspecific agitated state. The resident is given an antianxiety or neuroleptic drug, and the depression does not improve. A second common diagnostic error is the misdiagnosis of apathy as depression. Antidepressant drug therapy usually does not help people with severe apathy and loss of initiative due to brain damage or side effects of other drugs. A third common diagnostic error is failure to identify psychotic features, leading to a failure of treatment for depression, anxiety, or nonspecific behavior disturbances. Psychotic illness tends to respond best to regimens that include neuroleptic drugs and poorly to regimens that do not.
- For some of the tricyclic antidepressants and for all of the thymoleptic drugs, a therapeutic range for drug blood levels has been established for physically healthy people. Unfortunately, these ranges have not been validated for the frail elderly populations commonly treated in nursing homes. In general, published therapeutic ranges may be too high for residents who are malnourished, have low serum protein levels, are on multiple drugs, and have compromised cognition. Treat the resident and not the blood level. Blood levels can be helpful when prior experience has established a

blood level of a drug at which the resident does best. In residents in whom there is no such experience, a blood level can establish whether there is a potential problem with drug absorption or metabolism in a resident who has a unexpected response to a given dose of a drug.

- Adequate duration of a treatment trial is 6 to 8 weeks for antidepressant and antipsychotic drugs, 4 to 6 weeks for buspirone, 2 to 4 weeks for the thymoleptics, and 1 to 2 weeks for the benzodiazepines. If a correctly diagnosed resident does not respond to an adequate dosage of a psychotropic drug after these durations, the resident is unlikely to be a responder if treatment is continued. Therefore, try an alternative therapy.
- The steps to take after nonresponse to an appropriate treatment trial include:
  o Psychiatric consultation or reconsultation
  o Review of medical problems and other prescribed drugs that can cause or aggravate the mental problem being treated
  o Consideration of nonpharmacologic treatments, including psychotherapy and environmental manipulation
- If a second drug trial is tried in a nonresponsive resident who has not improved with a psychotropic drug regimen, consider using a drug of a different chemical class.
- If a resident responds partially but insufficiently to a drug trial, consider add-on therapy. In addition, reconsider nonpharmacologic therapies, and review potentially aggravating medical conditions. The two most common situations are partial response to antidepressant treatment and partial response to antipsychotic treatment.
- For residents responding partially to antidepressant treatment, add-on treatments to be considered include lithium, buspirone, stimulants if the resident is apathetic (e.g., methylphenidate [Ritalin]), and antipsychotic drugs if the resident has delusions or hallucinations. For virtually all of these combi-

nation treatments, ongoing psychiatric consultation is strongly advised.
- For residents with agitation and psychosis, in whom low-dose antipsychotic therapy has improved the psychotic features but left some residual agitation, treatment with a nonneuroleptic drug with antianxiety action is recommended. Popular alternatives include benzodiazepines, buspirone, and trazodone. These adjuncts usually result in fewer side effects than raising the antipsychotic drug dosage.

DOING WELL ON AN UNRECOMMENDED THERAPY

In most nursing homes there are residents who are tolerating, and apparently benefiting from, psychotropic drug therapies that are not currently recommended. Examples of such drugs include amitriptyline, a tricyclic with very potent anticholinergic effects, and substantial doses of long-acting benzodiazepines. Because of their association with an increased risk of falls, both of these therapies are currently regarded as undesirable, and high-dose benzodiazepine therapy is considered presumptively inappropriate according to new HCFA guidelines.

In approaching such situations, the critical question to ask is whether the resident is really doing well. If he or she has been taking the drug in question for a long time, psychotropic side effects may have come to be regarded as part of that resident's baseline.

However, if a rigorous and skeptical assessment of the doing well hypothesis supports a good response to a nonrecommended treatment, then follow these guidelines:
- Carefully document the resident's psychiatric diagnosis and history of response to the drug in question.
- Specifically and systematically assess the resident for adverse effects of the drug in question. For example, a resident receiving a long-acting benzodiazepine should un-

dergo testing of memory and testing of gait and balance (i.e., the ability to right oneself after a pull backward and to balance briefly on one foot). If the resident can pass rigorous tests of function in areas of concern, the doing-well hypothesis is supported. If not, a switch to a lower dose or less toxic medication is warranted.

- Often the doing-well hypothesis can neither be confirmed nor denied because the resident has an underlying progressive medical or neurologic condition that independently impairs function. In this situation, the decision to continue the resident on a nonrecommended therapy rests on assembling evidence that alternative therapies have been tried and found to produce a less satisfactory overall result, with all positive and negative effects considered. Whenever possible, an independent psychiatric consultant should review the assembled evidence and offer an independent judgment.

CASE EXAMPLE

Mrs. N., an 80-year-old woman with normal pressure hydrocephalus, moderate dementia, and urge incontinence (detrusor hyperre-

flexia), was treated for depression with imipramine, 75 mg at bedtime. Simultaneously, her urologist was treating her incontinence with oxybutynin (ditropan), an anticholinergic drug. A few days after the urologist started the bladder drug, the resident developed severe constipation, urinary retention, and delirium.

On assessment, Mrs. N. showed a rapid pulse and slightly dilated, poorly reactive pupils suggesting anticholinergic toxicity. Both drugs were stopped. Mental status improved, but depression and incontinence continued.

The resident was then treated for her depression with fluoxetine (Prozac), 5 mg/day, and a toileting program to empty her bladder. Fluoxetine has virtually no anticholinergic effect. On the new treatment program, Mrs. N.'s depression improved, and she regained continence.

This case shows a pharmacodynamic interaction between two anticholinergic drugs, and shows how alternative choices, including behavioral therapies, can avoid the interaction while still giving a good therapeutic result.

15
Psychosocial Well-Being

John N. Morris, PhD
Lisa Gwyther, MSW
Claire Gerstein, MSW
Katharine Murphy, RN, MS
David Levine, PhD

While conventional wisdom holds that cognitive and physical decline inevitably lead to social disengagement and lowered self-esteem, there is no simple cause-and-effect relationship. Despite changes in function, roles, and social community, life continues to hold meaning and value for most residents. Having good social relationships, a sense of control over one's life, and opportunities to engage in activities and routines that hold particular meaning for the resident are crucial factors in maintaining psychosocial well-being. Most residents are remarkably adaptive, most families stay involved, old values retain their meaning, and new relationships are established.

OVERVIEW

This chapter describes the strategies used to help residents who retain at least some cognitive skills for daily decision-making to revitalize their view of self, overcome negative expectations, circumvent disturbing relationships, and build on relationships that are supportive. Approximately one third of all residents have difficulties in these areas, half of which are usually found to have originated at some point in the prior 6-month period. In one multistate study of nursing home resi-

dents, about 20% appeared to have withdrawn from activities and daily interactions with others, and one quarter had unsettled relationships.

For most residents, these problems improve over a 6-month period with appropriate intervention. Approximately seven of 10 troubled residents will have better relationships and an improved view of self by the end of a 6-month follow-up period.

ASSESSMENT

The following sections describe how to assess residents for their psychosocial well-being.

Background Social History

All residents have a unique social history that should begin to be identified during the admission period. The assessment will be ongoing; new insights will evolve as relationships between caregivers and residents develop over time. The social history is based on conversations with the resident and at least one knowledgeable family member (if available) as well as information in referral documents. The assessment covers the following topics, documenting key factors in the resident's history, personality, preferences, habits, coping skills, and responses to daily life:

- Social roles, positions, and group memberships that give meaning to life:
  Family roles—parent, grandparent, spouse
  o Achieved status—education, work history, child rearing
  o Group identity—ethnic or religious identification, membership in a fraternal or civic organization, identification with a geographic area
  o History of limited social involvement— social life revolved around a person who is no longer present; activities limited largely to those things that the person could do on his or her own (e.g., watch television)
- Ability to relate to others:
  o Level of ability to make decisions of daily life—when to eat, who to interact with
  o Willingness to reach out versus distancing self from others—responds to small talk, unapproachable by all but closest family
  o Ability to communicate—functional hearing, vision, clear speech versus impairment that requires the staff to have a special understanding of the resident's communication style
  o Resident's physical appearance or cognitive status tends to limit opportunities for social exchange—resident is withdrawn, others shun or ridicule resident, resident has yet to adapt to recent changes in status
  o New difficulties interacting with others
- Relationships or activity preferences that can be a vehicle or focus of meaningful activities:
  o Family involvement in resident's care— frequency of visits, interest in working with staff, willingness to try new program ideas
  o Explicit preferences for distinct types of

social activities—small versus large groups, passive versus active activities, customary versus new types of activities, physical versus more sedentary activities
- Situational factors/personality traits that could limit social engagement options:
  o Grief or bitterness over admission into the facility—moving through grief versus inconsolable
  o The resident's foundation of trusting relationships with others—others have previously hurt the resident or failed to keep promises
  o Activity or social involvement options in the current facility that may be in conflict with the resident's prior lifestyle
  o The resident feels worthless, unworthy, punished by God; loss of interest in meaningful activities

Identifying Residents with Impaired Psychosocial Well-being

Consider a care plan follow-up when an intake or follow-up assessment indicates the presence of the following types of unsettled relationships or self-esteem problems. Focus on residents who have some residual cognitive capacity (e.g., those who can assume some role in making decisions).

- Covert or open conflict with staff or repeated criticism of staff—for example:
  o Chronic complaints about staff members to other staff members
  o Verbal criticism of staff members in therapeutic group situations
  o Criticism of staff communicated through families or another resident
  o Exhausting, never-ending lists of resident complaints (when one set of issues is addressed, new complaints always seem to emerge).
- Unhappiness with roommate—for example:
  o Frequent requests for roommate changes
  o Grumbling about roommate spending too long in the bathroom

o Complaints about roommate rummaging in one's belongings

o Fear of roommate's physical or verbal aggression

o Disgust with roommate's appearance, language, behavior, or visitors

o Statements such as, "My roommate doesn't like me."

- Unhappiness with residents other than roommate—for example:

  o Chronic complaints about the behavior of others

  o Poor quality of interaction with others

  o Lack of peers for socialization

  o Expressions of feeling different or superior to others

- Openly expresses conflict or anger with family or close friends—for example, expresses feelings of abandonment, ungratefulness, lack of understanding, or hostility toward family or friends

- Withdrawal from activities that once had meaning—for example:

  o Has suicidal thoughts

  o Resists use of crucial medications

  o Withdrawal accompanied by failure to eat or drink enough

  o Loss of interest in one's physical appearance and hygiene

  o No longer interested in wearing street clothes

  o Resists attending programs or participating in activities once enjoyed

- Perceives that daily routines and activities are very different from prior patterns in the community—for example:

  o Family no longer visits on a regular basis

  o Resident cannot make basic decisions on when to eat, what to watch on television

  o Much less active; doing little that was of value prior to coming into facility

SUPPLEMENTAL ASSESSMENT ITEMS

If the resident has a problem as specified in the previous section, it will be necessary to determine its cause and other associated factors. The section on background social history will be useful. The supplemental review in the following sections helps to place the problem into its broader context.

Situational Factors

Determine whether the problems are situational in nature, such as grief over the recent loss of family, friend, favorite staff, or functional ability. Try to determine if the problem can be remedied by environmental modifications or the simple passage of time. The issues to consider include:

- Is the resident new to the unit?

- Has the resident yet to be connected into meaningful roles or relationships—for example, resident has not seen children since transfer to the unit, minister has not visited?

- Is the roommate disruptive, domineering, or unreasonable? Does the resident being assessed exhibit these characteristics, all of which are likely to interfere with developing and sustaining a good relationship?

- Is the resident physically restrained, preventing socialization and participation in meaningful activities, for example, attending church services?

- Is the resident experiencing concurrent illness that serves to isolate the resident from others, for example, isolation for infection?

- Is the resident having difficulty adjusting to functional limitations related to a recent condition such as a stroke, myocardial infarction, memory changes?

- Is a particular staff member insensitive, abusive, unreliable, or unavailable to the resident?

- Do some direct care staff or family members interact more positively with the resident than others do? Could others learn from these experiences?

Long-Standing Problems

Determine whether the problem is reflective of long-standing personality characteristics, suggesting that resolution will be difficult or unrealistic. Consider the following issues:

- Is the family unit historically troubled, conflicted, hostile, or aloof with one another?
- Does the resident deny that relationship problems exist?
- Does the resident have a mental health problem (e.g., dementia, depression) that may preclude understanding and realistically perceiving the nature of the relationship?
- Is it a problem for staff, but not for the resident? If the resident does not see it as a problem, and it is not impacting other residents or families, is intervention warranted?
- Does the resident have resentment toward family specifically related to placement? Has the resident been left out of decision-making processes?

Mental Health Consultation

Consider a mental health consultation. Has there been a recent (within the last 6 months) psychosocial evaluation or consultation by a mental health professional—psychiatrist, psychologist, social worker, gero/psychiatric nurse?

Customary Routines and Preferences

Determine whether the problem is the result of a conflict between customary routines and preferences. Consider the following issues:

- Are current social activities and relationships in accord with the resident's preferences, values, and routines?
- What is the resident's characteristic mode of social interaction (e.g., has the resident always been a loner)?
- Are activities available in the resident's preferred activity settings?
- Are relationship opportunities structured around activities of interest?
- Are there residents living on the unit who would be appropriate peers? Have staff attempted to invite residents with common interests and functional levels to social activities?
- If the resident desires frequent contact with family/friends, is it happening?

Past Roles

Consider the issue of past roles. In the past, what has helped the resident hold on to a sense of being? Are such anchors (e.g., boss, caregiver, a lifelong hobby, job, or role such as an artist) now weak or lost? How might the care plan assist in retrieving or restoring continuity with past roles (in whole or in part)?

CARE PLANNING

This section discusses the strategies for addressing self-esteem and relationship problems. The first section discusses the utility of simultaneously treating both psychosocial and other problem conditions (e.g., mood). Specific approaches to care for such unsettled relationships or deterioration in self-esteem are then organized and discussed with respect to four problem areas:

- Absence of meaningful relationships or activities
- Isolation from family
- Absence of necessary environmental resources
- An indication that the resident is nearing the end of life
- The last section describes procedures for monitoring the care plan.

Strategies that Build on Other Care Plan Goals

In designing a program to address psychosocial problems, recognize that there are several classes of related problems around which a well-being care goal might be established, linking the well-being goal to other treatment strategies, including:

- Mood distress and problem behaviors
- Emerging deficits in communication or awareness
- Medical instability

Clinicians and direct care staff should plan

to use the time delivering physical care as an opportunity to observe resident interactions, to listen for grieving, to assist residents in verbalizing needs, wishes, and ideas, and to initiate actions that might help to improve a sense of well-being.

This type of care plan linkage is a primary strategy to address problems with relationships and self-esteem. Specific well-being treatment strategies are described in the next four sections.

Mood and Behavior Problems

Approximately 50% to 60% of all nursing home residents have mood distress (e.g., anxiety, depression) or exhibit problem behaviors (e.g., wandering, physical or verbal aggression, noisiness). For residents with psychosocial problems, the associated mood or behavioral symptoms are even more common—approaching 80% of all such persons. In treating these problems, the limited well-being treatment goals are as follows:

* Resident interactions will become more satisfying—conflicted interactions will become less frequent.
* The resident will build and expand on interaction opportunities with other residents, staff, and visitors.

Strategies to Create Opportunities for Relationships and Activities

The approaches to care included in this section are organized under a series of discrete treatment goals. In each instance, the staff's objective is to help the resident take small steps forward, rather than seek some sudden, dramatic improvement. Each small change for the better can help make a once untenable loss bearable, enabling the resident to find the strength and will to cope with other problems. The resident will be better prepared to enter into social situations that draw on their interest patterns. Each of the strategies presented offers the possibility of

reengagement, giving meaning to daily life, and reducing negative feelings associated with nursing home placement. When altering the resident's activity pattern to help establish new relationships of varying intensity, be sure to allow sufficient down time for privacy and reflections.

The approaches to create opportunities for relationships and activities are as follows:
* Ensure resident participation in meaningful activities:
  o To the extent physically and intellectually possible, bring the resident's daily schedule into accord with the customary routines before admission. This may require challenging existing facility routines and procedures. What were the resident's preferred habits and ways of organizing the day and spending time? For example, a resident who has a history of helping others may find satisfaction in reading to other residents, assisting in religious services, assuming the role of leader in group activities, or helping staff to prepare and distribute between-meal snacks. A resident who had many friends in the community may appreciate the opportunity to maintain connections with old friends or participate in community groups or activities.
  o Explore ways to enhance the resident's feeling of control and mastery. Increase the opportunities to make choices in matters of daily life, schedules, treatments, and so forth. Ensure that the choices provided remain within the resident's intellectual or physical capabilities. For example, for a resident who can initiate activities independently, provide a listing of the facility program alternatives, show the resident where activities take place, and introduce the resident to key group leaders (including staff, other residents, and volunteers). If the resident hesitates in initiating involve-

ment, have a nursing assistant and family members talk up the activity options and give reminders of specific activities scheduled each day.

- Link the resident into planned community-based activity programs at the facility. Examples include foster grandparents, joint child-resident day-care programs, day-care or exercise programs involving community-residing elderly, or a link to any local nursing or health care education programs. Also consider establishing a link with local schools; grade school classes can make holiday cards and bring them to residents at a joint social where food is served. For residents who desire greater involvement with community affairs, the staff can arrange for a member of a political party to speak to residents, the resident can be given the opportunity to volunteer, or members of a local Golden-Agers can arrange transportation to a meeting.

- Link more cognitively intact residents into a group activity. Depending on prior interests, residents can be channeled into a wide variety of social activities—e.g., political discussions, Bible reading, singing, current events discussion groups, ethnic socials, unit parties, and group trips outside the nursing home. One-on-one examples with other residents or visitors include card playing, walking, reading, reminiscing, and assisting a family member in considering the problems of the extended family unit.

- Introduce residents to others with shared interests. Try to make efforts to introduce the resident to others who may share some common bond (from the old neighborhood, or sharing enjoyment of a particular activity, or with a similar work history). Consider using a buddy help system.

Interventions to Enrich Family Visits

Consider the following strategies to enrich family visits:

- Work with the families to help improve the quality and adjust the frequency of their visits with residents. There are a wide variety of activity options that can enrich family visits and enhance the resident's feelings of well-being. The goals are to enrich the time spent together, and to provide better connections between the family and the facility (increasing the sense that the facility is a home in which family can be comfortable).

The frustration family can feel during visits often comes from the unrealistic expectations of residents, staff, and family. Sometimes families expect too much, sometimes too little. Unrealistic expectations may be based on a lack of information, incorrect information, or partial information. Families must be helped to recognize that new connections with the resident are necessary, that facility visits may never be like visits at home, and that progressive resident decline will call for new accommodations. Some families will come with extensive experience and information about nursing home care, but many will not. The goal is to help bring families to a common understanding of how visits may change as a result of the resident's changes in health and function. Suggestions for improving family visits are as follows:

o *Provide information to family visitors as follows:*
  * Group orientation meetings on a regular basis (e.g., monthly) at times that are convenient for families (e.g., evening or weekend). Invite the families of all newly admitted residents.
  * Provide orientation packets about the facility, residential unit, staff roles and responsibilities, names and titles of care team members, and all who can be called to discuss potential problems or request information.
  * Supplement written material with general conversations about expectations

regarding future resident change—functional loss, dementing illness, resident problems of behavior, feelings, and judgment—and how the family can respond to the resident.

* Include a list of typical family reactions to visiting nursing home residents. Family visitors learn more easily when they can identify with others in a similar situation.

* Provide a hot line or staff contact who will listen empathically to family complaints.

o *Improve the family visit.* Visiting implies a mutuality or reciprocity that is often beyond the capacity of the resident and family. Families may benefit from individualized discussion with knowledgeable staff in assessing strengths in the relationship, activities that can still be shared and enjoyed, and how to ensure that visits are meaningful for both resident and visitor. Most family visitors need specific guidance about how to help the resident feel like a host or hostess, or how to make visiting more reciprocal to reinforce the resident's self-esteem, identity, and connection to family. To improve the visits:

* Initiate these discussions at a mutually convenient time, or take advantage of times when family members seek out staff, or build this need to share information into the job description of direct care staff who may be in more frequent contact with families.

* Link each resident's family with a specific staff person (aide, social worker, activity staff, nurse) who will be their visit liaison. The family will want some feedback on how their relative does or does not anticipate or react to visits. A special staff person can monitor visits and make suggestions about alternate strategies.

o *Time visits to maximize resident responsiveness.* Residents have good days and bad days, and even better hours within the day. Suggestions for timing visits to coincide with resident routines, special events, and the resident's preferences will enhance the quality of visits from the perspectives of residents, staff, and families. Families will probably have an idea about their relative's best time for visits, favorite activities, and other habits. Ask regular family visitors about other commitments and when they are most comfortable visiting. Some education at this point is helpful. The special staff person previously mentioned may be helpful in pointing out opportunities or times that are best suited to the needs and wishes of both resident and family visitor. Also consider these factors when scheduling visits:

* Letting families know about the mealtime schedule and procedures, special events, down times, and gaps in activity programming may facilitate successful timing of the visits.

* For nonverbal or severely cognitively impaired residents, schedule visits so that the family may participate in care. This may help family visits become more meaningful (e.g., time the visit so the family can help the resident eat).

* Sometimes families need permission from the physician or nurse to limit their visiting, particularly if frequent visits impose excessive emotional stress on residents or family members.

o *Recruit family members who visit frequently* (i.e., more than once a week) to assume a central role in maintaining meaningful social interactions with the resident. For example:

* Suggest that family members continue to involve the resident in the life of the extended family—sharing gossip,

asking for resident input into decision making (e.g., "should we ..."), bringing the resident home at holidays, taking the resident out to eat or for day trips.

* The family can also play a useful role on the unit—grandchildren can visit, paid helpers can be recruited to visit or take the resident out of the nursing home on outings.

* For some residents, plan the family visits for times when the resident is most likely to be reassured by their presence (e.g., at bedtime).

* The family can provide the link that helps the resident bond or interact with other residents on the unit (e.g., inviting other residents to share ethnic foods from home or listen to the family member read a favorite story). Introduce the family members of other residents with the goal of establishing joint family visitation/activity groups (e.g., when a family member visits they will include other residents in the visit).

o *Discuss or demonstrate a suggested visiting activity* the first time a new visiting activity is attempted. Some families will need this individualized staff support to initiate changes in relating to their relative. Demonstrating may be more powerful than written or verbal suggestions.

o *Arrange for the availability of materials to promote visiting*—e.g., games, videos, short stories. Consider establishing an activity cart. Provide brief written instructions for use of materials that may differ depending on the extent of dementia.

o *Help families end visits gracefully*—families often have difficulty leaving without upsetting the resident who may not understand why the visitor is leaving. The staff can provide tips on strategies to smooth leave taking; visits that end successfully mean less disruption for other residents and staff and less discomfort for the resident being left.

o *Provide suggestions for family contacts and reminders between visits.* For example:

* Suggest that families leave reassuring messages on audio or videotape for use by residents when they become distraught.

* If the resident has immediate access to a phone, help the resident contact family or other loved ones outside of the home; also have distant family members phone or write letters on a regular basis. Phone calls can become burdensome on families, particularly if the resident with dementia calls frequently because he or she has forgotten recent telephone conversations. For this reason, carefully assess when to install automatic dialers on phones used by demented residents. Such devices can be quite useful for some demented residents and any cognitively intact resident who is also visually impaired.

* Have the family create a collage of pictures of familiar people, places, and important events that help to reaffirm the presence and continued love of family.

* Help families understand the importance of concrete reminders of future visits. Reminders like guest books, notes, gifts, treats, and pictures may reassure the resident that the visitor was there, will return, and that they are remembered and loved even when a family member is not physically present.

• Encourage sharing of feelings by resident and staff. As part of a movement toward an individualized approach to care, encourage staff to choose residents with whom to establish special relationships. Encourage the family to allow the resident to share expressions of grief over loss and reminisce about the past. The staff can use these indications of troubled relationships to help guide their formalization of these special relationships. Once established, inform the family of their existence. Plan time to talk with the resident, discuss subjects of interest, and ensure continuity. Keep the family informed of these discussions. The family is often crucial to understanding how the resident is feeling or even what the resident may mean.

- Address any issues of relocation trauma as the resident moves into the facility or moves between units in the nursing home. For example:
  o *Determine the process by which the resident and family made the decision for nursing home placement.*
    * Was the resident appropriately included as decision-maker? Has the resident had ample opportunity to articulate feelings about this major life transition?
    * What are the feelings that may have been unexpressed about the decision to come into care?
    * If the current resident-family relationship is strained, can it be modified by dealing with unspoken issues about admission to the facility?
    * Explore family members' feelings about resident's placement. Do family members have unarticulated feelings of ambivalence or guilt over the placement, making them less tolerant, more reactive, and confrontational with their relative?
    * If the resident must move to another unit within the facility, ensure that staff meet with the resident and family before the move. Schedule a visit to the new unit to meet staff, observe the program, and ask questions.

Strategies to Compensate for Environmental Barriers

Consider the following strategies to compensate for environmental barriers:

- Separate the resident from stressful environmental stimuli. Mood, behavior, and well-being problems often originate in immediate stresses in the environment—e.g., loud noises, crowded day rooms, noisy demanding roommates. Identifying and altering the stressful condition can lead to immediate positive resident outcomes. The presence of situational problems may be remedied by simple environmental modification or altered approach to resident care (e.g., create an altar or meditation place for a religious resident, better explain the flow of regular activity of the nursing home to a new resident). Relevant well-being goals include the following:
  o The resident will communicate with the staff about environmental factors (equipment, setup in room, roommate problems) needed to carry out an activity or special interest.
  o The resident will use the appropriate appliance to compensate for impairment—e.g., braces, eyeglasses.
- The following factors can cause stress:
  o Roommate incompatibility. The most immediate problem involves sharing a room with someone who is disturbing or troubling to the resident. If a room change is not possible in the short run (which is often the preferred solution) consider the following:
    * Separate the residents whenever possible
    * Identify and treat the underlying problems that cause distress for the residents that share the room
    * Increase frequency of staff monitoring
    * Identify events that trigger distressing

events and take steps to anticipate their occurrence

  * Sometimes it is helpful to have a meeting with the nurse or social worker and the roommates involved to air complaints and make some ground rules about problem areas (e.g., television volume [or use of headphones] or time spent in a shared bathroom)

  * Ensure that the resident is not endangered by others. Residents who are immobile (e.g., wheelchair-bound) and have restricted cognitive ability are often subject to verbal and physical aggression from other residents who are more mobile. Haphazard mixes of residents on units occur all too frequently. Physically separate these two types of residents.

  * Residents also may be disturbed by others who are noisy, less cognitively intact, or come from a very different cultural or socioeconomic background. In each instance the issue is one of resident mix. If there are many problems of this type, consider assigning residents to rooms and units using a more homogeneous placement model.

- Ensure the availability of the necessary mobility and communication appliances. For example:

  o Facilitate the resident's continued use of residual functional or intellectual capacities by providing necessary appliances and ensuring they are in working order—e.g., bring a leg brace each morning at a specified time to ensure that the resident can move about the facility and participate in activities of interest.

  o Facilitate alternative means of communication—e.g., ensure that the necessary hearing examinations have been completed and that adaptive appliances are present, in working order, and used ap-

propriately (see Chapter 16, Communication).

  o Alter environmental barriers where possible—e.g., provide access to safe areas previously off limits; provide access to safe outdoor areas; for the cognitively impaired, have family help personalize the room so that it seems less foreign and unfamiliar; place old pictures on the door to the resident's room to facilitate orientation and direction.

Strategies to Approach Care at the End of Life

When a resident approaches the end of life, there is a need to adapt the environment to ensure that family are welcomed as they may begin to increase their presence on the unit. The goal is to provide the opportunity for the resident and family to maintain necessary familial bonds and to help the resident retain positive self-esteem. The general approach to care can involve the following steps:

- If a hospice bed is present and the resident is stressed on the current unit, consider a transfer.
- If the resident is comfortable with the current unit staff, avoid pressure to transfer the resident inside the facility or to a hospital.
- Ensure that the staff are aware of the resident's wishes concerning the site of death and the presence or absence of family members.
- Provide an opportunity for family and relatives to stay with the resident during the terminal illness; help arrange for family transportation to the facility if necessary; orient the family about facility resources (e.g., the chapel, a place to be alone, the social worker schedule, what time would be best to talk to the nurse manager or nurse assistant, the location of phones and food machines).
- Help the family make decisions about how best to schedule and carry out resident visits. How long should they stay? What can

they do to make the resident more comfortable? Remember, there are no right answers. The goal is to be a sounding board for the family and the resident, and to provide accurate information and realistic suggestions. Be aware of their expectations. Help to bring the two together or ease the situation if it is advisable that they be apart.

- Provide the family with opportunities to ask questions about what to expect and what will happen.

Monitoring the Care Plan

At periodic intervals (at least monthly), evaluate progress toward the stated objectives and determine whether any changes in the psychosocial well-being care plan are warranted. Consider the following:

- Has the resident moved from settled to unsettled relationships, from a positive to a negative view of self?
- What is the evidence of the resident's increased control over life events—moving toward more positive view of self?
- How is the resident now dealing with grief or loss?
- Is the resident expressing pride or satisfaction with competence in self-care or coping?
- Is there any evidence of greater intimacy or companionship, concern for other residents or family?
- Is there any evidence of more appropriate concern for self or appearance?

Prepare the staff, especially the nurses and nursing assistants, to listen carefully to the resident and to be alert to statements (positive and negative) that the resident makes about him- or herself. Make sure the staff are aware of their responsibility under the care plan to nurture new relationships, praise the resident when goals are attained, and expand the range of short-term goals as proficiency is demonstrated.

CASE EXAMPLE

Mrs. L., a 65-year-old woman with an 8-year history of Alzheimer's disease, first entered the facility 3 months ago. She had resided with her husband of 40 years in an architecturally modified apartment in an elderly housing complex. She had become progressively more confused in the prior 18-month period. She had been hospitalized twice because of confusion, agitated behavior, and mild depression. Her physician had prescribed oxazepam for anxiety. She often became confused when challenged by a new situation, but with the help of her husband and extensive visits by her two children and sister, she had been relatively stable in the months prior to admission. Her husband helped her with most activities of daily living (ADLs). She would go walking in the neighborhood (usually with her sister) and would stop and talk with people she knew. She would smile at strangers. Her children also took her out for rides (stopping to get her ice cream and fried foods) at least twice each week. At the same time, there were periods when she became nervous and demanding. Her biggest fear was that her husband would put her in a nursing home. He would reassure her that this would not happen, and she would regain her more pleasant outlook.

Three months ago her husband had a stroke and died within a matter of days. At the time of the stroke, Mrs. L.'s children and sibling were unable to bring her into their homes. Her needs were seen to be too extensive, and they had never prepared themselves for such a placement.

On admission to this facility, Mrs. L. was aware that her husband had died. She cried about his death, and she cried about being in the nursing home. She felt abandoned and confused, and had periods of extreme agitation. Staff held extensive conversations with Mrs. L. and her two children about her history. Her children did not understand initially why Mrs. L. had become withdrawn. They blamed the staff, seemingly projecting their guilt at not being able to care for Mrs. L. in their homes. In response, the staff, too, became overly combative, and there was a 4-week delay in understanding that Mrs. L.'s loss and fears were not due to these factors, but rather to the sense of loss following the death of her spouse. Mrs. L. went to her husband's funeral. She seemed to hold up under the strain but cried for days after her return to the home. Only with time did the staff come to recognize her basically pleasant personality.

Once the staff and family were working together, Mrs. L.'s children and sibling made sure that someone visited her each day. The staff introduced her family to Mrs. L.'s roommate, a pleasant wheelchair-bound resident who had a mild stroke 2 years previously. Mrs. L. and her roommate seemed to be able to communicate with one another, and Mrs. L. enjoyed being with this person. Direct care staff were instructed to take the time to talk to Mrs. L., giving her the opportunity to do ADLs and care for herself. Attempts to introduce Mrs. L. to group activities were generally unsuccessful at first, with the exception that she was most willing to see her minister and join in a weekly prayer program. The staff were more successful in helping the family plan their visits. The family visited 5 days a week. They began each visit by asking the staff how Mrs. L. was doing, communicated their own impressions of her progress at the end of the visit, and to help encourage Mrs. L. to be involved in daily activities, they helped the staff identify strategies that had worked in the past.

Family members were encouraged to bring in sweets from the local ice cream parlor. Family also responded positively to the suggestion of offering Mrs. L.'s roommate treats. They decided on their own to take the roommate with them as they walked Mrs. L. on the grounds.

Mrs. L.'s children have helped her understand how the nursing home works. They have been brought into the care planning process, and are comfortable with staff. The staff know Mrs. L. as a person. They are actively working with and drawing on the insights of her children. Mrs. L. no longer cries for her husband. She has good relationships with her nursing assistant and roommate, and responds warmly to visits by her children and sister.

16
Communication

Rosemary Lubinski, EdD
Carol Frattali, PhD
Craig Barth, PhD

Nursing home residents face a troubling paradox. They live in a setting in which optimal functioning requires keen communication skills, while at the same time they may have serious difficulties communicating. Communication problems—pathophysiologic conditions that prevent residents from adequately receiving or expressing information vital to their physical, psychological, or social well-being—affect more than 50% of nursing home residents. These problems are typically associated with hearing loss, aphasia, dysarthria, apraxia, laryngectomy, dementia, reduced physiologic reserves, and depression. In addition, language, cultural, educational, gender, and ethnic differences between residents and caregivers may contribute to communication difficulties between either group.

This chapter discusses the most common communication problems exhibited in an elderly nursing home population. It provides techniques for identifying problematic situations and suggests practical strategies for facilitating communication with and among affected residents. Finally, the chapter notes the roles of the speech-language pathologist and audiologist in identifying and treating elderly residents with communication problems. These
services are often underused, and staff are encouraged to seek assistance from these professionals whenever communication problems are of a concern.

OVERVIEW

Communication between two or more individuals is a complex process that is conducted on many levels of awareness. It may occur receptively through vision and hearing, or expressively through speaking, writing, or gesturing. A communication problem prevents residents from adequately receiving or expressing information vital to their physical, psychological, or social well-being. The cumulative impact of such problems, especially in an institutional setting, can result in a heightened sense of isolation. Isolation, in turn, may become a primary cause of decline leading to problems such as depression. Communication difficulties can also be frustrating to caregivers, family, and other residents by affecting the quality of the therapeutic and social milieu, as well as interpersonal relationships.

There are many possible causes for the communication problems experienced by residents. Some are related to the aging process itself, while others are associated with conditions such as stroke, cancer, and progressive neurologic disorders. It is common to find more than one factor causing a communication problem in an elderly individual. For example, a resident may have sustained a stroke that resulted in aphasia and dysarthria, and may also be affected by a pre-existing hearing loss. A resident may have both dementia and a hearing loss. In addition, communication problems may be complicated by the resident's physical, psychological, and emotional status, as well as by environmental isolation that inhibits verbal interaction.

Receptive communication deficits may involve declines in hearing (i.e., acuity and/or speech discrimination ability), vocabulary comprehension, reading, and recognizing facial expressions. Expressive communication deficits may include reduced voice volume, changes in vocal quality such as hoarseness and harshness, difficulty in producing sounds (*dysarthria*), monotone inflection, and difficulty finding the right word, constructing sentences, writing, and gesturing. Environmental factors may also play a role, i.e., there may be few stimulating opportunities for a resident to converse with partners of choice, regardless of their communication skill level.

The communication problems found in an elderly nursing home population are usually associated with one or more of the conditions described in the following sections.

Hearing Loss

In addition to its effect on understanding speech or discriminating among environmental noises, hearing loss can complicate or exacerbate the diagnosis of disorders such as stroke and dementia. It can also have a profoundly negative effect on a resident's sense of self-worth and willingness to participate in conversation or social events, with resulting irritability, paranoia, confusion, fatigue, withdrawal, isolation, and sad mood. Hearing loss may also contribute to a resident's difficulty in performing activities of daily living (ADLs), taking medications, and following other therapeutic regimens. Hearing loss is the most socially isolating of the sensory losses.

The most common type of hearing loss associated with aging is *presbycusis*. While there are different kinds and degrees of presbycusis, typically the result in the older resident is a progressive, permanent, bilaterally symmetric hearing loss characterized by difficulty in discerning high-frequency sounds (e.g., s, th, sh, and f). This deficit may result in a reduced ability to comprehend speech, particularly in noisy situations.

The nature and extent of hearing loss depends on which part of the auditory system is affected. A conductive hearing loss results from disruption in the transmission of sound by a problem of the outer or middle ear. Possible causes include impacted wax in the external ear canal, middle ear infection (fluid), and loss of mobility in the middle ear bone structure (*otosclerosis*). A sensorineural hearing loss results from damage to the inner ear and/or auditory nerve, usually as a consequence of exposure to noise and normal aging. A mixed hearing loss is one that has varying components of conductive and sensorineural hearing losses.

Aphasia

Aphasia is an impairment in the ability to comprehend and/or express language that may affect some or all channels of communication, including listening and reading, speaking, writing, and gesturing. Aphasia is caused by damage to the language centers within the brain, usually specialized areas of the left hemisphere for most individuals. Some residents who are left-handed are right hemisphere-dominant for language. The most common cause of aphasia is a cerebrovascular accident or stroke, although it may also result from traumatic brain injury, tumors, hematomas, and infections of the brain.

The patterns of difficulty associated with aphasia result from where the brain damage has occurred (side and site of lesion) and the extent of the lesion. In general, damage to the left frontal portion of the brain results in a predominant pattern of difficulty in forming words and connecting words into complete sentences. An aphasic resident with damage to this area of the brain may use single words to express a larger idea (e.g., "water" for "Give me some water"); may be telegraphic, omitting the small function words of a sentence (e.g., "Daughter, Saturday, candy" for "My daughter came on Saturday and brought me some candy"); and may use incorrect grammar (e.g., "I sawn him" for "I have seen him"). Residents with this type of speech may sound like they are having difficulty planning how to say each word. In addition, this type of aphasic resident may have difficulty thinking of words (*anomia*) in that the resident knows what to say but cannot retrieve the precise word (e.g., "I want a cup of, cup of, oh, you know...." Finally, this resident may have some mild difficulties in auditory comprehension and associated problems such as dysarthria or apraxia of speech.

For residents with aphasia who have damage to the posterior portions of the brain, there may be a predominant pattern of difficulty in comprehension of auditory or visual information. These residents will have problems understanding what is heard or read, and will respond accordingly. For example, the resident may not understand lengthy, complex sentences or may not follow a conversation in which there are several alternating speakers. This resident may also have difficulty retrieving words or may use a wrong but related word (e.g., coffee for tea). Responses may sound inappropriate or jargonlike.

Some residents with aphasia have extensive damage to the language centers of the brain. These residents are considered to have global aphasia. They have major difficulties

in all communication channels, but there may be some ability to both understand and express ideas such as greetings, songs, prayers, counting, and other well-rehearsed items. Aphasia differs from the somewhat similar language changes associated with dementia in that aphasic residents are generally aware and frustrated by their communication problems, communication improvement can be achieved and maintained to some degree, and there is no further progression of the problem unless the resident suffers another stroke.

Dysarthria

Dysarthria is imperfect articulation of speech due to disturbances of motor control resulting from damage to the central or peripheral nervous system. It is characterized by any or all of the following difficulties:

- Reduced speech intelligibility
- Reduced ability to control loudness and voice
- Changes in voice quality, such as harshness, breathiness, loudness, and appropriate pitch
- Rate of speech
  Common causes of dysarthria include:
- Stroke
- Progressive neurologic disorders such as Parkinson's disease and multiple sclerosis
- Amyotrophic lateral sclerosis (ALS)
- Dementia (multiinfarct)

Impairment stems from neurologic damage to the central or peripheral nervous system, resulting in paralysis, weakness, or incoordination of the muscles involved in speech production.

Dementia-Related Problems

Dementia results in diffuse cerebral dysfunction to both hemispheres of the brain and in some cases to subcortical areas. It may be caused by numerous conditions, some of which are potentially reversible and others that are progressive. The most common causes of dementia among residents are Alzheimer's disease and multiinfarct dementia. Comprehension and expression of logical, coherent, and meaningful communication becomes increasingly difficult because of underlying difficulties in cognition. In early stages of dementia, the resident may have subtle difficulties in all channels of communication and may show some awareness of communication difficulties.

As the dementia progresses, difficulties in thinking of words, understanding, reading, and writing become more pronounced and detrimental to maintaining successful communication. In the final stage of dementia, all communication channels become severely compromised, and communication may be limited to understanding a few simple commands and expressing a very limited number of words.

Reduced Physiologic Reserve

Reduced physiologic reserve refers to any physiologic changes in the resident that may substantially weaken the integration of processes necessary for producing speech. For example, residents with congestive heart failure (CHF) or chronic lung disease may suffer *dyspnea* (air hunger) to the extent that they are unable to control their breathing long enough to generate normal sentences. Some residents may develop age- and disease-related physiologic impairments that reduce their capacity to produce speech. These impairments may compromise air flow through the vocal cords or may affect the cognitive and physical capacity to produce speech. For example, emphysema or CHF may diminish air flow; lack of respiratory muscle strength due to myasthenia can reduce a resident's ability to produce speech; rheumatoid arthritis may fuse the vocal cords; and stroke can impair the use of an assistive communication device.

Depression

Residents who have adequate ability to comprehend and formulate speech may still communicate infrequently or with diminished emotional content because of a prevailing mood disorder. Depression is frequently associated with aphasia, hearing loss, progressive neurologic disorders, institutionalization, and loss of significant others. All of these factors can manifest as communication problems. Dementia and depression can coexist.

Language Barriers

In some nursing home settings, there may be language, cultural, educational, and ethnic differences between caregivers and residents that result in problems of conveying information efficiently, effectively, and with sensitivity. Recent statistics indicate that the older minority population is growing at a faster rate than the older white population. In the next 25 years, about 15% of the elderly in the United States will be nonwhite. Currently, many nursing homes are staffed by minority individuals caring for white residents.

These two demographic trends have direct implications for communication in nursing homes. For example, while residents may be more comfortable communicating in English, nursing assistants who have recently immigrated from another country may have limited proficiency in English. Other residents may prefer to speak in their first language or may revert to another language when stressed or confused. Individual differences such as age, social class, and religious affiliation also influence how communication will be sent and received.

The content and style of messages are also dependent on cultural and ethnic heritage. Questions and comments about health and personal care are influenced greatly by this background. Lack of knowledge about and insensitivity to a resident's cultural and ethnic background may also lead to communication barriers and failure. Cultural and ethnic communication differences between caregivers and residents may lead to misunderstanding, social withdrawal, and noncompliance with or resistance to care.

IDENTIFYING THE RESIDENT IN NEED OF CARE

The assessment process begins with the completion of the Communication section on the Minimum Data Set (MDS). Residents who have been identified by this instrument to have a communication problem should be referred for a complete communication evaluation by a speech-language pathologist or a hearing evaluation by an audiologist.

If the problem existed before admission or has been ongoing at the facility, review the current approaches to care. For new admissions, secure this information from the attending physician, a family member, or the resident. If it is documented in records supplied at admission, review these records. For residents who have had the problem at the facility for a long time, review the facility record and talk with direct care staff. If there has never been a referral to an audiologist or speech language pathologist, or the resident's status has changed since the most recent referral, make a new referral. In any case, review and note how communication has been maximized in the past. Ask whether the family and staff have been sensitive to this issue. If there have been successful procedures in the past, they are a starting point for a future plan of care.

Nursing staff should look routinely to the speech-language pathologist or audiologist for help in deciding who are the best candidates for a more complete communication or hearing evaluation. It is not necessary to determine the cause or extent of the communication difficulty, but note that the resident is having difficulty in communication. In addition to the triggers on the MDS, consider the

following factors to determine the need for referral to a speech-language pathologist or audiologist. The following factors provide additional information about this need:

- Is the resident aware of or frustrated by his or her difficulties understanding or sending spoken or written messages?
- Does the resident have difficulty understanding a conversation or following instructions? Does the resident continually ask for words or sentences to be repeated, watch faces very carefully during interaction, complain of hearing difficulties, or mention that others do not speak clearly?
- Does the resident become anxious about participating in social activities? Does the resident refuse to participate? Is the resident more tired than might be expected after participating?
- Does the resident set the volume on a television or radio abnormally loud?
- Does the resident seem to miss the gist of simple conversations?
- Does the resident have difficulty expressing ideas in single words or short sentences?
- Do listeners have a difficult time understanding the meaning of what the resident is conveying?
- Do listeners have a difficult time understanding the resident's speech intelligibility (e.g., words sound unclear, mumbled, slurred, misarticulated)?
- Does the resident have an assistive listening device (e.g., hearing aid or portable amplifier)? Is the device used regularly during conversations or other social activities? Is it working properly?
- Does the resident have an assistive communication device such as an artificial larynx or a communication board? Is the device used regularly during conversations or other social activities? Is it working properly?
- Does the resident have adequate access to communication partners or activities that

generate an opportunity to communicate?
- Are staff receptive to the resident?
- Are staff, family, or significant others frustrated by their difficulties in communicating with the resident?

STRATEGIES AND TECHNIQUES OF THERAPEUTIC CAREPLANNING

In the nursing home population, communication problems may be of recent origin (e.g., due to a recent stroke or laryngectomy), associated with a progressive debility (e.g., Parkinson's disease or dementia), or represent a long-standing situation that has reached a plateau (e.g., previous stroke). Whatever the proximate cause, progression, or severity of the problem, the basic premises of therapeutic careplanning are the same. The general guidelines to help promote better communication are as follows:

- Approach communication with the resident in an adultlike tone and melody of voice and appropriate vocabulary level and sentence structure. Avoid an abnormally slow, sing-song melody and intonation, or an overly loud voice.
- Conduct communication in an unhurried fashion. Speak slowly and distinctly. Allow the resident ample time to think, talk, and respond.
- Establish and maintain eye contact with the resident while communicating.
- Monitor your nonverbal communication for signs of impatience and frustration (e.g., body language or tone of voice that signals impatience).

The general guidelines to enhance communication via the physical and social environment, are as follows:

- Eliminate or reduce competing noise when communicating (e.g., television, radio, group discussions).

- Ensure that the resident's access to visual cues is maximized during communication. Reduce glare and shadows in face-to-face communication. If the resident has unilateral vision or hearing impairment, approach and speak from the better functioning side.
- Provide an array of age-appropriate and stimulating activities for the resident's participation.
- Encourage the resident to take part in activities of choice, but recognize that some individuals benefit from watching rather than actively participating.
- Remove physical barriers that reduce communication opportunities (e.g., bring activities to the resident's floor, or provide rest stops along the way to activities that are distant from the resident's room).
- Encourage friendships among residents.
- Encourage and reinforce family visits and socialization with the resident. Educate visitors regarding communication and facilitating techniques.
- Sensitize staff to their vital role as communication partners for residents. Personal care activities are a perfect vehicle for establishing successful communication patterns. Other opportunities, including mealtime and social activities, are also opportunities for enhancing communication.
- Develop a problem-solving attitude among staff about ways to communicate effectively with residents.

The following sections describe care plans for communications problems.

Care Plan for Hearing Loss

Once hearing loss is identified, refer the resident to an audiologist for an assessment. Determination of hearing aid candidacy should be made by the audiologist, otologist, care providers, family members, and resident in a collaborative manner. The benefits of wearing a hearing aid vary greatly depending on numerous interacting factors including speech discrimination ability, personal motivation/choice, and presence and stage of dementia. Because of the many different types of aids available, the staff should consult with the audiologist or speech-language pathologist for information on how to assist residents with particular hearing aids.

For the resident who has a hearing aid, follow these guidelines:

• Encourage the resident to wear the hearing aid, particularly during prime socialization occasions (e.g., mealtimes, activities, visits, and routine daily care).

• Work with the audiologist or speech-language pathologist to learn how to:
  o Insert the ear mold properly
  o Place the hearing aid in the ear canal or behind the ear
  o Remove the ear mold and hearing aid
  o Turn the hearing aid on and off, and adjust it for telephone use
• Be sure the hearing aid is kept clean, supplied with fresh batteries, and switched off when not in use. Keep a record of the type of battery and replacement date in the resident's chart and check the battery as appropriate.
• When not in use, keep the hearing aid in a consistent place that is dry and secure, protected from spills or banging. Residents who

Table 16-1. Hearing Aids: Common Problems and Solutions

Problem	Cause	Solution
Whistling or howling noise	Earmold inserted improperly	Reinsert earmold
	cracked or loose tubing	Check or replace tubing
	Improper earmold fit	Have earmold replaced
	Hearing aid turned up too loud	Reduce volume
Scratchy sound; aid goes on and off	Defective cord (body aids only)	Replace cord
	Poor switch contact	Move switch back and forth several times
		Remove and reinsert plug body (body aid only)
Weak sound	Weak battery	Have ear examined
	Bent or blocked tubing	Check tubing
	Earmold inserted improperly	Reinsert earmold
	Excessive cerumen (wax) in ear canal	Have ear examined
No sound	Aid turned off	Turn to M or On
	Clogged earmold	Clean earmold
	Dead battery	Replace battery
	Battery inserted improperly	Reinsert battery correctly
	Corroded battery contacts	Clean contacts, if previously instructed
	Bent or blocked tubing	Check or replace tubing
	Cracked or broken cord (body aid only)	Check or replace cord

are independent in use of the aid should have easy access. To prevent loss or damage, hearing aids of demented residents could be maintained in a central, safe location (e.g., nurses' station).

Table 16-1 lists common hearing aid problems and solutions.

If the solutions in Table 16-1 do not solve the problem see the audiologist. Do not try to repair the hearing aid yourself.

For any resident with a hearing loss, follow these guidelines (regardless of the use of an assistive listening device):

- Reinforce family and significant others in using communication-facilitating strategies with hearing- impaired residents.
- Be sure the resident's ears are clear of canal wax and hair.
- Be sure the resident wears eyeglasses, if prescribed. A good view of the speaker's face facilitates communication.
- Gain the resident's attention before communicating by touching, coming into direct vision of the resident, or providing some type of signal that you are ready to talk.
- Be sure that there is adequate lighting for the resident to see the communicator's face. Do not talk from behind the resident or while standing in shadows.
- Reduce background noises while communicating (e.g., ask to turn off the radio or television; wait until corridor noise abates; close door). Such actions are especially important when communicating with residents who have reduced speech discrimination abilities.
- Speak with normal loudness and clear but not overarticulated speech. Never shout.
- Since most residents have impairments in high-frequency hearing, speak in a low-pitched voice. Most people raise both the loudness and pitch of the voice when speaking to a hard-of-hearing elder. Lowering the frequency of the voice is usually all that is

necessary.
- Pause frequently to check for comprehension. Pausing provides the resident with time to process information or ask for repetition or clarification.
- Avoid talking with hands near mouth or with food or gum in mouth.
- Individuals with beards or mustaches should monitor their speech when communicating with a hearing-impaired resident.
- If the resident is not a candidate for a hearing aid, consider using an assistive listening device. These devices can be obtained from the staff speech-language pathologist or audiologist. Assistive listening devices include:
  o *Telecommunication Devices for Deaf People (TDDs).* This device allows a resident to type a message and send it over regular telephone lines to another TDD where the message is then read.
  o *Telecaption decoders.* This device allows a resident to read rather then listen to dialog on television.
  o *Personal amplifier.* A portable device that includes an amplifier and headphone. This instrument enhances reception of one-to-one conversations.
  o *Room amplifiers.* These devices can be used in larger group situations. Specific types include audio loop, AM and FM, and infrared systems. Nursing homes should consider installing audio loops in auditoriums and large gathering areas.
- Continually monitor the resident's hearing ability for any change in status.
- Provide feedback to the audiologist or speech-language pathologist concerning progress or continuing concerns.

Care Plan for Aphasia

Residents with onset of dementia in the past year are in the prime period for the condition to improve spontaneously and are also most responsive to intervention by a speech-language pathologist. Appropriate therapy will not only maximize recovery but will also provide relief against withdrawal and frustration. Family, caregivers, and significant others will likewise benefit by learning productive communication techniques.

Use the MDS as the screening tool. Evaluation of the aphasic resident is typically begun by the nurse, who informally assesses the resident's ability to understand and express information related to the ADLs (e.g., to follow simple spoken directions, find words, use appropriate sentence structure, read and write). In addition, the staff should note the level and conditions under which the aphasic resident becomes frustrated when communicating. This assessment, along with any available information about the resident's prior communication/cognitive patterns, helps the speech-language pathologist to plan an appropriate comprehensive assessment of all communication abilities and a functional rehabilitation strategy.

Depending on the resident's needs, there may be individual or group therapy. In either case, the goal of rehabilitative therapy is to help the resident relate speech and language skills to everyday activities and interactions, and to support the resident's choices of communication mode, whether speech, gesture, writing, or an assistive device. Also, the speech-language pathologist should provide staff and family with suggestions on how to facilitate communication with the resident during rehabilitation and afterward.

Residents with long-standing aphasia (longer than 1 year) may not be as responsive to direct therapy, and continued monitoring by nursing staff is necessary to maintain the level of attained skill. Monitoring also helps to identify changes in communication ability that may foretell a new stroke or other confounding difficulties (e.g., the onset of dementia). The staff must assume primary responsibility for helping residents use their current

level of skill optimally. Again, consultation with the speech-language pathologist about the types of strategies is beneficial to staff.

Whether the aphasic condition is old or new, staff are likely to be the primary communication partners for most residents, so maximize their ability to communicate effectively. With proper training, the staff can develop useful techniques for facilitating the aphasic resident's understanding and expression. Incorporate the following guidelines in everyday communication:

- Face the resident at eye level when communicating.
- Use short, well-formed sentences and clearly articulated speech.
- Avoid saying words for the resident. Encourage the resident to think of similar words, descriptions, or associated ideas (e.g., ask what the object, person, or idea is like; where it is found; who uses it; what is its shape, size, color; what it is used for).
- Keep related ideas together (i.e., complete one topic before moving on to another). Inform the resident that the topic of the conversation is about to change.
- Pause frequently between utterances. This gives the resident time to comprehend or ask for clarification.
- Be alert to nonverbal cues from the resident signaling that a message has not been understood (e.g., a look of confusion or turning away from the speaker).
- Be prepared to repeat ideas (e.g., "You are going to the podiatrist, the foot doctor," while pointing to the resident's foot or shoe) but do not address the resident like a child.
- Encourage the resident to rephrase ideas that are unclear (e.g., "Tell me in a another way to help me understand better.").
- Repeat occasionally what the resident has said. This provides the resident with feedback that you have understood, or misunder-

stood, the conversation, and also helps the resident focus the conversation better.

- For the resident who has difficulty thinking of words quickly, provide an array from which to choose (e.g., "Would you like coffee, tea, or milk?").

- Ask yes/no questions rather than open-ended questions (e.g., "Would you like ice cream for dessert?" rather than "What would you like for dessert?").

- Occasionally, discuss the frustration either you or the resident is experiencing in communication. When done openly and gently, this often relieves the tension between communication partners.

- Encourage any aphasic residents who have a communication board to use the board during daily interactions. Keep the board visible and accessible. Communication boards should be individually designed or chosen for aphasic residents by the speech-language pathologist, and tend to be one of the following types: letter boards on which the resident points to letters to form words and phrases, word boards on which the resident points to whole words (e.g., Bed, Nurse), or picture boards on which the resident points to pictures depicting target words. Both word and picture boards focus on individual needs and ideas and are limited in their ability to convey a larger repertoire of ideas.

Care Plan for Dysarthria

Dysarthria is common among residents who have had strokes or have progressive neurologic disorders such as Parkinson's disease, multiple sclerosis, or ALS. The presence of dysarthria compounds aphasia, dementia, and other coexisting disorders. It can interfere dramatically with functional communication. Rehabilitation can successfully improve oral motor strength, range of motion, and coordination, which in turn may improve speech intelligibility at word, phrase, and conversational levels. For residents who cannot achieve speech intelligibility at a single word level, using compensatory strategies and assistive or augmentative communication devices will facilitate interaction with the staff, other residents, and family.

The following guidelines are useful in care planning for residents with dysarthria:

- Refer the resident for a communication evaluation by the speech-language pathologist. Since dysarthria is not just a problem in producing sounds clearly, a more comprehensive evaluation of respiration, voice, resonance, and articulation is necessary. The speech-language pathologist can make suggestions to facilitate communication.

- Ensure that confounding problems such as hearing loss, vision difficulties, and drug interactions are evaluated and treated.

- Reinforce formal treatment programs by helping the resident relate speech skills to everyday activities and interactions.

- Encourage the resident to speak more slowly with short phrases and pauses between phrases. Many dysarthrics need to inhale frequently because they feel they are going to "run out of air" while speaking.

- Ask the speech-language pathologist to provide the resident who speaks very softly with a voice amplifier to increase the perceived volume of the speaker. Nursing staff need to work with the speech-language pathologist in order to reinforce the resident's newly learned skills.

- Encourage the resident to self-monitor speech (e.g., "Mr. Jones, are you using your clear speaking skills?"). Ask the resident for feedback about newly learned techniques.

- Encourage the resident to use assistive communication devices such as a communication board or a computer. It is likely that with advances in current technology, improved portability, and decreased cost, computer-based communication assistive devices will become more common for residents to use.

- Encourage the resident to use gestures or other nonverbal means of communication during conversations.

Care Plan for Dementia

To ensure that the resident with dementia receives appropriate care, it is important first to identify any problem(s) that may be either confused with dementia or exacerbating to the situation. Such possibilities include differential diagnosis of dementia from transient ischemic attacks, left or right hemisphere strokes, hearing loss, visual loss, limited proficiency in English, depression, adverse drug effects, delirium, and a variety of potentially reversible systemic disorders. Consult the appropriate medical professional, speech-language pathologist, or audiologist for evaluation and optimal remediation/rehabilitation (*see* Chapters 10 and 11, Cognitive Loss and Delirium, respectively, for more detailed suggestions).

Most forms of dementia are progressive and characterized by increasing difficulty in communication. The staff will need to communicate with the resident regularly during all stages of the disorder in order to provide quality care. In turn, the resident will want to communicate during most of the course of the disease, despite serious language deficits in the areas of word retrieval and the ability to carry on a meaningful conversation.

In many cases, individuals with dementia will not profit from traditional speech-language pathology services. The role of the speech-language pathologist then becomes one of consultant to the staff about strategies they can use to facilitate communication with the resident with dementia.

The following guidelines may be useful in care planning for residents with dementia:

- Avoid information overload to the resident. Talk about one idea at a time. Make transitions between topics clear to the resident (e.g., "We have finished talking about the Thanksgiving holiday. Now we are going to talk about ...").
- Ask one question at a time.
- Be prepared to repeat ideas, and augment with nonverbal communication such as pointing and gestures.
- Add emphasis or intonation, but not loudness, to important words in a statement (e.g., "This is your *gout medicine*").
- Be concrete, not abstract, in statements and questions. Talk about things that the resident can see, hear, touch, or are otherwise immediately available or apparent in his or her environment. Avoid discussion that involves events or conceptualizations out of the current time frame (i.e., things "before," "later," "yesterday," "last week," and "tomorrow").
- Ask yes/no questions rather than open-ended ones (e.g., "Would you like cereal for breakfast?" rather than "What would you like for breakfast?").
- Avoid correcting misused words or faulty constructions. Instead, try to ascertain the topic and respond to the idea as a whole.
- Encourage the resident to repeat or "talk around" a topic. The additional content provided may help comprehension of what the resident is trying to communicate.
- There are times when it is best to tell the resident that you do not understand at this time but will come back to talk again in a few minutes. Repeated failure to communicate on the parts of both caregiver and resident only leads to frustration, resentment, and withdrawal. Sometimes a few minutes reprieve allows both communication partners an opportunity to calm down and focus on the intent of the message.
- When a resident leaves a topic, restate or summarize what you were discussing (e.g., "We were talking about your visit from Joan, your daughter").
- Use social communication frequently (e.g.,

"How are you?", "Please," "Thank you," "How is it going?").

- Incorporate appropriate humor and laughter into daily interactions with the individual. While the resident may not fully comprehend the intended meaning of humorous statements, the laughter generated may be relaxing and socializing.

- Ascertain when and with whom the resident communicates best. There may be a staff member who has a special rapport with the resident, or a situation in which the resident communicates more appropriately. Encourage or reinforce these interactions. Attempt to determine how and why these interactions are successful so that other staff may learn better communication techniques with the residents.

- Avoid placing the resident in difficult communication situations, such as large group events with strangers or new activities (field trips)—although individual preference for valued activity pursuits should be honored when possible.

- Provide as many opportunities as possible during daily care and activities for interaction with staff, other residents, and family.

Care Plan for Reduced Physiologic Reserves

A resident's general physical condition can significantly affect communication skills and opportunities, regardless of the nature or existence of a specific communication problem. To ensure that the resident is in the best possible physical condition to communicate, pay particular attention to respiratory function, arm and hand mobility, and any drugs that may be affecting receptive or expressive skills. Specifically:

- Monitor the resident's ability to produce phrases or short sentences at a comfortable loudness level. Does the resident inhale frequently within a word, phrase, or sentence? Does the loudness level decrease as the sentence progresses? Does the resident appear to give up talking because of respiratory difficulties or fatigue? If body control is a problem, turning and positioning orders should be emphasized.

- Encourage the resident to assume a body posture that facilitates adequate inhalation of air for speech purposes (e.g., avoid slumped-over posture, fetal position, and use of restraints around upper torso).

- Monitor the resident's motor skills, particularly arm and hand mobility and use. Adequate strength and range of motion of upper limbs are important in gesturing, using an assistive communication device, and inserting, removing, and adjusting the controls of a hearing aid. If deficient, prescribe range-of-motion exercises.

- Assess the resident's medication regimen to determine if any drugs are adversely affecting the ability to communicate (e.g., speech becomes slurred, resident becomes drowsy). (*See* Chapters 2 and 14, Polypharmacy and Psychotropic Drugs, respectively, for more explicit recommendations.)

- Consult the appropriate medical staff and professional speech-language pathologist if any of these conditions are noted.

Depression

Sad mood may either be a cause or a consequence of a resident's inability to communicate effectively. For example, hearing loss may result in depressive symptoms such as social withdrawal, suspiciousness, and irritability. Depression often accompanies communication problems resulting from stroke, dementia, and progressive neurologic disorders. Dementia and depression are frequently co-existing conditions, and they may exacerbate each other.

Whatever the cause-and-effect relationship in the given instance, the resident's mood is always an important factor in achieving effective communication. Depression, anxiety, apathy, and passivity due to a lack of motivation can negate the most carefully drawn therapeutic plans, undermine outcomes, and possibly result in loss of skills previously gained. (*See* Chapter 13, Depression, for more recommendations.) Several suggestions to facilitate communication with the depressed resident follow.

- Encourage staff, family, and other residents to interact as much as possible with the resident. Avoiding communication with depressed residents increases their problems.
- In conversation do not expect or demand responses, but rather look for nonverbal signs of comprehension to which you may in turn respond.
- Reinforce the resident for initiating and responding to interaction.
- Encourage the resident to participate in activities of choice and with desired communication partners.
- Identify a special significant other with whom the resident appears to have a positive relationship and encourage this individual to act as a primary communication partner for the resident.

Language Barriers

Caregivers must be sensitive to language, cultural, educational, gender, and ethnic differences between staff and residents, as well as among residents themselves. These differences are evident throughout verbal and nonverbal communication and eventually have an impact on communication between caregivers and residents of multicultural backgrounds. The guidelines for caring for residents with language, cultural education, gender and ethnic differences are as follow:

- Caregivers should be aware of residents' language, cultural, and ethnic backgrounds. For example, what is a resident's primary or preferred language? What information about health care needs might this individual be uncomfortable discussing with a caregiver or a person of the opposite gender? How does a particular culture value elders and long-term care?
- Caregivers should not presume a resident's cultural or ethnic preferences based on surname, address, or color. Many individuals with foreign names are acculturated into mainstream American society.
- Caregivers need to be sensitized to the vast array of language, cultural, and ethnic differences among residents. Of particular emphasis in educational programming for caregivers should be how the residents' value and communication systems compare and contrast with that of the caregivers.
- Caregivers should explore differences in nonverbal communication among resident groups. For example, some cultures (e.g., Arabic) do not encourage even informal direct physical contact among strangers or between individuals of the opposite sex (e.g., touching an arm, shaking hands). Other differences to explore include:
  o Eye contact—direct eye contact may be offensive in some cultures while appropriate in others. For example, in the African-American culture, eye contact is infrequent while listening and more frequent during speaking.
  o Distance—in general, in the United States most personal communication occurs about 1.5 to 4 feet away. Communication between a staff member and resident occurring closer than 1.5 feet may be considered uncomfortable. In other cultures, appropriate distance may vary.
  o Bodily movements—including facial expression, posture, and gestures. Again, all such movements are culturally bound and have different meanings. For example, offering a Moslem something with the left hand may be considered impo-

lite. Touching is common among Hispanic speakers but it is infrequent among Asians.

  o Vocal cues—many aspects of voice send nonverbal messages, including volume, pauses, rate, hesitations and silences. For example, speaking loudly is appropriate in Arab cultures while it signals aggression in others.

- Caregivers need to be sensitive to the types of questions they pose to residents of various cultures. For example, many Native Americans and African-Americans consider personal questions inappropriate or intrusive.

- Caregivers who speak with a foreign accent or dialect need to monitor how well others understand their speech. Older residents with hearing loss, comprehension difficulties, or less cultural experience with such caregivers may not understand the individual.

- Caregivers should also monitor their use of idiomatic expressions. Residents with limited proficiency in English may not understand such common expressions as "raining cats and dogs" or "bottoms up." In addition, limit the use of medical jargon such as "vital signs," "voiding," and "ADLs." Most lay persons do not know the meaning of such terms.

- Use of diminutive or childlike names is generally inappropriate with all older individuals regardless of culture or ethnic background. For example, referring to a resident as "Kiddo" might appear friendly but will be interpreted as offensive.

CASE EXAMPLE

From the moment she entered the facility, the staff had difficulty communicating with Mrs. W., age 70. This problem was noted by the staff at admission when she had been accompanied by her only son and daughter-in-law who appeared to be in charge. A widow

for several years, Mrs. W. had recovered well enough from two previous small strokes to live with her sister while her son maintained her home. After her third stroke, her daughter-in-law insisted that Mrs. W. move to a facility and that her home and possessions be sold to pay for her care. This stroke resulted in relatively severe expressive aphasia and right-side hemiplegia, and was complicated by other medical problems including diabetes.

In addition to the trauma of suffering multiple losses (functional independence, speech, and home), Mrs. W. experienced a very difficult transition to life in the nursing home. She not only lost a sense of control and continuity in her life, she had difficulty expressing her feelings and wishes.

The nursing facility was located in a large urban city, which was staffed primarily by minority nursing assistants. Mrs. W. was considered uncooperative by the nurse assistants because she refused to comply with nursing care routines, was emotionally labile and depressed because she frequently cried and refused to participate in any social activities, and abusive because she shouted obscenities at them in both English and Polish. Communication with Mrs. W. was difficult in that other than her repertoire of obscenities and several social phrases, she produced few intelligible words or phrases. Nursing assistants were particularly frustrated in communicating with Mrs. W., believing that she was more demented than aphasic. Mrs. W. received no friends or family visitors except on major holidays. Her son, in particular, felt uncomfortable coming to the facility.

The interdisciplinary team asked a speech-language pathologist to evaluate Mrs. W., who had no previous communication therapy. A communication evaluation revealed that in addition to a possible hearing loss, Mrs. W. had moderately severe expressive aphasia (Broca's type). However, her cognitive functions were intact. Speech-language therapy first focused on enhancing Mrs. W.'s good auditory comprehension skills and her functional ability to read, while improving her ability to say single words related to ADLs. The speech-language pathologist also designed a combination spelling and word communication board for Mrs. W. to use at times when she had particular difficulty expressing herself. These tools greatly enhanced communication between Mrs. W. and her caregivers, which reduced their frustrations. Some of each speech-language therapy session focused on taking Mrs. W. around the facility to acquaint her with other Polish residents, providing opportunities to maintain cultural and ethnic continuity. Discussing her interests helped to identify possible choices from the array of activities available in the facility.

The speech-language pathologist also worked with the nursing staff to change their way of communicating with Mrs. W. She encouraged staff to bridge ethnic and cultural differences by spending some time "just talking" with Mrs. W. about themselves and their families. Specific strategies to facilitate communication included monitoring their rate of speech without sounding childlike and encouraging Mrs. W. to complete phrases they had started. The staff were also encouraged to provide an array of responses from which Mrs. W. could indicate an answer. "Shake your head if you would like to drink coffee, tea, or milk." Staff were also given opportunities to use the communication board with Mrs. W. while the speech-language pathologist provided feedback on their techniques.

A team meeting with the nursing staff, social worker, and activities director resulted in the recognition that nursing assistants needed inservice training regarding the impact of communication difficulties and cultural and ethnic differences on older institutionalized persons. The social worker focused on ways to help the family cope more effectively with the institutionalization and provide Mrs. W. with more socialization. The activities director observed the speech-language pathologist's techniques for facilitating communication and worked with Mrs. W. to identify individual and group activities of interest to her. A referral to an audiologist was made and resulted in a hearing aid for Mrs. W.'s left ear. The speech-language pathologist and audiologist both worked with Mrs. W. and the nursing staff to understand how to insert, care for, and monitor the use of the hearing aid.

Mrs. W. has now resided in the nursing facility for 3 years. Her receptive communication is excellent and her expressive communication adequate for expressing her needs. She has become more accepting of carrying the communication board with her to meals and activities. While her family visits less frequently than hoped, Mrs. W. has made several friends among residents and nursing staff who provide her with conversation opportunities. She now willingly participates in group activities such as sing-a-longs, church, readings, and entertainment programs.

17
Vision

Elliot Finkelstein, MD
Katharine Murphy, RN, MS

Many people will experience age-related changes in visual acuity at some point in their lives. Some of these transformations are quite common, occurring as a result of predictable anatomic changes in the eye. However, never dismiss poor vision among older adults, i.e., visual loss that impairs independent functioning, as an inevitable consequence of aging. Medically evaluate the condition, which may be due to pathophysiologic changes such as cataracts, glaucoma, diabetic retinopathy, or age-related macular degeneration.

In the nursing home population, a resident who is experiencing deteriorating vision may also be sustaining losses in other sensory, functional, or social areas. The simultaneous occurrence of multiple deficits, including vision loss, can be devastating, affecting the resident's ability to remain independent in self-care, engage in satisfactory communication, and participate in formerly enjoyable activity pursuits. In addition, severe visual impairment places a frail elder at increased risk of falls, injuries, depression, and social isolation.

Changes in resident function, behavior, and affect may be apparent to caregivers and family members, but the ocular changes that may underlie them frequently go unrecognized by clinical staff. Instead, these changes may be attributed to the progression of a concurrent disease, such as dementia, or be perceived as a normal consequence of advanced aging. Thus, the opportunity to prevent visual loss by identifying, treating, and halting the disease process is often missed.

This chapter describes how to identify the resident in need of treatment, evaluate the major causes of visual impairment in the elderly, and develop care planning strategies for treating reversible conditions and maximizing residual visual capacity in residents with low vision.

OVERVIEW

The following anatomic changes in the eye occur with aging, and may be considered normal:

- The cornea generally remains clear, but may become thicker and more sensitive to glare.
- The lens invariably becomes more dense and less elastic, resulting in presbyopia, which is characterized by loss of accommodation (focusing power).
- The pupil generally becomes smaller, permitting less light to enter the eye and focus

on the retina. This can cause one's surroundings and printed material to appear darker and can cause a reduction in visual acuity. Pupillary changes can also reduce the older person's ability to adjust to changing levels of illumination, such as when moving between well-lit and darker areas.

- Changes in the integrity of the macula are common after 60 years of age.
- The retinal vasculature is subject to arteriosclerotic changes.

Despite the ocular changes associated with aging, most older people continue to enjoy good visual acuity with the aid of corrective lenses. However, millions of elderly individuals have ocular disease producing severe visual impairment that limits their independent functioning. According to current estimates, an elder with severe visual impairment is four times more likely to reside in a nursing home than in the community. The key to successful management of eye disorders in this group is early detection and remediation of treatable conditions, and interdisciplinary support that maximizes residual visual function and assists the resident in learning new ways to perform visual tasks.

Identifying the Resident Requiring Treatment

One of the major effects of vision impairment among nursing home residents is greater dependency in the activities of daily living (ADLs). In one study comparing residents with similar musculoskeletal problems and medical conditions, a significantly greater proportion of residents with poor vision were dependent on caregivers for ADL performance. In addition, depending on the severity of vision impairment, a change in visual function is often accompanied by changes in the resident's mood, behavior, or ability to function in social or activity pursuits. The resident may become depressed and withdrawn, ap-

pear more confused, or begin calling out for help.

The extent to which the resident may complain of changes in vision can vary greatly. The resident who is cognitively intact may report small, subtle changes so that early detection is possible, while the cognitively impaired resident may either be unaware of the changes or be unable to report adequately on what is happening. Also, in the nursing home setting there may be residents who are resigned to the misconception that their vision will deteriorate automatically as they grow older, and they may say nothing about a progressively worsening situation.

Deteriorating vision is never normal, so it is reasonable and desirable to educate residents, families, and staff about vision disorders. For example, convene groups of residents to discuss various ocular conditions, symptoms of common ocular disorders, and available treatments, which will encourage better reporting. Teach the residents to not neglect reduced vision, because in the majority of cases the condition can be treated or corrected.

Screen all residents upon admission and periodically thereafter for visual acuity and signs of deteriorating vision and other ocular disorders. Ask residents about any difficulties with their vision, interference with self-care (ADLs, medication management), and performance of activities they wish to pursue (e.g., walking, reading, card playing). This section highlights common functional changes and physical signs and symptoms that may be indicative of an ocular disorder. The presence of any of these conditions should prompt further evaluation.

Functional Signs of Deteriorating Vision

The following functional signs are commonly associated with deteriorating vision. Such changes are also common among other disorders. The key is to identify the functional change and determine if its cause is visually related.

- There may be a reduction in participation in visually intensive activities (e.g., reading, knitting, sewing). The resident may be observed asking another person to read a menu, greeting card, and so on.
- When the impairment is related to one part of the visual field, there may be difficulty ambulating without bumping into people and objects on one side. This may be accompanied by bruising or other signs of trauma on the extremities. At meals, the resident may regularly leave food on half the plate.
- When the visual impairment is in the inferior field, there may be problems walking and the resident may trip or fall over objects.
- The resident may have difficulty finding a specific location, and either limit travel altogether or restrict travel to familiar locations. The resident may get lost.
- The resident may misjudge placement of chairs when trying to sit down and subsequently either slip to the floor or position him- or herself at risk of falling.
- There may be poor eye-hand coordination, as evidenced by difficulty retrieving objects on a bedside table or utensils at the dinner table. The resident may spill food or fluids.
- Dressing and grooming abilities may change, as evidenced by deterioration in dressing skills, cleanliness, color coordination, application of make-up, and hair care.
- A male resident may begin to miss the toilet bowl while urinating.
- There may be unexplained withdrawal from favorite activities such as sewing, watching television, exercise, and dancing.
- There may be withdrawal from social activities such as dining with friends or participating in discussion groups.
- Behaviorally, a person with deteriorating

vision may develop new or exacerbated fears related to walking in crowded areas, taking elevators, or being alone at night. These fears may be exhibited as agitation, avoidance of or resistance to the activity, or repetitive complaints.
- Some people become more clingy and dependent on other residents, staff, or family for physical guidance or support in walking.
- Persons with dementia and other sensory impairments such as diminished hearing who also develop deteriorating vision may strike out at caregivers during personal care routines because they become startled and frightened.

Symptoms of Ocular Disorders

The following complaints are typically expressed by residents when there is an ocular disorder. However, some residents will not readily verbalize their complaints. Therefore, they must be asked during routine evaluations and whenever there is functional evidence of deteriorating vision or physical examination reveals an abnormality:

- Eye pain
- Burning of the eye(s)
- Discharge from eye(s)—mucoid, purulent, watery
- Foreign body sensation—something in the eye
- Decreased ability to see objects previously seen
- Diplopia (double vision)
- Reduced clarity or brightness of the environment
- Transient blurring of vision
- Appearance of vitreous opacities—floaters, spots, and other opacities
- Appearance of photopsias—flashes of light
- Progressive reduction in acuity
- Loss of part of the visual field

Signs of Ocular Disorders

The following signs are common indicators of ocular disorders:

Eyelid inspection:

- Redness, crusting, or discharge of lid(s)
  o Ptosis (drooping) of one or both lids
  o Turning in or out of lower lid(s)
  o Swelling of lid(s)
- Eye inspection:
  o Protrusion of eye not previously noted
  o Redness or other discoloration of eye(s)
  o Discharge from eye(s)—mucoid, purulent, watery
  o Change in pupillary size not attributed to new topical medication
  o Inability to close eye(s)
  o Crossing or turning out of the eyes not previously noted
  o Blood obscuring the iris

Vision Screening Tests by Nonophthalmic Professionals

This section describes the vision screening tests that may be performed by nonophthalmic professionals.

Amsler Grid Eye Test

The Amsler Grid is a symmetric pattern of squares with a central dot (Figure 17-1). Pattern changes noted with each eye signal possible maculopathy, retinopathy, or other visual pathway disturbance. To give the test, follow these steps:

1. Residents who usually wear glasses for reading should wear them for the test. Have the resident hold the grid at the same distance as for normal reading material.
2. Instruct the resident to keep both eyes open and to identify the dot in the center of the grid.
3. Instruct the resident to close or cover the eye with less acute vision while continuing to look at the dot. Ask, "Do the squares around the dot change shapes or disappear while your eye is covered? Do the lines on the grid appear to be broken, wavy, blurred, or not visible?" Record any changes on the grid.
4. Repeat the test, closing or covering the opposite eye.

Results. An affirmative answer for either eye may mean that macular or other pathology is present. However, unless a physician dilates the pupil and examines the macula, it is risky to draw conclusions from this test. Refer residents with a positive result on the Amsler Grid to an ophthalmologist for a complete retinal examination, which may include fluorescein angiography and macular visual fields as well as contrast sensitivity.

Other Vision Examinations

Nonphysician staff frequently ask what they can do to learn earlier in the course of vision-threatening diseases that something is wrong. Most staff members can be taught without much difficulty to determine the level of visual acuity. When residents complain that they do not see as well as in the past at either distance or near, vision testing can be a very ef-

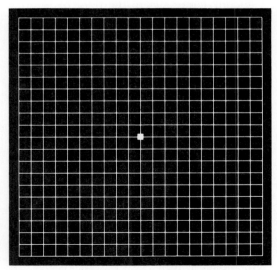

Figure 17-1. Amsler Grid eye test. Courtesy Keeler Instrument Company, Broomall, PA.

fective screening test. Additionally, tests to inspect pupil sizes and how they react to light can be performed. Testing intraocular pressure should be carried out by persons with the technical expertise and advanced knowledge of the implications of test results.

Medication and Vision Impairment

Periodically review the resident's medication orders. Some systemic medications can have a dramatic and irreversible effect on vision, while others may cause a transient fluctuation in visual clarity without structural pathology in the eye. Side effects can generally be avoided by reducing the dosage or substituting an equally effective but better tolerated drug. Common medications with side effects that may affect vision are given in Table 17-1.

CAUSES OF VISUAL IMPAIRMENT

This section highlights common causes of visual impairment that are found frequently in the nursing home population, and suggestions to treat them.

Cataracts

A *cataract* is an opacification of the natural lens of the eye or, alternatively, any lens opacity that interferes with vision. Cataracts are caused by metabolic changes in lens protein and fluid balance. The first sign of cataract development is, frequently, a myopic shift (i.e., an increase in nearsightedness) followed by significant opacification. Cataracts may also cause monocular diplopia (double vision in one eye), poor color discrimination, and severe problems with glare. In addition to age, they are frequently associated with diabetes mellitus, prolonged use of steroids, intraocular inflammation, trauma, and radiation.

Cataracts are often first noticed when vision begins to blur, i.e., the lens loses its clarity, making it more difficult to resolve and separate images. Increasing myopia may change the refractive state of the eye requir-

ing new glasses or even permitting some individuals to see at a distance or to read without correction. If left untreated, cataracts generally will lead to progressive diminution of visual acuity.

Treatment

For the resident who has been screened and found to have reduced vision and significant opacification of the lens, various treatment options are available depending on the severity of the impairment.

If there is a decrease in acuity, but the resident does not complain of visual difficulty and is able to perform ADLs, no surgery is indicated. Instead, observe the resident for changes in refractive error and density of the lens opacification. Consider surgery only when the degree of impairment warrants it, or when it is not possible for the examiner to see the retina or disk well enough to monitor retinal disorders or glaucoma.

If there is reduced visual acuity and a resultant inability to carry out the ADLs, perform an examination and refraction immediately to determine the cause of the problem. When vision cannot be improved adequately by refractive means, and the decline in acuity cannot be attributed to another ocular disorder, consider cataract surgery, but only after discussing the risks of the procedure and the prognosis with the resident and his or her family.

Surgical treatment of cataracts has evolved in recent years into one of the safest operations performed. The opaque lens is removed by phakoemulsification (ultrasound is used to remove the nucleus of the lens) or by expressing the nucleus. The remainder of the lens material is removed by aspiration. Following this, an intraocular lens (implant) is placed in the position of the lens that has been removed. Most people see well after the procedure if there is no preexisting disease.

Table 17-1. Action and Side Effects of Glaucoma Medications

Agent	Action	Side Effects
Timolol, levobunolol, metipranolol carteolol	Reduces aqueous secretion	Blurring, irritation, allergy, corneal anesthesia, punctate keratitis, bradycardia, heart block, bronchospasm, decreased libido, mood changes
Betaxolol	Same as above	Same as above, except fewer pulmonary complications
Epinephrine	Improves aqueous outflow	Irritation, adrenochrome deposits, allergy, rebound hyperemia, blurred vision, mydriasis, cystoid macular edema in aphakia, hypertension, extra systoles, headache
Dipivefrin	Same as above	Same as above, but prodrug structure makes systemic side effects less likely
Apraclonidine	Reduces aqueous secretion	Irritation, topical sensitivity, vasovagal attack
Pilocarpine	Improves aqueous outflow	Miosis, decreased night vision, variable induced myopia, brow ache, exacerbation of visual defect of cataract, cataractogenic, induced angle closure, retinal tear or detachment
Pilocarpine (Ocusert)	Same as above	Less intense miosis, less variability of myopia
Carbachol	Same as above	Same as above, but longer duration reduces variability; stronger, so miosis, myopia, brow ache, may be more intense.
Echothiophate, demecarium bromide	Improves aqueous outflow	Intense miosis, iris pigment epithelial cysts, induced myopia, cataract, retinal detachment, paradoxical angle closure, punctal stenosis, intense bleeding and inflammation with ocular surgery, abdominal cramps, diarrhea, enuresis, prolonged recovery from succinylcholine
Carbonic anhydrase inhibitors	Reduces aqueous secretion	Lethargy, parethesias, malaise, abdominal cramps, diarrhea, nausea, anorexia, renal stones, impotence, loss of libido, mental depression, hypokalemia, acidosis, aplastic anemia, thrombocytopenia, agranulocytosis
Hyperosmotic agents	Reduces vitreous volume	Congestive heart failure, diabetic ketoacidosis (glycerin), headache, subdural and subarachnoid hemorrhages

Reprinted with permission from American Academy of Ophthalmology, *Basic and Clinical Science Course,* 1995-1996, Section 10, Glaucoma, American Academy of Ophthalmology, San Francisco, 1995.

Glaucoma

Glaucoma is not a single disease entity but rather a group of diseases having certain common characteristics. These diseases usually involve elevated intraocular pressure resulting from impairment of aqueous fluid flow through the normal drainage passages, cupping and atrophy of the optic nerve head, and visual field loss. As an increasing number of cells is damaged or destroyed by increased pressure on blood vessels supplying the nerves, the visual field is reduced. This process generally begins at the periphery, resulting in a narrowed field of vision and ultimately, in severe cases, blindness. There are two major types of glaucoma: chronic open angle and angle closure.

In *chronic open angle glaucoma*, the angle formed by the iris and peripheral cornea is sufficient for the aqueous to access the drainage system. However, as a result of pathologic changes in the trabecular meshwork, there is resistance to the fluid passing through it. Intraocular pressure typically increases very slowly, and there is no pain or early change in vision.

In *angle closure glaucoma*, the iris-cornea angle is much more acute, and the peripheral iris blocks the aqueous from reaching the meshwork. This may cause the pressure to increase rapidly to high levels, thereby causing pain and reduced visual acuity.

The functional impact of glaucoma on the elderly is substantial. There may be constriction and altitudinal field changes while central changes are less common in the early stages. In cases in which the inferior field is depressed, the resident may have difficulty with ambulation because of problems seeing the ground. If the resident is on miotics (i.e., any agent that causes the pupil to contract), there can be great problems navigating in reduced illumination, a situation made even more troublesome if the resident has cataractous changes that further reduce the amount

of light reaching the retina.

Risk factors for the development of glaucoma include:

- Family history
- Age
- Race (African-Americans are at significantly greater risk)
- High myopia
- Narrow anterior chamber
- Systemic vascular disease
- Diabetes
- History of trauma
- Prolonged use of topical ocular corticosteroids

Early detection is essential to maintain vision. In most cases, chronic open angle glaucoma is asymptomatic until there is significant vision loss.

Treatment

The treatment of open angle glaucoma is generally medical. The most commonly used topical medications are beta-blockers, which act by increasing the rate of outflow of aqueous. However, these drugs may have a significant effect on the cardiac system and on the pulmonary system of residents with obstructive disorders.

Epinephrine-type drugs are also used frequently to reduce aqueous production, but since they may dilate the pupil, they should not be used when the drainage angle is very narrow. Also, as with beta-blockers, the cardiac system may be sensitive to these drugs, which will prevent their use.

The third frequently used topical medication is pilocarpine (cholinergic), which increases the outflow of fluid. The major problem with this drug is that it creates miosis (small pupil), often leading to reduced clarity of vision, the feeling that the environment is darker, and discomfort on instillation.

If these medications are not successful in

lowering intraocular pressure adequately, carbonic anhydrase inhibitors, both topical and oral, are often effective in reducing aqueous production, with the oral agent being more likely to cause electrolyte imbalance, renal lithiasis, and a general feeling of malaise. When medical treatment proves ineffective, laser treatment may be used to lower the aqueous pressure.

If the pressure in the eye cannot be maintained at a low enough level to prevent damage to the optic nerve with resultant visual field damage, filtering surgery is generally carried out. This surgery is risky because a passage is made from inside the eye to the outside so the excess fluid can drain out of the globe and be absorbed under the tissues that line the eye. There may be early problems with excessive or inadequate drainage or leakage of fluid, and failure to drain.

The preferred treatment for angle closure glaucoma is laser iridotomy. This is generally curative, and is accompanied by minimal morbidity.

Age-Related Macular Degeneration

Age-related macular degeneration (ARMD) is a disorder of the macula, which is the area of the retina responsible for the most acute vision. The condition results from a number of histologic changes in the deep macular area, and in some cases growth of new blood vessels (neovascularization) in the subretinal space. It is the leading cause of new blindness in the elderly in the United States. There are two major types of ARMD: nonexudative and exudative.

Nonexudative (dry) ARMD is the most common type, accounting for approximately 90% of cases. It is characterized by retinal deposits of drusen (yellowish, round opacities), atrophic changes, and pigment deposits, and it causes varying degrees of visual disability. There is no known medical treatment for nonexudative ARMD, which may or may not be progressive.

Exudative (wet) ARMD accounts for approximately 10% of cases but 90% of severe visual loss. It is characterized by serous exudate or bleeding of the subretinal vessels.

The key symptom of ARMD is blurred or distorted central vision, which may develop very gradually in the atrophic (dry) forms, or quite suddenly when subretinal vessels bleed or exude fluid. Prompt evaluation is critical, since new vessels can grow rapidly. Without treatment, the end result of exudative ARMD is usually poor, with vision ranging between 20/200 and the ability only to count fingers.

Treatment

Treatment is directed at the causes of exudative (wet) ARMD. Since laser therapy is of value only in the early stages, the resident should be seen immediately by an ophthalmologist whenever there are complaints of declining vision, central vision loss, or metamorphopsia (objects are seen as distorted in shape). A resident with ARMD in one eye may be given an Amsler Grid to observe on a regular basis and told to report any change in the appearance of the grid when viewed by either eye. In the late stages of the disease, only low-vision rehabilitative services are of value, but laser therapy may prevent a dense scotoma from enlarging.

Diabetic Retinopathy

Diabetic retinopathy (DR) results from a microvasculopathy whose origins are not fully understood. It is the leading cause of new blindness in the 20 to 64-year age group, and is a potentially devastating disease. After 7 years, at least 50% of diabetic individuals will have retinopathy, increasing to 90% after 20 years. Fortunately, fewer than 10% progress to the final stage (proliferative disease). There are three distinct stages:

• Background DR

- Preproliferative DR
- Proliferative DR

Background DR is characterized by a hyperpermeability and incompetence of the retinal vascular wall. The condition leads to capillaries with dotlike outpouchings (retinal microaneurysms) and veins that are dilated and tortuous. Dot- and flame-shaped hemorrhages are seen. Their shape is dictated by their depth in the retina. Edema also occurs and, if in the macula, may cause severe reduction of vision. When the serous fluid is resorbed, there often remains yellowish lipid precipitates, which are seen as hard exudates. Generally, there is no treatment at this stage unless the macula is involved.

As the disease progresses, *preproliferative DR* is characterized by microvascular occlusion, ischemia, and retinal microinfarcts (seen as soft exudates or cotton wool patches). There may also be gross venous abnormalities (e.g., loops, boxcar segmentation, dilated capillary beds, and shunts). Fluorescein angiography shows capillary nonperfusion in the midperipheral retina. It is important to confirm the presence of disease at this stage, because approximately 50% of cases will progress to proliferative disease within 12 to 24 months, and treatment may arrest it.

In *proliferative* DR, extraretinal fibrovascular proliferation results from widespread intraretinal capillary obliteration and ischemia. The process begins with superficial, fine vessels and little fibrous tissue, followed by an increase in the size of vessels and amount of fibrous material. Regression of the vessels may be accompanied by the formation of avascular sheets, which are liable to contract. On contraction, there is often bleeding and traction on the vitreous, which frequently leads to retinal detachment. There are also blood vessels that invade the vitreous and cause damage by bleeding and fibrotic contraction. Iris neovascularization resulting from chronic ischemia in the posterior segment of the eye may further complicate the situation.

Treatment

The treatment of DR depends on its stage. In background DR, there is generally no urgency to institute laser treatment unless macular edema is present with a threat to vision. It is worthwhile to control blood sugar and blood pressure at this time.

As the disease progresses to more ischemic changes, laser treatment is indicated. Panretinal photocoagulation is a procedure in which multiple laser applications are introduced in an attempt to reduce the metabolic demand of the retina that has caused the ischemia and edema.

In the later stages of the disease, there may be bleeding into the vitreous that obscures the retina, and this may necessitate a vitrectomy in order to improve visualization of the retina and to assess whether there are any retinal breaks or detached areas that require treatment. Laser treatment has been shown to reduce progression of retinopathy by 50% to 60%.

Retinal Vein Occlusion

There are two major types of retinal vein occlusion: branch occlusion and central occlusion.

Branch retinal vein occlusion is generally found in one of the temporal quadrants. It is characterized by superficial hemorrhages, retinal edema, and microinfarcts (cotton-wool spots). The affected vein is tortuous and dilated, and the site of the obstruction is generally at an arteriovenous crossing point. Histologic studies have shown that the common adventitia at these points binds the artery and vein together, and that the thickening of the arterial wall compresses the vein, leading to turbulence, endothelial cell damage, and thrombotic occlusion. Arterial changes secondary to systemic hypertension, diabetes, and arteriosclerosis may predispose to this condition.

Central retinal vein (CRV) occlusion may be nonischemic (i.e., having more venostasis than occlusion) or ischemic. Signs of the nonischemic type are seen in all four quadrants, and consist of dot- and flame-shaped hemorrhages, mild dilation and tortuosity of all branches of the CRV, and mild optic nerve head swelling. There may also be macular edema. Complete resolution occurs in up to 50% of cases, with almost half the remainder proceeding to total occlusion and the rest to partial resolution.

The ischemic type of CVR is characterized by retinal edema and hemorrhages in all four quadrants. There is also marked venous dilation and a variable number of microinfarcts. The visual prognosis is very poor, with no more than 10% of cases achieving 20/400 vision or better, and more than 50% of cases developing anterior segment neovascularization in less than 1 year if posterior segment ischemia is not treated.

Treatment

Visual prognosis is related to the extent of capillary damage and retinal ischemia. Progressive capillary closure results in edema, ischemia, and neovascularization, with poor prognosis. In eyes with intact foveal vascularity, retinal laser treatment is valuable in improving and retaining vision.

Ophthalmic evaluation is essential to proper diagnosis and treatment. Otherwise, there may be neovascularization of the iris and drainage angle with resultant glaucoma, which is difficult to treat and may cause severe pain.

Anterior Ischemic Optic Neuropathy

Anterior ischemic optic neuropathy is characterized by rapid onset of visual impairment ranging from slight to no light perception. There is also decreased color vision and, commonly, visual field defects. The physical signs are acute disk swelling, pallor, and often one or two splinter hemorrhages. As the process resolves, there is pallor of all or part of the disk and atrophy that may mimic glaucoma.

The condition is found most commonly in individuals over 60 years of age, and is due to changes in the posterior ciliary circulation. There is often concomitant hypertension and diabetes. Another cause is temporal arteritis, which may lead to a severe monocular or bilateral reduction in vision in a very short time. This is found most often in the elderly, and is associated with elevated sedimentation rate, possible painful, tender swelling of the temporal artery, pain on chewing, general malaise, anorexia, fever of unknown origin, and myalgias. It is important to consider temporal arteritis when diagnosing these symptoms, since this is one type of ocular disease that can be treated in the early stages with steroids, preserving vision.

Treatment

This disorder results from reduced blood flow to the optic nerve. Determine the emergency sedimentation rate, and if it is severely elevated (often above 75 mm), consider temporal arteritis as a diagnosis. It is important to determine whether this condition exists because vision can be lost irretrievably in hours to days if not treated rapidly and may be followed by loss of vision in the other eye. The most effective treatment is high doses of steroids. In cases with a high index of suspicion in which the sedimentation rate does not appear conclusive, do a temporal artery biopsy to determine if giant cell arteritis is present. However, do not delay treatment if suspicion is high and the biopsy will be delayed.

Herpes Zoster Ophthalmicus

Herpes zoster ophthalmicus results from the reactivation of the varicella-zoster virus. It is generally seen when the resident's immunity declines as a result of age or disease. The clinical syndrome is a consequence of the passage of the virus along the sensory nerves, with resultant eruption of the innervated dermatome. There are some cases that occur after reexposure to the virus.

Ophthalmic findings vary. They include early watery vesicles (blisters) and any or all of the following:

- Lid edema
- Late ptosis
- Conjunctival hyperemia
- Keratitis
- Intraocular inflammation with glaucoma
- Extraocular muscle palsies
- Optic neuritis

The cutaneous lesions generally clear within 3 weeks, but the intraocular changes may take many more weeks or months to heal. Postherpetic neuralgia, through which the resident experiences persistent or intermittent eye pain after the lesions have healed, may be difficult to manage.

Treatment

Treatment is generally directed at the sequelae of the disorder, with pressure reducing medications given for elevated pressure, topical medications for corneal problems, and acyclovir or famcyclovir for cutaneous disease. Topical capsaicin may also be beneficial with late pain.

Dry Eye

Dry eye, which is a common problem in the elderly, may be caused by an inadequate quantity and quality of tears or the inability to retain the tears in contact with the eye because of lid deformities. In many residents with dry eye, the tears evaporate more rapidly than they should, and dry spots can be seen on the cornea and conjunctiva. In some autoimmune disorders, there may be a marked reduction of tears.

In mild cases, the resident will complain of mild irritation, usually increasing as the day goes on or as humidity decreases (e.g., in dry atmospheres, during the indoor heating season). In more severe cases, there is increased discomfort and possibly some loss of clarity of vision as the corneal surface becomes less regular. In very severe cases, the resident will experience pain, may have difficulty keeping the eyes open, and may have changes in the corneal epithelium.

Treatment

Less severe cases can often be managed with artificial tears, instilled up to four times daily. If they are needed more frequently, use a preservative-free tear since prolonged, frequent use of drops with preservatives may cause superficial corneal inflammation. As symptoms become more severe, punctal occlusion and adaptation of glasses to moist chambers may be necessary.

Wet Eye

Wet eye, while not a serious medical problem, is very troublesome. It is generally caused by obstruction of the nasolacrimal system, by position of the lacrimal puncta, by ropion (inverted lid margin) with resultant rubbing of the globe by lashes and ectropion (everted lid margin) with the lid away from the eye, and by corneal and conjunctival foreign bodies. There may be chronic wetness of the eye that requires frequent wiping before tears run down the cheeks, or there may be tears running down the cheeks causing annoyance, embarrassment, and irritation of the skin. Treatment is generally effective when the abnormal condition causing it is corrected.

Treatment

Wet eye may be a very difficult problem to treat. If there is a malposition of the lid that causes the lower punctum to be away from the globe either from senile changes or previous trauma, this can be corrected surgically.

While laxity of the lower lid with *ectropion* is the cause, this can also be corrected, but it may be less effective in neurogenic cases due to a lack of muscle tone in the muscles of the involved lid. *Entropion* may cause severe tearing by irritating the globe as the eyelashes rub against the cornea and conjunctiva. This is also amenable to surgery with a high rate of success.

If the nasolacrimal system is narrowed or obstructed internally, the stricture can in some cases be bypassed by dilatation and probing. However, if this is not possible, it may be necessary to create a new pathway by performing a dacryocystorhinostomy (surgical incision between the lacrimal sac and the nasal cavity). Intranasal tumors can block the tears from reaching the nose.

Photopsias (Flashes) and Vitreous Opacities (Floaters)

Flashes and floaters result from liquefaction of the vitreous. This gel, which fills the posterior five sixths of the globe, is 99% water bound by long molecules. Some of these molecules lose their ability to bind the water and small lakes form, with the result that the vitreous gel becomes less stable. As the long molecules clump together, they may become large enough to see in certain circumstances (i.e., floaters). As the vitreous liquefies, it may move from side to side with ocular movement and strike the retina, causing mechanical energy to be changed to electrical energy by the photoreceptors, which is perceived as flashes of light.

While the vast majority of cases represent no serious ocular problem, flashes and floaters may also be present with retinal detachment, vitreous detachment, or vitreous hemorrhage. Have an ophthalmologist evaluate the resident when the condition first appears or if there is a significant change.

Lid Disorders

There are many disorders of the lids that affect the elderly. Some are cosmetic, others may cause discomfort, tearing, or drying of the eyes resulting in corneal exposure and possible ulceration. There are also tumors, both benign and malignant, which require surgery. The following subsections describe the lid disorders.

Lid Malpositions

There are three major types of lid malpositions: entropion, ectropion, and ptosis. In *entropion*, the lid margin turns in toward the eye, which is a result of reduced tone in the muscles of the lid or of scarring. This causes the lashes and skin surface to rub against the conjunctiva and cornea, causing pain, irritation, and, in some cases, corneal abrasion that may lead to mechanical trauma or severe infection. In *ectropion*, the lid margin turns out from the globe, resulting in tearing and drying of the eye. Both entropion and ectropion generally affect the lower lid.

In *ptosis*, the lid margin is lower than its usual position. The condition may be due to stretching and loss of elasticity of the structures holding the lid in position, malfunction of the levator muscle (which elevates the lid), or various neurologic disorders, or occasionally certain disorders in the chest, which interrupt the sympathetic nervous system. It is important to determine the cause before undertaking treatment. Treatment, if necessary, is surgical after determining there is no other disease involved. Procedures that raise the level of the upper lid margin to match that of the other side (or to match the two if there is bilateral disease) can be performed with the patient under local anesthesia. While there may be swelling, the pain in the postoperative period is generally not severe and residents may resume many of their activities that are not overly strenuous fairly quickly.

In *dermatochalasis* (pseudoptosis), there is

a loss of elasticity in the skin of the upper lid causing a dropping of the excess upper lid skin. The condition may be mild, presenting only a cosmetic problem, or severe enough that the skin hangs lower than the margin of the lid, resulting in visual impairment. Treatment is surgical and is indicated when the abundance of lid skin extends so far down that vision is impaired, generally temporally. Surgery consists of removing excess skin from the lids and suturing the edges together. It is done with the patient awake, and the postoperative pain is usually not overly severe. Residents may resume activities that are not too vigorous fairly early, e.g., using exercise bicycles or some aerobic exercises.

Lid Inflammation

Many types of inflammation affect the eyelids. The most common is *blepharitis*, which is characterized by crusting of the lashes and lid redness, and is often accompanied by marked conjunctivitis and pain. The condition may be chronic, beginning in childhood, and results from bacteria in the glands within the lids multiplying and causing infection. It is usually treated with topical antibiotics, warm compresses, and lid hygiene.

Chalazions (styes) may affect both upper and lower lids. They result from infection within the glands in the lid that have become occluded. The condition may be accompanied by marked redness, pain, and swelling, although a lid mass may appear without any apparent inflammation. They are generally self-limiting and respond to warm compresses. Large chalazions that do not get smaller may be incised and drained.

Lid Neoplasms

The most common type of lid neoplasm is the *papilloma*, which is a raised, generally irregular, nontender, often slightly pigmented lesion that may arise in several different sites. It is caused by a virus, typically remains small,

and may be single or multiple.

Basal cell carcinoma is a lesion of the lid that is generally smooth, may be cystic in a small number of cases, and grows slowly. While this type of carcinoma does not metastasize, it grows by direct extension and should be removed when small. Otherwise, there may be mild deformity, invasion of deeper tissue, and distortion of the lid margin.

Squamous cell carcinoma is also found on lids, may be very aggressive, and does metastasize. It should be evaluated when seen and excised early.

Conjunctival Problems

The most common problem involving the conjunctiva is *conjunctivitis*, which is characterized by inflammation of the transparent mucous membrane covering the eyeball and the inside of the lid. Various causative agents (e.g., bacteria, viruses, allergens, chemicals, and trauma) have been identified. There may or may not be purulence or watery discharge, and the level of discomfort varies greatly. Conjunctivitis presents nursing staff with a difficult infection control challenge, particularly among residents with dementia and poor hygiene habits. As with any other treatment or procedure involving bodily fluids, wear protective gloves when administering ocular medications or cleansing around the eye. In addition to antibiotic ophthalmic drops and ointments, include meticulous handwashing among staff and among affected residents in its management. Emphasize prevention by encouraging mandatory handwashing before and after administering any eye medications.

Another common disorder is *subconjunctival hematoma*, which is characterized by the appearance of a red area, which seems painted on the globe, that may be very small or large enough to block out all the white. It is caused in most cases by coughing, sneezing, rubbing the eye, trauma, or straining. While the appearance of the condition may look alarming, it generally has no adverse sequelae, and will most often clear within 7 to 10 days. Very infrequently, it may result from hypertension or coagulation disorders, which should be suspected with repeated episodes.

Corneal Disorders

The most frequent corneal disorders are corneal abrasion (i.e., scratched cornea) and corneal foreign body. *Corneal abrasion* is generally a painful injury, and may be caused by rubbing the eye when the lid has not closed completely, by inadvertently having the cornea struck by a piece of clothing, paper, hairbrush, another object, or a foreign body. This type of lesion is generally self-limited, and the resident is usually more comfortable with the eye closed until it heals. The cornea should be uncovered and observed at least once every 24 hours while it is healing.

Corneal foreign bodies may be any type of material that finds its way onto the cornea and sticks to it or becomes embedded within it. Removal of the foreign body is essential to reduce pain and to prevent the corneal tissues from becoming more inflamed or possibly infected. Conjunctival foreign bodies may be present under the lids and may cause irritation and damage to the cornea with movement of the globe. In the elderly, immunologically compromised resident, there may be keratopathy caused by herpes simplex or herpes zoster.

CARING FOR THE RESIDENT WITH AN OCULAR PROBLEM

The following sections describe how to care for a resident with an ocular problem.

Consultation

When evaluating the resident with an ocular problem, it is important to determine the rapidity with which the change in vision has occurred and to what extent the resident's normal acuity and visual field have been al-tered. If a marked change in acuity or visual field has occurred quickly (i.e., over minutes to several days), an immediate consult by an ophthalmologist is indicated.

Evaluate any pain in the eyes, lids, or surrounding tissues as soon as possible, especially if the pain is severe. Not only is eye pain debilitating, it may in some cases (e.g., angle closure glaucoma, corneal ulcers) be associated with vision-threatening disorders.

Conjunctivitis, blepharitis, chalazions, and similar infection problems generally do not constitute emergencies, and can often be treated by the primary care physician. If necessary, refer for ophthalmic care within several days. However, more severe infections of the lacrimal system (e.g., dacryocystitis), herpetic keratitis, cellulitis of the orbit, and corneal infections require immediate ophthalmic treatment.

Commonly Prescribed Medications

Commonly prescribed eye medications, geriatric doses, possible side effects, and recommended interventions are given in Table 17-2

Administration of Topical Medications

The following subsections describe how to administer eyedrops and ointment.

Eyedrops

Residents vary greatly in the manner in which they accept the instillation of topical medications. Some will put their head back and follow instructions without difficulty. Others will squeeze their lids tightly shut, push the caregiver away, slap, scream, and make markedly evasive movements. For the former, ask them to put their head back and look up while gently pulling down the lower lid to make a trough to accept the medication. It is generally advisable to have the resident close his or her eye for 1 minute after instillation to increase absorption and to prevent washing

Table 17-2. Common Antiglaucoma Agents

Agent	Group	Concentration	Dosing Frequency	Patients/Conditions for Whom it is Helpful	Concerns
Timolol	Beta-adrenergic blocker	0.25% to 0.5%	qd–bid	Young patients; cataract, hypertensive	Asthma, COPD, heart block, mental changes in elderly
Levobunolol	Beta-adrenergic blocker	0.5%	qd–bid	Same as above	Same as above
Metipranolol	Beta-adrenergic blocker	0.3%	qd–bid	Same as above	Same as above
Carteolol	Beta-adrenergic blocker	1.0%	bid	Same as above	Same as above
Betaxolol	Beta-adrenergic blocker	0.5%	bid	Same as above	Same as above, except fewer pulmonary complications.
Epinephrine	Adrenergic agonist	0.5% to 2.0%	bid	Young patients; cataract	Hypertension, aphakia, soft contact lens; narrow angles
Dipivefrin	Adrenergic agonist	0.1%	bid	Patients with systemic epinephrine problems or allergy	Similar to epinephrine
Pilocarpine	Direct cholinergic	0.5% to 4.0%	qid	Older patients with minimal cataract, aphakes	Central opacity, young patients, peripheral retinal pathology

Table continues

Table 17-2. Common Antiglaucoma Agents–*Continued*

Agent	Group	Concentration	Dosing Frequency	Patients/Conditions for Whom it is Helpful	Concerns
Carbachol	Direct and indirect colinergic	0.75% to 3.0%	tid	Same as pilocarpine	Same as pilocarpine
Echothiophate, demecarium bromide	Indirect cholinergic	0.125% to 0.25%	qd–bid	Aphakic, pseudophakic	General anesthesia, ocular surgery; retinal detachment, cataract
Acetazolamide	Carbonic anhydrase inhibitor	62.5 to 250 mg	qd–bid	When topicals fail; acute glaucoma	Lethargy, depression, weight loss, acidosis, renal stones, bone marrow depression
Acetazolamide capsules	Carbonic anhydrase inhibitor	500 mg	qid	Same as above	Same as above
Methazolamide	Carbonic anhydrase inhibitor	25 to 100 mg	bid	Same as above	Same as above
Mannitol	Hyperosmotic	1–2 g/kg	IV q 6–8 h	Very high pressure; acute glaucoma	Congestive heart failure, urinary retention
Glycerin	Hyperosmotic	1–2 g/kg	po q 6–8 h	Same as above; less likely to produce congestive heart failure	Worsens diabetes, nausea, vomiting
Isosorbide	Hyperosmotic	1–2 g/kg	po q 6–8 h	Same as above; diabetes	Diarrhea

Reprinted with permission from American Academy of Ophthalmology, *Basic and Clinical Science Course*, 1995–1996. American Academy of Ophthalmology, 1995.

out most of the drop by frequent blinking.

It is best for the resident who can cooperate a little (but is still difficult) to recline with the head back, and to look up over the head. Again, pull the lid down and apply the drop gently.

For the extremely combative resident, it may be necessary to get assistance from another person to distract, reassure, or comfort the resident while eye medications are being administered. Because there is a risk for eye injury in attempting to deliver these medications to a combative person, it is best to wait, withhold the medication, and try again later. Additionally, to avoid confrontation with frightened or cognitively impaired residents who typically resist eye medications, schedule medications to be administered while the resident is sleeping.

Ointments

Use the methods employed to apply eyedrops to administer ophthalmic ointments. The process can be made easier by holding the tube of medication in a loose fist without squeezing it. After approximately 1 minute it becomes very soft and runny because of the transferred heat and will flow out of the tube much more easily.

Treatment of residents with glaucoma is generally carried out according to the previous regimen. However, in residents who have had recent surgery for cataract or glaucoma, be very careful to put as little pressure on the eye as possible in the early postoperative period. Administration of ointments should be done most carefully.

Environmental Modifications

The following environmental modifications and techniques have been found to be helpful to visually impaired residents in a nursing home setting:

- Use large bright signs to identify the resident's room.

- Hang balloons outside the resident's door and along handrails.
- Create a consistent, predictable environment in the resident's room. Be sure that it is free from clutter, that personal articles are in the same place, and that everything is within reach.
- Create a consistent, predictable environment throughout the nursing unit. Minimize clutter in the hallways.
- Provide large-print books, large-number telephones, and large numbers on the resident's room door.
- Provide a large-screen television, if possible, in the common areas.
- Install a colored toilet seat in the resident's bathroom. They are easier to discern than a white seat in a white room.
- To enhance independence at mealtimes, use color contrasts in tableware (e.g., light colored dishes on a dark background). Inform the resident exactly what is on the tray and where. Use the clock system to indicate locations. For example, say, "meat is at 3 o'clock," dessert is at 12 o'clock," and so on. Be sure the tray setup is consistent, especially when there are hot liquids being served.
- To avoid startling a resident, always announce your approach. Speak directly to the resident in a normal voice tone, or if the resident is also hearing impaired, in a tone that maximizes his or her understanding of the conversation.
- When teaching, use task segmentation (i.e., break down procedures into a series of steps and teach one step at a time). Give full visual descriptions of the activities, objects to be used, and so on, and have the resident's sense of touch substitute for vision.
- Never touch a resident unless he or she knows you are there.
- Never move a urinal or commode without announcing your presence and intent.
- When walking with a visually impaired resi-

dent, have the resident hold your arm.

- To enhance safe mobility when walking with the resident, describe the area as you lead him or her to a chair. Place the resident's hands on the chair back or arms so that he or she can sit down.
- Orient and reassure the resident in strange surroundings. Schedule another person to accompany the visually impaired resident and describe the new area. Identify landmarks that are easy to detect and teach the resident to use them as reference points.
- Let the resident know when you are going to leave the room to avoid anxiety or fear.

Maintenance of Visual Appliances

The following recommendations have been found to be helpful in maintaining residents' visual appliances:

- Clean lenses with warm (not hot) water, and dry with soft, lint-free lens paper. Use the case provided when storing the glasses.
- Label each pair of glasses with the resident's name. If the resident wears one pair for distant viewing (i.e., beyond the reading distance) and another pair for near viewing, apply an adhesive strip to the frame stating the purpose of each.
- The only way to be certain whether glasses are for reading or distance viewing is to put them in a lensometer to determine the prescription of each. It is possible in many cases, if one is certain the two pairs of glasses belong to the same individual, to make a good guess. This can be done by asking the resident to read with one pair and then the other and see which one is better. Distance viewing can then be tested and the other pair of glasses should be better for that.
- Attach string cords to the frames to keep glasses around the resident's neck, if appropriate.
- Report any broken or missing glasses im-

mediately and arrange for replacements.
- Encourage the resident to wear the glasses as needed.

CASE EXAMPLE

Mr. K. is a 90-year-old man who has been a resident of a nursing home for 5 years. Prior to admission, Mr. K. had a 10-year history of periodic severe depression precipitated by two major losses: the deaths of his wife and daughter-in-law in the same week, and a sudden severe, permanent loss of vision in his right eye secondary to temporal arteritis. He was admitted to the nursing home following a difficult 10-month stay in a psychiatric hospital where he was treated successfully with antidepressants and electric shock therapy.

During the preadmission assessment the social worker learned that Mr. K. had many friends, and enjoyed watching television, reading, and walking two to three miles daily. Upon admission he was found to be cognitively intact, social, and independent in ADLs. Once oriented to his new environment, he was able to take long walks throughout the facility and outdoors using a cane. He continued to pursue his usual daily routines, and soon made a good adjustment to the nursing home where he met many old friends.

Four years after admission Mr. K.'s vision in his left eye had deteriorated markedly. Although he was still highly involved in self-care activities, he began requiring more cueing and supervision. He began to have difficulty negotiating hallways, especially turning corners. He became more socially withdrawn and stopped walking outdoors. The staff wondered if he were becoming depressed. One night, he became agitated and screamed, complaining that he saw the night nurse and two security guards go through his window. Although he appeared initially to be acutely confused (delirious), upon examination he was cognitively intact and quite coherent. After ruling out the possibility of a reaction to medications, his physician believed his illusions were secondary to deteriorating vision. He was referred to an ophthalmologist.

Upon examination by the ophthalmologist, Mr. K. was found to have a dense cataract in the left eye, and surgical removal was recommended. Since Mr. K. opted initially not to have surgery he was referred to an occupational therapist for low-vision evaluation and rehabilitation.

The occupational therapist found that Mr. K. had residual sight to discriminate light colors from dark ones (e.g., yellow from black) and to identify bright reds. He could see both 1-inch and 2-inch letters drawn in black. He could see reflections of light on the unit's floor and walk the hallways following the reflection of light. In self-care he continued to have many remaining strengths. He was independent in eating, but messy, and therefore restricted himself to the small unit dining room rather than the main dining room with his friends. He was independent in dressing and hygiene with verbal cues, setup, and structuring. Because he demonstrated good learning abilities and an ability to learn new light patterns, Mr. K. was considered an excellent candidate for low vision rehabilitation. His short-term goals were the following:

- To become reoriented to the elevator, the door leading outside the facility, and the courtyard
- To learn how to use a talking book
- To increase the number of people he speaks with for socialization

His long-term goals included being able to go independently to the main dining room, concerts in the facility auditorium, and outdoors; and become more independent in ADLs.

Mr. K. was seen by the occupational therapist five times a week for 1 month and accomplished his goals. By this time Mr. K. was feeling more confident and expressed a wish to have the cataract surgery. He was then admitted for day surgery.

For Mr. K., the results of surgery were dramatic. Sight in his left eye improved to the point that he could see colors and details of items of clothing, read normal print books, and read his own watch. He quickly resumed his usual level of involvement in social, leisure, and self-care activities.

18
Falls

Lewis A. Lipsitz, MD
Adam Burrows, MD
Douglas Kiel, MD
Margaret Kelley-Gagnon, RN

Falls are a common cause of morbidity and mortality among elderly nursing home residents. Forty percent to 50% of residents fall each year. Six percent to 10% of falls result in serious injury. Hip fractures account for approximately half of all serious injuries. In some residents, falls may cluster several weeks or months before death. In others, falling episodes may accompany functional decline and the development of delirium.

Syncope (fainting) is an important cause of falls. It is distinguished by a transient loss of consciousness and spontaneous recovery. Syncope may not always result in a fall to the ground, but it does interrupt postural control and is therefore a potential source of serious injury. It is also associated with functional decline. Approximately 25% of nursing home residents report a history of syncope over the preceding 10 years, and 6% of residents experience syncope each year. Of those who experience syncope, 30% suffer recurrent episodes, probably because their underlying medical conditions make them particularly vulnerable.

Falls not only have a major impact on the lives of the residents but also impose serious administrative and economic burdens on the institution itself. Nursing home staff spend considerable time treating the injurious consequences of falls, and the legal liability to the nursing home is substantial. In 1989 and 1990 falls involving elderly residents accounted for more than 40% of 946 claims reported by nursing homes insured by one major carrier and cost an average $13,000 to $26,000 per claim to resolve.

For all of these reasons, quality care for the nursing home resident depends on a systematic, effective approach to the prevention and management of falls.

OVERVIEW

Falls in any age population may occur as a result of extrinsic factors, e.g., a misplaced chair or a highly polished floor. However, in a frail elderly population the great majority of these incidents are due to underlying pathology in the individual who has fallen. In the nursing home setting, the staff should never assume a resident's fall to be a random, accidental event. Every occurrence should provoke a careful investigation of the possible underlying diseases or functional impairments.

The maintenance of postural stability in old age is highly dependent on:

- Healthy neurologic and sensory functioning to maintain postural control
- Sufficient muscle strength to permit functional mobility
- Blood pressure homeostasis to ensure adequate perfusion of the brain with blood

Falls in the elderly are usually a result of age-related changes in these bodily systems or disease-related factors that impair functional capacity, including medications and environmental hazards that overwhelm an individual's ability to compensate.

Gait and Balance

Healthy aging is associated with several neurologic and sensory changes that impair postural control. These primarily involve degeneration of neurons in the frontal cortex (resulting in difficulty initiating movement), in the basal ganglion (producing parkinsonian features of aging), and in the cerebellum (causing ataxia and impaired balance). In addition, there is an age-related loss of peripheral sensory receptors, including mechanoreceptors in the large joints (predominantly ankles, knees, hips, and facet joints of the cervical spine), which feed back proprioceptive information to the brain stem about the body's position in space. When this flow of information is diminished, the body's ability to correct its position when spatially perturbed is impaired significantly.

As a consequence of these various age-related changes, older people frequently manifest an increase in body sway. Body sway is most noticeable when the resident's eyes are closed, since the individual will have developed an increased dependence on visual input to maintain balance in order to compensate for the decline in other sensory mechanisms. Body sway is greatest in elderly people who are prone to falling.

Muscle Strength

Despite the conventional wisdom, a decline in muscle strength is *not* an inevitable consequence of normal aging. Rather, it is most likely due to the adoption of an increasingly sedentary lifestyle. Recent studies have shown that much of the decline in strength that is widely observed in older people is reversible through a regular program of resistance exercises. (*See* Chapter 29, ADL Rehabilitation, for more information.)

Blood Pressure Homeostasis

Maintaining a stable blood pressure while performing activities of daily living (ADLs) depends on reflex changes in heart rate and vascular resistance as well as an adequate intravascular volume. For example, the act of standing up or eating a meal threatens to reduce blood pressure by causing blood to pool in the legs or abdomen. In a younger, healthy individual specialized baroreflexes respond to reductions in blood pressure by increasing heart rate and vascular resistance, which keeps the blood pressure at a normal level.

However, in the course of normal aging, baroreflex function can become impaired, resulting in a blunted heart rate response to hypotensive stimuli. Consequently, elderly individuals are at increased risk of developing postural or postprandial hypotension, and they typically experience greater blood pressure reduction in response to hypotensive drugs such as nitroglycerin. In a recent study of elderly nursing home residents, individuals with a history of recurrent falls showed the greatest blood pressure declines during normal ADLs.

Normal aging is also associated with stiffening of the heart muscle, an abnormality that impairs cardiac ventricular relaxation and therefore impedes early diastolic filling of the heart with blood. As a consequence, the older heart is typically more reliant on atrial contraction to fill the ventricle and help generate an adequate cardiac output. If atrial fibrillation occurs, atrial contraction is lost and cardiac output can fall as much as 50%. The result may be a fainting episode (syncope) or a sudden fall.

A further consequence of impaired diastolic filling in advanced age is an increased dependence on ample blood return to the heart (preload) to fill the ventricle and generate an adequate cardiac output. Conditions that reduce preload, such as an upright posture, meal ingestion, and diuretic or nitrate medications, can cause hypotension and falls or syncope.

Although elderly people require ample blood volume to compensate for impaired diastolic filling, the influence of aging on other bodily systems may act to reduce blood volume. For example, aging kidneys tend to excrete excessive amounts of salt and water due to age-related reductions in the secretion of the hormones renin and aldosterone as well as an increase in atrial natriuretic peptide. Given the elderly individual's reduced sense of thirst and the likelihood that acute illness or functional impairment may limit access to food and fluids, the result often is rapid dehydration. (*See* Chapter 24, Dehydration, for more information.) A hypotensive fall while getting out of bed may be the first manifestation of dehydration in the elderly resident.

Disease-Related Factors

Various diseases become more prevalent with advanced age. Either alone or in conjunction with the age-related changes previously discussed, they further increase the risk of falling. Acute illnesses such as pneumonia, congestive heart failure (CHF), stroke, or myocardial infarction may present initially as a falling episode.

Common chronic disease conditions producing falls include neurologic illnesses (e.g.,

Parkinson's disease, strokes, peripheral neuropathies, autonomic insufficiency syndromes such as Shy-Drager syndrome, or pure autonomic failure), musculoskeletal problems (arthritis, skeletal deformities, myopathies, and so forth), sensory impairments (vision, hearing, proprioception, and vestibular dysfunction), cardiovascular disorders (valvular heart disease, arrhythmias, cardiac ischemia, carotid sinus hypersensitivity, and vasovagal reactions), and neuropsychiatric diseases (dementia, depression, impaired judgment). Each of these conditions may influence the development of falls by affecting sensory input to the brain, central processing of sensory information, or neuromuscular output to the muscles and joints that control gait and balance.

DRUGS

Drugs are also important disease-related causes of falls among the institutionalized elderly. Many drugs have sedative, hypotensive, or neuropsychiatric side effects. Common examples include:

- Neuroleptics, sedatives, antidepressants, antihistamines, and anticholinergics, which sedate the individual and impair motor reflexes
- Antihypertensives, cardiovascular medications, and psychotropics, which produce hypotension
- Analgesics, H_2 blockers, or any medication whose side effects may produce confusion.

Age- and disease-related changes in *pharmacokinetics* (decreased hepatic and renal clearance or increased volume of distribution) and *pharmacodynamics* (increased target organ sensitivity) may result in serious drug toxicity when these agents are given at customary doses for young patients. Therefore, any drug may be responsible for a fall in a geriatric patient. (*See* Chapter 2, Polypharmacy, for more information.)

Environmental Hazards

The combination of multiple age- and disease-related abnormalities impairs the ability of an elderly resident to compensate for common environmental hazards. Commonly encountered hazards include poor lighting, slippery floors, loose rugs, inappropriate use of canes and walkers, stairs, poorly fitting shoes, bed rails, rapidly closing elevator doors, and irregularities in floor surfaces.

Stair accidents are commonly caused by visual distractions such as patterned carpets or shadows that make it difficult for a resident to perceive where one stair ends and another begins. High beds may force short residents to slide or jump to the floor, which causes a loss of balance and fall. Beds and tables on wheels may also be hazardous if they slide away easily when a resident attempts to lean on them for support. Even a common hinged door may present a hazard to a resident who has difficulty making the necessary turns to close the door.

Behavioral and Cognitive Factors

Dementia is another important risk factor for falls, particularly in the nursing home population. In the early stages, impairments in judgment may cause demented residents to take inappropriate risks that result in falls. Such risks include climbing over bedrails, moving furniture, or carrying heavy objects. Later abnormalities in visuospatial perception may cause demented residents to walk into objects, miss the seat of a chair while sitting down, or try to walk outside through windows or locked doors. Wandering can increase the opportunity to fall, while agitation may perturb balance or responsiveness to environmental obstacles. In the late stages of Alzheimer's disease or in other dementing illnesses such as strokes or Parkinson's disease, neuromotor abnormalities often develop. These include the stiff, slow shuffling gait of basal ganglion degeneration, or the hesitant, *petit pas*, magnetic gait of frontal lobe dysfunction.

IDENTIFYING THE RESIDENT IN NEED OF ATTENTION

The clinician's responsibility is to:

- Identify those residents who are at risk of falling
- Treat those who have fallen

The goal in either case is to prevent future falling episodes and their adverse consequences—physical injury, limitation in activity, debilitating fear. Because residents who have already fallen are at highest risk, they must be given special attention in order to discover and treat any underlying pathology, which left untreated will cause them to fall again.

Nursing home residents who fall are:

- More cognitively impaired
- On more medications
- Weaker in the legs
- More unstable in gait and balance than those who do not fall

According to one study, if hip weakness, poor balance, and more than four medications are present simultaneously in a resident, then the likelihood of falling during a 1-year period is 100%. Medications most commonly associated with falls include psychoactives (antidepressants, antipsychotics, and sedatives), diuretics, and vasodilators.

The resident assessment protocol for falls in the HCFA Resident Assessment Instrument establishes a useful framework to identify residents at risk of falling. The trigger for *additional* falls is the occurrence of a fall within the previous 180 days. For an *initial* fall, it is two or more of the following triggers:

- Use of any psychoactive drug
- Impaired sense of balance
- Indicators of weakness in the legs (bedfast, hemi- or quadriplegia, or poor leg control)

Table 18-1 summarizes the risk factors for falls.

Residents who are nonambulatory (i.e., bed- or chairfast) are susceptible to falls during transfers or self-initiated attempts to move, so they are often physically restrained by well-meaning clinicians for reasons of safety. However, using physical restraints is not recommended for several reasons:

The risk of injury from falls in the absence of restraints is relatively low.

By restricting movement, physical restraints cause further deconditioning, pressure ulcers, and agitation, and may actually increase the risk of injury and falls.

Nonambulatory residents can usually be better protected by a well-coordinated individualized care plan including involvement in meaningful activities, comfortable positioning, regular toileting schedules, judicious use of medications, and close monitoring.

Evaluating the Resident Who Has Fallen

Evaluating the resident who has fallen begins with a careful history and physical examination, which in most cases is enough to identify the underlying abnormalities responsible for a fall. Try to determine whether the fall is an acute, isolated event or the manifestation of a chronic ambulation problem associated with multiple falls. If the cause is the former, start a careful search for an underlying acute illness (e.g., an infection) or an adverse medication effect that may first present as falling. The presence of a fever, pneumonia, dehydration, or other predisposing factor may easily be overlooked in the haste to treat the resultant injury. Consider any new onset of falling in a resident as a marker of underlying illness until otherwise confirmed. Also assess the possibility of injury due to the fall. A painful, foreshortened, externally rotated leg

Table 18-1. Risk Factors for Falls in the Nursing Home

Factor	Characteristic or other definition
Polypharmacy	More than four medications
Psychoactive medications	Antidepressants; antianxiety/hypnotics; antipsychotics
Lower extremity weakness	Difficulty rising from a chair
Gait impairment	Many steps (more than 15) to turn a circle
Peripheral neuropathy	Abnormal position sense in the great toe

may indicate the presence of a hip fracture.

Taking the History

The resident's history should document the sequence of events leading up to the fall and should consider fully the effect of any diseases or medications. Were medications or meals given before the fall? Was the resident walking, standing, transferring, reaching, using the toilet, or exercising? Were there hazardous conditions associated with the fall, such as foreign objects on the floor, poor lighting, or slippery floor surfaces? Associated symptoms often give important clues to the etiology. Syncopal falls should raise the suspicion of hypotension or a cardiovascular etiology. Falls caused by vasovagal reactions are often preceded by nausea, vomiting, dizziness, fatigue, emotional distress, or sweating. A seizure may be preceded by an aura and followed by a slow recovery marked by lethargy and confusion.

People who fall will report occasionally that their knees suddenly buckled, causing the fall. This sudden loss of postural control without loss of consciousness is typical of a drop attack, which may occur while walking or turning the neck, and sometimes results in a period of time during which the victim is unable to get up off the floor. Possible causes include vertebral basilar insufficiency, Parkinson's disease, hydrocephalus, seizure disorders, vestibular disease, carotid sinus hypersensitivity, or subclavian steal syndrome.

Physical Examination

Start the physical examination with an assessment for injury, and measure the vital signs at the time the resident is discovered. Usually this is done by the nurse or nursing assistant. It is essential to check the pulse for brady- or tachyarrhythmias and for irregularities that would suggest frequent ectopic beats or atrial fibrillation. Take the blood pressure and heart rate while the resident is supine, immediately upon standing, and then again 3 minutes after standing if circumstances permit. The standing position is most sensitive to immediate and delayed orthostatic hypotension, but sitting vital signs are also helpful in detecting orthostatic hypotension if the resident is unable to stand.

Tailor the remainder of the physical examination to the etiologic possibilities suggested by the history, but it must be comprehensive enough to identify underlying diseases that may present atypically as falls. Essential components of the examination include a search for skin lacerations, bruises, or areas of focal tenderness or deformity that may signify the presence of a fracture. A reduced level of alertness may indicate an acute intracranial bleed or subdural hematoma. Auscultate the heart and lungs for evidence of CHF or murmurs of aortic stenosis, mitral regurgitation, or hypertrophic cardiomyopathy. Examine the stool for blood to rule out the possibility of gastrointes-

tinal bleeding. Perform a careful neurologic examination to evaluate gait, balance, motor function, coordination, and sensation. Bedside tests of hearing and visual impairments are also helpful to identify these potentially remediable risk factors for falls.

Gait and Balance Assessment

The most important part of the clinical evaluation process is to observe gait and balance, particularly during the activity that was associated with a fall. Ask the resident to perform the following actions, if possible:
- Get up from a chair with the arms folded in front
- Stand still for the Romberg maneuver with eyes open and eyes closed, then with a slight sternal push (with eyes open)
- Walk 20 feet without any assistive device, then repeat using an assistive device, if the resident has one
- Climb stairs
- Turn in a 360 circle in each direction

Difficulty in rising from a chair without pushing off with the arms suggests significant quadriceps muscle weakness. Instability or difficulty in performing any of the other tests suggests postural incompetence as well as specific functions to target for therapy. A brief assessment of gait and balance can lead to the detection of unsuspected Parkinson's disease, hemiparesis, foot drop, ataxia, or joint pain.

Laboratory Studies

Various tests may be helpful to confirm the presence of underlying illnesses suggested by the history and physical examination. Table 18-2 summarizes these tests.

Figure 18-1 summarizes the key components of the clinical evaluation of the resident who falls chronically. The evaluation process depicted will rarely uncover a single diagnosis that explains recurrent falls, but will likely identify multiple contributors that can be mini-

Table 18-2. Tests and Procedures

Test	Purpose
White blood cell count and hematocrit	To detect occult infection or anemia
Electrolytes, urea nitrogen, and creatinine	To suggest dehydration or renal insufficiency
Serum glucose analysis	To rule out hyper- or hypoglycemia (since hyperosmolar dehydration due to hyperglycemia may first present as falling)
Electrocardiogram	To detect arrythmias, cardiac ischemia, or conduction disturbances
Head computed tomogram	For the resident with focal neurologic abnormalities such as hemiparesis, cranial nerve abnormalities, reflex changes or sensory loss on examination, to diagnose a stroke, subdural hematoma, brain tumor, or hydrocephalus
Magnetic resonance imaging	For the resident with suspected cervical myelopathy, lumbar stenosis, or sciatica, to detect compression of spinal cord or nerve roots

mized through treatment. By reducing the number or severity of conditions contributing to falls, the overall risk can be substantially reduced.

TREATING THE HIGH-RISK RESIDENT

Figure 18-1 describes the specific interventions for each of the major mechanisms of falls. The following sections discuss the steps necessary to treat residents with a high risk of falling.

Address Predisposing Pathologic Conditions

The first step in treating the resident at high risk of falling is to address all predisposing pathologic conditions that may be contributing factors. For example:

- The anemic resident may benefit from a vitamin supplement or a transfusion
- The resident with orthostatic hypotension may be helped by minimizing hypotensive

drugs, liberalizing salt in the diet, providing support hose, and elevating the head of the bed at night
- The resident with painful arthritis may walk more securely with analgesics, nonsteroidal antiinflammatory drugs, or assistive devices

Eliminate Environmental Hazards

The next step is to work with nursing home staff (e.g., administration, facilities' maintenance, and others) to eliminate any environmental hazards. Sometimes it may be necessary to use creative solutions for residents who fall recurrently, such as putting their mattresses on the floor of their rooms or padding their environments to prevent injury. Observing the resident during a fall-precipitating activity may reveal other creative ways to avoid falls, such as lowering the height of a bed, installing a sliding door in place of a hinged door, redesigning closets for safer access, improving lighting, providing secure step stools to reach

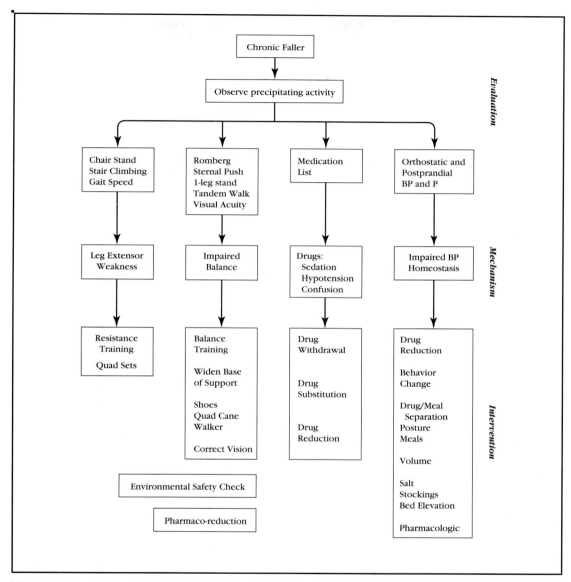

Figure 18-1. Key components of the clinical evaluation of the resident who falls chronically.

objects on shelves, or lowering shelves to within easy reach of residents.

Involve the resident in decisions about arranging furniture and other objects so that they are not obstacles but are still in safe reach. Make sure the traffic lanes are clutter-free. Ensure that the bathroom grab bars are secure and of proper height for the resident and located on both sides of toilets, showers, and bathtubs. Place nonskid mats or appliques in showers and tubs.

Institute Training Programs

For the elderly resident with leg extensor weakness, strength can be improved markedly through resistance training. A recommended training program involves lifting progressively increasing weights at the ankle by extending the knee. Three sets of eight repetitions for each leg should be performed 3 days a week, starting at 80% of the maximum weight that can be lifted at the ankle with one extension of the knee. The weight is increased in small increments weekly until a training effect is achieved. (*See* Chapter 29, ADL Rehabilitation, for more information.)

The resident with impaired balance may benefit from a balance-training program, which can be as simple as practicing standing on one leg alternately for progressively increasing periods of time. Other possibilities include special rocker platforms and tai chi exercises. Whatever the training method chosen, widen the base of support as much as possible with special shoes (athletic shoes are ideal), a quad cane, or walker.

For the resident with impaired vision, obtain an ophthalmology consultation for a diagnostic evaluation. Corrective lenses or cataract extraction should be prescribed as indicated. (*See* Chapters 17 and 29, Vision and ADL Rehabilitation, respectively, for more information.)

Pharmacoreduction

Where possible, consider withdrawing any drugs that are potentially related to falls though their sedating, hypotensive, or cognitive effects. As an alternative, seek less toxic substitutions or reduce the dose. Drug elimination or dose reduction is also important in residents with impaired blood pressure homeostasis and hypotensive syndromes who may likewise benefit from modifications to their daily routine or behavior (e.g., refraining from taking hypotensive medications at mealtimes; providing small, frequent meals; encouraging residents to lie down after eating; and teaching them to stand up slowly after dorsiflexing the feet a few times to restore circulation). Pharmacologic intervention with agents such as fludrocortisone (Florinef) is often necessary to treat orthostatic hypotension, but using fludrocortisone requires careful monitoring for adverse drug effects such as CHF and hypokalemia.

CASE EXAMPLES

The following cases describe two fall scenarios and how they were treated.

Case Example 1

Mrs. F. is an 88-year-old female resident with a history of hypertension, constipation, degenerative arthritis causing chronic pain in the hips and knee, and mild angina for which she was recently prescribed isosorbide dinitrate, 20 mg orally three times a day. Despite a painful gait requiring her to limp and use of a cane, she had no previous history of falling.

One morning at 9:00 AM, Mrs. F. was found on the floor of her bathroom, having fallen while standing up from the toilet. She indicated she had experienced dizziness before her fall. When found on the floor by the nurse, her blood pressure was 110/70 mm Hg with a pulse of 86 bpm. A brief examination revealed a left buttock hematoma but no other injury.

In retracing the circumstances before the fall, the nurse documented the following series of events. Mrs. F. awoke that morning at about 7:00 AM in her usual state of health, i.e., with arthritic pain but no other complaints. Her blood pressure, taken routinely each morning, was 160/90 mm Hg. At 8:00 AM she took her Isordil and sat down in the dining room for breakfast. She stood up after breakfast at about 8:45 AM, walked to the bathroom, and sat on the toilet to defecate. She usually has to strain to move her bowels. The last she remembered is standing up from the toilet when she fell.

The most likely cause of Mrs. F.'s fall was drug- and meal-related hypotension. Although her chronic arthritis placed her at constant risk of falling, she remained well compensated until the added hypotensive stresses of a new medication and a meal probably reduced blood pressure to the extent that it caused her to fall. Also, 1 hour after taking Isordil and eating breakfast (the time of their peak effects), the added hypotensive stresses of a Valsalva maneuver (straining) during voiding and subsequent posture change may have caused sufficient hypotension to compromise cerebral perfusion and interrupt postural control. Confirm this diagnostic possibility by measuring blood pressure on another day during the same series of events. If hypotension is documented, the logical treatment is separating meals and medications so that their peak effects do not coincide.

Case Example 2

Mrs. W., an 80-year-old female resident, fell 3 times in a 1-week period. She had a history of mild dementia complicated by nocturnal agitation, diabetes mellitus, and osteoarthritis. Her medications included haloperidol (Haldol), flurazepam (Dalmane), glyburide (Micronase), and ibuprofen (Motrin). Evaluation of her falls revealed a pattern of falling in the bedroom and bathroom, usually while changing position or reaching for personal articles.

An examination revealed sleepiness and inattention. Vital signs were normal without blood pressure changes on standing, and there were no signs of CHF. She exhibited hypertrophic knee changes, quadriceps muscle weakness, resting tremor, rigidity, and peripheral vibration and position sense loss. She had difficulty rising from a chair and her gait was stooped and hesitant. Lab results were notable for pyuria and bacteriuria.

Management was directed at both the acute and chronic problems. The urinary tract infection was treated with antibiotics. Flurazepam, a benzodiazepine with a prolonged half-life making her drowsy during the day, was discontinued. Parkinsonian features were attributed to haloperidol, which was also stopped. A referral was made to physical therapy for quadriceps muscle strengthening, hip and knee range of motion exercises, and gait support.

This case example shows the multifactorial nature of falls among nursing home residents. In this example, an acute problem (urinary tract infection and associated delirium) compounded polypharmacy side effects (benzodiazepine-induced sedation and neuroleptic-related parkinsonism) and chronic neuromuscular diseases (diabetic peripheral neuropathy, muscle weakness, knee osteoarthritis). The addition of an acute illness to a clinical picture of multiple neuropsychiatric and musculoskeletal risk factors was enough to precipitate recurrent falls in this frail elder. As is often the case, the falls provided the stimulus for a careful medical evaluation and led to multiple new diagnoses.

19
Hip Fractures

Anne Nastasi, MD
Hillary Siebens, MD
Pauline Belleville-Taylor, RN, CS, MS

Care of the resident with a hip fracture presents significant challenges to the nursing home staff. Surgical fixation techniques have advanced and mortality rates have continued to drop, but the functional outcome of treatment for hip fractures can be poor. Residents risk losing their self-care and mobility skills after hip fractures and some may require 24-hour help indefinitely, either at home or in a nursing home.

OVERVIEW

Hip fractures are a significant cause of morbidity and mortality in the long-term care facility. Significant risk factors include a history of smoking, alcohol abuse, and a sedentary lifestyle. Incidence increases with age, paralleling the loss of bone mass due to osteoporosis, with white women 85 years of age and over being at the highest risk. Postmenopausal estrogen, dietary calcium supplements, and exercise programs to improve weight-bearing capacity have all been shown to reduce the rate of osteoporosis and, thereby, fracture risk.

About 94% of hip fractures occur because of falls, which makes fall prevention extremely important. Readily correctable risk factors for falls include removing environmental hazards, reviewing the appropriateness of psychotropic medications with a long half-life (e.g., tricyclic antidepressants, benzodiazepines, and antipsychotics), and correcting lower extremity weakness. Evaluate residents with gait abnormalities for use of assistive devices or braces. Medically treat neurologic conditions (e.g., Parkinson's disease).

In studies of functional outcome after hip fracture, about one fourth of those surviving were able to return to their preinjury level of physical functioning by 1 year postfracture. Only one third were able to return to prefracture self-care status; one fifth were independent in activities of daily living (ADLs); and one fourth returned to their preinjury social role functions. Almost 10% of those residing in the community before the fracture became permanent nursing home residents.

This chapter describes the types of hip fractures and recommended rehabilitation strategies and techniques.

IDENTIFYING THE RESIDENT WITH A HIP FRACTURE

The resident with a hip fracture will usually have had a recent fall, with the site of impact over the greater trochanter. This resident may complain of pain with movement of the hip or weight-bearing, and the injured leg will tend to be shortened and externally rotated compared with the uninjured leg. However, undisplaced femoral neck fractures may show little deformity and little pain on movement. There may only be a bruise over the area of impact.

For any resident who has fallen on a hip, plain radiographs from two views (anteroposterior and lateral) are recommended, particularly if bruising is present. Radiographs will usually show a fracture clearly, but undisplaced fractures of the femoral neck can be missed. In such cases, if the resident continues to bear weight on the hip, the fracture will demineralize about a week after the accident, at which time it will be clearly evident on radiography. To avoid the risk of displacement of an undisplaced fracture, order a bone scan if plain radiographs are unclear and the suspicion of femoral neck fracture is high. Also avoid weight-bearing on and manipulation of the injured leg while transporting the resident to the acute care hospital via ambulance.

Surgical Goals and Treatment

The primary surgical goals for treatment of hip fractures, particularly in osteoporotic elderly persons, are to restore mobility and function as early as possible. The objective is to achieve a stable fixation that will allow the patient to bear weight early. Minimizing blood loss and preventing medical complications such as deep vein thrombosis and pulmonary embolus are also important objectives in elderly patients.

About 50% of hip fractures occur in the femoral neck region, and the other 50% occur in the intertrochanteric region. The location of the fracture is important not only for surgical treatment but also for assessing the risk of complications and determining the proper course of rehabilitation.

Femoral Neck Fractures

Femoral neck fractures usually heal with difficulty because they disrupt blood vessels within the joint, compromising blood supply to the femoral head. Displaced fractures frequently develop avascular necrosis even when adequate closed reduction and pin fixation are achieved. The incidence of nonunion, despite adequate treatment, is about 15%, and the incidence of avascular necrosis with symptomatic collapse is also about 15%. Figure 19-1 shows three types of femoral neck fractures: impacted, minimally displaced, and displaced.

Because of the high rates of complications in the treatment of significantly displaced femoral neck fractures, hemiarthroplasty partial joint replacement has become a common treatment modality for such fractures, especially in people over 70 years of age. In a hemiarthroplasty, the prosthesis is inserted and cemented into the femoral shaft with the femoral head attached. The bipolar prosthesis that is generally used incorporates a plastic weight-bearing surface over the femoral head. This device reduces wear on the acetabular cartilage, resulting in decreased complaints of pain and a reduced degree of subluxation of the prosthesis into the pelvis over a long period of time. It is generally preferable to the older

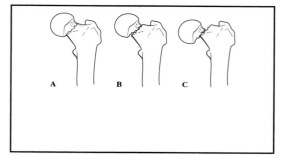

Figure 19-1. Three types of femoral neck fractures: (A) impacted (neck looks shorter with slight buckling proximally), (B) minimally displaced, and (C) displaced.

style prostheses (e.g., Thompson and Moore types), in which a bare metal femoral head is left in contact with acetabular cartilage. Figure 19-2 shows two types of hemiarthroplasty prostheses, an older style Moore prosthesis and a bipolar prosthesis.

The possible complications from hemiarthroplasty include loosening or breakage of the components, infection, and dislocation. Complication rates vary, but they are generally less than 5%. However, perioperative mortality is a bit higher than with the traditional pinning procedure. Because cement provides a stable fixation, patients can bear weight as tolerated postoperatively, which speeds up their return to previous functional levels.

Minimally displaced and impacted fractures of the femoral neck are fixed with multiple pins under radiographic guidance. This is relatively simple surgery since the joint capsule and hip muscles are not cut. These residents must remain touch-down weight-bearing, i.e., placing the foot on the floor *for balance only* for 6 to 8 weeks after surgery.

Intertrochanteric Fractures

Intertrochanteric fractures occur below the neck of the femur and outside of the hip joint capsule. Since there is an excellent blood supply in this area, nonunion and vascular necrosis are uncommon. However, because of the mechanical stresses placed on this area, the fracture often unites in a deformed position. The result is typically a varus and externally rotated hip, which produces shortening of the limb and weakness of the hip abductor muscles because of loss of mechanical advantage. Figure 19-3 shows an intertrochanteric femoral fracture.

The recommended operative treatment for an intertrochanteric fracture is a sliding compression screw type of device. Anatomic reduction, which is the alignment of all bony fragments, is important to minimize malunion deformities. The sliding compression screw will allow the fracture to compress slightly, encouraging faster bone healing and improving stability. With comminuted intertrochanteric fractures, frequently large fragments must be reduced and held with screws to stabilize the fracture. The postoperative weight-bearing status depends on the amount of reduction obtained and the stability of the fracture. It may be touch-down, partial, or full (as tolerated) weight-bearing, at the surgeon's discretion. Figure 19-4 shows two types of fracture fixation.

Evaluating Concurrent Illnesses

Thoroughly evaluate concurrent illnesses before taking the patient to surgery. In general, the most important presenting factor associated with a poor outcome in older patients is confusion or a recent change of mental status (*see* Chapter 11, Delirium, for more information). Other considerations include cardiac status, pneumonia, malnutrition, dehydration, and history of bowel obstruction, cancer, stroke, or psychiatric conditions.

Perioperative Care

In planning perioperative care, consider the following factors:

- **Drug regimens.** Review the drug regimen to determine if any medications are currently being prescribed that may have contributed to a previous fall (*see* Chapter 18, Falls, for more information). Review whether or not all medications are really indicated.
- **Postoperative skin care.** Avoid pressure on the sacrum, buttocks, and heels until the patient is able to move independently in bed (*see* Chapter 22, Pressure Ulcers, for more information).
- **Cardiovascular problems.** Patients with ischemic heart disease or abnormal electrocardiogram may need perioperative admission

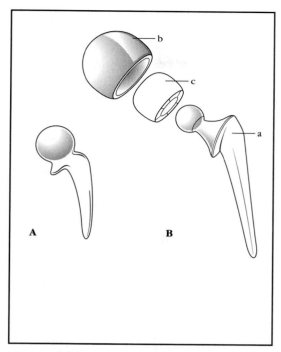

Figure 19-2. Hemiarthroplasty prostheses: (A) an older style Moore prosthesis and (B) a bipolar prosthesis, including a metal femoral component (ª), an outer head (ᵇ), and a polyethylene-bearing insert (ᶜ).

to the intensive care unit for close follow-up. Cardiac arrhythmias may require monitoring postoperatively to determine if they are hemodynamically significant.

- **Hypotension**. Even in cases in which there is a history of hypertension, hypotension, both supine and with standing, can result from bedrest, surgical blood loss, dehydration, and antihypertensive drug therapy. Hypotension may be a significant risk factor for a subsequent fall, particularly when the patient begins standing in physical therapy. Replace fluid appropriately in the preoperative and early postoperative periods.
- **Chronic respiratory conditions**. Patients with chronic obstructive respiratory conditions should have optimal bronchodilator therapy before surgery. Instruct all patients in deep breathing exercises as part of their mobility program.
- **Diabetes.** Closely monitor patients with diabetes during the postoperative period and adjust treatment regimens accordingly.
- **Long-term steroid therapy.** Patients on long-term steroids are at risk of hypoadrenalism during the postoperative period, and may require extra doses of steroids prior to surgery.
- **Gastrointestinal disturbances.** Peptic ulcer disease frequently flares after surgery. Manage these disturbances with antacids or H_2 blockers. Laxatives or bulking agents may be necessary for postoperative constipation, particularly after the use of opiate pain medications. Diarrhea may indicate the presence of a *Clostridium difficile* infection following a broad spectrum antibiotic given perioperatively.
- **Genitourinary problems.** Urinary tract infections (UTIs) commonly occur postoperatively if an indwelling catheter is used, and may present as delirium (acute confusion) in an elderly patient. Use an indwelling catheter only in certain circumstances. For example, a catheter may be used:
  o In patients with acute urinary retention
  o For purposes of closely monitoring fluid balance in a frail patient with an unstable medical condition
  o For a patient with a stage II or greater pressure ulcer in the sacral or buttock area
  o For a patient with uncontrollable pain
  o A preferred management program for postoperative urinary elimination is regular toileting of the patient using a fracture bedpan while the person is on bedrest, a bedside commode when the patient begins to transfer out of bed, and

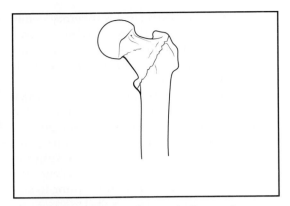

Figure 19-3. Intertrochanteric femoral fracture.

the bathroom after the patient is able to walk. If urinary retention develops postoperatively (or following indwelling catheter use), intermittent catheterization accompanied by mobilization of the patient is the best treatment method. The growth of asymptomatic bacteria should clear up after the indwelling catheter is removed, but symptomatic UTIs must be treated with antibiotics especially if a hemiarthroplasty implant was used in the hip.

- Incontinence. Incontinence is typically caused by difficulty with access to toilet facilities due to poor mobility. Bedside commodes and urinals are recommended. After a patient can be assisted to the bathroom, nurse assistants should encourage and assist in this activity. *See* Chapter 27, Urinary Incontinence, for more information.
- Neurologic conditions. Cognitive impairments that develop postoperatively must be evaluated to rule out UTIs, sepsis, cardiac failure, dehydration, or inappropriate medications. Postoperative pain and narcotic analgesics are common causes of delirium. Hyponatremia is also common in the post-

operative period, particularly if hypotonic fluids are administered. Patients with hepatic or renal insufficiency may have some confusional states resulting from the anesthesia, which will take longer than normal to resolve. Monitor the patient for subtle findings of concurrent strokes and assess diagnostically if present.

- Thromboembolic disease. Thromboembolic disease, a common adverse effect of orthopedic injury, surgery, and immobilization, is usually prevented by full anticoagulation with subcutaneous heparin or oral warfarin for at least several days until the patient is out of bed most of the time and progressing well with gait training. Intermittent compression devices applied to the lower extremities may be helpful in patients for whom heparin or warfarin is contraindicated. Elastic stockings do not prevent thrombosis but help manage dependent edema, which often develops in patients who are sitting for long periods.
- Nutrition. Give vitamin D (400 to 800 IU/

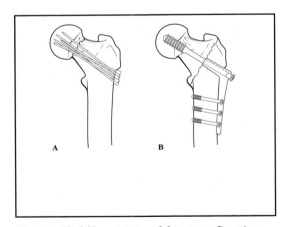

Figure 19-4. Two types of fracture fixation: (A) an impacted femoral fracture fixed with multiple pins, and (B) an intertrochanteric fracture fixed with a sliding compression screw.

day) and elemental calcium (1500 mg/day) to ensure an adequate calcium supply for bone healing. Vitamin C (500 mg/day) is recommended to aid collagen formation and enhance collagen cross-linking and strength.

POSTOPERATIVE THERAPY AFTER HIP FRACTURE

The goals of postoperative hip fracture therapy are:

- Pain-free, stable weight-bearing on the surgically repaired hip
- An adequate range of motion and strength for function
- A return to baseline ambulation with assistive devices
- A return to baseline function in self-care activities with or without assistive devices.

The following sections describe some therapy programs to help postoperative hip fracture patients.

Transfer Training from Bed to a Wheelchair

Start the rehabilitation program on postoperative day 1 or 2, with the patient sitting up in bed and starting active quadriceps and hamstrings exercises on both legs. The therapist should also instruct the patient on the appropriate range-of-motion exercises for the legs and strengthening exercises for the upper extremities. Patients with hemiarthroplasties should avoid flexion of more than 75°, adduction across the midline, or internal rotation because of the risk of dislocation. Encourage time out of bed and increase it as tolerated by the patient.

Early Gait Training

Depending on the type and status of the internal fixation device, start early gait training with protected weight-bearing. When the patient can lift the operated leg from the bed, start gait training with the walker. Patients who

have cemented hemiarthroplasties and those with stable compression screw fixation can bear weight to their tolerated pain level. Limit patients with pinned femoral neck fractures to touch-down weight-bearing for a period of 6 to 8 weeks. Touch-down weight-bearing means that the foot is placed on the floor for balance, with minimal weight on it (generally 10% body weight or less). If there is concern about the amount of weight a patient is putting on a pinned fracture, or if the patient complains of worsening pain in the groin or buttock, take follow-up radiographs to check the fracture alignment and hardware position.

Active Resistive Exercises of the Uninvolved Extremities

To assist with ambulation and transfers, perform active resistive exercises of the uninvolved extremities. The scapular depressor and triceps muscles should be specially targeted. Upper extremity and trunk strengthening exercises are particularly important for the patient who will be using a walker for mobility (e.g., one who cannot fully bear weight for several weeks). Resistive exercises for the scapular depressors are done by pushing up to a sitting position and extending the arms so that the weight of the body is held up by the arms. When sitting in a chair, the patient can push up on the arms or seat. The pushup is held for a count of eight and is repeated 10 times.

Leg extension exercises to strengthen the antigravity muscles are necessary to achieve a stable gait. Resistive extension exercises for the legs include hip and knee extension exercises. Hip extension exercises are done lying prone, tightening the gluteal muscles maximally for a count of eight. Knee extension, or quadriceps setting exercises, can be done sitting or supine by extending the knee fully, pushing the knee into the bed, and holding for a count of eight. These exercises should be done for 10 repetitions three to four times during the day.

Activities of Daily Living Evaluation and Training

Assess self-care skills such as grooming, dressing, bathing, and toileting with regard to the patient's weight-bearing status and hip precautions. Adaptive equipment, such as grab bars, raised toilet seats, and reachers can enhance a patient's independence as well as improve safety measures. Patients may be discharged to appropriate settings with rehabilitation as early as 7 to 12 days after a hip fracture. Unfortunately, they may have had only a few sessions of physical therapy and may not yet be able to stand independently or transfer without assistance. Continue therapy outside the acute hospital setting.

IMPLEMENTING THE REHABILITATIVE CARE PLAN

The following recommendations apply to the implementation of a rehabilitative care plan in the nursing home for the resident who has been discharged from the hospital with a repaired hip fracture:

- **Nutrition.** As previously noted, include physiologic doses of vitamin D at 400 to 800 IU/day and elemental calcium at 1500 mg/day in the resident's medication list. Vitamin C, 500 mg/day, may also be given as an aid to collagen healing. Adequate hydration and calorie intake are also essential. Rehabilitation is severely hampered when residents are dehydrated or malnourished.
- **Positioning.** Keep the resident's legs straight while lying in bed or sitting (using an ottoman, footrest, or other device). Do not cross the legs. The hip should not be rotated internally, nor flexed more than 90° for a pin fracture or screw fracture, or more than 75° for a hemiarthroplasty. Do not use low stools, low

chairs, or wedge seat cushions that hyperflex the hip. To avoid excess hip flexion and adduction, which could dislocate the hemiarthroplasty, place a pillow between the resident's legs when the resident is side-lying on the good side for the first 2 months after surgery. Hip precautions are usually maintained for the first 2 months after surgery. The hip precautions can go on for as long as 6 months if a dislocation occurs early in the postoperative period.

- **Transfers.** The proper way to transfer to and from an automobile is by sitting first and then swinging the legs in or out. Place the operated leg in front of the other when sitting or standing. Use armchairs so that the sit-to-stand transfer can be accomplished by pushing down on the arms safely.
- **Bathing.** A walk-in shower is preferable to a low bathtub. Grab bars may be necessary for security in a slippery tub or shower. A long-handled sponge is necessary for washing the lower legs and feet independently. A handheld shower and a tub seat may be useful for people who need to use a bathtub.
- **Shoes.** Flat-heeled shoes with nonskid soles are recommended.
- **Stairs.** When endurance is good (i.e., the resident is safely walking more than 100 feet on level surfaces), start stair training. When going upstairs, the resident advances the good (nonoperated) leg using the handrail on the operated side. When coming downstairs, the resident should step down with the operated leg first. Explain the mnemonic "Up with the good, down with the bad" to the resident.
- **Use of treadmills.** According to a recent study, gait training using a treadmill with parallel bars produced better results (i.e., higher mobility scores, greater hip adductor strength, and superior performance in

various gait parameters) than traditional training methods using a walker. The acquisition of necessary motor skills requires feedback and practice, and, according to researchers, this is more readily accomplished with a treadmill. In the study group, the treadmill was placed in front of a mirror so that residents could monitor how high they were lifting their legs, whether they were stepping with equal length on both legs, and so forth. Using a treadmill in rehabilitation following hip fracture/hip surgery is likely to increase in the future.

Rehabilitation Therapy Sequence

Beginning on the first postoperative day, physical therapy plans should include active exercises of both lower extremities using ankle pumps, ankle rolls, and quad set and gluteal set exercises. Ankle pumps consist of alternating ankle dorsiflexion and plantar flexion, either sitting or standing if possible. Ankle rolls consist of ankle range of motion through dorsiflexion, inversion, plantar flexion, eversion ranges, then reversing the direction. Instruct the resident in these exercises and encourage them to repeat the exercises up to four times an hour throughout the day. Also, deep breathing exercises are reviewed. During hospitalization, if the resident was sick or confused, participation in these exercises may have been minimal. However, all these exercises are feasible once the resident has stabilized, and should be carried out in the nursing home. Have the physical therapist train nursing assistants in instructing residents so they can consistently and appropriately encourage, cue, or assist residents in their rehabilitation efforts.

Start upper extremity exercises for scapular depressors and triceps strengthening 1 or 2 days after surgery. The first goal is independent sitting at the bedside, with the resident being able to dangle his or her legs over the edge. If there is a hemiarthroplasty, carefully observe and physically assist the resident as necessary to ensure that the 75° flexion limit is not exceeded.

When independent sitting at bedside is accomplished, the resident should then be sitting up in a sturdy chair with reclining capacities (e.g., cardiac chair) 30 minutes twice a day. Again, in cases of hemiarthroplasty, be alert to excessive hip flexion, adduction, or internal rotation. A pillow placed between the knees can help remind the resident not to cross legs or abduct. Gradually increase the sitting time to improve physical activity endurance.

Next, wheelchair transfers are started with the majority of weight being placed on the nonoperated leg. On the operated side, weight-bearing will be touch-down (for pinned femoral neck fractures and some intertrochanteric fractures with compression screws), 50% weight-bearing for other intertrochanteric fractures, or weight-bearing as tolerated for hemiarthroplasties.

When the resident can get out of bed, he or she can begin taking a few steps with a walker or using the parallel bars. Use the parallel bars if the fixation allows touch-down weight bearing only or if there is difficulty with weight-bearing due to pain or poor balance. At this stage, use of a walker is indicated only for residents with good balance who can bear weight as tolerated.

After the resident can walk a few steps with either parallel bars or a walker, gradually increase the walking distance. Follow residents who are ambulating independently while using the walker with a wheelchair initially in case they tire faster than expected. Depending on upper extremity strength and endurance progression, a resident who is on touch-down weight-bearing status can progress from the parallel bars to the walker if he or she has good balance.

When teaching bathroom transfers for residents with hemiarthroplasty, remember to use a raised toilet seat to avoid excessive hip flexion. Transfer training, including getting on and off the toilet, is generally done when the resident is safely able to perform a bed to wheelchair transfer following hip precautions. An ADL evaluation with an occupational therapist is often helpful to identify areas that may be improved with the use of adaptive equipment such as long-handled reachers. Residents can also benefit from learning how to conserve energy and use walkers during kitchen activities.

Communication among therapists and nursing staff about the resident's mobility status, progress, competency in the use of assistive devices, and motivation is crucial to help the resident regain function. Too often the resident is walking in the physical therapy sessions, but does not walk on the unit because the nursing staff is unaware of the resident's ambulatory status. All services must coordinate efforts to facilitate return to function in the resident's usual living environment.

If the resident is to be discharged home, perform an evaluation of the home living situation. Items such as shower chairs, a handheld shower nozzle, grab bars, and others can be ordered to provide safety in the bathroom. The goals for safe discharge of the resident to home are as follows:

- Stable lower extremity for weight-bearing
- Adequate range of motion and strength of the hip function
- Safe home ambulation with caregivers and an assistive device, if possible
- Independence in home exercise program (see Chapter 29, ADL Rehabilitation, for more information)
- Independence in self-care activities with or without self-care devices
- Understands and can maintain hip precautions
- Able to carry out safe car transfers, if feasible

For those residents who do not meet all of these goals independently, a discharge home will be determined by family, friend, or neighbor supports, as well as by the availability of home care assistance (formal and informal). Ultimately, the decision rests with the resident and family (see Chapter 34, Discharge Planning, for more information).

The goals for the resident remaining in the nursing home depend on the resident's balance, endurance, and motivation. They include the following goals:

- Maintain conditioning and strength with supervised ambulation on the unit
- Maximal independence with self-care activities and transfers
- For nonambulatory residents with adequate upper extremity strength, maximal wheelchair independence; the goal is to have the resident up in a chair for all meals
- Maintain functional range of motion of lower extremities
  o Full weight bearing after the fracture has healed
  o See Chapter 29, ADL Rehabilitation, for more suggestions

CASE EXAMPLES

The following case examples describe two hip fracture scenarios.

Case Example 1

Ms. C., an 82-year-old woman, was transferred to the nursing home 10 days after the pinning of an impacted right femoral neck fracture. The fracture occurred when she slipped and fell in her kitchen. She had significant pain in the right groin when arising and trying to walk. She was brought subsequently to the emergency room of a local hospital.

Her past medical history is significant for mild hypertension treated with diuretics and previous bilateral cataract surgery. She had lived alone in her own one-story home with a three-step entry, and has no family locally but is active in a seniors' group and at church.

She has a neighbor who visits daily.

Ms C.'s acute hospital course was complicated by episodes of confusion, especially in the evenings. These episodes resolved when sleeping pills and narcotic pain medications were discontinued.

Because of the pin fixation of her fracture, she is restricted to touch-down (10% body weight equals 12 pounds for her) weight-bearing on the right. Upon transfer to the nursing facility, she can perform lower extremity range-of-motion and deep breathing exercises independently. She can demonstrate a quad set but cannot hold her right leg up off the bed. She requires limited to extensive physical assistance for transfers to the wheelchair but can propel it independently for short distances. She can walk 10 feet in parallel bars with supervision while maintaining touch-down weight-bearing status.

Her rehabilitation program in the nursing home focused on exercises for strength and balance and improving her endurance. After 1 month, she was able to ambulate independently to the day room using a walker. Two months after surgery, her orthopedic surgeon cleared her to bear weight as tolerated. She was then able to progress to stair training. She was independent in her self-care, including showering, dressing, toileting, and kitchen skills. A shower chair, grab bars for tub and toilet, handheld shower nozzle, and stair rail were obtained, and she was discharged home after 3 months. She continued to use the walker for community ambulation, but she needed no assistive device for walking at home. Her neighbor helps her with marketing and drives her to doctor appointments.

Case Example 2

Mr. S., a 74-year-old nursing home resident with moderately severe Parkinson's disease, fell onto his left hip when transferring out of bed alone. The nurse noted that his left leg appeared shorter and the foot rotated outward, and Mr. S. complained of groin pain when the leg was manipulated gently. He was transferred to an acute hospital via ambulance. Radiography showed a displaced fracture of the femoral neck. His medical status was assessed carefully and found to be stable, and he underwent surgery the next day. A cemented left hip hemiarthroplasty was done because of Mr. S.'s Parkinson's-related gait and balance difficulties, and because of the displacement of the fracture.

Mr. S. was transferred back to the nursing home for further rehabilitation after a 12-day hospitalization. At that time, he was able to walk 25 feet in parallel bars with supervision, but he had slight pain in the lateral left hip. Some balance difficulty was noted during transfers and he had to be reminded not to cross his legs or sit with the hip flexed more than 75°. He also had to be cued for hip precautions during dressing and toileting tasks.

Mr. S. made steady progress in his rehabilitation program. Two months later, he was ambulating with a cane on the unit and used his adaptive equipment independently in performing his ADLs. His surgeon evaluated him and felt that his hip was stable enough to remove the hip range restrictions. He was then able to use a regular toilet seat and sit in a low chair at the dinner table.

20
Foot Care

Amy B. Katzew, DPM

Foot problems are a major cause of disability and decreased functionality in frail elders. They range from simple ailments (e.g., corns or ingrown nails) to more serious conditions arising from complications of diabetes mellitus and peripheral vascular disease (PVD). In addition, many painful foot disorders occurring in later life may be attributed to hereditary factors, years of strenuous activity, or abuse (e.g., ill-fitting shoes).

Symptoms and signs of systemic disease are often first noted in the feet. Therefore, the evaluation of foot problems requires attention to the resident's medical history (e.g., diabetes mellitus, cardiac disease, arthritis, hypertension, and PVD), along with any current treatment for these conditions.

Many foot problems involve the skin. Hyperkeratotic (overgrowth) lesions, bacterial infection, fungae, dry skin and ulcerations are commonly found in the long-term care facility population; signs of hypertrophy, mycotic infection, and changes in the color and continuity of the nail plate are also common. Always note any foot odor.

Evaluation of the foot also requires careful consideration of the resident's lifestyle, especially to the physical environment in which

they live and degree of ambulation. In every case, the goals of care planning should be to maintain and improve foot health, range of motion, and muscle effort; improve healing and reduce pain; encourage walking; and prevent further complications.

This chapter describes how to evaluate common foot problems in the elderly, how to implement appropriate care planning strategies, and when to seek podiatric consultation and care.

OVERVIEW

Foot problems are often manifested in the skin. Early signs may include a loss of hair due to a diminishing vascular supply, and the gradual appearance of brownish pigmentations due to venous stasis. Anhidrosis (diminished sweat secretion), dry skin, and fissures are common; and dryness, in turn, may lead to pruritus. Other problematic conditions include contact dermatitis, tinea pedis, and localized pyodermas (inflammations). Because these situations usually coexist with some form of PVD and, possibly, diabetes, an infection may develop, quickly leading to ulceration, necrosis, and the need for acute hospitalization.

Many systemic diseases produce serious foot complications. Osteoarthritis or degenerative joint disease is a major factor in walking limitations. Fixed deformities and inflammatory reactions to repeated microtrauma produce pain, stiffness, and swelling. Fasciitis (inflammation of the connective tissues), calcaneal erosions and spur formations, periostitis, and tendinitis are found commonly in elderly residents. Often, calcification is first discovered during a podiatric radiography.

DIABETES MELLITUS

Diabetes mellitus is a significant cause of foot morbidity in the elderly. The initial manifestation may be a foot ulcer. Other signs and symptoms may include paresthesias (burning, numbness, or tingling) sensory impairment, motor weakness, reflex loss, neuropathic arthropathy (Charcot's joint), muscle atrophy, dermopathy (e.g., small macules and papules of the extensor surface of the extremities that become atrophic and hyperpigmented), absent pedal pulses, and other clinical findings of peripheral vascular impairment. Neurotrophic or diabetic ulceration is related directly to the microangiopathy and neuropathy, with subsequent infection, necrosis, and terminal gangrene, unless there is early diagnosis and prompt treatment.

PERIPHERAL ARTERIAL INSUFFICIENCY

Peripheral arterial insufficiency appears in varying degrees in the long-term care facility resident. Overt indications of decreased arterial supply in the feet include muscle fatigue, cramps, claudication, pain, coldness, pallor, paresthesias, burning, atrophy of soft tissues, trophic dermal changes such as dryness and loss of hair, absent pedal pulses, and abnormalities in various vascular function tests. Pain that is attributed to mechanical causes in the feet may be ischemic in origin.

PEDAL ULCERATIONS

Pedal ulcerations associated with arterial insufficiency are painful, extremely slow to heal, and often lead to amputation. Edema, related to congestive heart failure, nephrosis, cirrhosis, or venous insufficiency, may result in shoes becoming tight, creating gait disorders, stasis dermatitis, skin breakdown, and ulceration.

ASSESSING THE RESIDENT AND DEVELOPING A CARE PLAN

The following sections describe how to assess the resident with foot problems.

Vascular Analysis of Pedal Blood Flow

Analyze pedal blood flow in the following sequence:
- Noninvasive physical assessment
- Noninvasive laboratory procedures
- Invasive arteriographic procedures

In many instances, it may only be necessary to do a physical evaluation. Noninvasive physical assessment of the resident's pedal blood flow should include palpation of the dorsalis pedis, posterior tibial, popliteal, and femoral pulses. The arterial blanch test consists of digital compression of the tip of the toe, then release, to allow blood flow to return. In a healthy elderly resident the skin should return to its normal color in 2 to 3 seconds. When blood flow is decreased, the skin will return to its normal color in 6 seconds or longer. To check venous filling time, the resident's feet are elevated to chest level for about 1 minute, until the veins are drained off. The leg is then lowered to dependency. The normal filling time is 6 to 10 seconds. A slower filling time indicates venous occlusive disease.

Absence of hair on the feet and legs, in combination with absent or weak pulses, may indicate decreased blood flow. Thickened, brittle, hypertrophic, mycotic nails may also indicate impaired circulation. Also, note skin pallor and skin temperature. Trophic changes in the skin, and lack of skin turgor, also provide important clues to impaired distal pedal blood flow. If possible, have the resident walk vigorously just before the examination for a more accurate indication of possible impediments to segmental arterial blood flow. Ask about the presence of claudication (cramplike pain in the calves caused by poor circulation). If appropriate, query the resident about night cramps, but note that the presence of burning night pain may also indicate a peripheral neuropathy.

Perform a noninvasive laboratory analysis if there is (are):

- Open lesions
- Indications of decreased blood flow
- Metabolic disease (e.g., diabetes) in combination with open ulcerations or infections
- Patchy foot or digital necrosis
- Gangrene

Analysis may include segmental pressure analysis, pulse wave analysis, and Doppler blood flow studies. Invasive (e.g. arteriographic) procedures are indicated only if the noninvasive tests indicate occlusion of major arteries and endarterectomy or bypass surgery are contemplated.

Neurologic Examination

Evaluation of peripheral neurologic status should include a sensory and motor examination. Local evaluation of the sensory nerves includes the use of a tuning fork at 128 vibrations per second, two-point discrimination, and pinch, prick, and temperature assessments. Patellar and Achilles reflexes are often absent in elderly people. However, loss of these reflexes from one examination to another suggests the development of a lower motor neuron lesion at the level of L3-4 if the patellar reflex is lost, or L5-S1 if the Achilles reflex is affected. An increase in these reflexes suggests an upper motor neuron lesion such as a stroke or cervical myelopathy. Examination of proprioception, muscle strength, and gait often yields additional useful information. Note at-rophy or wasting of any muscle or muscle groups in the lower extremity.

Radiographic Examination

Radiographic studies are indicated when unexplained severe discomfort is present for a long period of time, or following a fall or similar trauma. Radiographic examination of the foot should include anteroposterior, oblique, and lateral views. Take these views while the resident is standing, since misalignment of joints, erosions, bone loss, and other problems are often overlooked in non-weight-bearing radiographs. Additional studies may include special radiologic views, magnification views, magnetic resonance imaging surveys, and bone scans to detect fractures, spurs, or other bony abnormalities.

Dermatologic Examination

To perform a dermatologic evaluation of the resident, look for ulcerations, sinus tracts, fissures, hyperkeratotic lesions overlying bony prominences (e.g., soft and hard corns and calluses), and primary skin lesions, including hemorrhagic lesions. Systemic diseases possibly having dermatologic manifestations in the foot include:

- Erythema multiforme (inflammatory eruptions characterized by symmetric, erythematous, edematous, or bullous lesions)
- Psoriasis (sharp definable borders, red color, and silvery-white scale)
- Kaposi's sarcoma (reddish, bluish, black macules and patches that spread and coalesce to form large plaques or nodules)
- Scleroderma (fibrous degenerative changes in the skin and vascular abnormalities)
- Sarcoidosis (epithelioid granulomas)
- Fungal infections of the skin and nails are extremely common in the elderly. Minor skin or nail problems often become severe in elderly people, so careful assessment and treatment are necessary.

TREATING FOOT DISORDERS

The following sections discuss how to treat foot disorders.

Skin Disorders

Drying and thinning of the skin is common in elderly people and can lead to cracking, fissures, inflammation, and infection. Stasis dermatitis, skin atrophy, and diffuse keratosis are extremely common in facility residents, and ichthyosis (skin scaling) becomes more pronounced. Localized neurodermatitis may manifest itself on the dorsum of the foot; various skin cancers may also be found on the foot. Exfoliative dermatitis on the dorsum of the foot and distal portion of the leg may precede mycosis fungoides. The following list describes how to treat these skin disorders:

- Treatment of dry skin and fissures involves hydration of the skin. Good emollient skin lotions or petroleum jelly are frequently beneficial. Occlusion for one or two nights with petroleum jelly covered with plastic wrap is an excellent treatment for fissured heels.
- Local corticosteroid preparations are indicated for neurodermatitis and exfoliative dermatitis.
- Treat keratosis formation with gentle debridement, application of emollient creams, and use of pressure-reducing insoles made of plastizote or Spenco. An extra-depth shoe with removable insert may also be helpful.
- Treat fungal infections using an appropriate antifungal medication determined by culture studies.
- Treatment of stasis dermatitis involves the use of bland compresses (i.e., Burow's solution) once or twice daily. If this is not successful, an Unna Boot and elevation of the limb are often helpful.

If exfoliative dermatitis is severe, consider the possibility of an underlying lymphoma by checking for fever, weight loss, abdominal lymphadenopathy, or other signs of systemic illness.

Nail Disorders

The most common nail disorders among residents are onychocryptosis (incurvated nail borders), onychauxis (hypertrophy), onychogryposis (ram's horn overgrowth), and onychomycosis (fungal infection). Severely hypertrophic nails can cause nail bed ulcerations in the elderly. Incurvated nail borders can lead to irritation, inflammation, and infection (e.g., paronychia), and result in pain and complications.

Because inappropriate procedures on a poorly vascularized digit introduce a significant risk of infection, gangrene and, thus, amputation, keep the treatment of nail disorders in residents as simple as possible. Gently debride incurvated nails with or without the use of local anesthesia; surgical treatment is sometimes indicated. Have a podiatrist debride hypertrophic and mycotic nails with the proper instruments for nail cutting and grinding. Using sharp scissors is not recommended, since they may cause a puncture wound with accompanying bacterial infection. When subungual infections persist, the nail plate should be avulsed gently, under local anesthesia if the resident's circulatory condition is not compromised.

Lukewarm 5-minute soaks using Domeboro or saline solutions may aid healing of subungual infections if used twice daily until the area is healed, usually in 5 to 7 days. In diabetic patients, eliminate foot soaks and use a saline wash instead.

Corns (Clavi)

Corns occur in more than 50% of the geriatric population and can develop on or between the toes. There are two main types of corns: hard and soft. A hard corn occurs on a hammertoe over the proximal interphalangeal joint, on a rotated toe, or over a mallet toe, which is a plantar deviation of the distal phalanx that results in formation of hard hyperkeratotic tissue on the distal tips of the toes. These lesions can often become infected, with sinus tract formation sometimes extending down to the bone. A soft corn is a keratotic prominence between two toes that can be either firm or macerated and moist.

Treatment of both types of corns includes careful debridement and padding. Padding for hard and soft corns is best achieved by carefully applying felt or foam pads held in place by tape, self-adhering gauze, or lambs wool. Be careful not to decrease digital circulation with tape or gauze. Incision and drainage of a sinus tract, performed by a podiatrist, are often necessary, followed by padding. Follow-up treatment may include a saline wash and application of quarter-strength Betadine solution. If a resident has a severe reaction to Betadine, discontinue immediately. Obtain a culture and sensitivity test if a severe infection occurs, and introduce appropriate antibiotic coverage. Hospitalization may be considered in acute cases.

Encourage the resident with corns to wear wider and softer lace-up shoes. If distal clavi are present, use a soft insole or buttress pad. If simple treatments do not provide relief, surgical intervention by the podiatrist may be indicated, but only if the resident's circulation is not compromised.

Calluses

Callosities (e.g., plantar keratoses) often present a severe problem in the elderly. Progressive loss of toe function and fat pad atrophy associated with aging contribute to callus formation. Calluses may be found under any of the metatarsal heads, but the most common site is beneath the second and third metatarsal heads in conjunction with metatarsal phalangeal dorsal dislocation secondary to hallux valgus. Treatment using a cushion-soled shoe with the insertion of a one-eighth inch foam insole is often beneficial. Podiatric consultation for debridement and padding is indicated. Metatarsal pads may provide comfort, but avoid salicylic acid pads and plasters because they can lead to ulcerations and infections. In some cases, extra-depth shoes incorporating an insert with a metatarsal raise or an external metatarsal rocker bar may be indicated. Surgical interventions for metatarsal head lesions are not advisable because of the risk of recurrent calluses to an adjacent metatarsal.

Neuroma

Neuroma is often seen in combination with a chronic interdigital bursitis, and may also be associated with hallux valgus. It usually occurs between the third and fourth toes, but can also occur between the second and third toes. Pain may be present at any time, but it usually becomes worse when improper shoes are worn. Palpate the painful areas between the metatarsal heads. Nonoperative treatment includes injections of a steroid between the metatarsal heads, and wearing wide shoes, open-toed surgical shoes, or healing sandals, if possible. Orthotics with a metatarsal raise are often helpful. Temporary padding is achieved by placing either a one-eighth inch or one-quarter inch foam or felt pad slightly posterior to the metatarsal heads. When surgery is indicated, the neuroma is removed by various procedures determined by the surgeon on the basis of the anatomic abnormalities present.

Hallux Valgus (Bunions)

Bunions are more prevalent in women than in men. In the elderly resident, atrophy of muscles, ligaments, and tendons or improper footgear often complicate the problem. Progressive hallux valgus often leads to subluxation or dislocation of the second metatarsophalangeal joint, and consequently to severe hammertoe and callus formation. The deformity may be severe, but it may not be painful unless a callus or other pathology is present. Shoe fitting will often be a greater problem than pain because the resident may not want to wear "old women's" or "old men's" shoes. Proper shoes should provide the forefoot enough space both laterally and dorsally. Surgical treatment is indicated only if intractable pain and shoe-fitting problems persist after nonoperative treatment. Keep any procedure simple with the goal of providing ambulation as quickly as possible.

Heel Spurs (Plantar Fasciitis)

Heel spurs, which are usually localized to the inferior/posterior aspects of the heel, can be a source of great pain. In some instances, heel pain may be associated with systemic diseases such as rheumatoid arthritis or Paget's disease. In elderly people, the cause may be heel pad atrophy, inferior spur formation, or plantar fasciitis. The pain usually occurs early in the morning when arising, or after sitting for a long period, but gradually lessens after 15 to 20 minutes of walking. Pain may be inferior or posterior over the insertion of the Achilles tendon, which may be calcified.

Inferior heel pain may be treated with corticosteroid and local anesthetic injections directly into the most painful area. Two injections over a 3-month period are the maximum to give in a year. Injections given more frequently may cause increased atrophy of the heel pad. After the injection, support the plantar fascia with the appropriate padding or with a specially molded orthotic device with a padded heel. With this type of therapy, relief of inferior heel pain can be achieved in 85% of cases.

Posterior heel pain is usually treated with oral anti-inflammatory agents and heel elevation with a pad or orthotic. Avoid using corticosteroid injections in the posterior heel because of the risk of rupture of the Achilles tendon.

ARTHRITIC DISORDERS

The following sections describe how to treat arthritic disorders of the foot. For more information on arthritic disorders, *see* Chapter 8, Arthritis.

Osteoarthritis

Osteoarthritis in the foot commonly occurs in the first metatarsophalangeal joint, but can also occur in other areas of the foot, including the tarsometatarsal and the talonavicular articulations. Nonoperative treatment includes wearing a solid supportive shoe with, in about 50% of cases, an orthotic device or rocker bar, which limits motion of the first metatarsophalangeal joint.

Rheumatoid Arthritis

Rheumatoid arthritis frequently involves the forefoot, resulting in a symmetric, bilateral polyarthritis. The major structures involved are the metatarsophalangeal joints of the forefoot, but the subtalar and talonavicular joints may also be involved. Most residents with rheumatoid arthritis will eventually manifest some form of foot disease. Individuals with rheumatoid vasculitis, especially those receiving long-term corticosteroid therapy, may have skin ulceration and digital ischemia, with increased risk of infection.

Nonsurgical treatment usually involves the use of specially designed shoes (e.g., healing sandals), orthotics, and decompression padding. It can also include local injection of water-soluble cortisone and local anesthetic into inflamed areas.

Gout

Most residents with gout will, eventually, have an inflamed first metatarsophalangeal joint. Treatment includes systemic management with antiinflammatory drugs and xanthine oxidase inhibitors (allopurinol). Trauma can be an initiating factor, so direct nonoperative therapy involves controlling excess motion around the joint with the use of orthotics, surgical shoes (e.g., stiff-soled), or healing sandals. Consider surgical treatment if the resident has a painful and deformed joint, an open sinus tract to the joint, multiple urate crystal deposits, or severe joint deformity that renders shoe-wearing impossible or causes breakdown of the skin over the joint.

DIAGNOSING AND TREATING FOOT INFECTION IN DIABETIC RESIDENTS

Foot infections and their consequences are a common complication of diabetes, and frequently result in hospitalization. The risk of lower extremity amputation is many times greater in the diabetic than nondiabetic resident. However, many of these amputations could be prevented if residents and caregivers were more alert to the risk factors for foot infections and used appropriate methods of treatment and prevention.

While the pathophysiologic processes predisposing to foot lesions in diabetic residents are complex, three factors are principally responsible for foot ulcers and lower-extremity amputations: neuropathy, ischemia, and infection. Distal peripheral sensory neuropathy predisposes to foot injuries from even minor trauma, and often causes injuries to go unnoticed. Neuropathy affecting the motor nerves of the foot can cause changes in gait, alterations in pressure distribution, and foot deformities. Autonomic neuropathy may lead to skin dryness and shunting of blood away from the nutritive capillary beds.

Limb ischemia in diabetes may be caused by arteriosclerosis obliterans or other conditions that lead to cutaneous ischemia. Atherosclerotic changes usually involve the more proximal arteries. Cutaneous ischemia resulting from disease in small cutaneous vessels, or from local conditions such as tissue edema, may be a critical factor in delayed wound re-

pair. Impaired wound healing in diabetes may be a consequence of severe ischemia or infection, but commonly occurs without either.

While chronic hyperglycemia and other metabolic perturbations of diabetes may interfere with cellular and humoral responses to infection, the principal condition facilitating infection of the diabetic foot is the loss of the protective cutaneous barrier associated with foot ulcerations. Once microorganisms gain access through a cutaneous portal, they may cause only a mild cellulitis, which usually remains localized and indolent, but may progress to involve deeper tissues and more proximal portions of the extremity. The infection can usually be eradicated with appropriate treatment, but refractory or slowly healing ulcers may persist, providing opportunities for recurrent infection until healing and re-epithelialization occur. Deeper ulcers may allow penetration of bacteria into the underlying bone, causing a contiguous osteomyelitis.

Once a skin breakdown occurs, it is graded according to severity and should be treated appropriately. Table 20-1 shows the foot ulcer classification and recommended treatment regimens.

For the resident with diabetes, daily foot care involves the following common-sense approaches and practices:

1. Examine the resident's feet daily. Report any changes promptly.
2. Bathe the resident's feet with warm (never hot) water. Pat them dry. This must be done more frequently with incontinent residents.
3. Apply a gentle emollient skin cream, taking care to avoid the areas between the toes.
4. Refer the resident to a podiatrist to keep toenails trimmed neatly, straight across and even with the toes. Neither staff nor residents should attempt to trim toenails due to risk of skin puncture and infection.

Table 20-1. Foot Ulcer Classification and Recommended Treatments for Elderly Residents with Diabetes

Ulcer grade	Recommendation
Grade 0: No open lesions; healed ulcer with hyperkeratotic overgrowth	Treatment includes periodic debridement by podiatrist, use of padding, decompressive insoles, and custom-molded shoes.
Grade I: Superficial ulcer	Treatment includes debridement, incision, and drainage by a podiatrist, local and systemic antibiotic therapy, depressurization by casting or use of plastizote shoes, and occasionally, surgical intervention.
Grade II: Deeper ulcer; may penetrate through soft tissue to bone	Treatment includes debridement by a podiatrist and bed rest; secondary wound closure, skin grafting, or toe amputation are sometimes required and performed by a surgeon. Healing sandals are used when the resident is ambulatory.
Grade III: Complicated by presence of osteomyelitis	Treatment includes multiple deep cultures, as well as aggressive debridement and intensive systemic antibiotic therapy. Perform a quantitative wound culture and determine drugs to be used according to organism sensitivities. Repeated debridement of infected bone and soft tissue is often required by a surgeon or podiatric surgeon.
Grade IV: Digital gangrene	Treatment includes careful vascular analysis by a surgeon for determination of amputation levels. Wounds are often left open until quantitative wound culture methods show that the bacterial count is less than 10^5. Meticulous shoe fitting is necessary after single digital amputations or transmetatarsal amputation. After amputation of the foot at the ankle joint with removal of both malleoli, fit the resident with a special prosthesis to help maximize comfort.
Grade V: Total-foot gangrene	Treatment includes amputation below or above the knee.

5. Be sure the resident wears clean, white, cotton or wool socks or stockings daily. If socks get holes in them, discard them. Even small repairs can cause ulceration.
6. Be sure the resident wears shoes or supportive sneakers that fit well, and that there are no foreign objects (rolled-up socks, coins or other items, frayed or worn linings) present when the resident puts them on.
7. Avoid extremes of cold or heat, including the use of heating pads or hot water bottles.
8. Check for a loss of hair from toes or legs. Loss of hair often indicates loss of circulation.
9. Encourage the resident to rest the feet for brief periods throughout the day by removing shoes and elevating the feet.
10. Encourage the resident to exercise regu-

larly, and assist in maintaining an ideal body weight.

11. Use a bed cradle to keep the pressure of the sheet and blanket off severely impaired feet.
12. Strongly discourage the resident from going barefoot. Bare feet invite injury.
13. Discourage the resident from crossing legs when sitting.
14. Do not dig under the toenails or around the cuticles.
15. Discourage the resident from wearing the same pair of shoes and socks every day.
16. Don't allow the resident to wear wet shoes. If the resident is incontinent of urine, be sure that dry shoes and socks are available.
17. Discourage the resident from wearing plastic shoes.
18. Encourage smokers to stop. Smoking reduces circulation of blood to the feet.
19. Discourage residents from wearing garters or knotting stockings to keep them in place.
20. Survey the resident's room for obstacles (e.g., wheelchairs, walkers, or bed cranks) that can cause injury to the lower extremities or cause falls.

Table 20-2 gives local care recommendations for diabetic foot lesions. Adapt the prin-

Table 20-2. Local Care of Diabetic Foot Lesions Including Ulcers, Wounds, and Infections

Activity	Recommendation
Debridement by a podiatrist or surgeon	Remove debris and eschar initially and at daily or weekly follow-up. Sinus tracts may require surgical drainage. Use mild chemical debridement with a 50:50 mixture of normal saline and 3% hydrogen peroxide, as appropriate.
Cleansing	Cleanse daily with normal saline. Avoid soaking. Dry well, especially between the toes.
Dressings	Apply wet-to-dry dressings (normal saline or Dakin's solution). Discontinue as soon as exudation is minimal. Dress daily with a fine-mesh gauze to the wound surface, which is covered by a plain sterile gauze and Kling wrap.
Edema control	Elevate affected extremity as much as possible. If additional edema control is necessary, add elastic wraps or compression hose, if appropriate.
Activity control	Initiate complete bed rest, if possible. If not, limit to essential ambulation only.
Footwear	Use a protective temporary shoe with a molded insole, if feasible
Prevention	Institute preventive measures, including resident education, daily inspection, nail care, use of emollients, use of recommended footwear, and prompt reporting of problems. Be sure that the resident's feet are inspected by a physician at each visit.

ciples, as appropriate, to each case.

SUMMARY

Residents who complain chronically about their feet, who are noncompliant with footcare regimens, or who refuse to be treated, are at great risk of multiple functional complications as a result of foot problems. Identify at-risk residents and refer them for podiatric evaluation.

The relationship between the podiatrist and the resident is critical in determining the outcome of treatment. This relationship is usually established at the time of the initial interview. After the evaluation, the same podiatrist should see the resident at subsequent follow-up to ensure continuity of treatment and strengthen the patient-physician bond. The quality of the interview and its result often depend on the resident's hearing ability, attitude, mental state, and physical condition. The physician's attitude toward treating elderly residents with diminished capacities is readily detected by many residents. Therefore, it is incumbent upon the physician to be sympathetic, empathetic, understanding, and supportive during the examination process.

CASE EXAMPLE

Mrs. G. is an 86-year-old resident of a long-term care facility. She has been there for 2 years. The staff knew from her admission psychosocial history that she was strong-willed, a loner, and noncompliant with medical regimens. The nursing staff was aware that she would have problems because of her multiple medical diagnoses, which included long-term unstable insulin-dependent diabetes with both a neuropathy and retinopathy, PVD, hypertension, and chronic obstructive pulmonary disease. She was examined by a podiatrist when she first came to the facility and was found to have long, thick, mycotic nails with friable nail plates. She also had multiple corns and calluses on both feet. She refused to wear "old-lady" shoes, so her footgear consisted of tight, pointed-toed patent leather pumps, which she wore without stockings or socks. She resisted staff help with her activities of daily living and repeatedly declined podiatric care.

One day, after a bath when her feet were soft, she decided to pare the calluses with a razor. She cut too deeply, creating a hemorrhaging wound that she did not see because of the retinopathy, or feel because of the neuropathy. She placed her foot into the worn, soiled pump and did not inform the personnel on her unit about using the razor.

A week later, at her bath session, an aide noticed a foul odor coming from her left foot. Upon examination, a large draining ulcerated area was noted at the second and third metatarsals. When this was reported to her nurse, the podiatrist and physician were notified. The area was debrided by the podiatrist, who also obtained a culture and sensitivity test. Antibiotic therapy was ordered together with local treatment and bedrest.

Despite excellent care by the staff, the wound did not respond because the resident refused to stay in bed, take the medication, or allow local treatment to the area.

At a staff briefing it was decided to seek a meeting with the physician, podiatrist, and family. Following this consultation it was determined that Mrs. G. be hospitalized for intravenous antibiotic therapy and total bedrest. After an uneventful 1-week stay in the hospital, she returned to the facility. Her recovery was very slow, but with the team approach, which consisted of local treatment by the nurses, debridement of the area by the podiatrist, and the prescription of a healing sandal, oral antibiotics, and management of her medical problems by the physician, she avoided a further complication such as a below knee amputation.

The staff realized that she needed constant monitoring because of her noncompliance and that further problems with her feet could be anticipated.

21
Skin Disorders

Kathryn Bowers, MD
Christy Flory, RN, C

Skin disorders occur in persons of all ages and social groups. Some disorders respond quickly to treatment, while others defy cure. Some are amenable to traditional home remedies, while others require immediate professional help.

In the nursing home setting, certain types of skin disorders predominate, including nonpressure ulcers, dermatitis, scabies, pruritus, xerosis, herpes infections, and various types of skin cancer (basal cell carcinoma, squamous cell carcinoma, and malignant melanoma).

This chapter describes how to identify and treat various types of skin disorders, especially as they relate to an infirm, elderly nursing home population.

OVERVIEW

The skin, which is the largest organ of the body, is extraordinarily complex in structure and function. In the average person it measures more than 2 square yards and weighs about 10 pounds. In just 1 square inch of skin there are approximately 30 million cells, 100 fat glands, 600 sweat glands, 20 small blood vessels, 65 hairs, numerous muscles, and thousands of nerve endings. The skin ranges in thickness from 0.5 mm in the eyelid to more than 2 mm in the palms and soles.

The functions of the skin are many and varied. The skin protects the rest of the body from chemicals, injuries, the sun, and temperature extremes in the environment, while simultaneously keeping the body itself stable and in place. It helps regulate heat, transmits sensation, produces vitamin D, and--through its temperature, clarity, and color--provides information about both the physical and emotional states of the person.

In an infirm, elderly nursing home population, certain types of skin disorders are especially prevalent. Nonpressure ulcers are typically associated with hypertension, arterial ischemia, diabetes, vasculitis, and embolisms. Drug reactions resulting in skin eruptions are extremely common among the elderly. The incidence of xerosis and pruritus increases with age, as does the incidence of various types of skin cancers, which are often associated with chronic, lifelong exposure to the sun.

For some skin disorders, treatment involves finding and removing the offending agents, such as perfumed personal care products or troublesome drugs. For others, treatment involves choosing from complex medical and surgical options.

NONPRESSURE ULCERS

Nonpressure ulcers may occur for a variety of reasons, although they appear most commonly secondary to chronic venous hypertension.

Pathophysiology and Terminology

Hypertension and peripheral vascular disease affect both the large and small blood vessels. The lumina of the blood vessels become narrowed and restricted through plaque formation, aggregation of thrombi, thickening of vessel walls, or chronic fibrosis from venous insufficiency and chronic low-grade cellulitis. The consequent reduction of blood flow leads to ischemia and tissue necrosis with secondary ulceration. The presence of an ulcer implies the loss of both epidermis and dermis,

and indicates that the area will heal with scarring.

Causes of Nonpressure Ulcers

In an infirm elderly nursing home population, the presence of a nonpressure ulcer is usually a result of one or more of the following conditions:
- Venous stasis ulceration
- Arterial ischemic ulcer
- Diabetic ulcer
- Vasculitic ulcer (e.g., due to rheumatoid arthritis, lupus, or vasculitis)
- Embolic ulcers (e.g., due to cardiac arrhythmias, cholesterol, or neoplasia)
- Malignancy (e.g., due to squamous cell carcinoma or ulcerated basal cell carcinoma)

Table 21-1 contains information about arterial, venous, and diabetic ulcers.

Typical Presenting Example

Mrs. A., a 75-year-old resident, developed a new ulceration on the medial aspect of her left lower leg. She had a history of chronic hypertension, which was controlled with an

Table 21-1. Arterial, Venous, and Diabetic Skin Ulcers

	Visual Location	Pain	History	Physical Examination
Arterial	Distal extremities	+/−	Cardiovascular disease Claudication Smoking	Absent distal pulses No leg or foot hair
Venous	Medial ankle	+	Varicose veins Thrombophlebitis Cellulitis	Brownish discoloration of lower legs Inverted bowling pin configuration of lower legs
Diabetic	Pressure areas on foot	−	Diabetes Poorly fitting shoes	+/− Absent pulses +/− Absent hair +/− Neuropathy

+ = may be pressure variable; − = not pressure variable; +/− = may or may not be pressure variable.

angiotensin-converting enzyme inhibitor and diuretic, and a history of varicose veins, for which she underwent extensive vein stripping in the 1950s. During each of two pregnancies she developed thrombophlebitis of the lower leg. Over the last 15 years, she had almost yearly episodes of cellulitis requiring antibiotic therapy. On physical examination there was evidence of brown discoloration of her lower legs. Her skin was shiny and tense with minimal presence of hair. Her lower legs had the configuration of an inverted bowling pin. Multiple superficial and deep varicosities extended from the feet to the thighs. A clean-based, tender, 2-cm ulcer was present over the left medial malleolus. Her toenails and the soles of her feet had evidence of a chronic dermatophyte infection.

Identifying the Resident in Need of Treatment

Any resident who develops an ulceration in a nonpressure area, especially on the lower legs, is considered to require treatment.

Treatment Protocol

To establish the etiology of the ulceration, the clinician should ask the following questions:

- Is there a history of diabetes?
- Are pulses present? Is there a history of claudication or coronary artery disease?
- Is there a history of varicose veins, vascular procedures, thrombophlebitis, or cellulitis?
- What is the location of the ulcer? Medial leg tender ulceration is usually indicative of venous stasis disease. Diabetics will often have painless ulcers, typically over joint surfaces or weight-bearing areas. Arterial ulcers are usually located on the distal extremities; they are ordinarily painless, and the lower extremities have no appreciable pulses.

Once the etiology is established, do the following:

- Evaluate for the presence of purpura in areas of ulceration.
- Rule out the possibility of systemic vasculitis (the absence of purpura, arthritis, and renal disease, and a normal sedimentation rate).

Skin biopsies for routine histology and culture are helpful to establish the diagnosis of nonpressure ulcers. Perform a biopsy on all ulcerations that do not respond to standard therapy (*see* Chapter 22, Pressure Ulcers, for treatment procedures to close wounds) to check for an underlying skin cancer or vasculitis.

Treatment of ulcers consists of correcting the underlying problem if possible, debridement to remove dead tissue, regular cleansing of the lesions, systemic antibiotics if infection is present, elevation to prevent edematous fluid accumulation, and careful surveillance for healing or worsening. Generally, debridement, cleansing, and surveillance can be accomplished with wet-to-dry saline dressings every 8 to 12 hours (*see* Chapter 22, Pressure Ulcers, for more information). Arterial ulcers require very close attention since compromise of the blood supply to the area can result in necrosis, gangrene, and ultimately amputation. These lesions require surgical consultation.

CONTACT AND IRRITANT DERMATITIS

Contact dermatitis occurs in approximately 11% of the elderly. Irritant dermatitis is far more common, usually occurring in conjunction with an underlying xerosis, which predisposes the skin to be more reactive than normal to potentially irritating substances.

Pathophysiology and Terminology

Cell-mediated immunity and delayed hypersensitivity reactions to standard antigens decline with age, probably as a result of an age-related decrease in the number of Langerhans' cells. Delayed epidermal turnover time and consequent longer exposure of the antigen for sensitization leads to the continued rate of contact dermatitis in the elderly.

Allergic contact dermatitis requires immunologic sensitization to an antigen, which depends on interaction between an antigen, Langerhans' cells, and T lymphocytes. The initial exposure may not produce a skin reaction, but subsequent exposures will elicit an eczematous dermatitis within 12 hours to 2 days as a result of antigen stimulation of the memory cells.

Irritant dermatitis is the result of direct damage of the epidermis from a harsh chemical (e.g., soap). The reaction is nonimmunologic and no prior sensitization is required.

Causes of Dermatitis

Soaps are the most common cause of most cases of irritant dermatitis. The severity will vary depending on the hydration of the skin, occlusion (e.g., by an adult brief), or the presence of a preexisting dermatosis (e.g., venous stasis dermatitis). Irritant dermatitis associated with adult briefs is very highly prevalent among residents with incontinence.

The most common contact allergens are nickel, chrome, fragrances, and preservatives. Benzocaine, a topical anesthetic found in many creams and ear drops, may cause an allergic contact dermatitis, especially when applied to a chronically inflamed area such as venous stasis of the lower legs. Neomycin is the topical antibiotic most likely to cause allergic contact dermatitis, since an estimated 5% of the US population is previously sensitized.

Treatment Protocol

Establish the etiology of the contact or irritant dermatitis in order to plan treatment. The following treatment protocol is recommended:

- Identify the pattern of skin eruption. Does it appear only where a particular topical product has recently been applied?
- Check with the resident and his or her family about the contents of the resident's drawers and cabinets. Evaluate all personal care products that have contact with the skin.
- Discontinue the use of harsh soaps (e.g., deodorant soaps) and recommend mild unscented soaps (e.g., Dove, Tone, Purpose, Basis, Neutrogena) as replacements.
- Be alert to the involvement of fragranced products. Aftershave lotions, perfumes, colognes, and fragranced skin preparations are frequently found to cause dermatitis in the elderly.
- Treat the affected area with a topical steroid cream twice a day. Use hydrocortisone 1% to 2.5% on the face, groin, or sensitive skin creases. A fluorinated steroid (e.g., triamcinolone 0.05%) may be used in other areas.

SCABIES

Scabies is a contagious, pruritic infestation of the skin caused by the mite *Sarcoptes scabiei.* People of all ages and socioeconomic classes are susceptible. An elderly resident with scabies may evidence a nonspecific rash and minimal pruritus, making the diagnosis difficult.

Pathophysiology and Terminology

The adult mite, *S. scabiei,* has four sets of legs and measures 0.3 mm in length. The adult female digs a burrow in the stratum corneum of the epidermis of the skin, where fecal material and eggs are deposited. The deposited eggs hatch within 2 weeks. After initial inoculation, it takes 3 to 5 weeks to generate enough mites for the host to develop a very pruritic hypersensitivity reaction.

The clinical lesions of scabies are pinpoint vesicles or papules located predominantly in skin folds, the web spaces of the hands, wrists, flexural surfaces, the areola of the breasts, belt line, and the scrotum or groin. A minute black speck, which is the mite, may be present at the end of the burrow. The pruritus and inflammation represent an allergic hypersensitivity reaction. A peripheral eosinophilia may also be present, and resolves with treatment.

Norwegian scabies is a form often seen in severely immunocompromised or elderly residents. Very thick crusts and scales develop, with hundreds of mites present all over the body. This type of scabies is extremely contagious, and unless checked can be responsible for a large outbreak affecting many other residents, staff, and families at home.

Causes of Scabies

Outbreaks of scabies in long-term care institutions may be caused by visiting family members, new residents with an undiagnosed reason for extensive pruritus, or staff. The mite *S. scabiei* is the agent of infestation in humans, but a similar infestation occurring in dogs and cats may affect humans secondarily for a short period of time.

Typical Presenting Example

Mrs. C., an 83-year-old resident with a history of a stroke and aphasia, had recently been transferred to the nursing facility from another nursing home. She had an extensive eczematous rash below the neck, which appeared to be very pruritic, especially at night. There were crusts and scales noted on her breasts, in the web spaces of her hands, and in skin folds. One month later her roommate, the roommate's daughter, and one of the staff nurses experienced a similar, though less intense rash.

Identifying the Resident in Need of Treatment

A total skin examination is required immediately for any resident with extensive pruritus. Check for small burrows, especially in the web spaces, on the breasts, or in flexural areas. If burrows are found, scrape the top layer of skin with a #15 surgical blade, removing the top scale and crust. Place the material on a glass slide with a small amount of mineral oil and a coverslip. Evaluate the scrapings under low-power (10∞) magnification, looking for live mites, fecal material, or eggs. Several scrapings may be required, since an infected resident typically hosts only 20 to 30 mites at a time. A nurse can prepare the skin scraping for the lab to evaluate later.

Scabies should be strongly suspected in any resident with extensive pruritus of undetermined etiology.

Treatment Protocol

When scabies is confirmed or strongly suspected, the following treatment protocol is recommended:

- Trim the resident's fingernails and clean excess debris from underneath the remaining nails.
- Apply Elimite cream from the neck down, covering all cutaneous surfaces. A 30-g application is generally sufficient for the entire body. Use a Q-tip cotton swab to apply the cream inside the umbilicus and underneath the fingernails. Leave the cream in place for 12 hours, then remove by washing. Repeat the treatment in 7 days.
- Treat all persons having contact with the resident, including family members, other residents, and staff. It is not unreasonable to treat all residents and staff on the nursing unit if more than one person has been affected. Family members at home may also be at risk.
- Initially, the pruritus may be worsened by the Elimite treatment, but the resident's condition should improve over the next several days. Antihistamines may be required to help control itching (e.g., hydroxyzine [Atarax]), 10 to 50 mg orally every 4 hours,

as required).

- Consider oral antibiotics if there is evidence of suprainfection of skin lesions secondary to extensive pruritus.

SEBORRHEIC DERMATITIS

Seborrheic dermatitis is a chronic inflammatory disease characterized by moderate erythema, dry, moist, or greasy scaling, and yellow crusted patches, especially in areas of the body in which sebaceous glands are abundant (i.e., the scalp, face, chest, back, axilla, and groin) (Fig. 21-1). Seborrheic dermatitis is very common in the elderly nursing home population, especially in individuals with neurologic disorders such as parkinsonism, strokes, and multiple sclerosis.

Pathophysiology and Terminology

Seborrheic dermatitis is a disorder of increased epidermal proliferation and retention, leading to excessive scale. Dandruff is seborrheic dermatitis occurring on the scalp.

Causes of Seborrheic Dermatitis

A yeastlike organism, *Pityrosporum ovale*, is a likely cause or contributor to seborrheic dermatitis. It is unclear why individuals with neurologic disorders have an increased incidence.

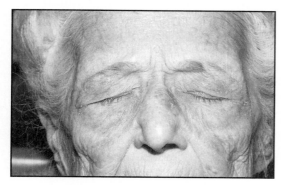

Fig. 21-1. *Seborrheic dermatitis involving the eyebrows and central face.*

Typical Presenting Example

Mrs. D., an 81-year-old woman with a 10-year history of parkinsonism, developed pruritus of the scalp, face, and anterior chest. Her only medications were levodopa, Colace, and hydrochlorothiazide. A trial of dandruff shampoo had been unsuccessful. On physical examination there was a thick, yellow, greasy, adherent scale over her eyebrows and nasolabial folds. Her scalp had a superficial white scale, and her chest had a well-demarcated erythematous plaque.

Identifying the Resident in Need of Treatment

Any appearance of a pruritic or nonpruritic scaling dermatosis on the scalp or face, especially in an individual with a history of neurologic disorders, may be seborrheic dermatitis and may require treatment.

Treatment Protocol

When seborrheic dermatitis is found, the following treatment protocol is recommended:

- Shampoo for 5 to 10 minutes each time three times a week with one of the following: selenium sulfide shampoo (2.5%); tar and salicylic acid shampoo; Nizoral shampoo (to decrease the amount of yeast).
- If the scalp is very pruritic and inflammatory, apply a midpotency topical steroid solution (e.g., Valisone, Synalar, Lidex) nightly or every other night; cover the head with a shower cap after application. Massage the liquid into the scalp, not the hair. Remove the shower cap and wash out application the following morning.
- For the face and chest, application of hydrocortisone cream 1% to 2.5% twice a day will decrease the erythema and scales. Since seborrheic dermatitis is a chronic disorder, long-term or intermittent therapy may be required.
- If mild topical steroids are ineffective, the addition of ketoconazole (Nizoral) 2% cream

may be beneficial.

• Seborrheic dermatitis is a benign disorder—not all residents (i.e., combative residents) require treatment. However, treatment improves the cosmetic appearance.

DRUG REACTIONS

Drug reactions manifesting in skin disorders are much more common in an infirm, elderly nursing home population, than in a younger age group. The likelihood of occurrence increases with the number of drugs prescribed.

Pathophysiology and Terminology

The following subsections describe common drug reactions in an elderly nursing home population.

Drug Exanthema

A drug exanthema, the most common allergic reaction to drugs, typically presents with small, erythematous, symmetric papules and macules that blanche and coalesce. The rash will usually begin within 2 to 10 days after the drug has been started. Antibiotics and allopurinol (e.g., Zyloprim) may produce a rash 2 to 3 weeks after the start of therapy. Drug exanthemas usually start on the trunk or dependent areas and spread toward the extremities.

The most likely etiology of a drug exanthema is deposition of drug antigen and antibody complexes in vessel walls (type II or III immune response).

Urticaria

Urticaria (hives), the second most common allergic reaction to drugs, is indurated erythematous, wheallike plaques that arise quickly and, typically, last less than 24 hours, although they may be present for several weeks after discontinuing the offending agent. There is no overlying scale in the epidermis; the erythema blanches completely with pressure; and there should be no residual pigmentary changes after the urticaria resolves. Le-

sions may be papular, arcuate, or annular. Occasionally, urticaria may be accompanied by other symptoms (e.g., wheezing, diarrhea, diaphoresis, and hypotension). Urticaria may be due to two factors:

• Immunoglobulin E (IgE)–mediated hypersensitivity with antibody stimulation of basophils and mast cells resulting in release of histamine and other substances
• Non-IgE–mediated direct release of histamine from mast cells and basophils

Erythema Multiforme

Erythema multiforme is a distinctive reaction pattern that is often secondary to drug ingestion. The skin lesion consists of annular, erythematous papules and plaques that may be urticarial. The hallmark sign is the presence of target lesions (i.e., resembling a bull's eye), which often start on the palms and soles. More advanced cases will have associated fever, malaise, and involvement of mucous membrane surfaces (Stevens-Johnson syndrome).

Toxic Epidermal Necrolysis

Toxic epidermal necrolysis (TEN) is an acute, extensive, blistering eruption involving both cutaneous and mucosal surfaces. It is a rare complication of drug therapy, usually associated with nonsteroidal antiinflammatory drugs [NSAIDs], antibiotics (e.g., trimethoprim-sulfamethoxazole [Bactrim]), barbiturates, phenytoin (Dilantin), and allopurinol (e.g., Zyloprim). TEN is a life-threatening disorder with a high mortality rate, especially in the elderly. It most likely represents an acute epidermal toxic reaction, and is probably an extreme variant of erythema multiforme. Immediately transfer residents with TEN to an acute care hospital for treatment.

Causes of Drug Reactions

Almost any drug can be responsible for a drug eruption, especially in an elderly nursing home population. The most common causative agents include:

- Antibiotics (especially penicillin and the sulfa drugs)
- Antiseizure medications (Dilantin, phenobarbital, Tegretol)
- Nonsteroidal antiinflammatory drugs
- Gold salts
- Hypoglycemic agents
- Phenothiazines
- Thiazides
- Quinidine
- Blood products
- Radiocontrast media
- Opiates

Typical Presenting Example

Mrs. E., an 84-year-old resident with a seizure disorder of longstanding duration, developed an acute urinary tract infection. Bactrim, one tablet orally twice a day, was prescribed. After 5 days of antibiotic therapy, she developed itching of her back and buttocks. A fine red, papular exanthema was noted. There were no blisters or ulcerations on the skin or mucosal surfaces. Her other medications included Darvon, Dilantin, and Colace.

Identifying the Resident in Need of Treatment

Any unexplained skin eruption, either pruritic or nonpruritic, should prompt a total skin examination, including mucous membranes. Also, review the resident's drug history, paying particular attention to any new drugs (i.e., those administered within the last 2 weeks) or long-term drugs that are commonly associated with drug eruptions. Also, consider possible underlying infection (e.g., could the condition be a viral exanthema?).

Treatment Protocol

The following treatment protocol is recommended:

1. Review all drugs that are currently prescribed.
2. Discontinue the possible offending agent.
3. If symptoms of wheezing, diaphoresis, diarrhea, and hypotension accompany a drug eruption, initiate fluid support and emergency intervention, as required.
4. Symptomatic treatment for itching or discomfort may include:
   o Aveeno or oatmeal baths
   o Antihistamines (e.g., hydroxyzine [Atarax]), 10 to 50 mg every 4 to 6 hours, as required)
   o Pramosone or Sarna lotion, as required
   o Cool compresses
   o Bland emollients (e.g., Aquaphor, Eucerin, Vaseline)
   o Topical steroids may help to decrease significant pruritus. Oral steroids are of no benefit except in the phenytoin hypersensitivity syndrome (i.e., drug exanthema with hepatitis and fever)
5. Monitor the resident over the next 2 to 3 weeks as the drug eruption resolves. Check for blisters or ulcerations, both on the skin and mucosal surfaces (i.e., mouth, genitals, anal mucosa).
6. Consult a dermatologist if the rash does not resolve or has atypical features.
7. Clearly document the drug reaction on the resident's chart and problem list. Include any chemically related compounds that could cause further reaction.

PRURITUS

Pruritus is a very common problem among infirm, elderly nursing home residents. It may be a component of a primary skin disease (e.g., eczema or psoriasis) or may be due to various physical or environmental factors.

Pathophysiology and Terminology

Pruritus is persistent itching of the skin. Xerosis refers to dry skin that may or may not have the symptom of pruritus. The itch sensation is secondary to stimulation of itch/pain receptors located at the dermal-epidermal junction of the skin. Histamine and other peptide mediators are responsible for propagation of the itch response.

Causes of Pruritus

In the nursing home setting, pruritus is generally worse at night, probably as a result of decreased mental and physical activity. Hot baths and frequent bathing will exacerbate pruritus, as will a decrease in environmental humidity. Specific causes include the following:

- Xerosis
- Infestations—scabies, head, pubic, or body lice, insect bites
- Metabolic diseases—hyper- or hypothyroidism, diabetes mellitus
- Hematologic disorders—polycythemia rubra, lymphoma/leukemia, paraproteinemia, cutaneous T cell lymphoma, iron deficiency anemia, mastocytosis
- Renal disorders—uremic pruritus, pruritus associated with hemodialysis
- Liver/gastrointestinal disorders—cholestasis, carcinoid syndrome
- Drugs (almost any drug may be a causative agent)
- Dermatologic disorders—bullous pemphigoid (Fig. 21-2), dermatitis herpetiformis, atopic dermatitis, psoriasis, contact derma-

titis, irritant dermatitis, fungal infection, folliculitis, urticaria, lichen simplex chronicus, lichen planus
- Psychogenic—delusions of parasitosis, neurotic excoriations, periods of emotional stress

Treatment for pruritus and xerosis (dry skin) is the same (*see* the section on treatment protocol). However, the medical etiology of pruritus needs to be evaluated and treated.

XEROSIS

Xerosis is a very common dermatologic complaint among the elderly. The incidence increases with age, and may affect as many as 80% of individuals over 80 years of age.

Pathophysiology and Terminology

As people age, there is a decrease in the water content of the top layer of the skin (the stratum corneum) and an abnormal maturation of the epidermal cells. The skin will have a fine superficial scale, usually without significant erythema (Fig. 21-3).

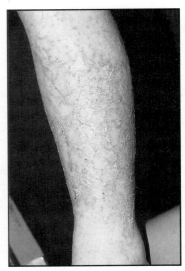

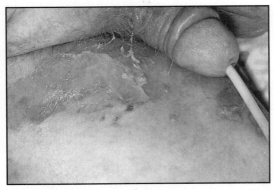

Fig. 21-2. Bullous pemphigoid of the groin. This eruption was preceded by intense pruitis.

Fig. 21-3. Eczematoles dermatisis and xerosis of the leg.

Causes of Xerosis

Xerosis may be caused by multiple internal and environmental factors. They include:

- Preexisting skin disease (e.g., eczema, psoriasis, ichthyosis)
- Use of drugs (e.g., diuretics, H_2 blockers)
- Metabolic diseases (e.g., diabetes mellitus, hypothyroidism)
- Frequent bathing, especially with hot water
- Harsh soaps
- Low environmental humidity
- Winter climate
- Aging skin with decreased water content, decreased lipid content, and diminished sweat gland function

Treatment Protocol

The objective of treatment for both xerosis pruritis is to hydrate the epidermis. Moisturizers increase the water content of the epidermis, and emollients fill the spaces between keratinocytes in the stratum corneum with lipids. The following treatment protocol is recommended:

1. Discontinue frequent bathing.
2. Use warm, not hot, water for bathing.
3. Use mild unscented soaps for bathing (e.g., Dove, Tone, Purpose, Basis, Neutrogena).
4. Apply a bland emollient cream (e.g., Eucerin, Moisturel, Lubriderm, Aquaphor, Vaseline, Theraplex) to the body after bathing and otherwise on a daily basis. After bathing, pat the skin with a towel until it is still a little moist. Apply cream to all areas to seal in moisture.
5. Use a room humidifier during the winter months to increase local air humidity.

HERPES ZOSTER

Infection of the skin with the varicella zoster virus is the most common cutaneous viral infection in the elderly. The first symptoms are numbness, paresthesia, or pain in the affected dermatome. The thoracic and cervical dermatomes are the most commonly affected. A fever may develop 2 to 4 days later, and then a rash appears consisting of red papules and vesicles in a bandlike or linear distribution ending at the midline. Isolated lesions may occur outside the dermatome. The vesicles become purulent, then crust off and heal with possible scarring; the typical course is 2 weeks.

Pathophysiology and Terminology

Herpes zoster is a reactivation of childhood varicella virus (i.e., chicken pox). The virus lies dormant in the dorsal root or cranial nerve ganglia and can be reactivated by illness, immunosuppression, or old age. As many as one third of the cases may develop postherpetic neuralgia, which can be very severe. Vesicles on the tip of the nose indicate involvement of the nasociliary branch of the ophthalmic division of the trigeminal nerve, with a strong possibility of an associated keratoconjunctivitis.

Causes of Herpes Zoster

Herpes zoster is caused by reactivation of the varicella virus within a nerve root. Individuals with immunosuppression and malignancies are at a higher risk of developing disseminated zoster.

Typical Presenting Example

Mr. G., a 75-year-old resident with a history of chronic obstructive pulmonary disease and asthma, developed a sharp, burning pain over his posterior back. No lesions were observed on physical examination. Twenty-four hours later a linear streak of erythema was noted at the continued site of pain. The following day fluid-filled vesicles developed, overlying the erythema. The resident complained of chills, loss of appetite, and extreme fatigue. His current medications included prednisone, 15 mg orally every other day, Lasix, and Theodur.

Identifying the Resident in Need of Treatment

The following procedure is recommended:
1. Identify the vesicular dermatomal eruption.

2. Conduct a total skin examination and evaluate for possible dissemination. Are there similar lesions outside the dermatome?
3. If the diagnosis is not clear, it can be confirmed by Tzanck cell test, culture, or rapid immunofluorescence studies.

Treatment Protocol

The objective of treatment for herpes zoster is relief of pain, prevention of infection, and prevention of dissemination. The following treatment protocol is recommended:
1. Apply cool compresses with 1:20 Burow's solution to the affected area 4 times a day.
2. Prescribe analgesics (NSAIDs initially) for pain. Opiates may be required for severe pain.
3. Culture the wound and institute oral antibiotics if there is evidence of suprainfection.
4. Prescribe acyclovir, 800 mg orally five times a day, if diagnosis is made in the early stages. Acyclovir reduces the duration and severity of the disease, and may also decrease postherpetic neuralgia.
5. If there is considerable pain, edema, swelling, or facial involvement, consider prednisone, 40 to 60 mg orally every day, with a taper over the following 3 weeks. Oral steroids may help to prevent postherpetic neuralgia, but evaluate the risk/benefit ratio for each resident individually.
6. If there is evidence of dissemination, transfer the resident to an acute care hospital. Isolate and prescribe intravenous acyclovir.
7. Obtain an ophthalmologic consultation for involvement of the tip of the nose or eye.
8. Staff who have not had chicken pox should not provide direct care to residents with draining zoster lesions as there is risk of contracting chicken pox.

ACTINIC KERATOSES

An actinic keratosis is a poorly demarcated, red- or skin-colored, flat or elevated, keratotic growth, which may develop into a cutaneous horn or a squamous cell carcinoma. Middle-aged or elderly individuals, especially those with fair complexion, are prone to developing actinic keratoses.

Pathophysiology and Terminology

Actinic keratoses (also called solar keratoses) are focal areas of atypical epidermal cells that form abnormal keratin. On physical examination, actinic keratoses appear as 1 to 10 mm pink or red macules with irregular borders or papules with an adherent white, gray, or yellow scale. They occur on sun-exposed areas of fair-skinned individuals, and are most commonly found on the dorsum of the hands and forearms, face, neck, and on the upper back and chest (Fig. 21-4).

Causes of Actinic Keratoses

Actinic keratoses are caused by frequent and prolonged exposure to the sun.

Typical Presenting Example

Mrs. H., a 79-year-old woman with a history of Parkinson's disease, was recently admitted to the nursing facility. During the admission physical examination, she was noted to have about 50 2 to 4 mm gray-white, rough, scaly papules scattered on her face and forearms, along with multiple solar lentigines and telangiectasias on her face.

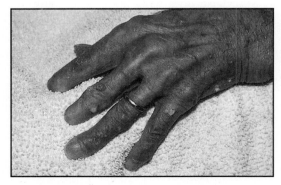

Fig. 21-4. Multiple actinic keratoses on the dorsum of the hand.

Table 21-2. Basal Cell Carcinomas

Type of Basal Cell Carcinoma	Description
Nodular	Commonly appears as a pearly papule, with central ulceration, telangiectasias, and the border of the lesion has a rolled edge
Pigmented	Characterized by a shiny blue-black papule, nodule, or plaque; the pigment can also be speckled
Superficial	A red, scaly, eczematous-appearing plaque that originates most frequently on the thorax
Morphisform (scarring)	The most aggressive type; it appears as a whitish, sclerotic patch with ill-defined borders, resembling a scar

Identifying the Resident in Need of Treatment

Perform a total skin examination at the time of admission. Any appearance of a skin tumor should trigger an immediate evaluation to determine the presence of premalignant or malignant conditions. Give any resident with a history of skin cancer a total skin examination annually.

Treatment Protocol

Prevention is the most effective form of therapy. Residents who have developed actinic keratoses or skin cancers should wear protective clothing and wide-brimmed hats outdoors and use sunscreen (at least SPF 15) on sun-exposed areas.

When a few actinic keratoses are present, cryosurgery with liquid nitrogen is recommended. When multiple actinic keratoses are present, topical chemotherapy is recommended, (i.e., 5-fluorouracil [5-FU] applied twice a day to affected areas), with treatment discontinued when the actinic keratoses become painful, crusted, and eroded (usually within 2 to 4 weeks).

In all cases, obtain a biopsy of thick and indurated actinic keratoses as a check for squamous cell carcinoma.

BASAL CELL CARCINOMA

Basal cell carcinoma is an epithelial tumor that seldom metastasizes but has the potential for local invasion and destruction; it is the most common type of skin cancer, constituting 65% to 80% of the 500,000 skin cancer cases diagnosed each year in the United States.

Pathophysiology and Terminology

Basal cell carcinoma may arise either from normal or sun-exposed skin. Its pathogenesis remains undefined. Table 21-2 describes the four types of basal cell carcinoma.

Causes of Basal Cell Carcinoma

Chronic, cumulative sun exposure and fair complexion (i.e., poor tanning ability) are prominent factors in the development of basal cell carcinomas. Previous therapy for acne (with radiation) greatly increases the risk, even in individuals with good tanning ability.

Typical Presenting Example

Mrs. I., a 70-year-old woman with a history of stroke, was admitted to the nursing facility. During the admission physical examination, a 3-cm erythematous, slightly scaly plaque with a whitish center was noted on the extensor surface of the right forearm. Her forearms and face showed photodamaged skin (senile lentigines, telangiectasias, and actinic keratoses). The family reported that the plaque on her forearm, which had been thought to be eczema, had never responded to the topical steroid that had been prescribed. A biopsy revealed superficial basal cell carcinoma.

Identifying the Resident in Need of Treatment

Perform a total skin examination at the time of admission. Any appearance of a skin tumor should trigger an evaluation to determine the presence of premalignant or malignant conditions. Give any resident with a history of skin cancer a total skin examination annually.

Treatment Protocol

Perform a biopsy on any lesion suspected of being a basal cell carcinoma to verify the diagnosis. Referral to a dermatologist for a shave or punch biopsy is recommended.

If the presence of basal cell carcinoma is confirmed, treatment is determined by the histopathologic type, size, and location, general health of the resident, and whether the lesion is primary or recurrent. Options include surgical excision, Mohs' micrographic surgery (specialized surgical technique that minimizes tissue loss by using multiple frozen sections), radiation therapy, cryosurgery, and electrodesiccation and curettage (a procedure in which the tumor is removed with a curette and the remaining tissue is electrocauterized). Topical 5-FV (Efudex) can be used to treat superficial lesions.

SQUAMOUS CELL CARCINOMA

Squamous cell carcinoma develops from the squamous epithelium; it is locally invasive and has the potential to metastasize, and represents 10% to 25% of all skin cancers diagnosed (Fig 21-5).

Pathophysiology and Terminology

Squamous cell carcinoma arises from atypical epidermal keratinocytes, as seen in actinic keratoses or on sun-damaged skin.

Causes of Squamous Cell Carcinoma

Chronic, cumulative sun exposure and a fair complexion are prominent factors for the development of squamous cell carcinoma. Other

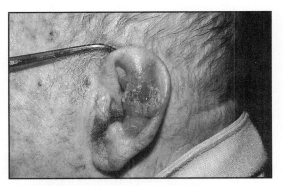

Fig. 21-5. Squamous cell carcinoma of the ear. This lesion metastasized to the lymph nodes of the neck.

predisposing conditions include:
- Exposure to radiation (accidental, therapeutic, or diagnostic), with a latent period of 15 to 25 years
- A history of phototherapy (psoralen-ultraviolet-high treatment)
- Arsenic ingestion
- Immunosuppression
- Organ transplantation

Most squamous cell cancers occur on sun-exposed areas, or in sites of chronic injury (e.g., burn scars, irradiated sites, erosive discoid lupus erythematosus, and osteomyelitis sinuses).

Typical Presenting Example

Mr. J., an 81-year-old man with a history of stroke, was admitted to the nursing facility from home. His past medical history included a history of prostate cancer treated with radiation therapy. On a routine physical examination he was noted to have a 2-cm shallow ulcer on the sacral area. His family reported that the lesion had been diagnosed and treated as a pressure ulcer for almost 5 months. A 4-mm punch biopsy was performed and a diagnosis of squamous cell cancer was made.

Identifying the Resident in Need of Treatment

Perform a total skin examination on admission. Any appearance of a skin tumor should trigger an evaluation to determine the presence of premalignant or malignant conditions. Give residents with a history of skin cancer a total skin examination annually.

Treatment Protocol

The treatment of choice for a squamous cell cancer is surgical excision. However, small well-differentiated squamous cell cancers on actinically damaged skin can often be treated with electrodesiccation and curettage. Excise poorly differentiated or large tumors.

MALIGNANT MELANOMA

Malignant melanoma is a cancerous neoplasm of melanocytes, arising de novo or from a preexisting benign nevus. It occurs most often in the skin, but may also involve the oral cavity, esophagus, anal canal, vagina, leptomeninges, and the conjunctivae or eye. Its incidence increases dramatically with age. The three principle melanomas found in whites are superficial spreading melanoma, nodular melanoma, and lentigo maligna melanoma.

Nonwhites represent approximately 8% of melanoma cases. Acral-lentiginous melanoma—the most common type seen in nonwhites—occurs on the palms, soles, or under the nails. The risk factors are poorly understood. Any dark discolored nail should be suspected to be a malignant melanoma.

Pathophysiology and Terminology

Malignant melanoma is a cancerous neoplasm of melanocytes and nevus cells. The majority of melanomas (80%) arise from normal skin, with the remainder arising from moles. The three principal types are:

- *Superficial spreading melanoma.* This is the most common malignant melanoma, representing about 50% of the cases. It is charac-

terized by a period of radial growth of atypical melanocytes in the epidermis. An immune host response may lead to partial or complete regression of the radial growth phase. Deeply invasive (vertical) growth is superimposed on the radial phase. While superficial spreading melanoma can occur anywhere on the body, it is most often found on the lower leg in women or back in men. The lesion can be various shades of red, white, blue, black, or brown. It can appear as a plaque or nodule, and may bleed or ooze. The border can be irregular and may be surrounded by a rim of pink inflammation or loss of normal pigment.

- *Nodular melanoma.* This type of malignant melanoma arises without a perceptible radial growth phase, most often occurring on the head, neck, and trunk. It typically presents as a uniformly pigmented, elevated, odd-colored nodule that enlarges rapidly and often ulcerates. It may arise de novo or from a preexisting malignant melanoma of a different type.

- *Lentigo maligna melanoma.* This cutaneous malignant melanoma is found most often on the sun-exposed areas of the skin, especially the face and forearms of the elderly. It begins as a circumscribed macular patch of mottled pigmentation, showing shades of dark brown, tan, or black, and enlarges by lateral growth before dermal invasion occurs. This type is the slowest growing, has the least tendency to metastasize, and seems to be the least aggressive form of malignant melanoma (Fig. 21-6).

Causes of Malignant Melanoma

A history of dysplastic nevi, congenital nevi, changing nevi, and melanocytic dysplasias are considered risk factors for the development of malignant melanoma. Other factors associated with increased risk include poor tanning ability, a history of blistering sunburns, freckles, fair skin, red or blond hair, blue or hazel

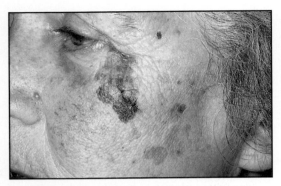

Fig. 21-6. *Lentigo maligna melanoma on the cheek*

eyes, and a family or personal history of melanoma. Sunlight is a major etiologic factor in lentigo maligna melanoma. Individuals with a history of lymphoma, leukemia, or a renal transplant appear to be at higher risk of developing a malignant melanoma.

Typical Presenting Example

Mr. K., an 83-year-old man, was admitted to the nursing facility for rehabilitation after sustaining a fracture of the left hip. Upon physical examination, he was noted to have a 2.1-cm serpiginous brown, gray, and black papule on the cheek. Half of the lesion was flat and half was raised. The family reported that Mr. K. had a flat brown lesion on his right cheek for at least 25 years, but over the last 5 years the color and shape had changed. A biopsy revealed lentigo maligna melanoma.

Identifying the Resident in Need of Treatment

Perform a total skin examination on admission. Any appearance of a skin tumor should trigger an evaluation to determine the presence of premalignant or malignant conditions. Have a dermatologist immediately evaluate any nevi or pigmented lesions having the classic "ABCDE" signs (asymmetry, border irregularity, color change, diameter greater than 6 mm, or elevation).

Treatment Protocol

Treatment of a melanoma includes surgical excision, a complete physical examination searching for evidence of metastatic disease, and a follow-up with a dermatologist every 3 to 6 months (or more often if warranted). Since there is a genetic predisposition to the disease, if a resident is diagnosed with a melanoma, notify family members so that they can commence appropriate screening.

22
Pressure Ulcers

Gary H. Brandeis, MD
Julia W. Powell, RN, MA

Pressure ulcers (i.e., pressure sores, decubitus ulcers, and bedsores) can occur at any site of pressure, most commonly the sacrum, coccyx, hips, heels, ankles, and buttocks. They affect 5% to 15% of nursing home residents, with an additional 60% or more residents at risk because of their health status or various environmental factors that increase their vulnerability. Costs of care for pressure ulcers occurring in nursing homes are estimated at over $355 million per year. However, pressure ulcers are treatable and preventable, and successful outcomes can be expected with appropriate care.

This chapter describes how to identify residents at risk for developing pressure ulcers and how to develop preventive care and treatment plans.

OVERVIEW

Pressure ulcers are localized areas of skin death and loss caused by excessive pressure being applied for a prolonged period of time. They typically occur when tissue is compressed between an exterior surface (e.g., a bed) and a bony prominence (e.g., the sacrum). The resulting decrease in blood flow deprives the tissue of needed nutrients and oxygen, resulting in skin death, sometimes in as little as 2 hours.

Table 22-1 shows the standard classification for pressure ulcer stages that is used in Health Care Financing Administration's Minimum Data Set (MDS) and Resident Assessment Protocols.

While pressure is requisite for the formation of pressure ulcers, various medical and environmental factors greatly increase the potential for occurrence. When assessing the skin, remember that stage I ulcers may be difficult to detect in an individual with dark skin. In addition, if the ulcer is covered with an eschar, the eschar must be removed before determining the stage. Any other covering, such as a bandage or a cast, must be removed, if clinically desired, to assess the skin. A thorough assessment of contributory factors is essential to effective care planning.

A resident is at risk for pressure ulcer development if:

- The skin integrity is compromised so that the skin cannot resist local forces such as pressure, shear, friction, and moisture. Shear and

Table 22-1. Standard Classification for Pressure Ulcer Stages

Stage	Description
Stage I	A persistent area of skin redness (without a break in the skin) that does not disappear when pressure is relieved
Stage II	Partial-thickness skin loss; presents clinically as an abrasion, blister, or shallow crater
Stage III	Full-thickness skin loss, exposing the subcutaneous tissues; presents as a deep crater with or without undermining adjacent tissue
Stage IV	Full-thickness skin and subcutaneous tissue loss, exposing muscle and/or bone, or other supporting structures

friction typically occur when a resident is dragged rather than lifted across the surface of a bed or chair. Moisture can macerate (soften, weaken) the skin, which makes it vulnerable to the consequences of pressure.

- Any of the following medical conditions are present: poor nutrition, urinary or fecal incontinence, diabetes, arteriosclerotic vascular disease, impaired mobility, or altered level of consciousness.
- Any of the following situational factors is present: resident is bed- or wheelchair bound, has suffered a recent hip-fracture, has a history of pressure ulcers, is physically restrained to a bed or chair, has impaired tactile sensory perception.

IDENTIFYING THE RESIDENT REQUIRING A CARE PLAN

The following sections discuss how to determine which residents require a care plan to treat pressure ulcers.

Background Clinical Review

Consider the following clinical factors in the assessment for pressure ulcers:

- Is a pressure ulcer present or does the potential for formation exist?
- What stage is the ulcer?
- How long has it been present?
- Is the resident infected?
- What risk factors for ulcer development or poor healing are present?
- What preventive measures or treatments are currently being used?
- If this is a recurrent lesion, what treatments have been effective in the past?

Try to establish a wound care team to recommend, institute, and direct care for pressure ulcers. This team can consist of any individual with an interest or expertise in this area. Potential members include the primary care physician, surgeon, nurse, enterostomal therapist, and nurse assistant.

Clinical Factors that Suggest a Need for Intervention

Consider implementing a pressure ulcer care plan if the resident already has a pressure ulcer or is at increased risk of developing one. The following items suggesting increased risk are readily identifiable from the MDS assessment instrument:

- Impaired transfer or bed mobility
- Bedfast, hemiplegia, quadriplegia
- Urinary or fecal incontinence
- Moisture (e.g., sweating from fever)
- Peripheral vascular disease (PVD)
- Insulin-dependent diabetes mellitus
- Recent fracture of lower limb
- Weight loss
- History of previous pressure ulcers

- Impaired tactile sensory perception
- Medications, especially drugs that impair cognition, the ability to turn or reposition, or the ability to detect pain
- Physical restraints
- Massage

Complicating Conditions and Treatments

Several conditions not only place a resident at high risk for developing pressure ulcers, but they may also complicate their treatment. Such conditions include:

- Alzheimer's disease and other dementias. An impairment in cognitive ability, particularly severe end-stage dementia, can lead to immobility (*see* Chapter 10, Cognitive Loss, for more information).
- Edema. The presence of extravascular fluid can decrease blood flow. If prolonged or excess pressure is applied to an area over a bony prominence with edema, skin breakdown may occur.
- Antidepressants, antipsychotics, and anti-anxiety/hypnotics. These medications can produce or contribute to confusion, lack of mobility, and incontinence (*see* Chapter 14, Psychotropic Drugs, for more information).

DEVELOPING A PREVENTIVE CARE PLAN

If a resident does not have a pressure ulcer and is not receiving skin care treatment, the clinician should evaluate for risk factors. Where the potential for developing pressure ulcers exists, a monitoring program (i.e., full visual inspection at least once daily) and an individualized preventive care plan are required. Figure 22-1 shows a treatment worksheet that the staff can use to remind them, and to record their responses to all the factors that need to be considered in treating pressure ulcers.

While all risk factors are important, it may be necessary to target certain areas depending on individual resident needs.

The following sections describe the recommended interventions for each risk factor category.

Impaired Transfer or Bed Mobility, Bedfast, Hemiplegia, Quadriplegia

The recommended interventions for impaired transfer or bed mobility are as follow:

- Establish a daily program to examine all possible pressure points in contact with a chair or bed, including the back of the head, shoulders, scapula, sacrum, ischial tuberosities (the bottom part of the pelvis area), and heels. Develop a monitoring protocol for each resident. For instance, during morning care or dressing activities, try to complete a skin assessment.
- Schedule position changes at least every 2 hours to reduce time spent on any particular pressure point. Reposition the resident to minimize the time spent on areas of increased risk, such as the trochanter when lying on the side.
- Try to teach cognitively capable chairbound residents to lift and reposition themselves on a scheduled basis. Establish proper positioning for each resident. When possible, establish a schedule with the resident and monitor for adherence. Provide regular reminders when necessary. Physical therapy for arm and leg strengthening can enhance resident self-care in repositioning.
- Keep the bed sheets clean and wrinkle-free to minimize friction and shearing forces.
- Where appropriate, use a pressure-reducing device (e.g., a foam mattress or pad, gel pad, water mattress or air support bed). When a resident is at risk, choose a device that is best suited to his or her clinical situation. For example, a gel pad with a plastic covering may be more practical and effective than a foam pad for an incontinent resident. In addition to padding environmental surfaces, it is important to relieve the pressure of one bone against another (e.g, tight knees, heel against buttock, elbow against rib cage). Soft wedges or pillows to keep

Pressure Ulcer Treatment Worksheet

Name: _____

Direction:
1. Date the top of each column
2. Using the appropriate code, complete the column. If a code does not exist, please write the appropriate information in the blank.
3. Use as often as needed.
4. Mark drawing for each ulcer; use a separate sheet for each ulcer.

Date					
a. Location					
b. # Sites					
c. Stage					
d. Picture					
e. Appearance					
f. Infection					
g. Antibiotics					
h. Dressing					
i. Turning					
j. Reduction/Relief device					
k. Debridement					
l. Nutrition					
m. Incontinence					
n. Mobility					
o. Resident education					
p. Change					

Figure 22-1. Pressure ulcer treatment worksheet.

Pressure Ulcer Treatment Worksheet

Name: _____

Direction:

1. Date the top of each column
2. Using the appropriate code, complete the column. If a code does not exist, please write the appropriate information in the blank.
3. Use as often as needed.
4. Mark drawing for each ulcer; use a separate sheet for each ulcer.

Date					
a. Location					
b. # Sites					
c. Stage					
d. Picture					
e. Appearance					
f. Infection					
g. Antibiotics					
h. Dressing					
i. Turning					
j. Reduction/Relief device					
k. Debridement					
l. Nutrition					
m. Incontinence					
n. Mobility					
o. Resident education					
p. Change					

Figure 22-1. Pressure ulcer treatment worksheet. (Continued).

knees, ankles, and other bony surfaces apart may also be useful, particularly if contractures are present. Remember that these devices *reduce*, but do not *relieve* pressure. They are useful adjuncts to the entire care plan.

- Use draw sheets, trapezes, or mechanical lifts to aid in positioning and reduce the shearing forces.
- Review the activities of daily living (ADLs) care plan for strategies regarding mobility and transfer (*see* Chapter 29, ADL Rehabilitation, for more information).

Urinary or Fecal Incontinence

Try to keep the resident dry to prevent skin maceration, which can lead to skin breakdown. Review the incontinence care plan for strategies (*see* Chapters 27 and 28, Urinary Incontinence and Bowel Disorders, respectively, for more information).

Moisture

Like urinary or fecal incontinence, perspiration or wound drainage can lead to skin maceration and breakdown. Prompt cleansing or application of barriers is indicated. Vigilance is also needed to avoid overdryness, which can predispose skin to cracking and breakdown.

Peripheral Vascular Disease

Peripheral vascular disease is usually caused by obstruction to blood flow, especially in the arteries and veins of the leg, and so presents an increased risk for pressure ulcers in the lower extremities. Therefore, focus monitoring on the legs, heels, and ankles. The resident should avoid wearing tight or worn shoes with ragged interiors. If leather shoes become hardened from exposure to urine, consider specially designed incontinence shoes that can be laundered regularly.

Peripheral vascular diseases can be either arterial, venous, or both. All increase the risk

of ulcer formation over an extremity. Arterial disease in the leg can be recognized by intermittent claudication, numbness, coldness, and pain at rest. Chronic venous disease rarely causes pain but can be recognized by chronic edema, scaly, itchy skin around the ankles, dark brown discoloration of the legs, and varicose veins.

Insulin-Dependent Diabetes Mellitus

Diabetes is a risk factor for pressure ulcers. No evidence exists correlating glucose control with the formation of pressure ulcers, but good medical practice should include close supervision and control of blood sugar.

The later effects of diabetes, such as decreased visual acuity and peripheral neuropathy, can also contribute to pressure ulcer formation by inhibiting the resident's awareness of skin pressure or breakdown. For example, a diabetic resident may not feel pressure on the heel while lying in bed and may not change positions to relieve the pressure, resulting in skin breakdown. Likewise, a resident with peripheral neuropathy and impaired vision may not be able to see or feel a foot ulcer developing. Therefore, all diabetic residents should receive a periodic skin assessment with particular attention to the feet. At the same time, examine their shoes for defects that can exert excess pressure, friction, or moisture on the foot (e.g., torn or cracked linings, a pebble under the sole, tight new shoes or straps).

Recent Fracture of Lower Limb

Follow the recommendations in the sections on impaired transfer or bed mobility.

Weight Loss/Malnutrition

Malnourishment decreases wound healing ability and increases the likelihood of skin breakdown. Weight loss is an indicator that the resident may be malnourished. If malnutrition is a problem, initiate a care plan in accordance with the recommendations given in Chapter 23, Nutrition.

History of Previous Pressure Ulcer

A resident who has had a skin breakdown in the past is at an increased risk, especially when other risk factors exist. A new ulcer may occur at the previous site because the skin over the old ulcer site is more fragile. When this occurs, reinstitute the prior pressure ulcer treatment program.

Impaired Tactile Sensory Perception

A resident who cannot feel pressure will be unaware of being in one position too long. For these residents, teach the cognitively capable to lift and reposition themselves on a scheduled basis. Other residents either must be reminded to change their position, or it must be done for them. Schedule the monitoring and cuing of residents to change position at least every 2 hours to reduce the time spent on any particular pressure point.

Medications

The side effects of many medications can exacerbate other risk factors. For example, medications can cause sedation, confusion, or decreased pain sensation, which can lead to more time in bed or sitting in a chair, increasing the chance of pressure ulcer formation. Review a resident's medication list for side effect implications. Be wary of antipsychotics, pain relievers (especially narcotics), antianxiety/hypnotics, and antidepressants.

Restraints

Follow the recommendations in the section on impaired transfer or bed mobility. *See* Chapter 31, "Restraint Reduction."

Shear or Friction

Shear or friction occurs when the surface skin and underlying tissues move in opposite directions, causing deep tissue damage (i.e., torn blood vessels). Elderly persons are particularly susceptible. *Shearing* often happens when the resident slides down in a bed or a chair or is dragged along the surface of the sheets or chair during repositioning. Avoid the shearing force by lifting the resident with a draw sheet to reposition. Reduce the angle of the bed or chair to prevent the resident from sliding in an attempt to find a comfortable position. While the resident is in bed, place the head of the bed at no higher than a 30° angle.

If the resident has a tendency to slide while seated in a chair, it may be a sign that the chair is too big, the seat cushion is uncomfortable, or that the resident has been sitting too long and needs to be repositioned. Look for and address the underlying problem (e.g., provide the resident with an appropriately sized, comfortable chair; try a recliner; alter the positioning schedule). Never restrain a resident who has a tendency to slide down in the bed or chair since this will place the resident at risk for strangulation, as well as pressure ulcers.

Friction occurs when two surfaces, such as skin and bed linens, rub against each other. The rougher the surface, the more the friction and the more damage to the skin. Again, lifting the resident with a draw sheet or teaching the resident to use a trapeze to lift off the bed during repositioning reduces friction. Sheepskin also reduces the effects of friction.

Although once believed to augment circulation, massage over the skin, especially the bony prominences, actually increases shear and friction, increasing the risk of pressure ulcer formation. Therefore, avoid massage in at-risk residents.

Assessment Scales

In addition to the MDS, scales such as the Norton Scale and Braden Scale assess an individual's risk for development of a pressure ulcer. The Norton Scale evaluates overall physical condition, mental condition, activity, mobility, and incontinence. The Braden Scale assesses sensory perception, moisture, activity, mobility, nutrition, and friction and shear. These scales are another method of quantifying risk of pressure ulcer formation. Examples of these scales are found in *Pressure Ulcers in Adults: Prediction and Prevention*, published by the Department of Human Services.

TREATING PRESSURE ULCERS

This section describes how to treat pressure ulcers in residents. Brand names are given for illustrative purposes and do not represent an endorsement.

Pathophysiology of Wound Healing

With an appropriate treatment program, the vast majority of pressure ulcer lesions will improve or be totally healed. However, the healing process takes considerable time, ranging from several weeks (stages I or II) to many months (stages III or IV).

While pressure ulcers are considered chronic wounds and do not heal as rapidly as acute wounds (e.g., surgical incision), like acute wounds they heal in three distinct phases:

• Inflammation phase. This is the body's first response to injury. The inflammatory response helps clean the wound and decrease the bacterial count in order to set the stage for further healing. Blood cells and other substances migrate into the wound and remove devitalized tissue and debris. New cells (fibroblasts) deposit a matrix so that surface (epithelial) cells can begin to grow or migrate from the outside of the wound toward the center. The ulcer and surrounding skin may be reddened, edematous, and warm to touch; often an eschar (dead tissue) forms over the ulcer. The inflammation phase lasts approximately 5 days.

• Proliferation phase. Fibroblasts are active and synthesize collagen, which is the predominant structural protein of connective tissue. Epithelial cells continue to migrate and new tissue is formed. New blood vessels begin to supply needed oxygen and nutrients. The combination of new blood vessels and cellular proliferation gives the ulcer bed a reddened appearance and is called granulation tissue. The proliferation phase peaks in several weeks, but can continue (though at a slower rate) for several months.

• Differentiation or maturation phase. Scar tissue previously formed is remodeled. Collagen fibers contract and the tissue becomes stronger. The differentiation or maturation phase can take as long as a year to complete.

For each of these three phases to proceed maximally, establish and maintain an optimum local environment. Keep the wound or ulcer clean, moist, and free of infection. Also, maintain the resident's overall nutrition and treat other conditions (e.g., diabetes).

Stage I Treatment Strategies

The following subsections describe the treatment strategies for stage I pressure ulcers.

Relieve Pressure

To relieve pressure on a pressure ulcer:

• Establish a turning schedule (e.g., every 2 hours).

• Use a pressure reduction device for the bed or chair (e.g., foam, water mattress, gel pad, air mattress).

Note that pressure reduction is helpful but it is not sufficient to eliminate a risk completely.

Relieve Friction and Shearing

To relieve friction and shearing on a pressure ulcer:

• Establish a program to lift (not drag) a resident from the bed. Physical or occupational therapy can help improve positioning techniques. When the resident is severely limited in bed mobility or transfers, use assistive devices (e.g., mechanical lift, trapeze, draw-sheet, or sheepskin).

- Keep the bed clean (i.e., no foreign objects, no food particles, no wrinkled sheets). Be alert for all sources of moisture, and change sheets and clothing as needed.
- Keep the head of bed at an angle of less than 30° unless contraindications exist (e.g., severe congestive heart failure or aspiration risk).
- Use a lubricant such as cornstarch on a bed-pan surface.

Treat Any Associated Factors

To treat any associated risk factors, follow the procedures discussed in the section on developing a preventive care plan.

Stage II Treatment Strategies

To treat stage II pressure ulcers, follow all of the stage I recommendations and the additional procedures described in the following subsections.

Wound Debridement

If an eschar or necrotic tissue is present, the choice of method for debridement depends on the expertise of the staff and clinical needs of the resident. For example, if the clinician believes the tissue under the eschar or necrosis is infected, mechanical debridement is the method of choice since it is most efficient. However, mechanical debridement requires the attention of someone adept at the process. In such a case, if expertise is not available, a surgical consultation is in order. Here are some methods to remove necrotic tissue or eschar:

- Mechanical removal of the necrotic (dead) tissue or eschar with a sharp blade for scraping is the most efficient method but the process may be painful. Premedication with an appropriate analgesic agent can minimize discomfort.
- Another method to accomplish mechanical

debridement is to use wet-to-dry dressings. Removal of devitalized tissue is possible with wet-to-dry *coarse* gauze changed at least every shift. These dressings allow the eschar or necrotic tissue to stick and the gauze to be removed when the dressings are changed. Administering analgesic medication before the dressing change may minimize discomfort. Other options for mechanical debridement include irrigation under pressure or whirlpool therapy.

- Use enzymatic removal of the necrotic tissue or eschar if the deeper tissue is not believed to be infected, mechanical means are not available, or the resident is unable to cooperate or has refused mechanical debridement. Examples of products that may be useful are collagenase (Santyl), sutilains ointment (Travase), fibrinolysin-deoxyribonuclease (Elase), trypsin (Granulex), and papain (Panafil).

Wound Cleansing (Noninfected)

To promote a healing environment, bacterial colonization should be minimized. Therefore, to clean a noninfected pressure ulcer:

- Use sterile normal saline (wet-to-damp dressings) three or four times a day or as required to promote an appropriate environment for healing. If the dressing becomes soiled or there is excessive discharge soaking through the dressing, more frequent changes are necessary.
- Avoid using antiseptics such as povidone iodine, iodophor, sodium hypochlorite, peroxide, or acetic acid, which impede epithelial cell growth.

Wound Cleansing (Infected)

In addition to cleansing with normal saline as described in the previous section, see the section on infection treatment strategies for directions on treating infection.

Dressings

The purpose of proper dressing is to create a favorable, physiologic environment (i.e., a clean and moist milieu that will encourage the growth of new tissue and prevent bacterial contamination). Selecting a type of dressing is often based on the amount and type of exudate present. For example, use a *coarse* mesh gauze wet-to-dry dressing for debridement of a wound covered with necrotic tissue; a *fine* mesh gauze wet-to-damp dressing is useful for maintaining the moist environment of a clean wound, and will reduce the amount of new tissue removed when the dressing is changed. The wound should be fully packed with the dressing to reduce any open areas. Take care not to pack the wound too tightly, which may generate additional pressure on the area.

Individualize the selection of tape (paper, plastic, adhesive) to secure the dressing. Some residents have allergies or sensitivities to certain tapes. If a history is not available, base the selection on trial and error, closely monitoring the skin at each dressing change. Try to keep the dressings intact until the next dressing change (to promote healing and to prevent contamination) to minimize the damage to surrounding healthy skin. Follow these procedures to dress draining wounds:

- If the wound is clean and draining minimally, use a dressing that is moisture vapor-permeable or transparent adhesive (Opsite, Tegaderm), or a hydrogel dressing (Vigilon, Geliperm).
- If there is necrotic material in need of debridement, use wet-to-dry sterile normal saline gauze, taking care to avoid maceration of the surrounding, intact skin.
- If the wound is draining moderately or an exudate is present, use a dressing with absorptive properties to decrease drainage yet maintain a moist healing environment (e.g., hydrocolloid or hydroactive particles [Duoderm, Restore]) or use alginate

(Kaltostat).

- *Note:* When a hydrocolloid dressing is working, the dressing may appear boggy. The staff may be tempted to remove it as the bogginess can be mistaken for excessive drainage or infection. Do not remove the dressing unless drainage is leaking around the edges, the dressing has lost its seal, or signs of surrounding cellulitis or pain are present.
- If the wound is draining heavily (i.e., more than one or two gauze pads are needed per dressing change), use dextanomer (Debrisan, Envisan) or copolymer starch (Bard absorption dressing), or use alginate (Kaltostat).
- Change the dressings as per the individual care plan schedule or sooner if:
  o The dressing becomes loose or ruffled
  o Excessive drainage or exudate is noted
  o Signs of infection are present (e.g., erythema [redness], induration [firmness], warmth, increased drainage)
  o Local pain or discomfort is noted

Monitor Wound for Healing

Monitor pressure ulcer wounds for healing as follows:

- Check for the formation of granulation tissue (i.e., tissue with a clean, pink, moist wound bed). If not present, either continue with the prescribed program giving it more time or consider another plan such as a different type of dressing.
- Photograph the ulcer every 2 weeks (minimum) at a fixed distance using the same camera and a marker (e.g., a ruler). If photographic equipment is not available, draw a picture of the wound on the resident's chart, showing its position and defining its measurements for length and width.

Stage III and IV Treatment Strategies

To treat stage III and IV pressure ulcers, follow all of the stage II recommendations and obtain an expert consultation. Consult with a physician, enterostomal therapist, or nurse (RN) who is well versed in wound care, or consult with members of the wound-care team if available. Consider:

- Debridement to remove necrotic tissue.
- Surgical evaluation (e.g., flap or repair, probing of the wound for the presence of sinus tracts).
- Specialized beds to relieve pressure (e.g., air-fluidized or low-air-loss beds).
- Dressing recommendations: Use loosely packed wet-to-damp normal saline gauze to provide a moist, healing environment or as per expert advisement. To prevent inadvertently losing the gauze in a large wound, use a long strip of gauze (e.g., Kling) instead of multiple gauze pads.

Expert consultation does not need to be limited to stage III and IV lesions. Therapy services can be consulted for positioning for all stage lesions. A nonhealing stage II lesion should invite expert consultation.

Infection Treatment Strategies

Follow the procedures in the following subsections to treat infected pressure ulcers. For more information on infection, *see* Chapter 3, Infection.

Infected Ulcer Without Surrounding Skin or Systemic Infection

To treat an infected ulcer without surrounding skin or systemic infection:

- Cleanse the wound. *See* the procedure in the section on stage II treatment strategies.
- Apply an antimicrobial ointment (e.g., silver sulfadiazine two to three times per day).
- Monitor the wound frequently (at least two or three times per day).

Infected Ulcer with Surrounding Skin or Systemic Infection

To treat an infected ulcer with surrounding skin or systemic infection (i.e., cellulitis—skin that is reddened, tender, warm, firm, with or without accompanying fever):

- Cleanse the wound. *See* the procedure in the section on stage II treatment strategies.
- Obtain a wound culture and sensitivities. Since all open pressure ulcers are colonized with bacteria, a swab of the surface does not necessarily culture the infecting organism. An aspiration or biopsy of the wound for quantitative culture will be more accurate. (*See* Chapter 3, Infection, for more information.)
- Administer oral or intravenous antibiotics to cover *Staphylococcus, Streptococcus,* anaerobes, and gram-negative organisms— usually a broad-spectrum antibiotic will suffice until the culture and sensitivity results are available. If a fever is present, use intravenous antibiotics, which may require transfer to the acute hospital (*see* Chapter 3, Infections, for more information).
- Monitor the wound frequently (at least two or three times per day).

Infected Ulcer that is Resistant to Therapy

If an infected ulcer is resistant to therapy, consider osteomyelitis or an underlying bone infection. This is difficult to detect and may require radiography or a bone biopsy to diagnose.

PSYCHOSOCIAL ISSUES

Preventing and treating pressure ulcers can be difficult, frustrating, and time-consuming, especially in the long-term care setting where the resident may have dementia and may not fully understand the rationale behind what is being done. It is essential that the resident, family, and direct care staff be kept informed of the purpose, rationale, and direction of the care plan. Without interdisciplinary communication among physicians, nurses, social workers, therapists, and the resident and his or her family, the care plan objectives will likely be compromised.

In educating the resident and family to the objectives of the care plan, emphasize the importance of maintaining good nutrition and changing position (e.g., getting out of bed to a chair, or shifting while in a chair) to keep body weight off the ulcer to the fullest extent possible. Where appropriate, give the resident some freedom about the direction and outcome of care by teaching him or her to inspect the skin with a mirror and to alert the nursing staff if incontinence has occurred. Consult with recreational therapy to explore ways to maintain resident engagement in leisure and social activities. If appropriate, provide supportive therapy or psychotherapy to help the resident (or family) deal with the frustration of chronic disease and distorted body image that is often associated with pressure ulcers.

CASE EXAMPLE

Mrs. M. is an 87-year-old woman with a history of Parkinson's disease and dementia with agitated behavior. She was recently admitted to the nursing home from an acute care hospital where she had a surgical repair of a left femoral neck fracture sustained in a fall at home.

On admission to the nursing home Mrs. M. was excessively drowsy. She had reduced spontaneity of movement, rigidity of all extremities, and impaired sensory perception in her feet. Mrs. M. required extensive assistance with bed mobility and transferring, and depended on others for wheelchair locomotion. In addition, she was incontinent of urine and feces. Her skin was dry and flaky. She had a 2 X 3 cm stage II pressure ulcer with clean granulation tissue over her sacrum and a 2 X 1 cm stage I ulcer over her right trochanter.

Nutritional risk factors associated with pres-

sure ulcer formation included anemia, low serum albumin, and a low total protein. She weighed 94.2 pounds–11 pounds below her ideal body weight based on her height, bone structure, and weight history.

Referral medications included lorazepam (Ativan), 0.5 mg three times a day, docusate Na (Colace), 100 mg twice a day, carbidopa/levodopa (Sinemet), 25/250 mg four times a day, aspirin, 325 mg/day, and a daily multivitamin.

Management plans were instituted and directed toward healing the two pressure ulcers and preventing further skin breakdown. Because clinicians and family members believed that lorazepam was chiefly responsible for her lethargy and decreased activity level, it was discontinued. As Mrs. M. became more alert, recreational therapy became involved and suggested activities that her devoted husband could start with her during his daily extended visits. Since the stage II ulcer was clean and free of drainage, wet-to-damp normal saline dressings were applied once a shift. Pressure-relieving devices (i.e., an air mattress for the bed and a gel cushion for a reclining chair) were provided. Position changes at least every 2 hours were also started. Physical therapy became involved to improve her ability to change position. The nursing staff assisted Mrs. M. to the toilet regularly and her continence improved. The staff also found that Mrs. M. had a good appetite but needed extra time and verbal cuing to complete her meals. The added support in addition to high-protein supplements with meals helped her to regain the lost weight. With such fastidious care the ulcers healed within 2 months.

23
Nutrition

Ann Gallagher, RD
Kathleen Pintell, RD
Gretchen Robinson, RD
Pauline Belleville-Taylor, RN, MS, CS
Susan Hartery, RD

Nutritional problems are common among elderly nursing home residents. Food intake levels may be insufficient, unplanned weight loss occurs, and some residents are significantly below (or above) their optimum body weights. Nutritional deficiencies reflect worsening health status, difficulties in following therapeutic diets, distressed mood, and intake of multiple medications; and they indicate that the resident may be at risk of sudden decline or complicating health problems. While all residents may benefit from a nutritional assessment, not all will benefit from treatment (e.g., medication management may represent a complex challenge or approaching death may preclude aggressive meal supplementation to regain lost weight).

Early recognition of the problem can help to ensure appropriate and timely nutritional intervention. For example, alter dietary prescriptions, introduce meal support services, prescribe nutritional supplements, and titrate medications. Design therapeutic programs to help a confused resident maintain a scheduled feeding routine or to assist the resident in
the use of adaptive utensils. As other health problems emerge, nutrition monitoring or changes may be crucial components to the overall therapeutic plan of care—e.g., for residents with pressure ulcers, edema, wounds, infection, nausea, constipation, muscle atrophy, diarrhea, or diabetes.

Oral feeding is always preferred, but if necessary tube (enteral) or parenteral feeding programs may be instituted. (*See* Chapter 26, Feeding Tubes, for more information.)

OVERVIEW

Nutritional status is the condition of the body resulting from utilization of the essential nutrients available to the body. Nutritional status depends not only on the intake of dietary essentials but also on the body's ability to use them. *Malnutrition* is a condition of the body resulting from an inadequate supply or impaired utilization of one or more of the essential food components. Malnutrition may be a predisposing factor or cause of deterioration related to other diseases.

In an elderly facility population, the ability

to take in or assimilate food is frequently effected by one or more of the following key factors, which are described in the following sections.

Mechanical Problems

The mechanical problems related to nutrition are as follows:

- Chewing problems. Poor oral care is often an unrecognized problem for many nursing home residents. (*See* Chapter 25, Oral Status, for more information.) Chewing problems may be caused by poor or missing teeth, ill-fitting dentures, mouth sores, mouth pain, or gum disease. Residents with these problems may not be able to eat enough food to meet their calorie and nutrient needs. A significant weight loss may result in poorly fitting dentures and infections, which can lead to additional weight loss.
- Swallowing problems. These problems may be the direct result of chemotherapy, radiation therapy, or surgery for malignancy in the area of the head or neck; fear of swallowing due to of chronic obstructive pulmonary disease (COPD), emphysema, or asthma; stroke; hemiplegia or quadriplegia; Parkinson's disease, Alzheimer's disease or other dementia; or amyotrophic lateral sclerosis.
- Reduced ability to feed self. This condition may be due to arthritis, contractures, partial or total loss of voluntary arm movement, hemiplegia or quadriplegia, vision problems, the inability to perform activities of daily living (ADLs), or coma.

Appetite Problems

The appetite problems related to nutrition are as follows:

- Decreased appetite. Constipation, intestinal obstruction, or pain may inhibit appetite. Shortness of breath (frequently seen with congestive heart failure and COPD) may be accompanied by a heightened fear of choking when eating or drinking, which links food with danger in the resident's mind.
- Drug-induced anorexia. The side effects from drugs are a major concern with this population (*see* Chapter 2, Polypharmacy). Reductions in appetite may be due to side effects such as constipation, drowsiness, diarrhea, nausea, and the altered ability to taste and smell food.
- Mental status. In some residents, malnourishment can have its origins in one or more mental disorders (e.g., dementia, depression, a paranoid fear that food is poisoned), all of which make it difficult for residents to track their own food consumption, to stay attentive to the task of eating, or to maintain energy levels. The presence of a cognitive deficit can also cause mechanical problems related to eating and feeding.

Increased Nutrient Requirements

Increased nutrient requirements (e.g., calories, protein, vitamins, minerals, water, and fiber) are a consequence of many diseases or medical conditions. The presence of diseases such as COPD increases calorie needs. Cancer therapies (chemotherapy, radiation therapy, surgery) require aggressive nutritional support to achieve their goal. For residents with incurable malignancies who are undergoing palliative therapy or are not responding to curative therapy, aggressive nutritional support is often medically inappropriate. Residents with pressure ulcers, surgical wounds, or traumatic wounds have increased nutrient requirements for calories, protein, vitamin C, and zinc in order to speed healing.

Adaptation to Special Diets

Residents may have to adjust to changes in their diet. Special diets can include the following:

- Diabetic diets

- Sodium- and potassium-restricted diets
- Increased or decreased fiber diets
- Increased or decreased protein diets
- Calculated diets for diabetes or weight gain or loss
- Renal diets
- Mechanically altered diets
- Lactose-free diets

Some of these diets can feel very restrictive to the resident. Familiar foods from home, or food that is traditional in the resident's culture or religion, may no longer be allowed.

Residents with food allergies generally have had them for a long time and have adapted to avoiding certain foods or ingredients.

Psychosocial Status

The following psychosocial factors have an impact on residents' nutritional status:

- Communication Residents with cognitive problems or language barriers may lose interest in eating due to the inability to communicate food preferences. If residents with individual, ethnic, or religious food preferences cannot make these preferences known, their food intake will be affected negatively.
- Environment Food is not only sustenance, but eating is a social event with broad cultural implications. Food stimulates feelings and memories. A resident may lose interest in eating for the following reasons:
  o The food is unappetizing or unattractively presented
  o The place in which meals are served does not lend itself to socialization among residents
  o There is inadequate staff assistance or time to feed residents or assist them in eating
  o There is an unrecognized need for adaptive feeding equipment for residents who can be helped to self-feed with such assistance
- Behavior problems Behavior problems

(e.g., persistent pacing or wandering, withdrawal from activities) are often accompanied by a refusal to eat, resistance to staff caregiving interventions, or a willingness to eat only a limited variety or amount of food. A resident with dementia may also be taking and eating food from another resident's plate, causing disruption at mealtimes.

- Mood problem Residents who are depressed or anxious may have severely decreased food intake, and may not be interested in food and mealtimes.
- Cultural issues A facility is often composed predominantly of one ethnic or religious group. The nutrition service departments of these facilities must provide culturally sensitive foods. In other facilities, where the mix of residents is more diverse, certain foods may be avoided by custom, cultural, or religious prohibition.

Many activities involving Catholic, Protestant, Jewish, and other religious and secular holidays include food. Special foods at holiday times can be something residents really look forward to and enjoy. Hispanic, African-American, and Native American residents enjoy their special foods and food-related social customs just as residents with Italian, Irish, and other national heritages do. Food preference will vary by geographic area. For example, a resident may have grown up in the south and always cooked the traditional southern dishes. Such a resident, now in a facility in the northeast, may have many complaints about the food being served.

CLINICAL AND ETHICAL CONSIDERATIONS

The nutrition treatment plan must be realistic and based on the resident's needs and preferences whenever possible. Quality of life should be the main focus for elderly residents. Only pursue an aggressive nutritional support program if the end result is an improvement in the quality of life and the resident desires it.

Unnecessary restrictions in the diet can also compromise the resident's quality of life. The interdisciplinary team, together with the resident and family (if possible), should monitor and adjust the nutritional plan of care according to mutually agreed upon priorities. For example, a resident on a diabetic diet is experiencing tissue breakdown, has a poor appetite, and had a decreased food intake during the past 2 weeks. The interdisciplinary team may decide to discontinue the diabetic diet temporarily. The resident's glucose must be monitored and any resulting hyperglycemia treated with a sliding scale insulin regimen. Then the resident may be placed on a high-protein, high-calorie diet with greater variety to improve intake. Review and adjust the nutritional plan as the resident's condition changes.

When oral intake is no longer possible or safe, more aggressive measures such as tube feedings are an alternative. If there is an advanced directive about the placement of a feeding tube, the resident's wishes must be respected and comfort measures alone may be the treatment of choice.

IDENTIFYING THE RESIDENT WHO REQUIRES TREATMENT

It is important to recognize that in many nursing homes, the registered dietitian is available only on a consulting basis. For this reason it is essential that the dietary staff work closely with the nursing staff to gather appropriate information, identify existing or potential problems, and communicate them to the dietitian. Assess residents with the following problems and conditions for a nutritional problem, and modify the care according to the nutritional issues identified:

- Unplanned weight loss (i.e., more than 5% in the last 30 days or 10% in the last 180 days)
- The resident leaves 25% or more of his or her food uneaten (even when substitutes

are offered) for at least two out of three meals
- A therapeutic diet is ordered to treat problematic conditions (e.g., calorie-specific, no added salt, lactose-free)

These factors will help clinicians recognize and treat problems that impact eating. The sections following these checklists discuss other factors to consider when conducting a nutritional assessment.

What are the resident's problems with eating? Check for:

- Poor acceptance of therapeutic diet
- Presence of longstanding eating problems such as food allergies and intolerances, or religious restrictions
- Loss of mobility
- Sensory problems related to alterations in sense of smell, taste, and appearance of food
- Breathing and swallowing difficulties
- Extreme confusion and forgetfulness
- Poor vision
- Poor appetite due to medications
- Poor dentition with decline in oral status
- Need for assistive devices to maintain independence
- Poor positioning, cutting, or placement of food
- Food not seasoned to resident's taste
- Improper food preparation
- Depression
- Bereavement
- Relocation to or within the nursing home
- Inconsistent programs for assistance with eating
- Feeding via syringe, or tube feedings

Have the resident's eating skills improved, or stayed the same? If not, then consider:

- Ability to chew or swallow
- Neurologic or muscular disease
- Opportunities for socialization at mealtimes
- Sufficient time and assistance provided at mealtimes

- Dining room environment
- Independence

Is the resident free from pressure ulcers?

If a pressure ulcer is present:

- Is the resident consuming an adequate diet and sufficient fluids?
- Is increased nutrient intake needed (e.g., protein, iron, folate, vitamin C, zinc, calories, and water)?
- Will the resident accept supplements of high nutrient density?

Medications

If a resident is found to have a decrease in food intake or a change in nutritional status, consider the possibility of a drug and nutrient interaction. In particular, residents taking (or overusing) any of the following types of medications may need adjustments to their nutritional care plan or a review of their medications for possible alternatives or reductions: antiparkinsonism agents, diuretics, cardiac glycosides (digoxin), antiinflammatory drugs, antacids, laxatives, psychotropics, and antibiotics.

Some drugs may cause gastric irritation or diarrhea from alteration in intestinal flora. Appetite may also be affected by some drugs. The resident may have symptoms of anorexia, nausea, vomiting, dry mouth, or a sore mouth. Drugs, or the interaction of multiple drugs, may cause an alteration of taste and smell, or produce an aftertaste. Nutrient metabolism as well as a decrease in the absorption of nutrients, may also be affected by medications.

Medical Evaluation Results

Review the residents' medical evaluations in depth and treat them on an individual basis. Many residents will have multiple medical problems. A single problem may not pose a significant threat to the resident's well-being, but a combination of medical problems may seriously jeopardize the resident's quality of life. The presence of an acute problem, or a history of chronic disease, will affect each resident differently.

If the medical evaluation reveals the presence of cancer, diabetes, hyperthyroidism, cardiovascular disease, fever, infection, other gastrointestinal problems, or any other diagnosis that may affect nutrient requirements, the nutritional care plan should reflect the resident's need and be reviewed routinely.

Laboratory Test Results

A thorough nutritional assessment should include a review of laboratory test results to determine whether or not a resident is at nutritional risk (Table 23-1). Use biochemical measurements to evaluate visceral protein.

Table 23-1. Selected Laboratory Values for Assessment of Nutritional Deficits

Lab Values	Normal values	Mild deficit	Moderate deficit	Severe deficit
Serum albumin (g/dL)	> 3.5	< 3.5-3.2	< 3.2-2.8	< 2.8
Transferrin (mg/dL)	> 200	< 200-180	< 180-160	< 160
TIBC (ug/dL)	> 214	< 214-182	< 182-152	< 152
TLC (per mm3)	> 1500	< 1500-1201	< 1200-900	< 900

Table 23-2. Normal Hematologic Values

Test	Male	Female
Hemoglobin (g/dL)	14-18	12-16
Hematocrit (%)	40-54	37-47
Serum Iron (ug/dL)	75-175	65-165
Ferritin (ng/mL)	15-300	12-150
Vitamin B12 (pg/mL)	160-1300	160-1300
Folate (ng/mL)	3-17	3-17

Serum albumin levels correlate with the degree of malnutrition and the increased risk for mortality and morbidity. This is the most common value used to assess nutritional status because it is readily available. It is usually part of the admission and annual laboratory workup. However, serum albumin is a late indicator of malnutrition and it is associated with chronic disease. Serum transferrin is a more sensitive indicator of nutritional status and is more reflective of acute changes. However, it is not as readily available as serum albumin. Serum transferrin may be determined directly or calculated using the total iron binding capacity (TIBC). The formula to calculate transferrin is as follows:

Transferrin (mg/dL) = 0.8 TIBC (ug/dL) - 43

The total lymphocyte count (TLC) is an indicator of immune function. It is not an absolute indictor of nutritional status, but it is often used to support an assessment. The TLC formula is as follows:

$$TLC = \frac{\% \; Lymphocytes \; x \; Total \; white \; blood \; count}{100}$$

Perform a hematologic assessment to determine whether there is an anemia and characterize its type and if there is a related nutritional deficiency. Certain blood cell tests may be useful in nutritional assessment. However, these tests are often influenced by other factors and not necessarily affected by nutritional intervention. *See* Table 23-2 for more information about normal hematologic values.

Specific laboratory values can be used to assess the resident's hydration status. Serum osmolality is indicative of hydration status and can be calculated by using the following formula:

$$Serum \; osmolality = (2 \; x \; Serum \; Na) + \frac{blood \; urea \; nitrogen}{2.8} + \frac{Blood \; Glucose}{18}$$

The normal values are 275-295 mOsm/kg. Values greater than 295 mOsm/kg indicate dehydration.

Urine tests are also indicative of hydration status. The normal values are as follows:

Specific gravity: Normal value = 1.005-1.030
Urine osmolality: Normal value = 38-1400 mOsm/kg H$_2$O (elevated levels indicate dehydration)

Other laboratory values may be significant to a comprehensive nutritional assessment on an individual basis but are not routinely evaluated. These values may be disease specific (e.g., those associated with renal function, diabetes, and heart disease). Evaluation is done to establish baseline values in order to monitor progression and control of disease. *See* Table 23-3 for examples.

Physical Factors

Anthropometric measurements are used to evaluate body energy stores and protein mass. These measurements include height, weight, and triceps skinfold.

Table 23-3. Some Laboratory Tests and Their Normal Values

Laboratory tests	Normal values
Blood glucose	70-110 mg/dL
Sodium	135-148 mEq/L
Potassium	3.5-5.0 mEq/L
Calcium	8.8-10 mg/dL
Phosphorus	2.7-4.5 mg/dL
Blood urea nitrogen	6-26 mg/dL
Creatinine	0.5-1.7 mg/dL
Cholesterol	100-200 mg/dL
Triglycerides	30-175 mg/dL

In the elderly, when a triceps skinfold may not be available or reliable, use a simple indicator of total body fat known as the body mass index (BMI). The formula is as follows:

$$BMI = \frac{weight\ (kg)}{height\ (m)^2}$$

The nomogram in Figure 23-1 suggests the most desirable BMI for a particular age. A BMI between 24 and 27 is considered normal for a healthy older adult. A BMI greater than 27 indicates obesity. A BMI less than 24 indicates that a potential problem may exist and further evaluation should be done.

Strategies for Completing the Nutritional Assessment

Note: Do not use any single piece of data as the sole indicator of nutritional status. Consider the following data to determine nutritional status:

- Upon admission, interview the resident and his or her family to obtain a diet history

(previous therapeutic diets, food allergies or intolerance, food preferences, cultural concerns). Try to get a 24-hour recall of a typical day's intake. Record and periodically update food preferences.
- Observe the current intake for several days.
- Evaluate the current therapeutic diet for appropriateness.
- Evaluate the present intake for adequacy based on needs as calculated by the Harrison-Benedict equation.
- Evaluate the weight in several ways. What is the resident's usual weight? What is the average weight for the previous year? What is the weight range for the previous year? Are there any significant changes? See Table 23-4 which uses material from the *Handbook for Clinical Dietetics* to evaluate weight loss. If a problem is suspected, calculate the percent weight change with the following equation:

Percent weight change =
$$\frac{(usual\ weight - actual\ weight)\ x\ 100}{usual\ weight}$$

- Check the resident's height. The highest stated adult height is generally appropriate when calculating needs.

Use Table 23-4 as a guide to nursing and nutrition services to evaluate the significance of weight loss.

ESTABLISHING A NUTRITIONAL CARE PLAN

All residents need to receive a thorough nutritional assessment by the registered dietitian upon admission to a facility. Document this nutritional assessment in the resident's medical record. The nutritional section of the medical record serves as a method of communicating vital nutritional information to all members of the interdisciplinary team. The dietitian or diet technician documents information on the nutritional status of each resi-

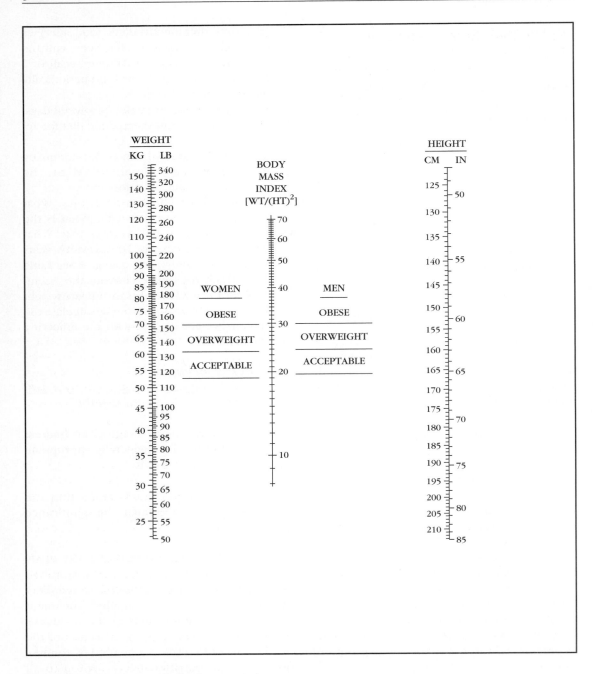

Figure 23-1. Nomogram for body mass index

Table 23-4. Evaluating the Significance of Weight Loss

Time interval	Significant weight loss (%)	Severe weight loss (%)
1 week	1.0-2.0	>2.0
1 month	5.0	>5.0
3 months	7.5	>7.5
6 months	10.0	>10.0

dent on a regular basis. Include in this documentation a thorough annual nutritional assessment with quarterly reviews. This documentation should also include an assessment of nutritional risk, goals for maintaining the resident in good nutritional status, and a plan for achieving these goals. Provide follow-up monitoring and recommendations as often as necessary.

Documentation can also include the following:
- How well the resident is using an adaptive feeding device
- Percentage of food consumed at each meal
- The resident's ability to eat independently, or with assistance, and type of assistance needed
- Type of cueing a resident needs
- Presence of a swallowing problem, and a description of how a resident is doing on a swallowing program
- Presence of depression or other mood problem and how this is affecting the resident's food intake
- Caloric and nutrient needs
- Special dietary considerations (e.g., lactose intolerance, diabetic, congestive heart failure [CHF], and so forth)

TREATMENT STRATEGIES

The following sections discuss some strategies to improve nutrition for residents.

Strategies to Enhance the Dining Experience

Try to promote the dining experience to enhance the resident's physical and mental well-being. The dining room should have a pleasant atmosphere, and a homelike environment. Mealtimes are a part of the social fabric of a resident's life, and can stimulate strong memories of home, family, and friends. It can be one of the few activities of the day that the resident can look forward to.

Try to seat residents with others of their own choosing whenever possible. Also, try to offer residents choices in seating areas. Facilities may offer a variety of seating times, too. Residents can be grouped according to similar cognitive levels. Encourage a climate of mutual respect. Try to encourage social interactions and conversations among residents, as well as between residents and staff members. As much as possible, avoid nursing procedures while residents are enjoying their dining experience.

Some nursing facilities have several dining areas, but smaller facilities may have only one area. Larger nursing facilities may have different types of services (waitress service, tray service, or a combination of both). For residents with intact cognition a dining room where residents select foods that are served by a dietary/waitress staff will enhance their choices and independence. Staff need to be aware of any resident embarrassment or frustration about the decreased ability to eat and feed oneself.

Lighting and decor in the dining room are important. Many activity departments in facilities successfully decorate the dining areas to follow holiday or other special themes.

Place furniture so that residents can walk or maneuver a wheelchair around the room easily. Acoustic ceiling tiles can help minimize

Table 23-5. A Sample Dining Card Format

Feeding strategies
Place one item in front of resident at a time
Needs plate guard
Uses adaptive utensils, specify type _____
Hand-over-hand approach
Needs frequent verbal cues
Identify all foods to resident
Other_____
Position per O.T._____

Particular Preferences	Significant Observations

Name _____

☐ Feeds self independently

☐ Needs Assistance

☐ Feed

noise. Do not play televisions and radios during mealtimes, since they can be distracting and upsetting to some residents with cognitive and sensory deficits. Pleasant background music can help to promote a calm, relaxed atmosphere.

In dining situations in which residents are more debilitated and less able to make their own meal selection at the table, tray service is practical. However, for those with certain types of cognitive problems, residents may need to be presented with one item at a time from the food tray.

The nursing staff work together with the resident to ensure the maximal level of independence in eating activities for that resident. Eating activities may be the last area in which the resident can still have some functional independence. Working with a resident to help improve or maintain feeding abilities is a time-consuming task. Staff who are unfamiliar with the resident, such as float or agency staff, may be uninformed or unable to carry out the resident's usual feeding care plan. An innovative nursing and medical staff, together with the dietitian, occupational therapist, and speech therapist, can develop procedures and tools to help the nurse assistants to meet the resident's feeding and nutritional goals.

Coordinate the arrival of the meal trays with the Food Service Department so that the residents are prepared for eating. Use a Kardex, rolodex, notebook, or bulletin board as a tool to assist in preparing the resident for a meal or to actually feed or help feed a resident. *See* Table 23-5 for a sample card format. The float or agency staff can use this dining tool to ensure the continuity of a resident's eating and feeding program.

Specific Interventions For Different Nutritional Problems

The following subsections discuss the specific interventions for different nutritional problems.

Mechanical Problems

The specific interventions for mechanical nutrition problems include the following:

- Chewing problems. Residents with either a chewing problem or a poor oral status that interferes with nutritional intake need an oral assessment. A member of the nursing staff can start this. A nurse assistant may notice a resident spitting out hard-to-chew foods at mealtimes, or, when a resident's tray is collected, the staff may see that the resident has eaten around the hard to chew food. Nursing staff may start to notice a pattern of choking episodes around mealtimes, too. A change in usual habits, such as a resident refusing food that would have been enjoyed a few weeks ago, can indicate chewing problems or other problems in the mouth area. It may take the resident longer to eat food than was the previous pattern. Have a dental hygienist or dentist conduct a dental examination to determine the fit of any existing dental appliances, the need to adjust an existing appliance, or the need for a new dental appliance. *(See* Chapter 25, Oral Status, for more information on this subject.) A mechanically altered diet

(soft, ground, or pureed food) may need to be initiated. Sometimes a change in diet alone can solve the problem. Monitor the adjustment to the mechanically altered diet. If the cause of the resident's chewing problems has been fixed, the resident may resume the previous diet.

- Swallowing problems. Consult a speech therapist to evaluate a resident for a suspected swallowing problem. The nursing staff may notice that the resident forgets to chew and swallow food once it is in the mouth. Cueing the resident to chew and then swallow food may be beneficial for this type of problem.

Staff may notice a new problem or an increase in choking episodes involving food or fluids at mealtimes. Residents who are being weaned off tube feedings or who have experienced a cerebrovascular accident (CVA) will need to learn to chew and swallow again. The speech therapist, dietitian, and nursing staff need to work together to make this happen. Keep suction apparatus in the dining area or near the bedside. The texture of the food may need to be changed. Solid foods may have to be ground or pureed. In particular, residents with a history of CVA may have a residual dysphagia that causes an inability to manage their liquids. In such cases, thicken their liquids with a commercial thickener.

After a resident learns the swallowing techniques, the speech therapist needs to teach the nurse assistants how to cue the resident in specific adaptive devices the resident needs to eat with and how the resident should use these adaptive devices. The staff should question the resident and get feedback. For residents with communication problems, the staff need to observe for nonverbal clues on how this resident is adapting to the new device.

For residents with problems of dry mouth due to a reduction in saliva, a side dish of applesauce may be very helpful for swallowing. Cranberry sauce can also be served with

meat meals to help relieve dryness.
- Reduced ability to feed self. There are two ways to involve the nursing staff with residents with a reduced ability to feed themselves:
  o Provide a clean adaptive feeding device
  o Ensure that the resident is using it correctly and consistently

The occupational therapist can be instrumental in assessing the resident for adaptive feeding devices, such as built-up utensils, weighted plates, nosey cups, plate guards, and other devices. The therapist can also demonstrate and teach the resident how to use the adaptive feeding devices. The nurse assistants can be taught by the therapist to follow through with the resident's use of these devices at mealtimes and at activities where food and drink will be present.

Appetite Problems

The specific interventions for appetite problems include the following:
- Food preferences. Ensure that the food provided conforms to the resident's food preferences. Evaluate the intake needs and assess the nutritional risk. Constipation, diarrhea, and intestinal obstruction need to be identified and treated by the staff clinicians. (*See* Chapter 28, Bowel Disorders, for specific interventions.) As these conditions improve or cease, the resident's appetite should return to previous levels.

The presence of pain in the gastrointestinal tract or elsewhere can greatly interfere with a resident's appetite. The cause of the gastrointestinal pain needs to be identified and the condition treated. As the clinician conducts the workup, the diet is reviewed. Nursing staff monitor the changes in appetite and, together with the dietary staff and other members of the interdisciplinary team, make necessary changes based on preferences and symptoms. Pain anywhere in the body may cause anorexia, nausea, dizziness, or vomiting. For a resident experiencing anorexia or nausea, review the medications for possible effects on appetite or alteration in the resident's ability to taste or smell.
- Multiple meals. Offer six small meals at intervals throughout the day and evening to residents with a loss of appetite. The staff may need to offer one food item at a time and praise residents for their efforts. It may also be useful to ensure that snacks are not eaten too close to mealtimes, and residents may need to be discouraged from drinking large quantities of liquids before or during meals, especially low-calorie or noncaloric fluids.
- Exercise. Consult a recreational or a physical therapist to provide increased physical activities between meals. This may help to stimulate the appetite.
- Mental status. The interdisciplinary team needs to work together with the resident and the family to identify mood problems and treat them appropriately. As the mood improves appetite and intake should increase. (*See* Chapter 13, Depression, for more specific information.
- Paranoia and fear. Some residents have fears that their food is poisoned or contaminated. The staff should spend time establishing a sense of trust with the resident. When food is served:
  o Identify all the food items placed in front of the resident
  o Make positive statements about the food
  o Serve the food in the original containers
  o Open the containers in front of the resident
  o Use a separate utensil and taste the food first in front of the resident to show that the food is safe
  o Do not mix medications with food
  o Establish a consistent mealtime routine that all staff follow and that is comfortable for the resident (a change in routine could lead to suspicion)

Increased Nutrient Requirements

The specific interventions to increase nutrient requirements include the following:

• Weight loss. The dietary and nursing staffs need to talk with the resident, family, and other staff to evaluate appetite and intake. The dietitian and clinician need to work closely to alter the meal plan to provide additional nutritional supplements. Teach the staff to become aware of special food preferences, and the times when the resident is more receptive to a snack. Provide high-calorie liquids instead of liquids with low or no nutritional value.

• Wound healing. A resident with inadequate nutritional intake is not receiving the nutrients necessary to prevent skin breakdown from the presence of pressure ulcers, skin tears, or disorders of the skin. Calories, protein, vitamins, minerals, and fluids are all important in the prevention and healing of pressure ulcers. Adequate calories, based on height, weight, and health conditions, are essential for energy. When a resident does not take in enough calories, the body starts to break down fat and protein stores for energy. The loss of body fat increases the risk of pressure ulcers.

Protein is essential for the repair and growth of body tissues. The normal requirement for protein is 0.8 g/kg of body weight. For the repair of tissue, a ratio of 150 calories per 1 g of nitrogen is recommended. Vitamin C (ascorbic acid) is particularly important in preventing and healing pressure ulcers. The normal requirement for vitamin C is 60 mg/day. A resident with a pressure ulcer may require 200 mg/day. Zinc is essential to wound healing, and the normal requirement is 15 mg/day. A resident with a pressure ulcer may need to take 25 mg/day.

A good fluid intake is necessary to prevent dehydration, which is one of the main causes of skin breakdown. A resident should receive 1500 to 2000 mL of fluid over each 24-hour period, unless medical contraindications exist. Usually this is best accomplished by taking fluids in every 1 to 2 hours while the resident is awake. (*See* Chapter 24, Dehydration, for more information.)

• Nitrogen balance. Skin integrity and other physical signs indicate whether or not a resident is in a catabolic state. In a catabolic state, the resident's body is in a destructive state of metabolism, making wound healing and the build-up of new tissue impossible. Perform a test known as the nitrogen balance test to confirm the condition. This test can also be done to monitor a treatment plan that has been established to reverse catabolism and promote anabolism.

The following example describes how to calculate the nitrogen balance for a resident. A dietitian will be the most likely person to determine the resident's actual state of nitrogen balance. This sample calculation is described to help understand all the components involved in determining nitrogen balance.

The dietary, nursing, and medical staff consult on the need to obtain a nitrogen balance value. However, this test is not routinely done in facilities. The dietary and nursing staff need to collect a calorie/protein count for a 24-hour period. If the resident attends activities or goes off the unit, then the activities staff or others need to be notified of the calorie/protein count process. From the information collected over 24 hours, the dietitian determines whether this resident has taken in 72 g of protein. Next, a 24-hour urine collection is carried out and sent to the laboratory to determine the amount of urea nitrogen in the urine. Here are the calculations:

o 24-hour protein intake = 72 g

Formula:

$$\frac{\text{\# g protein}}{6.25} = \text{Nitrogen intake (\# of g N)}$$

$$\frac{72 \text{ g}}{6.25} = 11.52 \text{ g N}$$

o 24-hour urine collection reveals a urine urea nitrogen (UUN) = 5.2 g nitrogen

Formula:
Nitrogen intake (g N) - (UUN + 4 g N) =
Nitrogen balance

Example:
11.25 g N - (5.2 g N + 4 g N) =
+2.05 Positive nitrogen balance
This resident's nitrogen balance is positive with a value of +2.05. Medical, nursing, dietary, activities, laboratory services, and other facility staff or service providers need to work together to go through all the steps to calculate nitrogen balance for a resident.

Adaptation to Special Diets

Keeping quality of life as the main focus, diet restrictions should be as liberal as possible. A sodium-restricted diet generally does not need to be stricter than a no-added-salt diet (3 to 4 g Na$^+$) unless there is a life-threatening diagnosis such as CHF or renal failure. Flavor enhancers such as lemon, vinegar, or sugar and seasoning mixtures of various herbs and spices can be provided to the resident to help replace the taste of salt. It is difficult to eliminate salt if the resident is accustomed to heavy use, but the taste buds do adjust.

The standard diabetic diet should be a regular diet with no concentrated sweets. Restrict the diet only if the blood glucose level is very difficult to control within an acceptable range.

If a resident is overweight and weight reduction will be beneficial to his or her quality of life, try a regular diet with controlled portion sizes and no between-meal snacks or high-calorie foods with little nutrients before instituting a stricter diet.

High-fiber diets can often cause excess flatulence and constipation if enough fluid is not consumed. Encourage residents to introduce additional fiber in their diet on a gradual basis and remind them to consume adequate fluid. It is very helpful to establish a goal for the resident (e.g., 12 oz of fluid at each meal and 8 oz between each meal). It is common for residents not to get enough fluid because of a decreased thirst sensation in this population. Some residents will void fluids because they are on diuretic therapy and do not want to void frequently.

Lactose-restricted diets are usually not a problem for the resident. The resident is probably accustomed to the diet from years of intolerance. Rarely is someone completely intolerant of lactose. Therefore, treat milk and milk products with enzymes that break down the majority of the lactose. These products are usually tolerated and well accepted by the resident. The clinician may want to prescribe enzyme tablets for lactose-intolerant residents.

In most nursing homes, the majority of modified therapeutic diets are not restricted diets but rather they consist of increased nutrient diets such as high-protein and high-calorie diets and diets modified in texture by chopping, grounding, or pureeing. These diets pose a challenge to the food service department.

In the elderly nursing home resident, try to concentrate as many calories and nutrients in as small a volume as possible. Many residents are volume-restricted, tire easily from eating, or require much nursing time to feed.

When food texture is modified, food appearance is also modified and becomes less appealing. Serve ground foods with sauces and gravies. Blend pureed foods until they are smooth and then scoop them into different shapes to make them appear like whole foods.

Feeding Strategies

Evaluate residents for chewing and swallowing problems. If the resident wears dentures, check to see whether they fit properly. If a problem is identified, consult the speech therapist and dental staff. Make sure the resident is positioned properly in the dining room chair, wheelchair, gerichair, or bed. Try to encourage residents to eat while sitting up in a chair, if they are able. However, for those residents who must eat while in bed, make sure the head of the bed is elevated at least 90 (unless there are positioning restrictions), and that the head of the bed remains up for 30 to 60 minutes after the meal has been completed.

Avoid using a large spoon overloaded with food. Allow the resident adequate time to chew and swallow between bites. For the resident with a dry mouth, provide sips of fluid between bites, unless he or she has difficulty swallowing thin liquids and is at risk for aspiration. Allow the resident adequate time to eat the meal (approximately 30 to 45 minutes). If a resident tends to bite down on utensils or keeps the mouth tightly closed, the staff need to promote relaxation by encouraging or soothing conversation and by holding the resident's hand.

Loss of Sense of Taste

If a resident loses the sense of taste, review the medications being given. Make sure that good oral hygiene is being maintained. Try serving highly seasoned foods (but, be aware that these foods may cause gastric distress). Adding salt to the food is contraindicated if the resident has CHF or hypertension.

Lemon juice can be added to food to enhance flavor but may give the food a bitter taste. Many elderly residents enjoy sweet tastes. If allowed, try using an artificial sweetener, sugar, honey, jams, or jellies to enhance the taste of food as appropriate. Another way to enhance the taste of the food is to vary temperature (i.e., foods that are normally served hot could be served cold).

CASE EXAMPLE

Mrs. B. is a 93-year-old woman admitted to a nursing home 3 years ago from her own apartment. She is 5 feet tall. On admission she weighed 90.25 pounds. During her first 2 years

as a resident, her weight remained relatively stable. Over the past year, however, she began to lose weight gradually. The staff noticed a decrease in intake as well as an increase in energy expenditure due to wandering. Her albumin was 3.4 g/dL, indicating decreased visceral proteins. She had ill-fitting dentures, so a dental consult was ordered.

She was also noted to have an increase in her cognitive impairment and was incontinent at times. She developed a superficial decubitus on her buttocks due to incontinence. A calorie count was done for 3 days to compare her actual intake to needs. Food preferences were again discussed with Mrs. B. but she offered no suggestions for menu alternatives. Small, frequent feedings were instituted to meet her needs. A nutritional supplement was added between meals, but was not well-received by the resident. The decubitus healed with appropriate skin care.

A regular toileting program was started, which helped with Mrs. B.'s incontinence. Recently, she developed a temperature with a respiratory infection and was noted to have increased confusion. She developed pneumonia and her appetite continued to decrease with additional weight loss. Due to the increased confusion, she needed to be fed. Aspiration was ruled out as a cause of her pneumonia. Once antibiotics were instituted, her temperature decreased and the pneumonia resolved.

Mrs. B. often became combative when she was encouraged to eat. A number of different techniques were tried. Placing one item in front of her at a time was successful. This information was noted on the Dining Room Kardex so that any member of the nursing staff could follow the procedure that was most successful. Finger foods were also noted to be better received because she prefers to feed herself. She is very fond of desserts and loves ice cream. The staff noticed that Mrs. B. ate the nutritional supplement if ice cream was added to make a frappe. She also accepts high-calorie, high-protein puddings between meals. Her weight stabilized and she slowly began to gain the weight she had lost.

24
Dehydration

Loretta C. Fish, RN, MS, CS
Kenneth M. Davis, MD, MS
Kenneth L. Minaker, MD

Without water, adults can live only about 4 days. Water is necessary for countless complex processes including mechanical support of tissues, distribution of nutrients to cells, elimination of wastes, and regulation of body temperature. When a person is dehydrated—i.e., when there is a net decrease in total body water—it is more difficult to maintain adequate blood pressure, deliver sufficient oxygen and nutrients to cells, and eliminate wastes. Many distressing symptoms may result from dehydration, including dizziness on sitting or standing, confusion or a change in mental status, decreased urine output, decreased skin turgor and dry mucous membranes, pooling and hardening of secretions, and constipation.

Dehydration also is associated with significant morbidity and mortality. Hospitalized elderly persons with dehydration have a mortality rate ranging from 17% to 48%. Morbid consequences of dehydration include decreased functional ability, predisposition to falls because of orthostatic hypotension, fecal impaction, predisposition to infection, fluid

and electrolyte disturbances, and untimely death.

Residents are particularly vulnerable to dehydration. Visual, cognitive, or motor impairments may make it difficult or impossible to access fluids independently. The perception of thirst may be muted. The aged kidney has a decreased ability to concentrate urine (i.e., conserve fluids). Acute and chronic illnesses can also alter fluid and electrolyte balance.

Unfortunately, many symptoms of dehydration do not appear until a significant amount of fluid has been lost. Early signs and symptoms tend to be unreliable and nonspecific in elderly residents.

When dehydration is identified, treatment objectives focus on restoring normal total body water, preferably orally. If the resident cannot consume between 2500 and 3000 mL (the amount required for replacing daily needs and repairing a deficit) in fluids and/or foods every 24 hours, water and electrolyte deficits will have to be made up by other routes. Administer fluids intravenously, subcutaneously, or by enteral tube until the resident is adequately

Table 24-1. Typical Sources and Average Daily Intake of Fluids

Source of intake	Amount of daily intake (mL)
Water in food	800-1000
Water or liquids in beverages	1500
Water produced by metabolic processes	300

Table 24-2. Typical Sources and Average Daily Output of Fluids

Source of loss	Amount of daily loss (mL)
Eliminated from kidneys as urine	1500
Eliminated through skin and lungs as insensible water loss	500-1000
Eliminated in feces	100

hydrated and can take in and retain sufficient fluids orally.

The best defense against dehydration is prevention. To prevent dehydration effectively, identify residents at high risk for dehydration, monitor their fluid balances closely, and establish institutional policies and programs to ensure that all residents receive adequate hydration.

OVERVIEW

Dehydration may occur any time fluid loss is greater than fluid intake. Tables 24-1 and 24-2 describe the typical sources and average daily intake and output of fluids, respectively.

Clinical Consequences

Dehydration is the most common fluid and electrolyte disorder among residents. It's clinical consequences depend on the extent and compartment of fluid loss and derangements in blood supply and electrolyte concentrations.

When the extracellular compartment is depleted of significant volume, *hypovolemia* (decreased blood volume) occurs, which can have serious clinical consequences. The effects of hypovolemia include:
- In the brain, the symptoms are dizziness on standing
- In the heart and peripheral vascular system, the symptoms are decreased cardiac output, cardiac ischemia, and orthostatic hypotension (with an associated predisposition to falls)
- In the kidneys, the symptoms are decreased urine output (with an associated predisposition to urinary tract infections [UTIs]), and kidney failure
- In the intestine, constipation, fecal impactions, and bowel ischemia may occur

When individual organs lose fluid volume, often associated with changes in ionic equilibrium, serious consequences can also occur, as follows:
- In the brain, the typical symptoms are malaise and confusion
- In the lungs, pneumonia resulting from poor mobilization of thick bronchial secretions
- In the skin and mucosa, pressure ulcers (bedsores) and dry mucous membranes
- In glands and organs with secretory ducts, stasis with precipitation of hard secretions, for example, parotid duct obstruction, renal stones, and cholelithiasis

Throughout all the affected tissues, the efficiency of enzymatic processes is depressed.

Pathophysiology and Terminology

In the extracellular fluid compartment of the body, *osmolarity*—the concentration of salt (primarily sodium) in water—is closely regulated by a series of neuroendocrine, cardiac, and renal responses. When osmolarity rises, vasopressin is released from the pituitary gland in the brain. This hormone causes the kidney to resorb water, resulting in a concentration of urine and dilution of blood serum. If osmolarity continues to rise because fluid losses exceed the kidney's water reabsorption capacity, the thirst mechanism is stimulated, which causes the resident to drink more fluids, thereby preventing further rises in blood osmolarity.

Dehydration occurs when one or more aspects of this regulatory mechanism are slow or fail to respond to fluid loss and/or a decrease in fluid intake. Dehydration can present in three forms:

- *Hypertonic dehydration* (also called hypernatremic dehydration), caused by loss of more water than salt, which results in high serum sodium levels and high serum osmolarity
- *Isotonic dehydration*, with loss of both water and salt, which results in normal serum sodium levels and normal serum osmolarity
- *Hypotonic dehydration*, loss of more salt than water, or isotonic dehydration with replacement of only water, which results in low serum sodium levels and low serum osmolarity

In all three forms there is a decrease in the amount of total body water.

Whatever the form, dehydration must be identified and treated promptly to avoid any serious consequences. A protocol to identify residents in need of a care plan is discussed in the section on identifying the resident who requires a care plan. Note, however, that virtually any deterioration in functional or mental status may be the first clue to the presence of dehydration. Indeed, such a change may itself be a precipitating factor in developing dehydration, especially if the resident is now dependent on caregivers for fluid intake.

PREDISPOSITION OF THE ELDERLY TO DEHYDRATION

Several age-related physiologic changes in fluid regulation predispose the elderly to dehydration by decreasing the adaptability of the fluid regulatory system to respond to changes in fluid balance. An older kidney cannot produce concentrated urine as well as a younger kidney. Therefore, older people are less able to reduce the amount of water excreted by the kidney when eliminating body wastes. This also means that when fluid intake is inadequate, or fluid losses are increased (as occurs during fever), the older kidney may not be able to retain sufficient amounts of fluid to prevent dehydration.

Thirst sensation also decreases with age. Because older people tend not to feel as intensely thirsty, they may not drink enough to replace lost fluids. Hormones that help to maintain body fluid volume, such as renin, aldosterone, and angiotensin, are also decreased with aging.

The ratio of muscle to fat in the body decreases with age. Since more water is present in muscle than in fat, older people have less total body water. Therefore, the percentage of total body weight made up by water decreases with age. Furthermore, in older people each liter of fluid loss results in a greater percentage loss of total body water than in a younger person. For example, 1 L of fluid loss in a 60-kg elderly woman represents a 3.7% total body water loss versus a 2.8% total body water loss in a 60-kg young man who lost 1 L of fluid. The elderly woman will be more severely dehydrated than the young man.

Table 24-3 shows water as a percentage of total body mass and the amount of total body water in individuals weighing 70 kg.

Causes of Decreased Fluid Intake

Any condition that causes decreased fluid intake or increased fluid loss may result in dehydration. In residents, the following con-

Table 24-3. Water as a Percentage of Body Mass and Total Body Water in a 70-kg Individual

Water as a percentage of Total Body Mass (%)		Total Body Water in a 70-kg Individual (L)
Young men	60	42
Elderly men	55	39
Young women	53	37
Elderly women	45	32

ditions are typical causes of decreased fluid intake:

- Limited access to fluids: physical restraints are in use, restricted mobility, poor vision
- Fluid restriction (self-imposed, therapeutic, or iatrogenic): prolonged period of NPO (nothing by mouth) status while waiting for procedures; withholding of fluid to prevent incontinence, nocturia or aspiration; therapy for edema, hyponatremia, or congestive heart failure; insufficient amounts of fluid offered to dependent residents throughout the day
- Altered sensorium: decreased consciousness level (sedatives, neuroleptics, narcotics, structural and metabolic central nervous system [CNS] insults, febrile illness); decreased level of awareness (dementia, delirium, mania, psychosis, depression)
- Gastrointestinal disorders: swallowing disorders, bowel obstruction
- Alteration in thirst: primary adipsia (absence of thirst); medication-related—any medicine that causes anorexia (e.g., digoxin, amphetamines); focal CNS pathology (stroke)

Causes of Increased Fluid Loss

In residents, the following conditions are typical causes of increased fluid loss:

- Chronic or acute infections: fever causing excess loss from skin and lungs, increased metabolic rate
- Gastrointestinal losses: vomiting, nasogastric drainage, laxative abuse, bowel preps for procedures, diarrhea, ileostomy
- Excessive urinary losses: diuretic misuse, glucosuria (glucose in urine), diabetes insipidus, lithium treatment (one cause of diabetes insipidus), high-protein tube feedings (excess protein in the blood is excreted by kidneys causing excessive fluid loss)
- Environment-related fluid loss: heat wave, hyperthermia

IDENTIFYING THE RESIDENT REQUIRING A CARE PLAN

The following sections describe items from the Minimum Data Set-based resident assessment to identify the resident who is at high risk for dehydration.

Two or more of the following conditions suggest dehydration:

- Deteriorated cognitive status
- Deteriorated activities of daily living (ADL) status
- Failure to eat or take medications
- UTI
- Dehydration diagnosis
- Diarrhea, fever, or internal bleeding
- Dizziness/vertigo
- Vomiting
- Recent weight loss
- Did not consume all liquids provided
- Leaves 25% or more of food uneaten
- Parenteral/intravenous (IV) or feeding tube
- Taking a diuretic

Assess the resident for the presence of dehydration by gathering information from the physical examination, caregiver observations, and laboratory testing.

Physical Examination

The following physical examination findings suggest the diagnosis of dehydration:

- First, perform a cardiovascular assessment to determine whether the resident is hypovolemic. A depressed level of consciousness (marked by lethargy or stupor), delayed capillary refilling, tachycardia, tachypnea, poor urine output, and hypotension are the most severe clinical signs of hypovolemia. This requires immediate treatment with intravenous fluids.
- An unintentional recent weight loss of more than 2 pounds—2.2 pounds (1 kg) equal 1000 mL of water. Note that a recent weight loss of greater than 10% requires immediate IV fluid replacement to restore adequate blood volume.
- Note orthostatic blood pressure changes—a drop of 20 mm Hg or more in systolic pressure and/or a drop of 10 mm Hg or more in diastolic pressure upon sitting or standing; or blood pressure lower than usual (*see* Chapters 1 and 18, Vital Signs and Falls, respectively). Note that these findings may be due to the side effects of medication.
- Note orthostatic symptoms: a drop of less than 20 mm Hg in systolic blood pressure but accompanied by symptoms of dizziness upon sitting or standing. Note that these symptoms may not be due to dehydration.
- Note an elevated pulse when the resident is supine and upon sitting or standing. This may not be present in a resident because of the loss of cardioacceleratory response to sympathetic nervous system stimulation.
- Note elevated respirations, which indicate an increased water loss via the lungs.
- Look for flat neck veins while the resident is lying supine.
- Note a decrease in urine volume and/or more concentrated urine than usual. Inspect the urine for decreased clarity and foul odor, which suggest infection.
- Look for dry and sticky oral mucous membranes, which may be confounded by medication side effects (e.g., anticholinergic drugs) or mouth breathing.
- Note poor skin turgor measured over the forehead or sternum. Note that this is often difficult to assess in residents due to the normal aging loss of skin elasticity.
- Note whether the tongue is furrowed or swollen.
- Note an elevated body temperature. Residents may, however, not always become febrile in response to infection.

Caregiver Observations

The following caregiver observations can indicate the presence of dehydration:

- Change in mental status: increased confusion, lethargy, and agitation
- Recent decline in functional abilities (e.g., weakness)
- Decrease in fluid intake (less than 1500 mL/24 h)
- Anorexia often parallels a decrease in fluid intake; anorexia is also significant in itself, since approximately one third of daily fluid requirements are obtained from water in food
- Excess fluid output from vomiting, diarrhea, polyuria, diaphoresis, tachypnea, and excessive sputum; vomiting and diarrhea will also cause loss of salt and water
- Presence of constipation or fecal impaction; hard, dry stools indicate dehydration; diarrhea may occur with a fecal impaction or infection (e.g., *Giardiasis, Clostridium difficile, Salmonella, Shigella, toxigenic Escherichia coli, Campylobacter, or Yersinia*).

Laboratory Testing

Perform laboratory tests to:

- Confirm the presence of dehydration and determine the type and severity of fluid loss
- Determine the source/cause of fluid loss

Laboratory results will provide data with which to monitor the resolution of a resident's

Table 24-4. Types of Dehydration and Their Clinical Characteristics and Common Causes

Type of dehydration	Clinical characteristics	Common causes
Hypertonic Dehydration (water loss)	High serum sodium levels (> 145 mEq/L) Elevated hematocrit Elevated blood urea nitrogen/creatinine ratio (> 25:1) High serum osmolarity (> 295 mOsm/L) High urine osmolarity	Diabetes insipidus Diabetes mellitus Tachypnea Fever
Isotonic dehydration (water and salt loss)	Normal serum sodium levels (135-145 mEq/L) Elevated hematocrit Elevated serum protein Normal serum osmolarity (280-295 mOsm/L)	Vomiting Diarrhea Inadequate food and fluid intake Excessive sweating Overuse of diuretics
Hypotonic dehydration (salt loss)	Low serum sodium levels (< 135 mEq/L) Low serum osmolarity (< 280 mOsm/kg Low urine osmolarity	Same causes as isotonic dehydration but with ongoing replacement of water without the necessary salt

dehydration. A change from the baseline can indicate fluid loss or gain even when the absolute value is still in the normal range. For example, a resident with dehydration may have a hematocrit of 44%, but a previous hematocrit of 40%. Both values are normal, but a short-term increase of 4% can reflect recent fluid loss.

To determine the type of dehydration, its most likely cause, and the appropriate treatment, order serum electrolytes, glucose, urea nitrogen, creatinine, osmolarity, hematocrit and urine osmolarity. Table 24-4 will help to interpret the laboratory results.

Try to distinguish dehydration from the syndrome of inappropriate secretion of antidiuretic hormone (SIADH). SIADH is a common cause of *hyponatremia* (low serum sodium) without dehydration. Residents with SIADH secrete an excessive amount of vasopressin

(ADH), which causes the kidney to reabsorb water. This dilutes the blood and results in low serum sodium (less than 135 mEq/L) and low serum osmolarity (less than 280 mOsm/ L) levels. The way to distinguish hypotonic dehydration from SIADH is to examine urine osmolarity. In hypotonic dehydration urine osmolarity is very low. SIADH urine osmolarity will be inappropriately elevated above a maximally diluted urine, often above serum osmolarity. Treatment for SIADH involves water restriction. SIADH can only be diagnosed in a resident with normal blood volume, i.e., not dehydrated.

Treat elevated serum glucose levels of greater than 300 mg/dL. Rehydration will usually bring an elevated glucose level into a more acceptable range. Check urine ketones if glucose is greater than 300 mg/dL. If ketones are present, insulin therapy may be required. Ketoacidosis is uncommon in elderly residents. In contrast, a hyperosmolar nonketotic diabetic state is a common cause of dehydration in elderly residents.

Conduct laboratory testing to determine the illness responsible for dehydration as follows:

- Culture the suspected sites of infection: urine, stool, sputum, blood, and skin lesions.
- Dipstick urine for leukocytes. Leukocyte esterase is a component of white blood cells that indicates the presence of a UTI. A positive result for nitrates indicates the presence of bacteria.
- Test stool for blood. Send the stool sample for a *C difficile* toxin titer if prolonged diarrhea is present.

DEVELOPING A CARE PLAN FOR THE DEHYDRATED RESIDENT

The following care planning strategy is recommended for residents who have been diagnosed with dehydration.

Oral Rehydration Therapy

Oral rehydration is the preferred route of hydration. It is more physiologic, less expensive, and feasible in a long-term care setting. The primary risk is aspiration of fluid into the lungs in residents with swallowing difficulties and/or altered consciousness. In such cases, oral rehydration solutions may be administered temporarily by feeding tube (*see* the section oral rehydration guidelines for suggested rehydration fluids and plan of administration). Oral rehydration may also be supplemented with subcutaneous rehydration (*see* the section on subcutaneous fluid administration protocol).

To help guide fluid replacement, estimate the fluid deficit using the following procedure (for more information, *see* the section on estimating fluid deficit):

- In the first 24 hours, replace up to one half of the estimated fluid deficit, plus ongoing fluid losses (from output records), plus the

normal maintenance fluid of at least 1500 mL/day.

- During the next 48 to 72 hours, recalculate the fluid deficit and replace the remainder of the fluid deficit plus maintenance fluids (*see* the section on maintenance therapy for more information).
- The contraindications to oral rehydration are as follow:
- Hypovolemic shock (*see* the section on physical examination for an assessment of hypovolemia)
- The resident has greater than 10% recent weight loss.
- Absent bowel sounds may reflect an ileus or bowel blockage
- Hard, tender, or rigid abdomen may indicate peritonitis or need for surgical intervention.
- Excessive fluid loss, e.g., severe, persistent vomiting and/or diarrhea, to the extent that the resident's oral intake cannot replace output and the degree of dehydration becomes more severe.
- Refusal or inability to drink 800 to 1000 mL/8 hours or about 2.5 L/24 hours.

Maintenance Therapy

When the resident is medically stable, maintain hydration at 1500 to 2000 mL/24 h. This is best accomplished by administering prescribed fluids every 1 to 2 hours while the resident is awake. Continue this treatment until clinical signs are normal. Maintenance fluid amounts equal the usual daily output (1500 mL) plus excess losses occurring as a result of current acute illness (losses will be recorded on output records, except for insensible losses from the lungs and skin).

If resident cannot drink 800 to 1000 mL/8 h (or about 2.5 L/24 h), administer IV fluids or subcutaneous hydration therapy. (*See* the sections on subcutaneous fluid administration protocol and intravenous fluid replacement guidelines for more information.)

Monitoring Status of Resident During Therapy for Dehydration

To monitor the status of residents during therapy for dehydration, follow these steps:

1. Weigh the resident daily until the weight is stable, then once a week for 4 weeks, and then weigh monthly. It is preferable to get a fasting weight, which can be compared most consistently from day to day. Use the same scale at the same time of day, with the resident dressed in clothing of comparable weight. Balance the scale before each weighing to avoid measurement errors. Record what the resident was wearing when weighed. Clothes and shoes can weigh up to 5 pounds.

2. Start an intake and output record. Continue the record until the resident is medically stable and the condition causing dehydration is resolved. To facilitate accurate recordings, provide caregivers with a list of the milliliter contents of common containers. Post reminders on the chart and Kardex, in the utility room, and in the bathroom.

3. Measure and record orthostatic blood pressure and pulse daily until adequate hydration is restored.

4. Inspect oral mucous membranes, tongue, and skin turgor over forehead or sternum every day.

5. Monitor and record stools.

6. Monitor mental status. Confusion resulting from dehydration may persist for several weeks after fluid and electrolytes are returned to balance (see Chapters 10 and 11, Cognitive Loss and Delirium, respectively).

7. Follow the laboratory results of serum sodium, osmolarity, urea nitrogen, creatinine, hematocrit, and glucose as indicated by the severity of dehydration and route of fluid replacement. Laboratory results may be omitted if the resident can drink 2500 to 3000 mL/24 h, the dehydration is resolving, and the weight loss is less than 3%. However,

the cause of the dehydration should still be investigated, which may require laboratory testing.

Determining Reasons for Dehydration

Determine the reason for dehydration and make the appropriate care plan changes or referrals as follows:

- Infection—Treat according to the recommendations in Chapter 3, Infection. Monitor vital signs until they return to baseline.

- Excess fluid loss—Treat the underlying cause to alleviate abnormal fluid loss. Record the response to the treatment.

- Decrease in food or fluid intake—Does the resident need assistance to access fluid? If so, provide assistance not only at mealtimes but also between meals. Consult occupational therapy, as appropriate, for adaptive devices to enhance independence in eating and drinking.

- Observe the resident eating a meal. Does the he or she spill a lot of food or fluid, perhaps indicating a hand-to-mouth coordination deficit, shaking hands, or weak hand grasp? Does the resident consistently leave food or fluid untouched on one side of the tray (e.g., left-sided neglect with hemiplegic stroke perhaps indicating that the resident is unaware of food on left side of tray)? Is the resident encouraged and helped to consume meals? (See Chapter 23, Nutrition, for more information.)

- Fear of urinary incontinence—Is the resident intentionally restricting fluids? If yes, instruct resident, staff, and family about the importance of regular, adequate hydration. (See Chapter 27, Urinary Incontinence, for more information). Symptomatic UTI can be a cause of transient urinary incontinence. Dysuria and urgency may defeat the resident's ability to reach the toilet in time. Urine is a good culture medium. Studies show that high fluid intake, frequent voiding, and emptying the bladder (low residual volume) effectively wash bacteria out of the bladder.

- Fear of dysphagia and aspiration—Is the resident or caregiver intentionally restricting fluids? Determine the cause of the feeding disorder. Thicker fluids, such as flavored gelatin or pureed soup, may be easier to swallow than thin liquids. Position the resident upright when giving food and fluids.
- Review medications—Could side effects be contributing to dehydration? Anorexia is a common side effect of digoxin. Evaluate sedating side effects, drugs causing anorexia or nausea, anticholinergics producing dry mouth, and drugs requiring extra hydration (e.g., lithium). Evaluate laxative use. Are laxatives causing frequent bowel movements or watery stools? Are diuretics being overused? Is the dose too high? Withhold diuretics while the resident is dehydrated. Evaluate the therapeutic intent and dose of diuretics before re-administering this medication to the rehydrated resident.
- Educate the resident and family about hydration goals. Involve the family in meeting these goals with the resident. Provide a written hydration plan of care to prevent dehydration in the future.

ORAL REHYDRATION GUIDELINES

Oral rehydration (either by mouth or by feeding tube) is the preferred route of hydration. Most residents with dehydration have lost both water and salt. Therefore, rehydration fluids should include both water and salt. Past studies have shown that a small amount of glucose added to these rehydration solutions facilitates absorption of the salt and water. There are many commercial preparations of rehydration solutions that range from low-sodium (50 mEq/L) to high-sodium (90 mEq/L) concentrations. Some of these preparations are currently under study to determine whether

they more quickly restore water and electrolytes to the body than the usual fluids available in institutions.

Types of Solutions

Like water, most juices (orange, cranberry, apple, grape), contain very little sodium, but have the advantage of providing some calories. Tomato juice, vegetable juices, and broth made from bouillon have high concentrations of sodium (greater than 150 mEq/L).

Caffeine has a mild diuretic effect, so try to avoid giving dehydrated residents caffeinated fluids such as tea, coffee, and caffeinated soft drinks. Hot beverages, such as decaffeinated tea and coffee, however, may be preferred by the resident. Milk, while providing protein and containing sodium, tends to cause feelings of fullness, which may discourage adequate drinking. Be aware of the high sugar content of many juices, soft drinks, and gelatins, which may cause diarrhea or be contraindicated in the diabetic resident. Avoid alcoholic beverages because alcohol inhibits vasopressin release, which results in a water diuresis.

Implementing and Monitoring Oral Rehydration Plans

To implement and monitor oral rehydration, write a fluid prescription or make up a flow sheet so that caregivers on all shifts will be diligent about administering oral fluids every 1 to 2 hours while the resident is awake. The actual amount, time, and type of fluid administration should be individualized for each resident, and will require consultation with both the physician and a registered dietitian. This needs to be incorporated into a written plan of care so that everyone (including the family) is aware of hydration goals.

It is important to recheck dehydrated residents frequently with vital signs, physical examination, signs of fluid status, and periodic blood studies of serum electrolytes. For those dehydrated residents who cannot take maintenance fluids (1500 mL/day plus replacement fluids of approximately 1500 mL/day in oral solutions), consider supplemental IV or subcutaneous fluid administration. Oral hydration may need to be combined with subcutaneous hydration for residents who cannot drink 2500 to 3000 mL/24 h.

ESTIMATING FLUID DEFICIT

The following two formulas provide educated estimates of fluid loss to guide fluid replacement. They may have significant error, but they still provide a good general estimate of fluid loss. Ongoing assessment of the resident during fluid replacement is necessary to evaluate effectiveness of treatment.

Formula Weight Comparison

If there is record of a recent predehydration (preillness) weight, estimate the fluid deficit with the following formula:

Preillness weight (kg) – current weight (kg) = fluid deficit in liters (L)

This formula is based on the fact that 1 L of water weighs 1 kg. Since a recent, rapid body weight loss more likely represents fluid loss than muscle or fat loss, the kilogram loss can be converted to liters to estimate fluid loss.

Note that this formula depends on the accuracy of the weight measurement and assumes that resident was weighed with similar weight clothing, balanced scale, and so on. To the extent that this is not so, the margin of error in estimating fluid deficit is greater.

For example, Mrs. Jones' preillness weight was 46 kg. Her current weight is 44.6 kg. Using this formula:

> *46 kg - 44.6 kg*
> *= 1.4 kg*
> *= 1.4 L or 1400 mL fluid deficit*

To determine what percent total body water loss this deficit represents, multiply 46 kg by 0.45 (for the percentage of water in the body for an elderly woman, *see* Table 24-3) to get the preillness total body water (20.7 L). Divide the estimated fluid deficit 1.4 L by 20.7 L, which equals a 6.7% fluid deficit, representing a significant dehydration.

Replace this fluid deficit with hypotonic (low in salt) fluids if the resident has hypertonic dehydration, or isotonic (similar to normal body salt concentrations) fluids if there is isotonic dehydration. Residents who have hypotonic dehydration need additional salt in their fluid replacement.

Free Water Deficit Formula

To estimate free water deficit (hypernatremic dehydration), use the following formula. This formula assumes a loss of water without a loss of sodium.

Fluid deficit (L) equals total body water (TBW, in liters) – the current TBW
Current TBW: In elderly men, equals 0.5 x body weight in kg
In elderly women, equals 0.45 x body weight in kg
Desired TBW equals [measured serum sodium (mg/dL)/140] x current TBW

In young people, water comprises 60% of the body weight as compared with only 50% in elderly man and 45% in the elderly woman. This proportional decrease in water is secondary to the increase in fat and decrease in lean body mass with aging. Most of the body water is in muscle. There is little water in fat.

Consider the following example based on this formula:
Mrs. Jones' current weight is 44.6 kg
Her *current TBW* = 0.45 X 44.6 kg = 20.07 L
Mrs. Jones' serum sodium = 148 mEq/l
Her *desired TBW* = 148/140 X 20.07 = 21.2L

Mrs. Jones' *fluid deficit = desired TBW* (21.2) *– current TBW* (20.07) = 1.1 L fluid deficit

This represents a 5% water deficit (1.1 ÷ 21.2), which is a mild dehydration. Replace the missing fluids with hypotonic fluids, such as water and fruit juices.

SUBCUTANEOUS FLUID ADMINISTRATION PROTOCOL

Subcutaneous fluid administration, called *hypodermoclysis*, can be useful in the long-term care setting for hydrating elderly residents for whom oral rehydration is not an option and intravenous access is difficult or undesirable. When isotonic solutions are used, they are safe and easily started and maintained by caregivers. This avoids costly transfer to acute care settings.

Residents for whom subcutaneous fluid administration is contraindicated include:

- Residents who refuse fluid support or will not benefit from it.
- Residents with severe blood coagulation disorders who bleed into the skin very easily.

The procedure for subcutaneous fluid administration is as follows:

1. Explain the procedure to the resident. Cleanse the site with 10% povidone-iodine solution (the preferred sites are the lateral abdomen, lateral and anterior thighs, and upper hips).
2. Clean off the povidone-iodine with an alcohol solution.
3. Insert an 18 to 20 gauge needle, using sterile technique, in the subcutaneous tissue by pinching the skin between the thumb and forefinger. Insert the needle at a 45 angle. There should be no blood return upon needle insertion. The needle should be lying free and movable between the skin and muscle. Needles can be placed at two sites simultaneously.
4. Attach the needle to IV tubing.
5. Secure the needle by covering it with a transparent dressing (e.g., Op-Site). Secure the IV tubing with tape.
6. Use isotonic IV fluids (normal saline or 5% dextrose and 0.45% sodium chloride).
7. Run infusion at 60 to 100 mL/h through each needle for the prescribed volume. If the resident needs more than 100 mL/h of fluid, begin a second infusion on the opposite side of the body, with each running at 60 to 100 mL/h. The fluid should infuse readily without pain or lumps.
8. It may be useful to inject 100 U of hyaluronidase (Wydase) through the IV tubing before starting the infusion. Then add hyaluronidase, 150 U, to each liter of fluids. Hyaluronidase breaks down some of the tissue barriers and may speed up the absorption of fluid into the tissues.
9. Stop the infusion if the resident complains of pain at the infusion site, has excessive infusion site tissue swelling or bruising, develops redness or irritation around the infusion site, or has signs of fluid volume overload (pulmonary edema).
10. Infusion tubing can be capped, with a sterile technique, and the needle left in the subcutaneous tissue between infusions as long as there is no infusion site redness or irritation. Change needles and infusion sites every 48 to 72 hours to prevent infection.

INTRAVENOUS FLUID REPLACEMENT GUIDELINES

Intravenous fluid replacement is best reserved for settings in which the dehydrated resident can be monitored closely. Follow these guidelines:

1. Correct hemodynamic collapse, manifested by hypotension, orthostasis, and decreased urine output. The initial therapy is to rapidly infuse normal saline until these parameters of volume status stabilize. The goal during rapid fluid replacement is to reduce serum osmolality to 300 mOsm/kg at a rate that reduces serum osmolality by no more

than 2 to 3 mOsm/kg or serum sodium by no more than 1 mEq/L Na+ per hour. Follow this with a gradual infusion to correct the total osmolar deficit over the next 48 to 72 hours. In the resident with hypernatremic dehydration, replace 25% to 50% of the fluid deficit within the first 24 hours. The intravenous solution should be *isotonic*.

2. The hemodynamically stable resident should have replacement of one half of the fluid deficit over the first 24 hours, with the remaining volume replaced over the next 48 to 72 hours. The replacement fluid for these patients during this phase will be 5% dextrose and 0.45% sodium chloride solution. Residents with isotonic dehydration (normal or low serum sodium) should have normal saline (0.9% sodium chloride solution) or 5% dextrose and 0.45% sodium chloride solution as replacement fluid.

3. In addition to correcting the fluid deficit, ongoing fluid losses must be replaced. These losses average 1.5 to 3 L/day in the healthy person and may be significantly greater in illness.

4. Continually reassess the fluid status, including the measurement of intake and output, weight, blood pressure, pulse, serum chemistries, and osmolarities. These must be done daily to ensure appropriate fluid replacement. The fluid deficits of dehydration may be corrected safely over 72 hours, yet the associated mental status changes may persist for as long as 2 weeks.

5. *Warning:* Overzealous IV rehydration, such as replacement of the entire fluid deficit over 24 hours, may result in death from cerebral edema. Dehydration of brain cells is prevented by the generation of osmotically active solute (idiogenic osmoles), which sets up an osmotic gradient to maintain intracellular water in the face of systemic hyperosmolarity. If plasma hyperosmolarity is corrected too rapidly, there may be excessive movement of water into the brain, which will cause cerebral edema and possible death.

DEVELOPING A CARE PLAN FOR THE RESIDENT AT HIGH RISK FOR DEHYDRATION

Identifying residents at high risk for dehydration allows for close monitoring of fluid balance, prophylactically hydrating residents, and intervening early to decrease the number of risk factors for dehydration. The Resident Assessment Protocol for dehydration in the HCFA Resident Assessment Instrument provides a useful framework for identifying residents at risk for dehydration.

A research study examined risk factors in nursing home residents and found that women over 85 years of age with more than four chronic illnesses, taking more than four medications, and requiring assistance with mobility were at greatest risk for dehydration. Another study observing fluid intake identified the *semi-independent resident* as more likely to have an inadequate fluid intake than independent and dependent residents. Semi-independent residents are defined here as those who are cognitively unaware of their needs yet have mobility and those who are physically impaired in mobility but are cognitively aware.

Dehydration risk factors can be categorized in terms of whether they decrease fluid intake or increase fluid loss. The higher the number of factors, the greater the risk of dehydration (*see* the sections on causes of decreased fluid intake and causes of increased fluid loss for more information). Ongoing fluid loss through the lungs and skin occurs at a normal rate of approximately 500 mL/day. Therefore, decreased fluid intake for any reason can lead to dehydration. With few exceptions (residents on dialysis or a diagnosis of SIADH), one cannot over hydrate residents with oral isotonic fluid administration.

Approaches to Care for High-Risk Residents

To care for residents at a high risk for dehydration:

1. Keep a list of residents at high risk for dehydration in the nurses' stations and other strategic locations on the unit to remind staff, families, visitors, and volunteers to monitor the consumption of fluids. Update this list frequently.

2. Start a fluid intake record. Record the daily intake for at least 24 hours. If the intake is less than 1500 mL/24 h, assess for the presence of dehydration (*see* the section on identifying the resident requiring a care plan for more information). Decreased intake is a common but subtle cause of dehydration, especially in the elderly. An intake record is easier to obtain and usually more accurate than an output record, and as such can be a very useful tool for early identification of at-risk residents.

3. Identify residents who need assistance to obtain and drink fluids. Provide assistance not only at mealtimes but also between meals. Contact the occupational therapist as appropriate for adaptive devices to enhance independence in eating and drinking. Notify family, visitors, and volunteers who help with feeding.

4. Prophylactically hydrate residents who will be undergoing procedures that require bowel preps, use of radiographic dyes, or food restrictions. Radiographic dyes used in intravenous pyelograms and cardiac catheterizations are hyperosmolar solutions. They can produce cellular dehydration by causing water to exit cells in order to dilute the hyperosmolar intravascular space.

5. Establish hydration protocols to be instituted immediately when acute symptoms or illness (e.g., fever, diarrhea, vomiting, polyuria, anorexia) threaten fluid and electrolyte homeostasis. A hydration protocol should prescribe a minimum of 120 mL fluid intake per hour while awake and, depending on the type of fluid loss (i.e., primarily water, or water and salt), should indicate the type of oral hydration to be given. Do not view vomiting as a contraindication to oral rehydration. If there is no evidence of bowel obstruction, frequent administration of small amounts of oral fluids in addition to antiemetic medications is an effective treatment for dehydration or early prevention of dehydration, except in rare cases of intractable vomiting.

6. Monitor the weight of residents on diuretics at least weekly. Review for possible dehydration if the weight drops more than 2 pounds.

Institutional Approaches to Care for At-Risk Residents

In a broad sense, *all* nursing home residents, by virtue of needing protected care, are at risk for developing dehydration. The following institutional policies to hydrate all residents can reduce the incidence of dehydration:

1. Schedule routine fluid administration at least three times a day between meals, e.g., midmorning, midafternoon, early evening. Older people better tolerate the frequent administration of smaller quantities (150 to 250 mL) of fluid than infrequent large quantities.

2. Offer at least a full glass of fluid with medications. Studies have shown that residents tend to drink the entire amount of fluid offered.

3. To maintain hydration, establish the resident's preferences for type and temperature of fluids, and individualize the oral hydration plan accordingly to encourage compliance.

4. Instruct the resident, staff, and family members about the importance of regular, adequate hydration to prevent dehydration. Involve the resident and family in establishing and meeting hydration goals. Evaluate

whether and why the resident or family is restricting fluids.

5. Consider providing a choice of liquid refreshments at group activity programs. Assign a staff member to encourage and monitor intake. Because the thirst sensation is decreased with age, fluid needs to be offered and encouraged, not simply made available.

6. Arrange for residents to eat meals and have snacks with others. Residents typically consume more food and fluids in a social setting than in isolation.

7. Provide good oral hygiene to enhance the consumption of food and fluids. Be sure the resident's dentures are clean and fit properly.

8. Instruct the staff to use a direct, positive approach when administering fluids to residents. Say, e.g., "Here is some juice for you," or, "It is important that you drink this water now." Avoid asking the resident if he or she wants something to drink. Residents may not feel thirsty in response to volume depletion, and may not recognize their need for fluid.

9. Explore cultural attitudes toward food and fluids. Explain, as appropriate, that alcohol and caffeine contribute to water loss through the kidneys.

10. Review the resident's medications to assess the possible impact on fluid and electrolyte balance. Consider the possible side effects that cause decreased intake or excess output beyond the therapeutic intent. Be especially alert to laxatives, which are used by 40% to 60% of elderly nursing home residents. Discontinue diuretics when residents become ill or have limited access to fluids (e.g., before procedures).

CASE EXAMPLE

A nursing assistant reported to the charge nurse that Mrs. J. is complaining of feeling very tired and "washed out" and does not want to go to the dining room for lunch. The nursing assistant thought that Mrs. J. did not "seem herself."

Mrs. J. is an 86-year-old woman who has resided at the nursing home for the past year and a half. She has three stable medical problems: hypertension, mild renal insufficiency, and coronary artery disease. She fractured her hip in a fall 2 years ago and has used a walker since that time. She dresses and toilets independently and eats meals in the dining room. Although Mrs. J. is a quiet person, she participates in bingo games and attends craft classes in the nursing home. Her medications are hydrochlorothiazide, 25 mg/day, and a nitroglycerin patch. Her usual weight is 46 kg.

On physical examination, Mrs. J.'s pulse is 74 bpm, and blood pressure is 136/70 mm Hg with no orthostatic change. However, her usual blood pressure is 140 to 150 mm Hg systolic over 70 to 80 mm Hg diastolic). Her oral temperature is increased at 100.8°F, and respirations are 22/min. Her weight is 44.6 kg. She has some nasal congestion; her lungs have increased secretions and rhonchi; and her abdomen is soft with bowel sounds present. She had urinated a small amount at least 4 hours prior to the examination.

On further questioning, the nurse found that Mrs. J. did not attend the bingo game the previous evening because she was too tired. She left most of her breakfast uneaten and had left over half of her previous evening meal uneaten. Mrs. J. denied feeling hungry or thirsty. She is oriented to person, place, and time, but seems slightly lethargic.

Several factors indicate that Mrs. J. is becoming dehydrated, probably secondary to an upper respiratory infection. She has had a change in her mental status and her activity level has decreased. Her oral intake has decreased, while her output has increased due to an increased respiratory rate (insensible losses via lungs). Also, her weight is lower than usual.

The nurse examined Mrs. J. and determined that she is a candidate for oral rehydration therapy. Mrs. J.'s slightly lower blood pressure from her baseline could represent hypovolemia, but she does not appear to be in hypovolemic shock since she does not have orthostatic changes. Her recent weight loss of 1.4 kg is most likely fluid loss. The nurse estimates a fluid deficit of about 1400 mL (1.4 L) [1 kg water = 1 L]. Compared with Mrs. J.'s preillness estimated total body water (46 kg x 0.45 = 20.7 L), this fluid deficit is approximately 6.7% (1.4 liters/20.7 L).

Decreased salt and water intake with increased water loss leads to hypertonic dehydration. Mrs. J.'s laboratory results were notable for increased serum sodium (148 mEq/L). Free water deficit can be estimated using the current serum sodium value. Estimating free water deficit using the serum sodium equals a 1100 mL water deficit (1.1 L). This represents a 5% fluid deficit.

Management is directed at replacing fluids and treating symptoms of an upper respiratory infection. The diuretic is held while Mrs. J. is dehydrated. Her fluid deficit is approximately 1.1 to 1.4 L (1100 to 1400 mL). Half of this should be replaced in the first 24 hour plus a 1500 mL usual daily output plus an estimated increase of 500 to 700 ML/day excess output via the lungs from tachypnea and elevated temperature. This equals approximately the 2550 to 3000 mL fluid intake required during the first 24 hours.

The nurse established an oral rehydration plan that includes hydration with water and fruit juices and soups at lunch and supper. Approximately 120 to 150 mL of fluid is administered every hour while Mrs. J. is awake, with about 250 mL given at meals.

This case shows that decreases in function and nonspecific changes in mental status can be indicators of dehydration. Caregivers and family members who know residents well will notice changes that others can miss easily. It is important that rehydration therapy be started early, while oral fluids are easily administered.

25
Oral Status

Michael Griffiths, DDS, MSPH
Pauline Belleville-Taylor, RN, CS, MS

Proper function of teeth or dentures is important for nutritional adequacy. Clean and attractive teeth or dentures can promote a positive self-image, which enhances social relationships with family, staff, and other residents. Good oral health can decrease the risk of oral discomfort and, in some instances, systemic illness from oral infections or cancer.

Residents who have multiple medical conditions and medications, functional limitations in self-care, and communication deficits are at greatest risk for problems of the oral cavity. Also at risk are more self-sufficient residents who lack motivation or have no lifelong pattern of performing oral health functions. Residents with a history of alcohol or tobacco use have an increased likelihood of developing chronic oral lesions.

The oral health care plan corrects, improves, or stabilizes the oral health status of the resident. The plan should indicate the prevailing dental health problem and necessary corrective actions. All residents should have a thorough oral health evaluation within 90 days of admission and yearly thereafter to rule out the possibility of life-threatening or debilitating oral conditions. The goal should be the highest attainable oral health status, given the resident's medical, psychological, and dental status. The personal wishes of the resident should also factor into this evaluation. Specifically, counsel those residents who have dental phobias and historical problems with dental care to allay their concerns about modern dental care. In those instances in which the cure for an oral problem could compromise the resident's total well-being, delay or modify dental care.

There are two federal programs to reimburse geriatric dental care services: Medicare and Medicaid. The Medicare program does not pay for dental services other than those provided by an oral surgeon related to severe medical problems. Reimbursement in the Medicaid program varies from state to state. The clinician needs to confer with the local consulting dentist or dental association chapter about the availability of services for the elderly.

OVERVIEW

Every resident should have an individual oral health care plan. The goals of the plan are to:
- Eliminate active disease
- Restore the resident's oral cavity to the highest attainable level of functionality, given constraining factors such as medical status and medications, psychological status, and structure and function of the upper and lower jaws or masticatory complex

To develop care planning for residents, oral health problems are divided into the following four categories. Each represents a chronic or acute condition, jeopardizing the resident's total well-being.

1. *Dental caries (cavities)* refers to the destruction of the enamel dentin and cementum, and can lead to infection in the nerve structure of the tooth. In older residents, root surfaces may be difficult to restore. Typical treatment options include fillings (white or silver), crowns, extraction, and root canal.
2. *Periodontal disease (gum disease)* refers to the destruction of the supporting structures of the teeth, and presents as red, bleeding gum tissue. This disease is increasingly prevalent in the latter stages of life, and may not be detected by casual inspection. Typical treatment options include:
   - Scaling and root planning—With hand or mechanical devices, hard deposits are removed from the teeth and soft tissue is removed from the area of the gum tissues adjacent to the teeth.
   - Tooth extraction.
   - Splinting—Connecting two or more teeth together with a movable or fixed splinting device.
   - Irrigation—Through a mechanically driven pulsating device or through mechanical rinsing, antimicrobial agents are placed near the natural teeth above and below the gum line.
   - Brushing and flossing—The only proven

means to control bacterial plaque and prevent calculus buildup. Using the proper cleansing agent can protect the teeth from progressive gum disease and cavities along the root surfaces of the teeth.
3. *Pathology of the hard and soft oral structures* refers to oral lesions, many of which have benign consequences if diagnosed and treated promptly. The presenting problems may be compounded by other health conditions or medications. Typical treatment options include biopsy and surgical removal.
4. *Temporomandibular dysfunction* refers to dysfunction of the temporomandibular (jaw) joint, which can inhibit adequate nutrition. Typical treatment options include removable bite splints, surgery, and medications.

IDENTIFYING RESIDENTS IN NEED OF DENTAL REFERRAL

The following sections discuss the manifestations of oral disease and the need for a prompt response.

Mouth Pain or Sensitivity

The causes of mouth pain or sensitivity may be minor and easily treatable (e.g., gum irritation from ill-fitting dentures, localized periodontal problem, or other conditions) or serious (e.g., oral abscess, cancer, advanced tooth decay, or periodontal disease). Residents with cognitive impairment or communication problems are difficult to assess. They may not complain specifically of mouth pain, but may refuse to eat or change their usual patterns of behavior. An acute change in behavior can indicate the presence of mouth pain in a nonverbal resident.

The primary method by which a nondentist can evaluate the presence of mouth pain is to observe the quantity and types of food consumed by the residents. When evaluating a resident with mouth pain, review the medical record to see if a dentist has examined the resident since the problem was first noted. Was the current problem addressed? Were the recommendations followed?

LESIONS, ULCERS, INFLAMMATION, BLEEDING, SWELLING, OR RASHES

The cause of these problems may be minor (e.g., irritation from wearing dentures 24 hours a day) and easily treatable (e.g., a combination of mouth care and removing dentures), or serious and potentially life-threatening (e.g., infection). Minor local treatments include the use of glycerin swabs, rinsing with 3% hydrogen peroxide, removing dentures for a time, limited change to a soft diet, and the use of other topical and or systemic antifungal (Nystatin) antibacterial/antimicrobial agents (tetracycline, amoxacillin).

Contact the facility dentist to write specific orders and or recommendations. If the problem does not resolve with specific local treatment after 1 or 2 days, or if the signs are accompanied by pain, fever, lymphadenopathy (swollen glands) or other signs of local infection (e.g., redness), chewing or swallowing problems, or changes in mental status or behavior, consult a dentist.

Check the mouth for ulcerative areas in residents who have one or more of the following diagnoses: stroke, Alzheimer's disease, Parkinson's disease, anxiety disorder, depression, diabetes, or septicemia. Candidiasis, a common infection in these residents, is characterized by white areas, especially on the tongue, that appear to be removable and leave ulcerative areas.

Broken, Loose, or Carious Teeth

While not usually indicative of an emergency situation, broken, loose, or carious teeth may progress to more severe problems (e.g., dislodging a decayed tooth and swallowing or aspirating it), so consider consulting a dentist.

Lack of Dentures

If a resident has lost some or all of the natural teeth and is not currently wearing dentures or partial plates, the staff should assess whether the resident has the cognitive ability and motivation to wear dentures. Additionally, determine whether a dentist has evaluated the resident for dentures. Ask the following questions:

- Why are dentures or partial plates not being used?
- Are the dentures in good repair?
- Do the dentures fit well?
- Are the dentures comfortable to wear when eating or talking?
- Does the resident like his or her appearance when wearing dentures?

There are no standard rules to use in selecting the resident most likely to benefit from dentures. Consider the following issues:

- If the resident has dentures: Does the resident wear them? Are they used for eating most of the time? Are dentures in good shape, or are new ones needed? The final question to be asked and the most important is: Can the resident's functioning and self-image be improved by fabricating dentures?
- If the resident does not have dentures: Does the resident want dentures? Does the resident have a terminal prognosis that will reduce the likelihood of benefit from dentures? Does gum deformity preclude the construction of dentures? Is the resident too cognitively impaired to become accustomed to dentures?

The decision to fabricate dentures may require repeated discussions among the resident, family, and staff. Many residents and their families have preferences that are based on ideal desires and not on the reality of the resident's current physical and emotional state. Therefore, the final decision should rest with a dentist who has significant clinical experience to determine the feasibility of dentures.

When all of the acute problems are stabilized, focus the oral health care plan on preventive maintenance, which is key to rehabilitation of the resident. The plan typically should include an ongoing intervention strategy to control or eliminate chronic, complex oral health conditions such as periodontal disease and dental caries. Consult a dental hygienist for recommendations about regular oral hygiene care.

DENTAL TREATMENTS

The following sections discuss the background factors of dental health considerations, and the diagnostic treatment relating to dental health.

Background Factors

Two groups of residents need to be identified:
- Individuals with oral hygiene problems
- Individuals with oral/dental health problems who may benefit from dental evaluation

Consider the following clinical factors in the assessment:

- *Impaired cognitive skills.* Does the resident need reminders to clean his or her teeth or dentures? Does the resident remember the steps necessary to complete oral hygiene? Would the resident benefit from task segmentation or supervision?
- *Impaired ability to understand.* Can the resident follow verbal directions or demonstrations for mouth care? If the resident has language difficulties, does he or she know what to do when handed a toothbrush and toothpaste and placed at the bathroom sink?
- *Impaired vision.* Is the resident's vision adequate for gathering or selecting oral hygiene equipment?
- *Impaired personal hygiene.* Did the resident receive supervision or assistance with oral/dental care during the last 7 days? Has an assessment been done to determine whether the resident can perform hygiene tasks independently? Does the resident have partial or total loss of voluntary arm movement or impaired hand dexterity that interferes with self-care? What therapies would the resident require to become more independent?

- *Motivation and knowledge.* If the resident is independent in oral/dental care but still has debris in the mouth or performs care less than daily, is the resident brushing adequately? Does the resident know it is important to brush near the gum line? Does the resident need to be shown brushing techniques or be given reinforcement to maintain good oral hygiene?
- *Adaptive equipment.* Many residents lack the motivation, knowledge, and physical ability in the area of oral health care and the specific type of adaptive equipment that would benefit. The toothbrush can be built up by using long-handled extensions or by increasing the bulk on the handle. Consider using an electric toothbrush, or a suction brush, for cleaning some residents' teeth. If the resident has dentures, are denture cleaning devices (e.g., denture brush, soaking bath) available?
- *Resists assistance with activities of daily living (ADLs).* Does the resident resist assistance in mouth care? Why? Does the resident want to perform his or her own mouth care? Does the resident feel pain in the mouth? Is apathy related to depression? Is there no experience in caring for teeth or mouth due to cultural factors? Is the staff's approach sufficiently supportive? Is the resident fearful?
- *Dry mouth from dehydration or medications.* Are the resident's lips, tongue, or mouth dry, sticky, or coated with film? Is the resident taking enough fluids? Is lip balm being applied to cracked or bleeding lips? Is the resident taking any medications that can cause dry mouth (e.g., decongestants, antihistamines, diuretics, antihypertensives, antidepressants, antipsychotics,

antineoplastics)? If these medications are necessary, has the resident tried saliva substitutes to stimulate moisture? Glycerine and lemon may dry the mucosa over the short- or long-term.

Dental Health Considerations

The oral health care plan for treating an indicated oral/dental problem is based on the following considerations:
- Is the source of mouth pain localized (e.g., a specific tooth) or generalized (e.g., the gums, the jaw)?
- Is the problem related to oral pathology (e.g., lesion, ulcer, rash, swelling, or other conditions)?
- Is the problem life-threatening or does it present an immediate threat to use of the mouth?
- Are some or all of the natural teeth lost, and has a determination as to suitability for dentures been made and documented?
- Does the care plan provide for infection control and relief of pain?
- Does the care plan provide for treatment of dental problems that arise?

Assess a resident's ability to undergo simple to complex dental procedures periodically by the health care staff using a risk-benefit strategy. If the anticipated benefit of treatment is greater than the risk of consequences from inaction, then the procedure is generally indicated. In reality, the risk/benefit analysis is never so clear. There are usually several intervention alternatives with varying risks. The decision may be to choose a less risky path (e.g., remove the teeth and use dentures rather than do a root canal to save the teeth).

Nursing Management of Oral Hygiene

Nursing staff are responsible for assisting residents in the maintenance of daily oral hygiene. A specific oral management plan must be in place for each resident. Residents who are more cognitively and functionally intact will assume most of the responsibility for their own oral hygiene. For these residents, staff input is limited to a periodic oral status assessment and regular monitoring to ensure that necessary dental hygiene supplies are available.

For residents with cognitive or functional deficits in oral hygiene activities, the nursing staff will take a more active role. Involve the nurse assistants from all three shifts in incorporating oral hygiene and maintenance into their daily plan of resident care. For example, some residents will brush their teeth before breakfast, and (where necessary) the night shift nurse assistant should be instructed to help set up needed equipment. Nursing-based oral care activities involve the following activities:
- Labeling and maintaining the dental appliance. Develop the plan to label the resident's dental appliance with his or her name.
- Monitoring to ensure that residents have adequate oral hygiene equipment and supplies at the bedside or in the bathroom.
- Identify the need to provide and train residents in the use of adaptive equipment to perform oral hygiene.
- Demonstrate oral hygiene techniques to cognitively impaired residents.
- Determine whether resident involvement in oral hygiene can be maintained partially through a task segmentation program. The staff might set up equipment and remind the resident to perform hygiene actions. The resident may then be able to brush and floss teeth.

Oral Hygiene

The goal of oral hygiene is to remove microbial dental plaque from the teeth, gingiva, and oral mucosa at least once a day. Many dentists and dental hygienists recommend that this be done twice a day.

When using a soft toothbrush, position the bristles on the gingival area nearest the tooth. Clean the tooth surface and the marginal gingiva using circular and short back and forth (horizontal) strokes, taking special care to brush carefully along the gum line. Daily flossing is the best way to remove plaque from between the teeth. Using a fluoride rinse at bedtime is an effective means of reducing dental caries.

Edentulous (toothless) residents should clean their mouths twice a day. Again, use a soft toothbrush on all oral surfaces, especially those that support a dental appliance. If necessary, apply dental adhesive cream or powder to a denture to help keep it in place. Remove and rinse dentures after meals and clean them once a day with a brush. Dentures and removable dental appliances should be removed once a day for a few hours. Many residents prefer that this be done while they sleep. Place the dental appliance in clean water or a standard denture cleanser when it is out of the mouth.

Nurse assistants need to assess the resident's oral cavity on a regular basis. Quickly address any problems with the fit of a dental appliance. When debris on teeth, gums, and oral tissues is found to be accumulating, and is not removed at least once per day, a follow-up investigation by the interdisciplinary team is warranted.

Dental Procedure

Whenever dental work is indicated, review the medical record for treatment history and other possibly relevant factors. For example, is the resident on anticoagulants (e.g., coumarin, heparin, or derivatives) that would put him or her at risk for bleeding? Does the resident have valvular heart disease or a prosthesis (e.g., heart valve, hip prosthesis, or other type of prosthesis) that make the resident highly susceptible to life-threatening infection; or does the dental procedure itself represent a greater risk to life? In residents at risk of developing bacterial endocarditis, use prophylactic antibiotics. Residents at risk include those

with the following conditions:
- Prosthetic cardiac valves
- Previous bacterial endocarditis
- Congenital cardiac malformations
- Rheumatic and other acquired valvular dysfunctions
- Hypertrophic cardiomyopathy
- Mitral valve prolapse
- Valvular regurgitation

The standard protocol for residents at risk of infection is as follows:

1. Give amoxacillin, 3.0 g by mouth, 1 hour before the dental procedure. Then administer amoxacillin, 1.5 g, 6 hours after initial dose.
2. If the resident cannot take medication orally, then administer ampicillin, intravenously (IV) or intermuscularly (IM), 2.0 g 30 minutes before dental procedure. Administer ampicillin, 1.0 g IV or IM, 6 hours later.
3. If the resident is allergic to these medications.
   - Administer erythromycin ethyl succinate, 800 mg by mouth, or erythromycin stearate, 1 g by mouth, 2 hours before the dental procedure, and then administer one half the original dose (erythromycin ethyl succinate, 400 mg, or erythromycin stearate, 500 mg) 6 hours later.
   - Or administer clindamycin, 300 mg by mouth, 1 hour before the dental procedure, and then administer clindamycin, 150 mg by mouth, 6 hours later.

If the resident is allergic to the above medications and cannot take medications orally, administer clindamycin, 300 mg IV or IM, 30 minutes before the dental procedure, and clindamycin, 150 mg IV, 6 hours later.

The protocol for high-risk residents (e.g., those with a prosthetic heart valve) is as follows:

1. Administer ampicillin, 2 g IV or IM, and gentamicin, 1.5 mg/kg (up to 80 mg), 30 minutes before the procedure, followed by amoxacillin, 1.5 g by mouth, 6 hours after

the initial dose.

2. For residents who are allergic to ampicillin, gentamicin, and amoxacillin, administer vancomycin, 1 g IV, slowly over 1 hour; beginning 1 hour before the dental procedure. No repeat doses are necessary.

Diagnostic Conditions and Treatments Related to the Oral Cavity

The following oral conditions may require input from a dentist, oral surgeon, or other consultant. They are often indicators of underlying systemic disease. They must be diagnosed, treated, and recorded in the resident's chart as a part of the overall health assessment.

Oral Cancer

Oral cancer represents over 6% of all cancers in men and 3% in women, and is more common in older than younger persons, and in persons with significant smoking or alcohol histories. When diagnosed late, it is one of the deadliest cancers; when diagnosed early, it is one of the more curable. Both edentulous and dentate residents of nursing facilities should have an annual oral examination by a physician and a dentist, and all oral lesions (including suspected denture ulcers) should be referred immediately to an otolaryngologist, oral surgeon, or dentist for evaluation.

Oral cancer is most often found on the floor or the mouth (under the tongue) or on the posterolateral border of the tongue and may present as a mass, an ulcer, or leukoplakia (white plaque). A preliminary oral cancer screening can also be performed by a dental hygienist. Treatment consists of radiation and/ or surgery. Each of these alternatives presents long-term maintenance problems that can pose difficulties for the nursing staff. Specific instructions should be made by the oncologist or dentist for mouth care during and following therapy.

Tardive Dyskinesia

Tardive dyskinesia is an iatrogenic extrapyramidal disorder that can be produced by long-term administration of antipsychotic drugs. It is characterized by oral/lingual/buccal dyskinesia that usually resembles continual chewing motions with intermittent darting movements of the tongue; there may also be abduction (flexion movements of the extremities). The disorder is more common in women than in men and more common in the elderly than in the young. The incidence is related to drug dosage and duration of treatment.

In some residents, symptoms disappear within several months after antipsychotic drugs are withdrawn; in others, the symptoms may persist indefinitely. The nursing staff should monitor residents on psychotropic medications with strong extrapyramidal effects (e.g., haloperidol, chlorpromazine, thioridazine, thiothixene) for early intervention. Only use these drugs when clearly indicated.

Herpes Simplex

Herpes simples is a transmissible, recurring infection characterized by red, ulcerative, crusting lesions. Herpes infections can cause decreased fluid and nutritional intake due to the painful ulcers present in the mouth. Therefore, symptomatic relief of pain and supportive therapy are important. Treatment consists mainly of using topical and oral antiviral agents (acyclovir). In some cases, broad-spectrum antibiotics have proven to be palliative when applied topically.

Aphthous Stomatitis (Canker Sore)

Aphthous stomatitis (canker sore) is an inflammation of the oral mucosa, often with an altered immune response as the predisposing factor. Deficiencies in iron, vitamin B_{12}, and folic acid may exist, and emotional stress can also precipitate an outbreak. Screen residents with lesions for diabetes mellitus, inflammatory bowel disease, liver function abnormalities, as well as dietary alterations such as an increase in the acidic foods in the diet. Treatment is symptomatic using topical agents such as viscous xylocaine or benadryl. For more severe cases, dissolve the contents of a 250-mg capsule of tetracycline in 50 mL of water and use as a rinse.

Candidiasis

Candidiasis, usually caused by *Candida albicans*, is a common, opportunistic oral infection often associated with radiation therapy to the head/neck area or long-term use of antibiotics, corticosteroids, or cytotoxic agents. It is a common complication of HIV infection. Any continued or abrupt change in the oral cavity can contribute to its occurrence. Chronic oral candidiasis can be a sign of impaired T-lymphocyte function. Candidiasis is also common in diabetics, those who wear dentures, and anyone with a chronic dry mouth (*see* the section on xerostomia), and in residents using inhaled corticosteroids. Treatment with topical nystatin oral suspension 4 to 6 mL held in the mouth for several minutes before swallowing (four times per day), is effective.

Denture Sore Mouth and Epulis Fissuratum

These conditions are often associated with poor fit or the constant wear of prosthetic appliances. Epulis fissuratum is hyperplastic tissue that can develop beneath a denture. Candidiasis also exacerbates sore mouth caused by dentures. In the debilitated elderly, remove the appliance at night or for several hours during the day to prevent this problem. When the condition cannot be alleviated through adjustment, relining, and/or periodic removal, or when continued trauma has induced overgrowth of redundant tissue, the tissue needs to be removed. Such intervention requires a thorough assessment and treatment plan by a dentist.

Xerostomia

Xerostomia can be either acute or chronic and has as its clinical sequelae the reduction of salivary flow. The physician or dentist should make efforts to determine the etiology of the decreased salivary flow (e.g., drug therapy as in tardive dyskinesia, mechanical salivary duct blockage, Sjogren's syndrome, diabetes, radiation therapy, and so forth). Treatment should consist of using saliva substitutes (Xerolube, oral balance) and hydration.

Residents receiving chemotherapy or with a diagnosis of myasthenia gravis can have their salivary function disturbed. In these severe cases, use salivary stimulants. Some of the cholinesterase inhibitors have been used with some effect to increase salivary function (neostigmine bromide, neostigmine methylsulfate). Any treatment regimen should always include daily fluoride therapy when natural teeth are present.

Dysphagia

Many of the effects of xerostomia can contribute to a swallowing problem (dysphagia). However, among nursing home residents, dysphagia is usually due to other causes such as a stroke, presbyesophagus, diverticulae, esophageal narrowing due to gastroesophageal reflux, or more serious disease. The dentist, working with a speech/language pathologist, can sometimes devise methods to help afflicted residents swallow, thus avoiding tube feeding. Have the staff dentist consider the use of intraoral devices to support and control the soft palate.

Angular Cheilitis and Cheilosis

Angular cheilitis and cheilosis are fissured lesions in the corner of the mouth that have been associated with mixed organisms, including *Staphylococcus*, *Streptococcus*, and *C. albicans*. Nutritional deficiencies in the B vitamins have also been implicated, as have dentures that need to be replaced. Treatment consists of medications such as antibiotics, B vitamin supplements, nutritional augmentation, and reline/construction of the false teeth.

Periodontal Disease

Periodontal disease is a chronic infection of the supporting structures of the teeth. It is one of the most prevalent oral health problems of nursing facility residents. The symptoms most readily apparent include a foul odor to the mouth, bleeding or swollen gums, and loose teeth. The resultant loss of teeth can lead to decreased nutritional intake, swallowing problems, and dyspepsia. Consider periodontal treatment, such as local anesthetic-assisted root planning and curettage, in most situations involving a chronically ill resident. Saving the teeth of a debilitated resident should be the overriding goal when the dental treatment required is not prolonged or potentially life-threatening. Pursue any treatment involving extraction of teeth with the total well-being of the resident in mind, including the consistency of the diet and short- and long-term planning for oral rehabilitation.

Rampant Tooth and Root Surface Decay

In residents with natural teeth, periodontal disease may lead to increased exposure of the root surface, which can become highly susceptible to dental decay. Any decrease in oral fluids combined with the lack of oral hygiene also contributes to advanced decay, often necessitating tooth extraction. Routine preventive procedures, including the use of fluoride and other therapeutic rinses, may forestall or avert the condition.

Lichen Planus

Lichen planus presents as a whitish lesion in the posterior buccal mucosa. It is thought to be an autoimmune response possibly initiated by emotional stress, debility, hypersensi-tivity to drug therapy, bacterial or viral infection, or an inherited predisposition. Treatment includes antiinflammatory agents and collateral treatment of secondary fungal infections as required. Consider treating with aspirin before moving to more aggressive interventions such as steroids. If the resident is allergic to aspirin, use ibuprofen.

Burning Mouth or Tongue Syndrome

The etiology of burning mouth or tongue syndrome is varied, ranging from neuritis to nutritional deficiencies (pernicious anemia). It has a strong psychogenic component, and requires a thorough diagnostic work-up. The discomfort associated with this syndrome typically results in decreased dietary and nutritional intake, so symptomatic relief is important. Treatment can include topical medications and systemic medications (viscous Xylocaine as needed before meals). Vitamin supplementation, specifically a high B-complex diet, and reduction of anxiety and emotional conflicts can often alleviate the condition. Some of these cases can be intractable.

Pemphigus and Pemphigoid

Pemphigus and pemphigoid are oral lesions similar to those occurring on the skin. The lesions present as bullae and frequently rupture when found in the mouth. Oral lesions most frequently are the primary site for this condition. The diagnosis is confirmed by biopsy. Treatment options are limited to palliative measures. However, corticosteroid and antibiotics for secondary infections have often produced dramatic remissions of the disease.

Dilantin Hyperplasia

Residents with seizure disorders who are taking phenytoin sodium (Dilantin) have shown a propensity for overgrowth of gingival tissue next to teeth. Such residents require a scrupulous oral hygiene regimen to control the potential problem and avoid surgical removal of the excess tissue.

Taste Disorders

Taste disorders can be caused by neurologic (e.g., stroke) and physiologic changes, diseases, nutritional problems, and drug therapy. The papillae of the tongue may atrophy and clinically produce the appearance of a red, raw, smooth, and shiny surface, but most commonly the tongue appears normal. Peripheral neuropathy of the trigeminal nerve associated with diabetes is the typical cause of neurologically induced taste disorders. Deficiencies in trace elements (e.g., zinc) are frequently associated with changes in a resident's eating habits and nutritional intake. The underlying problem must be diagnosed and treated accurately.

Drug Reactions

The lesion produced by a drug reaction usually consists of ulcerated borders. However, it can present in a variety of forms. In addition, although rare, some dental substances such as free mercury and free monomer from acrylic resins not polymerized before insertion in the mouth have produced local reactions. The medical record should contain information about a resident's allergies, and dental input should be provided as appropriate.

Cerebral Abscess, Bacterial Endocarditis, Osteomyelitis, and Septicemia

Cerebral abscess, most notably frontal lobe abscess, can occur due to blood-borne infection or local spread of an infection, such as from teeth, paranasal sinuses, or endocarditis. Regular oral examinations, oral health and dental care, and the use of prophylactic antibiotics as appropriate before dental care can reduce the likelihood of occurrence substantially.

Table 25-1. Procedure to Construct Dentures

Procedure	Resident Characteristics
Impressions	The resident needs to be able to hold his or her head up and not gag when materials touch the soft palate.
Bite registration	The resident should be able to follow *specific* instructions about opening and closing the mouth.
Try-in phase	Same as bite registration.
Delivery of dentures	The resident needs to be able to tell the dentist where the prothesis hurts and any feelings about keeping the dentures in the mouth.
Long-term considerations	The resident should not have demonstrated a propensity to lose things like glasses, teeth, and other removable protheses.

CASE EXAMPLE

Mr. J. was admitted recently to a nursing facility with uncontrolled diabetes and diminished mental capacity. He has periods of good humor, but is not always cooperative. He lost his upper denture last week. He has had a decrease in food intake.

Mr. J. should be evaluated by a dentist trained in the care of elderly residents. This dentist needs to determine Mr. J.'s suitability for replacement of the lost upper denture. The specific recommendations should include consideration of his medical, dental, and psychological ability to undergo the procedure with a positive outcome. Specifically, in this example, will Mr. J. be cooperative enough to have a full upper denture constructed? Is his mouth anatomically suitable for successful completion and use of a full denture? Is there any medical diagnosis, medication, or psychological characteristic that will prevent the successful fabrication and use of the maxillary denture? Record any specific enabling or disabling conditions, progress, and other related information in the resident's medical record. The common procedures and requirements for denture construction are hard to standardize, but Table 25-1 provides an outline for the procedure.

The overriding aim of this process is to fabricate and maintain dentures that assist Mr. J. in chewing his food and to provide esthetic results that enhance his self-image. Do not construct dentures solely to satisfy family desires. Make every effort to evaluate the resident's suitability for dentures based on objective clinical information that takes into account the resident's medical, psychological, and dental health.

26
Feeding Tubes

Myles N. Sheehan, MD
Pauline Belleville-Taylor, RN, MS, CS
Maria Fiatarone, MD
Susan Hartery, MS, RD

In the nursing home setting, feeding tubes may be placed temporarily or permanently when residents are unable to ingest enough fluid or calories to prevent dehydration or malnutrition. Short-term use of feeding tubes may also be warranted as a trial therapy or to provide supplemental nutrition when there is a need for increased calories, such as before surgery or during the perioperative period. Because of the ethical issues involved, nursing homes should develop an institutional policy about the placement of feeding tubes as well as the withholding and withdrawal of artificial nutrition. Such policies need to balance the traditional obligation to provide food and water to the sick, the benefits and burdens of tube feeding for the individual resident, the possibility of complications related to tube placement and feeding, and the informed wishes of the resident or the resident's proxy.

Feeding tubes may be placed because of a particular condition that makes it difficult or impossible to ingest adequate calories and fluid, or because of a nonspecific functional decline accompanied by poor nutrition and

hydration. In nursing home residents, tube placement is frequently related to cognitive decline, stroke, swallowing disorders, and intercurrent illness. Swallowing dysfunction may be a consequence of a stroke, a degenerative illness that affects the central nervous system (e.g., Parkinson's disease), or a disease process that directly affects the oropharynx, esophagus, or proximal stomach. Feeding tubes may be placed in these situations because of a mechanical blockage or because the swallowing problem causes aspiration of food into the lungs. However, feeding tube placement does not eliminate the possibility of aspiration.

The conditions associated with cognitive decline, such as Alzheimer's disease and multiinfarct dementia, may result in feeding tube placement because of poor nutritional status consequent to the resident's inability to swallow or because of agitation or resistance to feeding.

Inadequate oral intake due to transient factors (e.g., intercurrent illness such as pneumonia, or increased metabolic stress because of a fracture or surgery) may be improved by temporary placement of feeding tubes.

This chapter discusses the use of feeding tubes, describing the decision-making process about tube placement, as well as the strategies for tube feeding, maintenance, and dealing with complications.

OVERVIEW

This section discusses the causes of decreased oral intake and the clinical considerations of tube feeding.

Causes of Decreased Oral Intake

When evaluating nursing home residents for the possible use of a feeding tube, carefully consider the causes of decreased oral intake. Eating and drinking are highly coordinated acts that may be impaired due to a number of physical, social, or psychological reasons. Resolving these problems can prevent the need to use a tube. The goal is to determine why the resident is eating or drinking poorly. When a factor appears to be relevant, ask whether efforts have been made to reverse correctable conditions. The problems are as follows:

- Physical impairments, including altered level of consciousness, sensory impairment (e.g., inability to see, smell, and taste foods and fluids), functional deficits (e.g., the inability to cut food, transfer food to the mouth, to chew, and to swallow), and impaired nutrient absorption may interfere with intake and adequate nourishment. In addition, extremely low levels of physical activity are associated with decreased appetite.
- Medical illnesses. Review for stroke, delirium, progression of dementing illness, conditions that affect swallowing (e.g., Parkinson's disease) worsening of heart failure, lung disease, and cancer.
- Almost any medication that can cause gastrointestinal distress (e.g., digoxin, theophylline) may interfere with appetite and food intake.

- Illnesses that cause shortness of breath (e.g., congestive heart failure [CHF], pulmonary disease) may limit eating by interfering with chewing, swallowing, and the stamina it takes to complete a meal.
- Depression is an important, but often missed, cause of anorexia and weight loss.
- Agitation may limit the resident's ability to eat or to be fed.
- Dental problems. Check the resident's mouth for lesions and properly fitting dentures; refer to a dentist if necessary.
- Poorly prepared food, meals that are cold, and inadequate attention to the resident's dietary preferences can hinder adequate nutrition.
- Poor intake may be related to unpleasant circumstances at mealtime. Such interferences may include dining with individuals who are noisy, aggressive, or incontinent during meals, or dining in isolation or in a hurried institutional atmosphere.

Clinical Considerations

Before placing a feeding tube, review the following factors:

- Is the gastrointestinal tract capable of absorbing nutrients? If yes, proceed with tube feeding assessment. If no, consult with the gastroenterologist.
- Is there clear recognition by the resident, family, and staff of the treatment goals to be accomplished by tube feeding?
- Is the tube placement to be permanent or temporary? Is there full awareness by the resident, family, and staff of the complications and risks associated with tube use (e.g., aspiration, diarrhea, skin breakdown at the tube site, dehydration, inadequate nutrition, and vitamin deficiencies)?
- Has the site of the planned tube placement (i.e., nasogastric or nasoenteral, gastric, jejunal) been established?
- Has the method of placement (i.e., nasal tube, surgical gastrostomy or jejunostomy,

percutaneous endoscopic gastronomy or je-junostomy, or radiologically guided place-ment) been established?

- Have the type of feeding (i.e., the choice of formula) and the method of feeding (i.e., intermittent or continuous) been estab-lished?
- Is there full awareness by the resident, fam-ily, and staff of the complications and risks associated with tube placement (e.g., infec-tion, pulmonary placement of nasoenteral tubes, tube displacement, and potential problems associated with endoscopy or surgery)?
- When will the baseline indicators of nutri-tional status be assessed (biochemical and anthropometric), and when will the timepoints for periodic reassessment be determined?
- Will feeding tube placement lead to an in-creased use of limb restraint to prevent the resident from pulling the tube out?
- What are the institutional policies on start-ing and stopping tube feeding?

Consider the placement of a feeding tube only after addressing each of these issues sat-isfactorily.

IDENTIFYING THE RESIDENT REQUIRING TREATMENT

This section describes how to identify a resident requiring treatment with a feeding tube.

Background Clinical Review

Note: Obtain informed consent from the resident before tube placement if he or she is capable of making a decision. Review the ad-vance directive or consult with the surrogate decision maker before placing the feeding tube if the resident cannot participate in the deci-sion-making process.

The following clinical factors are pertinent not only to assess residents for possible tube placement, but also to monitor the effective-ness of tube feedings and to consider whether to continue or discontinue tube feedings in residents who may be able to eat normally:

1. Has there been recent weight loss, or is there evidence of malnutrition or dehydration?
2. Have calorie counts been done, and is the resident receiving adequate nutrition (i.e., at least 30 kcal/kg of body weight per day)?
3. Is there a clear reason for the weight loss, and what can be done, other than the use of a feeding tube, to correct the causes?
4. Are other nutritional approaches in place or have they been tried (e.g., dietitian re-view of resident's dietary preferences, nu-tritional supplements between meals, assis-tance with eating)?
5. Is there evidence of complications related to nutritional and hydration status?
6. What might be the complications with a resi-dent related to the placement or continued use of a feeding tube (e.g., using restraints on an agitated resident, or fluctuating blood sugars in a resident with severe diabetes)?

Indications for a Feeding Tube

Consider a feeding if the Resident Assess-ment Instrument (RAI) indicates that the resi-dent:

- Is comatose
- Has experienced a cerebrovascular accident
- Resists care (e.g., feeding)
- Has oral problems (e.g., a chewing and/or swallowing problem, mouth pain)
- Has marked weight loss
- Is dehydrated
- Has poor food intake
- Regularly complains of hunger

Establish a feeding tube care plan if the resident is already on a feeding tube.

Further Assessment

To conduct further assessment, make the distinction between those residents being evaluated for initial placement of a feeding tube and those already receiving tube feedings.

Residents Being Evaluated for Initial Placement of a Feeding Tube

During the physical examination of residents being evaluated for the initial placement of a feeding tube, look for the following conditions or factors:

1. Weight loss (greater than 5% in any 3-month period)
2. Low weight for height (e.g., body mass index:weight in kg/[height in m]² less than 22 m]
3. Inadequate caloric intake to maintain nutrition
4. Reduced ability to feed self
5. Impaired ability to chew and swallow food
6. Impaired ability to smell and taste, which interferes with adequate intake
7. Pressure ulcers

A medical evaluation for a feeding tube should look for the following conditions or factors:

1. Evidence of temporary cognitive impairment, such as delirium, that will worsen intake
2. Evidence of depression
3. Medications that may cause anorexia or nausea and limit food intake (e.g., digoxin, theophylline); almost any medication can cause gastrointestinal distress and lead to poor food intake
4. Review laboratory and other testing for the following:
   a. Serum cholesterol less than 160 mg/dL
   b. Serum albumin less than 4.0g/dL
   c. Unexplained anemia
5. A nutritional review by the dietitian
6. A swallowing consult from occupational therapy, possibly with videofluoroscopy

Residents Already Receiving Tube Feedings

A physical examination prior to initiating a feeding tube should look for the following conditions or factors:

- Weight gain or loss
- Presence of edema

- Measurement of the midarm circumference (see the section on task 3: review the efficiency of maintenance feeding)
- Respiratory rate and evidence of respiratory distress
- Pressure ulcers
- Skin integrity at the tube site
- Changes in bowel habits (e.g., diarrhea, constipation, abdominal pain)
- Integrity of the feeding tube (e.g., cracked, clogged, kinked)

A clinical evaluation prior to initiating a feeding tube should look for the following conditions or factors:

- A resident's behavioral reaction to tube feeding (e.g., repeatedly tugging at the tube, verbal complaints of discomfort)
- Evidence of temporary cognitive impairment, such as delirium, that will worsen intake
- Evidence of depression
- Medications that may cause anorexia

Laboratory and other testing should include the following conditions or factors:

- Calorie counts
- Residual material in the resident's stomach after gastric feeding
- If diarrhea is present and other causes have been ruled out, check the stool culture for *Clostridium difficile* toxin.
- Serum glucose, electrolytes, blood urea nitrogen, creatinine
- Serum albumin, cholesterol, hemoglobin, or hematocrit
- Radiographs for aspiration pneumonia, verification of tube placement

DEVELOPING A CARE PLAN

After evaluation, some residents being considered for feeding tube placement may be found to have reversible conditions that can be remedied by other means. Other residents with feeding tubes already in place may be able to regain the ability to eat and drink normally. Carefully consider whether a feeding tube is really needed. Always consider whether the nutritional goals can be met by hand feeding or by nutritional supplementation rather than by resorting to a feeding tube. It makes no sense to use a feeding tube when the resident can swallow but only needs additional food or assistance in eating.

People become malnourished when nutrient intake does not keep pace with nutrient needs for energy, vitamins, or minerals. To bring nutritional intake into balance with nutritional requirements, three possibilities exist:

1. If the resident has abnormally elevated nutritional requirements, treat the underlying condition to decrease metabolic requirements (e.g., treatment of infection or hyperthyroidism).
2. Increase the nutrient density of foods offered (e.g., substitute whole milk for tea, strained meat for broth, adding ice cream to shakes, and so on)
3. Increase the amount of food eaten by giving oral supplements between regular meals.

It may be possible to prevent or reverse malnutrition by using these three methods. Consider a feeding tube only when these methods have failed or are clearly impossible (e.g., in the case of a massive stroke).

In all cases, the clinician should proceed as follows:

1. Assess the resident's eating behavior and nutritional status. Be sure to involve a dietitian in this process.
2. Simultaneously treat all potentially reversible causes of poor oral intake.
3. If calorie counts and fluid intake return to acceptable levels, monitor weight and watch for continued improvement.
4. If irreversible illness is present or weight loss continues despite alternative treatment, determine the goals of placing a feeding tube (i.e., maintaining life, treating a specific condition), and obtain informed consent or refusal for tube placement.

For residents whose need for tube feedings is confirmed and from whom informed consent has been received, select the appropriate task and continue the care planning process in sequence:

- Task 1: Choose the type of tube.
- Task 2: Begin tube feeding.
- Task 3: Review the efficiency of the maintenance feeding.
- Task 4: Review for serious complications that may accompany feeding tube use.

The following sections discuss these tasks in more detail.

Task 1: Choose the Type of Tube

- The type of feeding tube used will depend on:
- The length of time the tube may be in place
- The possibility that the resident will pull the tube unless restrained
- The possibility of aspiration of retained feeding
- The availability of a physician with the skill required to perform the indicated placement procedure

Placement for 2 to 4 weeks.

For the resident who will have a short trial period of tube feedings (i.e., less than 2 to 4 weeks), a nasogastric or nasoenteral feeding tube is frequently used. Never use a large nasogastric tube intended for gastric lavage or decompression for feeding. These tubes can cause irritation and erosion of the nose, nasopharynx, and esophagus. If the resident is agitated or confused and likely to pull the tube, gastrostomy or jejunostomy tubes are better alternatives. These types of tubes are less obtrusive, cause less discomfort, and can be disguised successfully with a covering. Confused residents usually do not need to be restrained when a gastrostomy or jejunostomy tube is in place.

Placement for longer than 4 weeks.

For the resident who will be tube fed for

longer than 2 to 4 weeks, or is likely to be tube fed permanently, place a gastrostomy or jejunostomy tube. For those residents who are able to swallow, but cannot meet all of their nutritional needs orally, using one of these tubes avoids the unesthetic appearance of a nasal tube, and allows the resident to socialize and enjoy mealtimes and activities without a visible tube that can lead to embarrassment and isolation.

The use of jejunostomy tubes is controversial. It seems reasonable that placing a tube beyond the pylorus will limit the rate of aspiration pneumonias, but many of these pneumonias are due to the aspiration of oropharyngeal secretions rather than the regurgitation of gastric contents. Jejunostomy tubes have been associated with a high rate of other complications and have not decreased the rate of aspiration pneumonia over gastrostomy tubes.

Physician availability

The method of tube placement, i.e., surgical, endoscopic, or via radiologically guided procedures, depends on the specific condition of the resident and the availability of a physician with the skills required to perform the technique.

Task 2: Begin Tube Feeding

After placing a feeding tube, make the following preparations for tube feeding.

Verify tube placement

This is very important with nasoenteral tube feedings. Confirm placement with a radiograph of the abdomen to show that the tip of the feeding tube is in the proper position. Tubes can coil in the pharynx, respiratory tract, and upper esophagus and must be repositioned before feeding can begin. Other methods of verifying placement of the tube are fallible. They include checking aspirates for pH and appearance (an acid pH; e.g., a pH level of

less than 4 suggests gastric placement, but a higher pH reading does not prove that the tube is not in the stomach), listening for gurgling noises over the stomach when pushing air through the tube, and checking for air bubbling when the end of the tube is placed in water.

Since it is impossible to obtain a radiograph each time a resident is fed, the clinician must rely on these techniques, recognizing that they are not perfect. In checking that a previously placed nasogastric tube remains in place, a reasonable approach is to use more than one of these methods for confirmation. However, obtain a radiograph each time a nasoenteral tube is placed, replaced, or the previous clinical methods of confirming placement with an established feeding tube give conflicting results.

Properly position the resident

Nasogastric and gastrostomy tubes can deliver a large amount of feeding solution to the stomach, creating the hazard of reflux, regurgitation, and aspiration. The risk cannot be eliminated, but minimize it by positioning the resident's head at a 45 angle at all times during, and for at least 1 hour after, each feeding. In residents with gastrostomy tubes or nasogastric tubes, especially those who frequently have high residuals of retained food in the stomach (*see* the next section), keeping the resident on his or her right side with the head elevated may help feedings to pass from the stomach into the small intestine, lessening the risk of aspiration.

Determine the type of feeding to be used

A wide variety of commercial formulas are available for tube feeding. Have the staff dietitian recommend an appropriate type depending on the needs of the resident. Factors to consider include osmolarity and caloric density of the formula. In most cases, an isosmolar, lactose-free formula that delivers 1 kcal/mL of fluid is a reasonable choice. Hyperosmolar fluids and those that contain lactose increase the risk of diarrhea.

There are special solutions available for individuals with malabsorption problems or for those requiring special diets because of liver or kidney disease. Residents with prolonged malnutrition and severe hypoproteinemia may have edematous intestinal mucosa, which limits nutrient absorption, and could require formulas with predigested protein sources. However, it is possible to refeed slowly in these instances using an isosmolar formula and carefully checking the resident for diarrhea as well as electrolyte and metabolic abnormalities.

Determine the feeding method, rate, and schedule. The use of feeding tubes requires that you determine:

- Whether the feeding will be given intermittently or continuously
- How fast to give the feeding
- How long or how many times a day to give the feeding

Nasoenteral and jejunal tubes usually require continuous feeding over approximately 18 hours a day. Continuous does not mean around the clock, but rather refers to a continuous drip of formula over the time of feeding. Most facilities avoid feeding around the clock, since feeding for 24 hours not only limits mobility, it may also elevate insulin levels and create a risk of hypoglycemia if the feeding is interrupted for some reason.

Intermittent feedings, where a large amount of feeding formula is delivered through the tube over a few minutes, are possible with gastrostomy tubes, but the large bolus creates an increased risk of aspiration. For residents able to participate in activities, a continuous method of feeding may permit flexible feeding schedules, with the time and rate of the feeding adjusted as much as possible to accommodate the resident's preferences. Stop the feeding during these activities and restart them on return. Usually, continuous feedings can be administered at night without disturbing the resident's sleep.

In starting feedings, isosmolar formula can be started at full strength and dripped at about 25 mL/h for 18 h/day. The rate may be increased to meet the resident's caloric needs (i.e., 30 kcal/kg/day). When beginning feedings, the rate may be either decreased or the formula diluted in the event of cramping or diarrhea.

Note: Do not assume that abdominal cramping or diarrhea is caused by tube feeding until all other potential sources of the problem have been eliminated.

With nasogastric or gastrostomy tube feedings delivered by drip, check the residual amounts of feeding retained in the stomach every 4 hours. The tube feeding is held, a syringe is placed on the feeding tube, and the retained material is aspirated and measured. If the residual is 10% to 20% greater than the hourly rate, hold the feeding, slowly return the residual to the stomach, and recheck the residual an hour later. Contact the physician or dietitian and reduce the drip feeding rate if the residual remains high. Alleviate prolonged retention of material in the stomach by repositioning the resident and using motility agents such as metoclopramide (e.g., Reglan) cautiously. In some cases it will be necessary to advance the tube beyond the pylorus. Decisions about tube repositioning and motility agents depend on the physician's assessment.

Intermittent feedings can proceed with small amounts initially, then increase to approximately 240 mL of formula (i.e., the contents of the can) given every 4 hours. Adjust the timing of the feeding to accommodate residents who can participate in activities. Perform a gastric aspiration through the gastrostomy tube before giving a feeding, and hold the feeding if more than 100 mL remains. Return to the stomach the retained feeding that is aspirated. Check the residual again in an hour. If less than 100 mL is aspirated, administer the tube feeding. As with continuous feedings, large amounts of retained feeding formula in the stomach may require repositioning, pharmacologic therapy, or a changeover from an intermittent method to a continuous method feeding. If these do not work or are not practical for the resident, you may need to reposition the gastrostomy tube beyond the pylorus.

Regular flushing of the tube to lessen clogging is an important part of the care plan. Usually, a minimum of 30 mL of water is used to flush after each intermittent feeding and after checking for residuals. For those who have continuous feedings, flush the tube with at least 30 mL of water every 4 hours when the residuals are checked. The physician and dietitian may determine that additional amounts of fluid should be given depending on the resident's individual needs (*see* the next section).

Determine the amount of formula to be given daily

To maintain weight, give approximately 30 kcal/kg/day. To increase weight, or in the presence of metabolic stress factors (i.e., surgery, infection, fractures), increase the requirement to 35 to 40 kcal/kg/day. For a 70-kg man to maintain his weight, for example, he should receive 70 kg x 30 kcal/kg/day or 2100 kcal/day. If he is receiving a formula containing 1 kcal/mL, he will need 2100 mL of formula day. Calculate the drip rate by dividing the amount to be received (2100 mL) by the number of hours (typically, 12 to 18 hours per day) that the feeding will be dripped. With an 18-hour drip, this will be about 115 mL/hour. A similar calculation can be done for intermittent feedings. (Dietitians and other specialists in nutrition use a more sophisticated method of determining caloric needs, which uses the Harris-Benedict equation. *See* protocol 3 later in this chapter.)

Task 3: Review the Efficiency of Maintenance Feeding

Review tube feedings initially at least weekly for their efficacy in maintaining the resident's nutritional status and hydration. Consider the following issues:

Calories

The caloric goal of 30 kcal/kg/day for weight maintenance can be difficult to achieve if tube feedings are frequently diluted because of diarrhea, or interrupted because of tube plugging or high gastric residuals. Do not assume that diarrhea is caused by tube feeding. (*See* the section on evaluation of diarrhea in tube-fed residents.) Frequent tube plugging or high residuals may require tube replacement beyond the pylorus.

Fluids

Monitoring intake or output of fluids is especially important whenever:
- Tube feeding is started
- Changes are made in the formula or rate of feeding
- There are intercurrent illnesses that may place the resident at risk for dehydration or fluid overload

Dehydration can be a problem in tube-fed residents who cannot increase their free water intake. In hot weather or for residents with a fever, osmotic diuresis, or diarrhea, it is important to add water to the tube feeding to prevent dehydration. Hyperosmolar feedings can create dehydration by drawing off water into the gut. Water intake should be about 25 to 30 mL/kg of body weight, or about 1 mL/kcal of ingested formula per day.

Most isotonic tube feedings are 85% water. Therefore, for a 70-kg resident on a weight maintenance feeding at 30 kcal/kg/day, 2100 mL of the isotonic feeding will provide 1785 ml of free water. Make sure that at least the additional 315 mL of free water is given daily in tube flushes. This is an adequate fluid intake assuming that the resident is sedentary and there are no reasons for increased fluid loss. If the resident receives a concentrated feeding formula, add the water so that a total of 2100 mL of free water is given per day.

In addition to hyperosmolar feeding formulas, residents who receive a formula with added fiber (e.g., Jevity or Isocal with fiber) may need to have additional water to avoid constipation. Residents receiving a fiber formula should have 1.0 to 1.25 mL of water per kcal of tube feeding. Since most isotonic formulas are 85% water, 240 mL of formula (the contents of one can) provides 250 kcal, containing 204 mL of free water. The water requirement for 250 kcal is 250 to 312 mL. Since 204 mL of free water is already in the feeding, an additional 46 to 108 mL of water must be added per 240 mL of formula to meet this additional requirement.

Determining the fluid prescriptions for each resident depends on other concurrent medical conditions (e.g., CHF, kidney function, diabetes, or other medical conditions).

Other nutrients

Most tube feedings provide adequate vitamins when given in amounts over 1500 kcal/day. Residents with evidence of specific deficiencies usually require supplemental vitamins; others may require intravenous supplements if the vitamin deficiency is a consequence of failure of gut absorption of the vitamins.

Weight gain

In cases in which tube feedings are started due to weight loss and poor nutritional status, the resident should achieve a weight gain if feeding is adequate. Check the weight at least once weekly and document the change over time.

In some cases, weight gain may not be evidence of adequate nutrition but rather a sign of fluid overload and CHF. Include a physical assessment to check for edema and ausculta-

tion of the lungs for evidence of fluid. Some peripheral edema is common in tube-fed residents, especially those with protein-calorie malnutrition and low albumin. Serial measurements of the circumference of the arm midway between the acromial process (i.e., close to the shoulder) and the olecranon (elbow) will show evidence of gains in body mass unrelated to fluid retention. This is a low-cost test of low burden to the resident and nursing home staff. The only requirement is a flexible tape measure marked in centimeters. Document the serial measurements on a flow sheet in the resident's medical record. To increase the accuracy and reliability of measurements, it is recommended that the same person do the measurement each time. This is an easy way to monitor nutritional gains with feeding and helps differentiate these gains from fluid overload.

Laboratory parameters

When beginning tube feedings, frequently check the glucose and electrolytes (i.e., sodium, potassium, chloride, bicarbonate), probably daily for most residents, until the tube feeding regimen is stabilized. Residents who are severely undernourished may need their electrolytes checked more than once a day because of potentially lethal abnormalities associated with refeeding. Performing checks of the electrolytes, glucose, calcium, phosphorus, magnesium, and albumin in all residents on tube feedings is crucial, but they are especially important in those with the most severe nutritional deficiencies.

For residents with diabetes, tube feedings may require adjusting insulin regimens and frequent monitoring of blood sugars. The frequency of the testing depends on the severity of the diabetes and the change in glucose levels. When tube feedings are withheld either because of illness or tube dysfunction, change the insulin dosage and monitor the blood sugar.

After stabilizing the tube-feeding regimen, laboratory testing remains an important part of monitoring response to treatment. A monthly check of electrolytes is reasonable in residents who are doing well and on a stable feeding schedule. Albumin, cholesterol, and other nutritional indices should, depending on the reason for tube feeding and the severity of the malnutrition, improve to normal levels over time. For residents who were anergic initially (i.e., unable to react to an antigen such as tuberculin or candida), repeat skin testing after several months may show a reaction to antigens.

Returning to self-feeding or assisted feeding without the use of tubes

Except for residents who are comatose, include in the care plans the need for continual reassessment of tube feeding and evaluation of the resident's potential to ingest adequate food and fluids without a tube. For residents with swallowing difficulties, a swallowing evaluation and videofluoroscopy can yield crucial information regarding the safety of beginning oral feedings. Residents who continue to aspirate food and fluids should have tube feedings maintained. For other residents (e.g., those who began tube feeding because of failure to thrive, unexplained weight loss, or serious illness), a return to normal eating is an important goal. Continue to have solid food and supplements provided to these residents at mealtimes throughout the period of tube feeding. Ideally, they can receive their favorite foods.

Encourage residents to increase their oral intake to the point that the tube can be withdrawn. Refeeding by tube may reverse the anorexia of starvation and improve, rather than replace, oral intake. If possible, time the tube feedings so that they are administered at night or between normal meal times, in order to encourage normal eating. However, residents who resist feeding efforts, have difficulties in chewing, or experience mouth pain when eating may be unlikely candidates for return to oral feedings.

For care of a tube site, and tube blockage, *see* protocol 1. For residents receiving tube feedings who are experiencing diarrhea, *see* protocol 2.

Task 4: Review for Serious Complications

Monitor residents for delirium, agitation, anxiety, depression, and lung aspiration. Other conditions to watch for include:
- Removal of the tube by the resident or inadvertent displacement
- Blockage of the feeding tube
- Aspiration of feeding formula, with resultant respiratory distress and infection
- The side effects of feeding, such as diarrhea, constipation, fluid overload, dehydration, and abdominal pain
- Leakage around the tube site with skin breakdown
- Mechanical irritation of the gastrointestinal tract by the tube, causing esophagitis, gastritis, or gastric ulcers, perforation, or gastrointestinal bleeding

Table 26-1 describes other complications related to tube feeding.

CASE EXAMPLE

Mr. J. is a 78-year-old man with a 5-year history of Parkinson's disease. He was admitted to the nursing home 2 years ago weighing 160 pounds (at 6 feet tall). In the year following his admission, he had difficulty eating and increasing problems with swallowing. His physician attributed his swallowing difficulties to the Parkinson's disease. The rigidity and slow movements characteristic of Parkinson's disease impaired Mr. J.'s ability to feed himself. He had frequent episodes of coughing while eating and had two bouts of pneumonia within 6 months. During his first year of residence, he lost 20 pounds, his albumin fell to 3.2, and a stage II pressure ulcer developed

Table 26-1. Some Complications Related to Tube Feeding

Complication	Actions	Rationale
Alteration in mental status	Auscultate the lugs Inspect the feeding tube site If ordered, check laboratory studies	The resident may be anxious, confused, or lethargic due to: • Possible abnormality in electrolytes or glucose related to feeding • Hypoxia due to aspiration • Fever or infection related to aspiration or infection at the tube site • Dehydration from inadequate free water given with feedings
Aspiration	Suction the nasopharynx Place the resident on the right side Check vital signs If the resident is without pulse or respirations and is to be resuscitated, begin cardiopulmonary resuscitation If the resident is less critically ill, treat with supplemental oxygen, antibiotics, and obtain a chest radiograph	The resident may be noted to be in severe respiratory difficulty or have less dramatic presentation with fever, alteration in mental status, wheezing, increased respiratory rate, and tachycardia Aspiration can occur by two methods: (1) aspiration of oropharyngeal secretions or (2) reflux and aspiration of stomach contents. Placement of a feeding tube does not eliminate the risk of either. Aspiration can be associated with large amounts of retained feeding or improper positioning.
Feeding tube removal or displacement	Halt feeding Replace tube Obtain radiographs before restarting feeding when a nasoenteral tube is replaced	Tube removal may be due to resident agitation Frequent displacement of a nasoenteral tube is an indication for gastronomy tube placement

Table continues

over his coccyx. Assistance in cutting food and hand feeding by the staff was instituted but did not result in a weight gain because he continued to have swallowing difficulties. Calorie counts done on 3 successive days showed an average intake of 800 kcal/day.

An occupational therapy consult was requested for the swallowing difficulties. The recommended videofluoroscopy swallowing study revealed severe discoordination of swallowing with aspiration, which is consistent with Parkinson's disease.

A discussion was held with Mr. J. about the findings. The nursing home had a policy that favored the use of feeding tubes except in situations in which the resident was imminently dying, but it respected the informed desires of those residents who refused tube placement. The physician recommended tube placement in Mr. J.'s case, feeling that it would

Table 26-1. Some Complications Related to Tube Feeding–*Continued*

Complication	Actions	Rationale
Gastrointestinal bleeding and abdominal pain	Check vital signs, including orthostatic blood pressure and pulse Palpate abdomen for tenderness	Resident may present with vomiting blood or coffee ground material *or* with guaiac-positive stools, or dark, tarry bowel movements May be related to tube irritating the gastrointestinal tract and causing ulcers Tubes can often perforate the gastrointestinal tract, causing bleeding and infection Abdominal pain can also be caused by an improperly placed gastronomy or jejunostomy tube, with feeding entering the peritoneum In residents with diarrhea and abdominal pain, the cause may be too little blood flow tto the intestines or an infection process like *C.difficile*
Fluid overload	For acute pulmonary edema and respiratory distress, sit the resident up in bed, obtain vital signs, and treat CHF. To monitor fluid status: • Monitor weights at least weekly • Check for peripheral edema • Measure midarm circumference to see if weight gain is due to fluid or improved nutrition	Residents can experience fluid overload because of CHF or from being given too much fluid. Fluid overload may present as an emergency-like pulmonary edema with cyanosis, respiratory distress, and large amounts of pink-tinged frothy sputum, or it may occur over time with increasing edema and weight gain.
Dehydration	Check for weight decrease Obtain vital signs, especially orthostatic vital signs Monitor input and output Change the amount of water given by tube	Residents may experience dehydration due to not having enough fluids being given. Dehydration due to an increase in fluid loss can be atributed to fever (increased sweating, increased respiration), diuresis, severe diarrhea, and vomiting.

improve his nutritional problems, lessen the progression of pressure ulcers, and improve his well-being and level of function. Mr. J. agreed with the recommendation. A permanent feeding tube was placed via a percutaneous endoscopic gastrostomy.

With the assistance of the dietitian, Mr. J.'s feeding requirements were determined as follows. First, the dietitian used the Harris-Benedict equation to calculate the basal energy expenditure (BEE).

1. For a man (see protocol 3 for the formula for a woman and sample calculations), the equation is:

$$66 + (13.7 \text{ x weight in kg}) + (5 \text{ x height in cm}) - (6.8 \text{ x age in years}) = \text{BEE (kcal)}$$

Mr. J. weighs 140 pounds. This is converted to kilograms by dividing by 2.2. At 6 feet tall, he is 72 inches. This is converted to centimeters by multiplying by 2.54. Therefore, he weighs 63.6 kg and is 183 cm tall. His BEE is now calculated:

$$66 + (13.7 \text{ x } 63.6) + (5 \text{ x } 183) - (6.8 \text{ x } 78) = \text{BEE}$$
$$66 + 871 + 915 - 530 = \text{BEE}$$
$$1322 = \text{BEE}$$

2. The next step was to estimate Mr. J.'s total energy expenditure (TEE). This can be done in one of two ways. One method is to use the following formula:

$$\text{BEE (kcal) x (activity factor) x (injury factor)} = \text{TEE (kcal)}$$

The activity factors and injury factors are numbers that provide an estimate of how much energy is needed above the basal expenditure. (The factors are given in protocol 3.) In Mr. J.'s case, an activity factor of 1.3 was chosen because he is ambulatory, and an injury factor of 1.3 was chosen because of recent surgery (tube placement) and the pressure ulcers. The TEE is calculated as follows:

$$1322 \text{ kcal x } 1.3 \text{ x } 1.3 = \text{TEE}$$
$$2234 \text{ kcal} = \text{TEE}$$

(Alternatively, estimate the TEE by multiplying the BEE by 1.22 for normal conditions, 1.54 for stress, and 1.76 for situations in which the resident is losing weight and protein. In the case of Mr. J., multiplying the BEE by 1.76 gives an estimate of 2326 kcal for TEE.)

3. The third step was to calculate Mr. J.'s estimated protein needs. As a rule, for every 150 kcal of energy, 1 g of nitrogen is required. Calculate the total amount of nitrogen needed by dividing the TEE by 150. Nitrogen is a part of protein, and the amount of protein required can then be determined by multiplying the amount of required nitrogen times 6.25. In this case, Mr. J.'s TEE is 2234 kcal. Dividing by 150 kcal/g nitrogen gives the result that 14.9 g nitrogen are required daily. This 14.9 g nitrogen multiplied by 6.25 g protein/g nitrogen results in an estimate of Mr. J.'s daily protein needs of 93.1 g of protein.

The dietitian collaborated with the staff to determine a good schedule for continuous feeding. After talking with Mr. J., a schedule was arranged that allowed him to be disconnected from the tube feedings from noon to 6 PM so he could participate in activities and go out on trips. The dietitian next checked to see which formula would provide the needed calories and protein. The formula selected contains 1.06 kcal/mL and 10.5 g protein per 240 mL. Calculate the amount of formula needed to meet caloric needs by dividing the TEE in kilocalories by the caloric density of the formula.

The rate of feeding is determined by dividing the amount of formula needed by the time in minutes when the resident will receive the continuous feeding. For Mr. J., 2200 kcal will be delivered by 2200 kcal/1.06 kcal/mL of formula. This means that about 2100 mL of formula must be delivered over 18 hours. The rate for Mr. J.'s continuous feeding over 18 hours was calculated by dividing 2100 ml by 18 hours, or 117 mL/h. This can be rounded off to 120 mL/hour over 18 hours. The amount of protein was determined by dividing the amount of formula received per day by the amount of protein in the formula. In Mr. J.'s case, the formula selected has 10.5 g protein per 240 mL of fluid. Dividing the amount of formula given per day (2100 mL) by 240 mL and multiplying by 10.5 gives the result of 92 g of protein. This is close to the calculated 93.1 g of protein per day.

Finally, the dietitian determined additional fluid requirements. For every kilocalorie of formula, there should be 1 mL of free water. Most isotonic feedings are 85% water. Mr. J. receives 2100 mL of formula to deliver 2200 kcal/day. This means he receives 1870 mL of water (2100 x 0.85). The dietitian explained to the nursing staff that, at a minimum, they should make sure Mr. J. received an additional 330 mL of water in tube flushes.

Several weeks after tube placement, the staff had difficulty flushing the tube before beginning a feeding. Gentle irrigation with water resulted in the tube reopening. Three days later the problem recurred but failed to respond to irrigation with water. After conferring with the physician, Mr. J. was transferred to the local emergency room where a surgeon replaced the gastrostomy tube. The original tube was blocked with pill fragments, notwithstanding efforts by the staff to crush the pills adequately. To prevent this from recurring, the staff mixed the pills in custard and administered them orally with success.

In the 6 months following tube placement, Mr. J. regained 15 pounds and his pressure ulcer completely healed. However, shortly thereafter, he became incontinent of diarrhea, with up to six liquid movements per day. He developed a low-grade temperature of 100.4°

and some slight abdominal cramping. Blood pressure and pulse were 120/80 mm Hg and 70 bpm, respectively, without postural change.

The nurse reviewed the medication list for drugs that could cause diarrhea or elixir forms that contain sorbitol. No drug source was identified. Since a resident who had recently returned from the hospital and with whom Mr. J. shared a bathroom was having similar problems, the physician ordered that a stool specimen be sent for *C. difficile* toxin. Interim tube feedings were to be continued and vital signs checked every shift. The physician was to be called for a temperature higher than 101°, systolic blood pressure less than 100 mm Hg, or a postural drop greater than 15 points systolic, or pulse greater than 90 bpm. Mr. J. remained stable over the next 2 days with four to six stools a day. The *C. difficile* toxin returned positive, and the physician ordered metronidazole (Flagyl), 500 mg three times a day for 10 days. She also requested that Mr. J. and his roommate be placed on enteric precautions. Mr. J. improved on the metronidazole and a repeat stool specimen obtained after finishing the metronidazole was negative for *C. difficile* toxin.

An uneventful year followed with an additional 10-pound weight gain and some slight decline in functional status due to his increasing difficulty with Parkinson's symptoms. One evening, Mr. J. was noted to be lethargic about an hour after being fed. His respiratory rate was 40 breaths per minute, blood pressure 100/60 mm Hg, and pulse 100 bpm. He was poorly responsive and had gurgling respirations and was transferred to the acute hospital for presumed aspiration pneumonia. On return 10 days later, Mr. J. was noted to have large residual volumes prior to the next feeding. Feedings were delayed and volumes reduced, but the problem persisted over the next week. A gastroenterologist was consulted who diagnosed a motility disorder related to Parkinson's disease. To solve the problem, Mr.

J.'s gastrostomy tube was replaced by a jejunostomy tube advanced beyond the pylorus under fluoroscopy.

Summary

This case presents several features for review:

1. The resident has several indications for feeding tube placement: weight loss, evidence of malnutrition (low weight for height, decreased albumin, development of a pressure ulcer), pneumonias related to aspiration, and inadequate calorie counts despite assistance with eating.

2. The decision to place a feeding tube represented the resident's informed choice, which was made after the appropriate clinical evaluation and was consistent with his values and the policy of the nursing home.

3. A percutaneous endoscopic gastrostomy (PEG) tube placed because of the long-term necessity of enteral feedings made a nasoenteral tube a poor choice.

4. The use of a drip method of feeding rather than intermittent feeding depends on a number of factors. It is often easier to adjust continuous feedings rather than intermittent feedings around the activities of an alert resident. However, intermittent feedings can be given to suit a resident's schedule.

5. Tube clogging is a frequent annoyance with tube feedings. Ideally, only use a feeding tube to administer formula. Allowing Mr. J. to take his medications crushed in custard involves a risk of aspiration. This should be done only in alert residents with residual swallowing ability and requires attentive nursing care, a nearby suction machine, and monitoring for productive coughs and fevers indicative of aspiration pneumonia. An alternative would be to administer elixir forms of medication through the tube. Unfortunately, many medications do not come in elixir form and, for those that do, sorbitol (a common cause of diarrhea) is often used as a vehicle for the elixir. Sometimes, the staff must resort to crushed pills and deal with recurrent clogged tubes. However, not all medications can be crushed safely. Check with a pharmacist.

6. Diarrhea due to *C. difficile* is a common problem in nursing facilities. *C. difficile* is easily spread and can be difficult to eradicate from nursing homes. The points to be emphasized in this case are threefold:
   - Not all diarrhea in tube-fed residents is caused by the feeding.
   - *C. difficile* is transferred easily from resident to resident.
   - Good handwashing and careful cleaning are important measures in preventing the spread of infection in nursing homes.

7. Aspiration pneumonia and the revision of the feeding tube into a PEG-J tube does not mean Mr. J.'s problems with aspiration are over. He is at less risk for massive aspiration given that the feeding is now delivered distal to the pylorus, but there remains the risk for aspiration of oropharyngeal secretions. Given his Parkinson's-related swallowing difficulties, this is likely to be an ongoing problem.

PROTOCOL 1: CARE OF A TUBE SITE

A. Nasogastric Tube Site

Remove old tape and cleanse the skin at least once per day. Clean the skin with soap and water (unless otherwise indicated) and thoroughly pat it dry. Apply new tape to a different area on the resident's skin than was used previously. Change the tape as needed. Residents with nasogastric tubes need meticulous oral hygiene and good nasal care.

B. Gastrostomy Tube Site

Remove the old dressing, and gently wash around the site with soap and water. Inspect the skin, looking for any signs of skin irritation or breakdown, drainage, or exudate. Swab with a Betadine swab, then apply Betadine ointment to the site and cover with a sterile dressing.

For gastrostomy sites that are leaking, keep the skin around the site as clean and dry as possible. Use an appropriate protecting cream or ointment. You may need to obtain a culture of the site for laboratory analysis. It may also be necessary to apply a wafer of stomahesive around the site. If the drainage is severe, consider applying an ostomy appliance to collect it. However, this type of drainage, and skin breakdown or irritation, are an indication to further consultation. Keep the tube clamped off when the resident is not receiving tube feeding or medications. Gastrostomy tube retraction can occur, leading to leaking from the site. If this occurs, monitor the tube's placement and notify the attending physician.

If the skin problems and drainage are severe and intractable, consider closure of the gastrostomy site and placement of a jejunostomy tube at a different site.

C. Jejunostomy Tube Site
Follow the procedure for the gastrostomy tube site.

D. Tube Blockage
Tube blockage is a problem that occurs with all types of tubes. Try to obtain all of the resident's medications in liquid form or in capsules that can be opened and then dissolved in fluid and poured down the tube. Unfortunately, not all medications come in these forms. Inevitably, the staff needs to crush pills, which leads to pill fragments and other residue adhering to the sides of the tubes, producing a blockage. However, not all medications can be crushed safely. Check with the pharmacist. These tubes will need to be changed periodically.

If a blockage does occur, gently try to aspirate on the tube. If this does not work, try to instill a small amount of warm water. Try to work the fluid back and forth inside the tube. Be careful not to apply undue pressure since this pressure may go through into the resident's stomach. Sometimes a small amount of normal saline can be used to unclog a blocked tube. If all such measures fail, make arrangements for a new feeding tube to replace the blocked tube.

If you are successful in your efforts to clear the tube, check the placement of the tube before instilling any tube feeding, medication, and so on.

Follow the steps in Table 26-2 to eliminate diarreah and ensure adequate nutrition.

PROTOCOL 3

Calculation of Basal Energy Expenditure (BEE)
To calculate BEE, use the following Harris-Benedict equation:

Men:
$$66 + (13.7 \times \text{weight in kg}) + (5 \times \text{height in cm}) - (6.8 \times \text{age in years}) = \text{BEE}$$
Women:
$$655 + (9.6 \times \text{weight in kg}) + (1.7 \times \text{height in cm}) - (4.7 \times \text{age in years}) = \text{BEE}$$

To convert the weight in pounds to weight in kilograms, divide the weight in pounds by 2.2. To convert height in inches to centimeters, multiply height in inches by 2.54.

Calculation of Total Energy Expenditure (TEE)
To calculate TEE, use the following equation:

$$\text{BEE} \infty (\text{activity factor}) \infty (\text{injury factor}) = \text{TEE}$$

Activity factors are 1.2 for bedridden and 1.3 for ambulatory residents. *Injury factors* are 1.2 for surgery, 1.2 to 1.35 for skeletal trauma, 1.3 to 1.6 for sepsis, 1.5 to 1.7 for trauma, and

Table 26-2 Protocol 2: Diarrhea in Residents Receiving Tube Feedings

Approaches to Care	Explanation
Step 1: Acute Care	
• Perform a rectal examination to rule out fecal impaction. If the resident is impacted, see the section on fecal impaction management.	Tube feedings can cause constipation (because of low-residue formulas) and diarrhea. In the event of diarrhea, it is important to rule out liquid oozing around an impaction.
• Check diarrhea sample for occult blood.	Diarrhea may be due to a number of causes that are not related to enteral feedings.
• Send the sample to the laboratory for C. difficile toxin test.	Evaluate the resident for bleeding, infection, or other serious conditions that may cause diarrhea.
Ä Check for fever, tachycardia, postural blood pressure, abdominal pain, or tenderness.	While evaluating the cause of diarrhea, monitor the resident for hemodynamic stability, fluid balance, and urine output. Extra water may need to be added to tube feeding.
• Monitor fluid intake and output	
6. Review for easily reversible causes of diarrhea: medications (sorbitol in elixir forms), hyperosmolar formulas, too rapid delivery of formula, lactose in formula.	
Step 2: Treatment for underlying causes	
• Consult the dietitian.	The dietitian can make decisions about changes in formula, rate of feeding, change in medications that may be contributing to diarrhea, and can also consult the physician about necessary laboratory studies.
• Follow the treatment order: (1) Alter the tube feeding order (decrease the rate, dilute the formula, or switch to an alternate formula that contains fiber; do only one procedure at a time) (2) If diarrhea persists despite the previous measures, and is not related to infection, consider using kaolin pectate, opiates (deodorized tincture of opium), recognizing risk of confusion, respiratory depression, and so on. (3) Treat *C. difficile* infection if titer returns positive. (4) If diarrhea persists, consider venous alimentation since decreasing feeding rates, diluting formula, and so forth will likely lead to an inadequate intake of calories and protein.	

For more information, see Wilmore DW, Van Woert JH: Enteral and parenteral nutrition in hospital patients. In Rubenstein E, Federman DD, eds: Scientific American Medicine, New York, 1992.

2.0 to 2.1 for burns. Estimating the exact number chosen depends on the severity of the injury.

The following is an alternate, simplified method of estimating TEE:

For normal conditions: BEE x 1.22
For residents under metabolic stress: BEE x 1.54
For residents with marked weight loss: BEE x 1.76

Calculations of Protein Requirements

To maintain and replenish visceral protein stores, protein is required. Protein contains nitrogen (there is 1 g nitrogen in 16 g protein). To estimate protein requirements calculate on the basis of a ratio of each 150 kcal of energy requiring 1 g nitrogen. This 150 kcal:1 g nitrogen ratio allows you to determine the amount of protein required as follows:

Divide TEE by 150 kcal. This will give you the grams of nitrogen.

To determine the amount of protein required, multiply the number of grams of nitrogen by 6.25.

Examples of Calculating BEE and TEE

See the case example in this chapter for a male resident. The following example is for a female resident. Calculate the TEE for an 85-year-old female resident in your nursing home. She is 5 feet tall and weighs 110 pounds. She is bedridden and has frequent infections, but rarely requires hospitalization.
Calculate the BEE. The Harris-Benedict equation for women is:

655 + (9.6 x weight in kg) + (1.7 x height in cm) −

(4.7 x age in years) = BEE (kcal)

Using the metric system, determine the resident's weight and height in metric terms:

Weight = 110 lbs/2.2 lbs/kg = 50 kg
Height = 5 ft = 60 inches = 60 inches x 2.54 cm/inch = 152 cm

Place these metric values into the Harris-Benedict equation:

655 + (9.6 + (9.6 x 50))
x 50) + (1.7 x 152) - (4.7 x 85) = BEE
655 + 480 + 258 - 400 = BEE
993 = BEE

Calculate the TEE as follows:

BEE x (activity factor) x (injury factor) = TEE
993 kcal x (factor for bedridden) x (factor for mild sepsis) = TEE
993 kcal x 1.2 x 1.3 = 1549 kcal

Alternatively, you can estimate the total energy expenditure by using only one factor:
BEE x factor = TEE

Normal conditions: 993 kcal x 1.22 = 1211 kcal
Stressed conditions: 993 kcal x 1.54 = 1529
Severe weight loss: 993 kcal x 1.76 = 1748 kcal

Table 26-3 contains information about six common formulas, their caloric content, nutritional content, and recommended use.

Table 26-3. Tube Feeding Formula: Content Breakdown

Tube feeding	Isocal[a]	Isocal HN[b]	Ultracal[c]	Jevity[d]	Osmolite HN[e]	Osmolite[f]
Cal/mL	1.06	1.06	1.06	1.06	1.06	1.06
Nutritionally complete	Yes	Yes	Yes	Yes	Yes	Yes
Calories (mL) to meet 100% US RDA vitamins (mL)	1890	1180	1180	1400 cal (1321 mL)	1400 calories (1321 mL)	2000 calories (1886 mL)
Calories	250	250	250	250	250	250
Protein (g)	8.2	10.6	10.6	10.5	10.5	8.8
Carbohydrates (g)	33	29.8	29.5	35.9	33.4	34.3
Fat	10.6	10.8	10.8	8.7	8.7	9.1

[a]Isotonic; low residue; nutritionally complete to provide total dietary needs of most tube-fed residents; unflavored.

[b]Isotonic; low residue formula for residents who require nutrient-dense, high nitrogen feeding; bland unsweetened taste.

[c]Isotonic formula containing oat and soy fiber, which aids in normalizing bowel function.

[d]Standard isotonic tube feeding formula with fiber (3.4 g/8 oz); helps maintain normal bowel function; useful in management of tube feeding intolerance, i.e., constipation and diarrhea; high nitrogen and vitamin/mineral content; good for geriatric population; if gravity drip, use 10F tube or larger; with pump, smaller tubes adequate.

[e]High-nitrogen isotonic; low residue for residents with caloric requirements of less than 2000; well-suited for geriatric population or for residents with high nitrogen requirements; mild taste, useful as an oral supplement for residents with altered taste perception.

[f]Isotonic; low residue; due to lower nitrogen and nutrient content requirements, greater volume of feeding to meet requirements; not as well-suited for geriatric population as Osmo HN or Jevity; mild taste, useful as an oral supplement for residents with altered taste perception.

Information from Mead Johnson, Ross Laboratories.

27
Urinary Incontinence

Neil Resnick, MD
Margaret Baumann, MD

Urinary incontinence—the inability to control urination in a socially appropriate manner—affects over half of all nursing home residents and is the source of considerable morbidity and expense. It can cause skin rashes, falls, and pressure ulcers, and may lead to the use of indwelling catheters, which have their own set of problems. In addition, it may affect psychological well-being and social interactions, and its cost is enormous: US nursing homes spend over $4 billion per year in managing incontinence. However, incontinence in the majority of residents can be improved or even cured, and safer and more comfortable approaches are often practical for residents with indwelling catheters.

OVERVIEW

Comprehensive care planning for incontinence goes well beyond traditional bladder training. Such an approach not only has a much higher chance of success, but also will identify treatable sources of morbidity beyond the urinary tract. This chapter presents a structured approach to such care planning. The first two sections provide the background necessary for understanding the causes of incontinence. The third section outlines the techniques to detect and treat both the reversible and persistent causes of incontinence, and demonstrates how to segregate patients into clinical groups that facilitate formulation of a care plan. The last section provides details for each therapeutic intervention.

PHYSIOLOGY

The lower urinary tract consists of the bladder, the urethra, and the two urethral sphincters. During the storage phase, the bladder remains relaxed, while the proximal and distal urethral sphincters remain closed tightly enough to prevent leakage during maneuvers such as coughing, standing, or sneezing. During the emptying phase, the bladder contracts while the urethral sphincters relax sufficiently to permit the unobstructed flow of urine. The coordination required to orchestrate urine storage and evacuation is mediated by central nervous system (CNS) control of the parasympathetic, sympathetic, and voluntary nervous systems. The parasympathetic system innervates the bladder, while the sympathetic and

376

somatic nervous systems supply the urethral sphincters.

The largest volume that the bladder can hold is referred to as the *total bladder capacity*, while the volume that remains in the bladder (normally less than 50 mL) after voiding is termed the *postvoiding residual volume* (PVR); the difference between total bladder capacity and the PVR is known as the *functional bladder capacity*.

Pathophysiology and Causes of Incontinence

Continence depends on many factors both within and outside the urinary tract. Urinary tract factors include a bladder that can store and expel urine and a urethra that can open and close appropriately. Important factors outside the urinary tract include fluid balance, constipation, use of a wide variety of medications, and functional integrity of the CNS, spinal cord, and peripheral nerves. Other determinants include locomotion sufficient to reach the toilet on time; dexterity sufficient to remove undergarments; cognitive function and social awareness sufficient to realize when and where to void; and motivation sufficient to care.

Urinary tract dysfunction is an important risk factor for incontinence, but it is only one of many such factors commonly found in institutionalized elderly. The optimal approach to incontinence in such residents requires understanding the four ways in which the urinary tract can malfunction:

- The bladder contracts when it should not. This is the most common lower urinary tract cause of incontinence, found in nearly two thirds of cases. Formerly known as the spastic or uninhibited bladder, its correct name is *detrusor overactivity* (DO). It can be termed *detrusor hyperreflexia* when associated with an upper motor neuron lesion, and *detrusor instability* in the absence

of such a lesion, but it is referred to as DO in this chapter because the etiology is usually unclear even when an upper motor neuron lesion is present. Regardless of the cause, however, DO results in an abrupt gush of urine, usually accompanied by a sensation of urinary urgency—an *abrupt* and *strong* desire to void. In half of such people, the bladder is strong and empties completely, resulting in soaked clothes and puddles on the floor. In the other half, it is weak and fails to empty completely, resulting in rapid refilling and more frequent incontinence; this condition is known as D*etrusor* overactivity (or H*yperactivity*) with I*mpaired* C*ontractility* (DHIC).

- The bladder fails to contract when or as well as it should. Accounting for less than 10% of cases, and formerly known as the atonic bladder, this condition's correct name is *underactive detrusor (UD)*. The bladder that completely fails to contract can also be termed detrusor areflexia (when the cause is believed to be neurogenic) or *acontractile detrusor* (when the cause is unknown), but the generic term UD is used in this chapter for the same reasons outlined for the use of DO. In patients with UD, urinary retention may develop and overflow incontinence ensue.

- Urethral resistance is too high owing to obstruction (e.g., prostatic compression or urethral stricture in men, or a large cystocele or postsurgical stricture in women). While this is the second most common lower urinary tract cause of incontinence in men; it rarely occurs in women. In its most severe form, obstruction may result in overflow incontinence. Initially, however, obstruction frequently causes bladder overactivity and resultant urge incontinence. In this case, the use of bladder relaxant medications to treat men with urge incontinence may cause urinary retention. It is important to realize that postvoid dribbling is not a specific symptom for obstruction and is found in men without obstruction as well.

- Urethral resistance is too low (urethral incompetence). This results in leakage associated with coughing, sneezing, straining, or motion, a condition termed *stress incontinence*. Stress incontinence is the second most common lower urinary tract cause of incontinence in older women.

In summary, incontinence in nursing home residents usually has *multiple* causes, including many that are readily reversible, a few that are associated with serious underlying disease, and a majority of which are due to persistent abnormalities of the structure or function of the lower urinary tract. Therefore, a thorough assessment is a prerequisite to effective care planning.

EVALUATION AND TREATMENT PRINCIPLES

To maximize success, the approach to treating incontinence must be stepwise, systematic, and sensible. The following list summarizes the steps to this treatment approach:

1. Assess incontinence (24-hour voiding record).
2. Identify and treat the reversible causes.
3. Identify and treat the serious conditions, if appropriate (even if incontinence improves or abates).
4. Group residents for a targeted therapy.
5. The following sections describe these steps in greater detail.

Step 1: Assess Voiding Pattern and Behavior

The voiding record (Table 27-1) is essential for several reasons. First, it legitimizes the problem, assuring the resident, family, and staff that incontinence is viewed as abnormal and worthy of evaluation. Second, it provides clues to the causes or the contributing factors of

incontinence (e.g., polyuria due to diabetes mellitus). Third, it establishes the baseline frequency of voiding and incontinence, and facilitates formulation of therapeutic interventions.

Complete the record for 2 to 3 days and note the time of each incontinent episode and void, as well as the volume, if possible. The cognitively intact resident may be able to record the information as it occurs or report it to nursing staff. Otherwise, check the resident every 2 hours, recording continence status (wet or dry), as well as the amount voided into a commode or urinal (if the resident needs to void). Finally, note whether the leakage occurs in relation to an associated event (such as lifting the resident, or shortly after the resident suddenly indicates an abrupt urge to void).

Step 2: Identify and Treat Reversible Causes

The eight potentially reversible causes of incontinence can be recalled using the mnemonic DIAPPERS (Table 27-2). Like the serious conditions listed in the next section, all should be detectable by a targeted clinical evaluation, supplemented when necessary by simple laboratory tests; expensive and highly technical procedures are usually not required. Simultaneous treatment of all identified conditions is recommended.

The following subsections describe how to identify and treat the reversible causes of incontinence.

Delirium (Confusional State)

IDENTIFICATION

Delirium is characterized by inattention, an altered sleep-wake cycle, fluctuating confusion, and either increased or decreased activity patterns.

MECHANISM

The delirious resident is less aware of the need to void and the location of the toilet.

Table 27-1. Voiding Record

Name

Time	Wet or dry? Severity (damp/soaked)	Associated events	Intentional void (mL)

Table 27-2. The Reversible Causes of Incontinence[1]

Delirium

Infection

Atrophic urethritis

Pharmaceuticals

Psychological

Excessive urine

Restricted mobility

Stool impaction

[1]Adapted from Resnick NM: Urinary incontinence in the elderly. Medical Grand Rounds, 1984; 3:281-290.

Incontinence will usually abate with proper diagnosis and treatment of the underlying cause of delirium.

TREATMENT
See Chapter 11, Delirium.

Infection (i.e., Symptomatic Urinary Tract Infection)
IDENTIFICATION

The diagnosis of urinary tract infection (UTI) is based on signs and symptoms, urinalysis, and urine culture. The hallmarks of symptomatic UTI-associated incontinence are dysuria, frequency, or urgency—with or without the presence of fever and delirium—and new or worsened incontinence. Confirmatory tests include a urinalysis positive for greater than 5 white blood cells/high-power field, and a positive urine culture. Note that the clinical signs can be caused by other conditions (such as atrophic urethritis or sensory abnormalities

of the urethra), and that asymptomatic bacteriuria—present in 30% to 40% of nursing home residents—does not cause incontinence. However, although disease can present atypically in elderly people, it is often difficult to determine whether incontinence represents the only atypical symptom of a UTI in an otherwise asymptomatic resident. Therefore, it is prudent to administer one course of antibiotics and watch for improvement. If incontinence is unchanged, record the result and withhold further antibiotic therapy unless new symptoms develop.

MECHANISM

Dysuria and urgency due to symptomatic UTI may defeat the older person's ability to reach the toilet in time. As noted above, although it is much more prevalent, asymptomatic infection does not cause incontinence.

TREATMENT

Chapter 3, Infection, describes how to treat the *symptomatic* infection.

Atrophic Urethritis and Vaginitis
IDENTIFICATION

Atrophic urethritis is associated with concurrent vaginitis so often that it usually can be identified by simple examination of the vagina; stirrups and special tables are not necessary. The resident need only bend her knees and let her legs drop to the side—the same position used for catheter insertion in women. After spreading the labia with a gloved hand, look for vaginal mucosal dryness, erythema, or friability, which manifests as broken blood vessels (telangiectasia or punctate hemorrhages) or bleeding from the minimal trauma of spreading the labia. Another useful sign is pain during catheterization.

MECHANISM

Because the female urethra shares embryonic origin with the vagina, the urethral lining may atrophy as estrogen levels decline after menopause and expose the underlying tissue to the irritant effects of urine. This may result in inflammation that can extend to the bladder base (or trigone), where it can cause symptoms identical to those of a UTI. The inflammation may also cause or exacerbate urge incontinence, as well as dysuria, dyspareunia, urgency, and agitation (in demented patients). However, even without associated inflammation, urethral atrophy can impair sphincter closure mechanisms and exacerbate stress incontinence.

TREATMENT

Treat with conjugated estrogens (*see* the section on treatment specifics).

Pharmaceuticals

Since so many prescribed and nonprescribed drugs can cause or exacerbate incontinence, carefully review the medication list (Table 27-3).

Sedative Hypnotics and Alcohol

MECHANISM

Long-acting benzodiazepines, such as flurazepam and diazepam, may accumulate and cause confusion and secondary incontinence. Alcohol, occasionally used by nursing home residents (even without knowledge of the staff), can cause incontinence by clouding the sensorium, impairing mobility, and inducing a diuresis.

TREATMENT

Cautiously withdraw these agents, tapering doses slowly to avoid inducing withdrawal syndrome, a rebound of anxiety, or precipitation of depression.

Anticholinergic Agents and Opiates

Many agents have anticholinergic side effects. These include nonprescribed drugs, such as antihistamines used for insomnia, coryza, pruritus, and vertigo, as well as prescribed agents such as disopyramide, some antispasmodics (dicyclomine and Donnatal), antipsychotics, antidepressants (not selective serotonin reuptake inhibitors [SSRIs] such as fluoxetine, sertraline, paroxetine), opiates, and some anti-Parkinsonian agents (trihexyphenidyl and benztropine mesylate, but not Sinemet or deprenyl).

MECHANISM

Anticholinergic agents cause or exacerbate incontinence by a number of mechanisms. They can depress bladder contractility sufficiently to cause urinary retention with associated urinary frequency and overflow incontinence. Even in the absence of overt urinary retention, they may exacerbate incontinence related to other causes, particularly if they reduce functional bladder capacity by increasing residual urine volume more than they increase bladder capacity. In addition, most anticholinergics can cause dry mouth, which may prompt increased fluid intake and excretion. Finally, many of these agents have additional effects that can predispose to incontinence; for example, antipsychotic agents such as thioridazine and haloperidol may cause sedation, rigidity, and immobility, and antidepressants may cause sedation and confusion.

Opiates can also depress bladder emptying efficiency and induce mouth dryness and confusion. In addition, they interfere with sensory pathways so that the resident becomes less aware or even unaware of bladder fullness.

TREATMENT

Review the indication for each agent, especially since symptoms for which they are prescribed are often side effects of other drugs that might be adjusted or discontinued. If treatment is still indicated, determine whether the dose can be reduced or an agent with less or no anticholinergic effects can be substituted.

Table 27-3. Commonly Used Medications that May Affect Continence

Type of medication	Examples	Potential effects on continence
Sedatives/hypnotics	Long-acting benzodiazepines (e.g., diazepam, flurazepam)	Sedation, delirium, immobility
Alcohol	—	Polyuria, frequency, urgency, sedation, delirium, immobility
Anticholinergics	Dicyclomine, disopyramide, antihistamines	Urinary retention, overflow incontinence, delirium, impaction
• Antipsychotics	Thioridazine, haloperidol	Anticholinergic actions, sedation, rigidity, immobility
• Antidepressants	Amitriptyline, desipramine	Anticholinergic actions, sedation
• Anti-Parkinsonians	Trihexyphenidyl, benztropine mesylate (not levodopa/selegiline)	Anticholinergic actions, sedation
Narcotic analgesics	Opiates	Urinary retention, fecal impaction, sedation, delirium
Alpha-adrenergic antagonists	Prazosin, terazosin	Urethral relaxation may precipitate stress incontinence in women
Alpha-adrenergic agonists	Nasal decongestants	Urinary retention in men
Calcium-channel blockers	All	Urinary retention
Potent diuretics	Furosemide	Polyuria, frequency, urgency
Angiotensin-converting enzyme inhibitors	Captopril, enalapril, lisinopril	Associated cough may precipitate stress incontinence in women and in some men with prior prostatectomy
Vincristine	—	Urinary retention

For example, haloperidol is much less anti-cholinergic than chlorpromazine, and desipramine is much less anticholinergic than amitriptyline; trazodone and SSRIs such as sertraline are not anticholinergic.

Alpha-Adrenergic Agents and Antagonists

These include sympathomimetics (decongestants) and sympatholytics (e.g., prazosin, terazosin, and doxazosin).

MECHANISM

Because the proximal urethra and sphincter contain numerous alpha-adrenergic receptors, sphincter tone can be decreased by alpha antagonists and increased by alpha agonists. An older woman whose urethra has shortened and weakened with age may develop stress incontinence when prescribed an alpha antagonist for hypertension. An older man with an enlarged prostate may develop acute urinary retention and overflow incontinence if he takes a multicomponent cold capsule, most of which contain both an alpha agonist and anticholinergic agent, especially if he takes a nasal decongestant and a nonprescription hypnotic (i.e., an antihistamine) as well.

TREATMENT

Consider alternative agents. For women, consider another type of antihypertensive medication, such as a thiazide. For men with a large prostate, avoid combination cold remedies that contain alpha agonists or antihistamines.

Calcium-Channel Blockers

Calcium-channel blockers are used to treat angina pectoris, hypertension, and congestive heart failure (CHF). Common drugs in this class include diltiazem, nifedipine, and verapamil.

MECHANISM

Calcium-channel blockers can reduce smooth muscle contractility in the bladder and occasionally cause urinary retention and over-flow incontinence. Similar to anticholinergic agents, however, these agents can exacerbate incontinence even in the absence of overt urinary retention by increasing residual urine more than they increase bladder capacity. However, do not consider these agents the cause of incontinence in residents whose residual urine is less than 50 mL.

TREATMENT

Consider using an alternative agent, such as nitrates or beta blockers, for coronary artery disease or a thiazide diuretic for hypertension.

Potent (Loop) Diuretics

MECHANISM

The brisk diuresis induced by loop diuretics (furosemide [Lasix], bumetanide [Bumex], ethacrynic acid) can cause polyuria, urgency, and frequency, which can overwhelm the ability of a frail older person to get to the toilet in time.

TREATMENT

Since diuretics are most appropriate to treat CHF, first determine whether CHF is present. If so, determine whether it is due to systolic dysfunction. If it is instead due to the equally prevalent diastolic dysfunction, treatment with drugs other than digitalis drugs and diuretics (e.g., calcium-channel blockers) may be preferable. For residents with systolic dysfunction, consider whether diuretics may be given in the morning, when additional staff are available to assist with toileting. For residents who have peripheral edema in the absence of CHF, nondiuretic treatment may be preferable. Alternatives include sodium restriction ($\pm$), pressure gradient stockings, Ace bandage wrapping, and daily leg elevation. In addition, edema may respond to *discontinuing* many medications, such as potent nonsteroidal antiinflammatory agents (e.g., indomethacin) and dihydropyridine calcium-channel blockers (e.g., nifedipine, nicardipine, israpidine, felodipine).

Angiotensin-Converting Enzyme Inhibitors

Angiotensin-converting enzyme (ACE) inhibitors are often used to treat residentes following a myocardial infarction, and also to treat hypertension and CHF. Exmples of these drugs include captopril, lisinopril, and enalapril.

MECHANISM

The dry cough that sometimes accompanies treatment with ACE inhibitors can exacerbate or even precipitate stress incontinence.

TREATMENT

Switch to another agent if the cough cannot be controlled.

Psychological

The following subsections describe how to identify and treat the psychological factors of urinary incontinence.

IDENTIFICATION

Depression is often a factor in urinary incontinence. The signs and symptoms include psychomotor retardation or agitation, decreased appetite, lack of interest in surroundings, and sleep disturbance. There are a number of depression scales for older persons that can greatly help in identification.

MECHANISM

Severely depressed residents may lack the motivation to maintain personal hygiene and proper toilet habits.

TREATMENT

See Chapter 13, Depression, for more information.

Excess Urine Production

IDENTIFICATION

The voiding record in Table 27-1 will reveal an output of greater than approximately 2L/day. Alternatively, it may identify large-volume excretion at night (e.g., greater than 600 mL). To be relevant, however, the increased output must correlate with the problem; it is of little value to treat excess nocturnal excretion in a patient who is continent at night but incontinent during the day.

MECHANISM

In residents with impaired mobility or mentation—and especially in those who also have DO—excess urine output may overwhelm the ability to get to a toilet in time. There are many causes of excess excretion. Excess intake is a common cause; if present, check whether it is due to mouth dryness induced by an anticholinergic medication. Consider expanded volume states when there is peripheral edema or when the voiding record reveals excess nocturnal excretion; such conditions include CHF, venous stasis, and low albumin states, as well as the use of medications that cause peripheral edema (e.g., indomethacin and some calcium-channel blockers). The other major causes of polyuria are endocrine conditions that cloud the sensorium.as well: hypercalcemia, hyperglycemia, and diabetes insipidus (especially in residents taking lithium).

TREATMENT

Identify and treat the specific cause. Do not restrict fluid intake before determining the cause of excess excretion, since dehydration may result from many of these conditions (e.g., hyperglycemia).

Restricted Mobility

The following subsections identify and treat the causes of restricted mobility.

IDENTIFICATION

Residents who have difficulty getting to the toilet.

MECHANISM

For residents in whom lower urinary tract dysfunction is prevalent, adequate mobility is essential for the maintenance of continence. Therefore, incontinence will often improve or remit following treatment of the underlying cause of impaired mobility (e.g., arthritis, poor eyesight, Parkinson's disease, or orthostatic or postprandial hypotension).

TREATMENT

Identify and treat the specific cause or institute a program to maintain mobility status (*see* Chapter 29, ADL Rehabilitation, for more information). If a cause cannot be identified or treated, a urinal or bedside commode (augmented with scheduled toileting if necessary) will often be sufficient to improve or resolve the situation.

Stool Impaction

The following subsections describe how to identify and treat stool impaction in residents with urinary incontinence.

IDENTIFICATION

Although fecal impaction alone can cause urinary incontinence, always suspect it in a resident with both urinary and fecal incontinence, especially if the feces are loose and the bladder is also overdistended on abdominal palpation. A digital rectal examination is usually sufficient to identify stool impaction. However, plain abdominal radiography is often necessary since significant impaction may be present in the sigmoid colon or higher, even with a negative digital examination or documentation of daily bowel movements.

MECHANISM

The mechanism is poorly understood, but it appears that colonic overdistention inhibits spinal cord–mediated detrusor contraction. Therefore, residents with stool impaction generally present with overflow urinary incontinence.

TREATMENT

Disimpaction restores continence. Be careful not to underestimate the severity of the impaction. For frail residents, it is wise to use a large-volume enema (250 to 1000 mL), repeated on alternate days as necessary. Following disimpaction, address the precipitants of impaction and institute a bowel regimen (*see* Chapter 28, Bowel Disorders, for more information).

Step 3: Identify and Treat Serious Conditions

Although uncommon, serious conditions may underlie urinary incontinence. Identify and treat them since, in addition to their effect on continence, these conditions may have a significant adverse impact on quality and length of life. However, in some residents who are entirely dependent in ambulation, have little or no cognitive function, or are terminally ill, identifying and treating serious conditions may improve neither incontinence nor quality of life; such residents need not necessarily be assessed for these conditions. These conditions are summarized in Table 27-4 and described in more detail in the text that follows.

1. Bladder cancer or stones. Suggested by gross hematuria or microhematuria (greater than 5 to 10 red blood cells/high-powered field from a noncatheterized specimen) in the absence of current or recent UTI. Use urine cytology to pursue bladder cancer further. Use a fresh sample rather than a first morning urine specimen. The utility of

Table 27-4. Serious Incontinence-Related Conditions

1. Bladder cancer or stones

2. Prostate cancer (in men)

3. Neurologic lesions

   • Brain lesion

   • Spinal cord lesion

   • Herniated disc

   • Vitamin B12 deficiency

   • Plexopathy

4. Poor bladder compliance

5. Hydronephrosis

6. Tabes dorsalis

further evaluation, including intravenous pyelography (IVP) and cystoscopy, will depend on the clinical considerations previously listed.

2. Prostate cancer. Suggested by increased prostate firmness or nodule on rectal examination; obstructive symptoms and hematuria are usually not present. Prostate cancer detected solely by an elevated serum prostate-specific antigen (PSA), without clinical evidence of cancer, is unlikely to be the source of voiding symptoms or incontinence.

3. Spinal cord lesion/herniated disc. Suggested by increased or decreased reflexes, leg weakness, foot drop, loss of sacral reflexes, perineal sensory impairments, or a decreased sensory level. However, the abnormalities may be subtle. Damage to the

lower motor nerves supplying the bladder may cause UD and even lead to urinary retention. Conversely, impingement of the spinal cord above the conus medullaris (usually located at the level of the second lumbar vertebra) can cause DO or a more complex condition called *detrusor-sphincter-dyssynergia*, in which DO is accompanied by simultaneous sphincter spasm. This condition is rare in nursing home residents.

4. Decreased bladder compliance. Results in elevated bladder pressure during filling that can cause damage to the kidneys. Suspect this condition in residents with a history of pelvic radiation therapy, abdominal/pelvic resection, significant spinal cord lesion, or radical hysterectomy or prostatectomy.

5. Tabes dorsalis (tertiary syphilis). Treatable with antibiotics.

6. Hydronephrosis. Ureteral dilation that extends to the level of the kidney; caused by blockage anywhere in the urinary tract and often associated with renal failure. Since serum creatinine may be normal in older persons even in the presence of hydronephrosis and serious renal damage (because of the decreased muscle mass that accompanies aging), screen men whose PVR exceeds 150 to 200 mL for hydronephrosis by renal ultrasound. Because urethral obstruction is rare in women, renal ultrasonography is usually not necessary in women. Since incontinence may respond to symptomatic treatment while hydronephrosis persists, perform screening whether or not incontinence resolves.

Step 4: Group Residents for Targeted Therapies

For residents whose incontinence persists after reversible causes are treated, the next

After re-evaluating for the presence of reversible causes, do a bladderstress test, observe and measure void, and determine the bladder volume (PVR) immediately after a void. Group according to the combined results of the stress test and PVR.

Stress Test Negative

Group #1 PVR less than 100 ml DO more likely than DHIC; BOO (rare)**	Group #2 PVR 100–500 ml DHIC more likely than DO; BOO (rare)**	Group #3 PVR greater than 500 ml UD, DHIC; BOO (uncommon)
1. Behavioral therapy for DO 2. Add medications for DO, if necessary If incontinence persists: 3. Refer, if clinically appropriate 4. Intentionally induce urinary retention and initiate intermittent (if available) of indwelling catheterization 5. Undergarments 6. Indwelling catheter	1. Behavioral therapy for DO 2. Behavioral therapy to improve emptying 3. Medications: Estrogen; then, if PVR less than 250 ml, add bladder relaxants 4. Refer, if clinically appropriate 5. UTI prophylaxis* If incontinence persists: 6. Intermittent catheter 7. Undergarments 8. Indwelling catheter	1. Bladder decompression with an indwelling catheter for 2–4 weeks 2. Behavioral therapy to improve emptying 3. UTI prophylaxis* If incontinence persists 4. Refer, if clinically appropriate If not: 5. Intermittent catheter 6. Undergarments 7. Indwelling catheter

Stress Test Positive

Group #4 PVR less than 200 ml (stress incontinence likely, mixed incontinence possible)	Group #5 PVR greater than 200 ml SI + UD or SI + DHIC likely; overflow (UD greater than DHIC possible
1. Behavioral therapy for SI and for DO if necessary 2. Add medications: First: estrogen Second: alpha agonists Third: bladder relaxants 3. Devices (see test) If incontinence persists: 4. Refer, if clinically appropriate If not: 5. Undergarments 6. Indwelling catheter	1. Behavioral therapy to improve emptying If incontinence persists: 2. Refer, if clinically appropriate If not: 3. Intermittent catheterization 4. UTI prophylaxis* 5. Undergarments 6. Indwelling catheter

NOTE: Within each group, diagnosis are listed in order of likelihood. Details of each therapy are found in the Specifics of Treatment section
*Only for recurrent symptomatic UTIs and only if an indwelling catheter is not being used.
**BOO is rare in women without prior bladder neck suspension (for example, Marshall-Marchetti, but not including anterior colporrhaphy or anterior repair)
Abbreviations: [DO=Detrusor Overactivity, DHIC=DO with Impaired Contractility, BOO=Bladder Outlet Obstruction, SI=Stress Incontinence, UD=Underactive Detrusor]

Figure 27-1. Stepwise treatment approach for women with persistent incontinence.

step is to determine the most likely type of urinary tract dysfunction that is contributing. As previously discussed, there are only four basic abnormalities—DO, UD, urethral incompetence, and urethral obstruction. Unfortunately, these abnormalities frequently coexist, frustrating the ability to establish a precise diagnosis without sophisticated and largely unavailable testing. However, knowledge of the precise diagnosis is usually not necessary unless invasive intervention such as surgery is desired and appropriate, as it probably is in only 5% to 15% of cases. Instead, empiric therapy can usually be prescribed based on the results of the voiding record, stress test, and PVR determination alone.

The results of these tests enable residents to be assigned to one of eight clinically relevant therapeutic groups, as shown in Figures 27-1 and 27-2. The section on treatment specifics provides details of each therapy. However, no group is homogeneous; each contains residents with more than one diagnosis, as described here. The initial therapeutic approach outlined for each group is appropriate, regardless of the underlying pathophysiology, but consider referring residents for further evaluation when the risk of empiric therapy exceeds the potential benefit, when empiric therapy has failed or might be improved by more precise assessment, or when surgical therapy would be clinically appropriate if a correctable condition were found.

Therapies for Women

In women, the first step is to determine whether stress incontinence is present by using the bladder stress test, and to determine the amount of urine that remains after voiding by measuring the PVR. Theses two tests allow women to be divided into five therapeutically relevant groups. The following subsections decsribe these groups.

BLADDER STRESS TEST

In this test, check for leakage that accompanies an increase in abdominal pressure. Perform the test when the woman has a full bladder, but *not* when she has a sudden or strong urge to void. She should assume a position as close to upright as possible, relax, and either transiently strain or produce a *single* vigorous cough. A positive test is defined as an *instantaneous* spurt of urine that ceases the moment she stops coughing, and that reproduces her symptoms (in a demented woman this may be determined by asking the staff whether she leaks instantaneously when lifted); delay of more than a few seconds or failure to replicate symptoms has the same significance as a negative test. After the test, have the resident void into a receptacle to measure the voided volume. Immediately catheterize the woman for a PVR determination. If the combined volume of the void and the PVR total less than 200 mL—*and* the stress test was negative—fill the bladder with sterile water to at least 200 mL while the catheter is still in place. Remove the catheter and repeat the stress test, since the previously performed test may have been spuriously negative due to an insufficiently filled bladder.

There are several caveats to remember: false-negative tests may occur when the bladder is insufficiently full (i.e., less than 200 mL), when the pelvic floor is not sufficiently relaxed (best checked by observing the resident's buttocks; if they are not sagging, they are not relaxed), when the cough or strain is not vigorous, and when the resident is not upright. False-positive tests tend to occur when the resident experiences a strong urge (a symptom of DO), when a series of coughs is provoked (instead of a single *vigorous* cough), and when delayed leakage is counted as a positive test.

PVR

Because the PVR is the amount of urine that remains in the bladder after a void, it can be measured *only if voiding occurs*. The volume obtained by random catheterization has no significance if it is less than 600 to 700 mL, since a normal bladder may contain that much urine. Optimally, the PVR is measured within 5 to 10 minutes of a void. It is better to obtain the PVR after an intentional void, but measurement after an episode of incontinence is acceptable. Using a sterile technique, a catheter is inserted into the bladder. Gentle pressure over the suprapubic area helps the bladder drain. Do not rush; it can easily take a few minutes to empty the bladder, depending on the caliber of the catheter. Once the flow stops, ask the resident to sit up if possible or to cough or bear down until flow restarts; this is useful because in many elderly people the bladder may be oddly shaped or have diverticula that can hold 50 mL or more. When flow again ceases, slowly withdraw the catheter, pausing each time flow resumes. The risk of introducing an infection from a single catheterization is 2%. Antibiotic coverage is indicated in the presence of cardiac valvular disease, a large joint prosthesis, and when there is a history of endocarditis.

Group 1

Women in this group are most likely to suffer from DO. The small PVR suggests that their overactive bladder is also strong, but a small PVR may be found in women with an overactive but weak bladder (DHIC) if they strain to void. The final consideration, bladder outlet obstruction, is found in no more than 1% to 2% of women in this group; especially at risk are women who have undergone a previous bladder neck suspension (e.g., Stamey, Pereyra, Marshall-Marchetti-Krantz, or Burch procedures, but not an anterior colporrhaphy [also termed an anterior repair or Kelly procedure]).

The cornerstone of treatment for DO is bladder retraining or prompted voiding, depending on the patient's cognitive status (*see* the section on treatment specifics). If this fails or is only partially successful, bladder relaxant therapy may be added. Given the possibility of urethral obstruction, consider referral if a woman develops urinary retention when treated with a bladder relaxant, particularly if she had a prior bladder neck suspension.

For refractory cases of DO, intentionally induce urinary retention bu using larger doses of bladder relaxants; empty the bladder using intermittent or continuous catheterization. This technique frequently works well in community-dwelling elderly, but it is much less well tolerated in the nursing home setting due to the frequency of drug side effects and the unavailability of staff-administered intermittent catheterization. Unless urinary retention has been induced intentionally, an indwelling catheter is relatively contraindicated because it usually exacerbates bladder spasms.

Group 2

The list of possible causes in this group is the same as in group 1, except that DO with a strong bladder is less likely, while DHIC and bladder outlet obstruction are more likely; if used, empiric treatment with bladder relaxant medications must proceed more cautiously. However, whether or not bladder relaxants are employed, augmented voiding techniques may improve bladder emptying and increase the functional bladder capacity in many of these women. If augmented voiding techniques fail, intermittent catheterization can ensure complete emptying and may greatly decrease incontinence. Because the residual urine is not large enough in these women to cause overflow incontinence, catheterization need not be done several times daily; instead, tailor the frequency to the individual's needs.

For instance, if nocturnal incontinence is the most bothersome symptom, a single catheterization at bedtime may be sufficient. Prophylaxis against UTIs is indicated if there are frequent symptomatic infections and an indwelling catheter is not being used.

Group 3

If the PVR was performed immediately after a void, then the markedly elevated PVR most likely is due to DHIC or UD; obstruction is more likely to be present than in the previous two groups, but is still rare in the absence of prior bladder neck suspension. Because it is usually difficult to determine whether the urinary retention is subacute (and therefore potentially due to a reversible precipitant), and because overdistention may further impair bladder function, decompress the bladder with an indwelling catheter for 2 to 4 weeks . After eliminating all precipitants of retention (e.g., anticholinergic medications and fecal impaction), reassess the resident. Refer women with prior urethral suspensions for further evaluation if surgical decompression is clinically appropriate from other standpoints.

Regardless of the cause of the patient's retention, bladder relaxant therapy is contraindicated by the large PVR. If behavioral techniques to improve emptying do not improve symptoms sufficiently, consider intermittent catheterization. If feasible, it is extremely useful, but it usually must be performed several times daily to keep total bladder volume below 400 to 600 mL. An indwelling catheter is the last resort.

Group 4

Most of the women in this group have "genuine stress incontinence," but as many as half may have "mixed incontinence," in which genuine stress incontinence coexists with "urge incontinence" caused by DO. It is useful to differentiate symptomatically between these two groups because the best initial

therapy for women with mixed incontinence is probably that outlined for group 1. For women with stress incontinence alone, several approaches are available, including exercises, medications, and surgery. These approaches also apply to women whose mixed incontinence has not responded to treatment for DO.

The optimal candidate for pelvic muscle exercises is the woman who is cognitively intact and self-motivated; over half of such patients will improve substantially with these exercises, and better results may be possible with the addition of biofeedback or weighted vaginal cones (for the patient with mixed incontinence, add behavioral therapy for DO). Medications that increase urethral alpha-adrenergic tone are of some benefit, as are bladder relaxants for women with mixed incontinence. Other options include tampons and diaphragms, which can increase urethral resistance in some women, and a pessary for women who have uterine prolapse in addition to stress incontinence. Electrical stimulation is still in the experimental stage. If these conservative measures fail, consider surgery since many newer procedures can be performed through a vaginal incision with little morbidity.

Group 5

The most common cause of incontinence in this group is stress incontinence coexisting with a weak bladder. Other possibilities include overflow incontinence (due to bladder weakness or obstruction) and stress incontinence combined with urge incontinence (due to DHIC). Regardless of the cause, maneuvers that reduce the elevated residual urine are often helpful. If the patient can void, she should augment her stream by straining (the Valsalva maneuver) or by pressing on her abdomen (the Crede maneuver). This should be done *only during voiding*. Use of intermittent catheterization will also help emptying, but the frequency of catheterization can be less than that used in group 3 if stress incontinence is present. Women in whom the PVR can be kept below 200 mL are treated like those in group 4, but the risk of exacerbating urinary retention is higher if surgery is performed; the actual risk has not yet been determined.

Therapies for Men

Stress incontinence is very uncommon in men, and causes characteristic leakage when present. Therefore, lower urinary tract dysfunction is generally caused by DO, obstruction, and UD. However, once stress incontinence is ruled out, the approach in institutionalized men depends more on the PVR than on the actual type of dysfunction present (Figure 27-2).

Group 1 (Stress Incontinence)

From a practical standpoint, stress incontinence occurs only in men who have had a previous prostatic resection, and it is unlikely even in these men. In a man, stress incontinence causes a steady drip similar to a leaky faucet when he is in the upright position with a full bladder; overflow incontinence must be excluded by measruring the PVR. If stress incontinence occurs at bladder volumes below 200 mL, the only options are referral or condom catheter draininage. For those who can hold more than 200 mL, conservative management—which requires minimizing the challenge to the sphincter by reducing the PVR (if elevated), increasing voiding frequency, or decreasing excretion—is possible. Exercises to strengthen the sphincter are theoretically useful, but the sphincter is usually so damaged in men with stress incontinence that exercises rarely help. If conservative management fails, consider referral.

Group 2 (PVR Less than 100 mL)

A PVR below 100 mL excludes overflow incontinence, leaving as possibilities only DO and compensated outlet obstruction (with or without DO), in which the PVR is low because the bladder is still able to compensate. Because behavioral intervention is effective for either diagnosis, it is recommended as the first step. If postvoid dribbling incontinence is present, further benefit can be derived from allowing a longer time to void, double voiding (voiding twice each time), and gently milking the urethra after voiding.

If necessary, medications can augment (but not replace) behavioral treatments. However, because of the possibility of obstruction, try using drugs that decrease urethral resistance before other agents in men who have an intact prostate; alpha-adrenergic antagonists are preferable to drugs that induce prostate shrinkage (e.g., 5 reductase inhibitors) because they are at least as effective, and their benefit is apparent in days rather than 6 to 12 months.

If the resident is a candidate for surgical relief of obstruction, refer him for definitive diagnosis and therapy. If he is not a candidate, or if a further drug trial is desired, consider using bladder relaxants. If used, prescribe them in low doses and give them with the realization that urinary retention may ensue, especially in obstructed men. However, retention in such men usually develops over days to weeks and should be detectable early with regular assessment. Accomplish this by bladder palpation or percussion after the resident voids (any degree of palpability is abnormal), corroborated whenever possible by assessment of PVR by catheterization or ultrasound techniques (portable ultrasound machines are available). If symptomatic urinary retention is precipitated before incontinence is adequately controlled, reconsider referral for decompression if an operation would be appropriate should an obstruction be found. If surgery is inappropriate, urinary retention can be perpetuated pharmacologically and accompanied by regular decompression using intermittent or indwelling catheterization. As noted for

First, check for stress incontinence when the patient's bladder is full. Then, observe and measure a void, and immediately determine the residual bladder volume (PVR). If the PVR exceeds 150–200 ml. an ultrasound of the kidneys is *strongly* recommended to rule out hydronephrosis. If present, the resident requires either a referral to a urologist or a permanent indwelling catheter to prevent kidney damage. If there is no hydronephrosis, proceed as below:

Stress Test Positive	Stress Test Negative	Stress Test Negative
Group #1 **Stress Test Positive**	**Group #2** **Men with PVR Less Than 100 ml**	**Group #3** **Men with PVR Greater Than 100 ml,** **Stress Test Negative** **No Hydronephrosis**

If occurs, only at bladder volume greater than 200 ml; decrease bladder volume:
1. To lower PVR if elevated (improving emptying)
2. Increase voiding frequency, if feasible, or
3. Decrease urine production (for example, by fluid restriction but not below 1000 ml per day)
4. Refer, if appropriate
 	
If leakage occurs at lower bladder volume:
1. Refer, if clinically appropriate
2. Condom catheter
	1. Behavioral therapy for DO
	2. Add medications, if necessary:
	  First: alpha blockers
	  Second: bladder relaxants
	
	If incontinence persists:
	3. Refer if clinically appropriate
	
	If not:
	4. Undergarments
	5. Condom catheter
	6. Indwelling catheter
		1. If total bladder volume is greater than 800 ml, or PVR is greater than 500 ml, decompress with indwelling catheter for 2-4 weeks
		2. Refer, if clinically appropriated
		
		If not:
		3. Behavioral therapy for DO
		4. Add medications, if necessary:
		  First: alpha blockers
		  Second: if PVR is less than 200, bladder relaxants but not urecholine
		
		If incontinence persists:
		5. Behavioral therapy for emptying
		6. Intermittent catheterization
		7. Condom catheter
		8. UTI prophylaxis*
		9. Undergarments
		10. Indwelling catheter

Note: Details describing each therapy are in found in the Specifics of Treatment section of the text.

Figure 27-2. Stepwise treatment approach to men with persistent incontinence.

group 1 women, indwelling catheterization is generally inappropriate in the absence of retention.

Group 3 (PVR Greater than 100 mL)

The PVR exceeds 100 mL in only a minority of men, but it suggests that the detrusor is weak, in isolation, or in association with urethral obstruction or DO. Because the risk of urethral obstruction is higher for men in group 3 than in group 2, and because obstruction predisposes to hydronephrosis and renal failure, the first step is to use renal ultrasonography to exclude hydronephrosis in men whose PVR exceeds 150 to 200 mL, especially those with PVRs greater than 250 mL and an unexplained elevation of blood urea nitrogen and creatinine. If hydronephrosis is present, refer the resident for definitive surgical decompression, if appropriate, or have an indwelling catheter placed indefinitely.

The next step is to search for bladder overdistention. Since the bladder normally holds less than 600 to 700 mL, if the total bladder volume (PVR + volume voided) exceeds 800 mL, decompress it for 2 to 4 weeks with an indwelling catheter. This allows bladder strength to recover, permits a search for reversible precipitants (e.g., anticholinergic agents, alpha-adrenergic agonists, and fecal impaction), and facilitates urodynamic testing for men in whom retention persists and such knowledge would be helpful. Guidelines for removing the catheter, following the resident, and referral are found in the section on treatment specifics.

The absence of hydronephrosis and bladder overdistention does not exclude the presence of urethral obstruction, but it permits consideration of a broader range of options:
- Surgical decompression, including less invasive procedures such as transurethral incision of the prostate and insertion of an intraurethral stent
- Bladder retraining and medications (as for men in group 2)

- Intermittent catheterization
- Indwelling catheterization (least desirable because of the increased risk of infection)

Consider UTI prophylaxis for men with a high PVR and frequent symptomatic UTIs. Due to the selection of drug-resistant organisms, UTI prophylaxis is not indicated in the presence of an indwelling catheter.

TREATMENT SPECIFICS

This section details the treatments outlined in the previous section and referred to in Figures 27-1 and 27-2, and it also assumes that serious underlying conditions and transient causes of incontinence have been addressed. It is important to realize that treatment of the nursing home resident must be individualized, not only because factors outside the lower urinary tract so often impact on therapeutic feasibility and efficacy, but also because symptomatic improvement in some residents may be more important than a cure. For instance, although both may have DO, a severely demented and bedfast woman must be treated differently from one who is ambulatory and cognitively intact. Finally, it cannot be overemphasized that successful treatment of established incontinence must be multifactorial, especially in institutionalized elderly.

Behavioral Therapy

There are four types of behavioral therapy: two for DO (depending on the patient's cognition and motivation), a third for stress incontinence, and a fourth for improving bladder emptying (augmented voiding). Some methods, such as bladder retraining, require more effort by the resident, while others, such as prompted voiding for cognitively impaired patients, require more effort by the staff.

Behavioral Treatments to Reduce Detrusor Overactivity

The cornerstone of treatment for DO is behavioral therapy, of which there are two types. For cognitively intact residents, use *bladder retraining*, the goal of which is to increase the voiding interval to 4 hours or more while decreasing the frequency of incontinence or eliminating it entirely. For cognitively impaired residents, use *prompted voiding*. This technique relies on the staff to prompt the resident to void at intervals short enough to preempt leakage.

BLADDER RETRAINING

For cognitively intact and motivated residents, the goal of bladder retraining is to reestablish normal volumes and patterns of voiding by restoring the ability of the brain to control the bladder. This is accomplished by teaching the resident to resist the sensation of urgency, thereby averting leakage and increasing bladder capacity. Continence or major improvement has been achieved in up to 85% of cognitively intact and motivated individuals, but maximal benefit can take up to 2 to 4 months. For residents who experience initial success but relapse in the context of acute illness or depression, use prompted voiding until they recuperate sufficiently to resume bladder retraining.

Success depends on timing as well as resident and staff motivation. Before beginning treatment, residents should have recovered from any intervening acute illnesses, and medications that might interfere with mobility, motivation, or mentation should be discontinued. In addition, the staff need to understand that the goal is to extend the period between voids. This is crucial in the case of residents who require help to toilet because even physically impaired residents can succeed with staff help.

BLADDER RETRAINING PROCEDURE

The steps to bladder retraining are as follows:

1. Examine the voiding record to determine the longest interval between voids that is reproducibly associated with remaining continent; for most residents, this will be between 1 and 3 hours.
2. Instruct the resident to void at this interval, regardless of whether a need is perceived. This should be done *during waking hours only*.
3. Between scheduled voids, residents should suppress precipitant urgency since rushing to the bathroom makes controlling urination more difficult. Instead, they should sit quietly and try to resist the urge. Several methods may help, including relaxation techniques such as deep, slow breathing with eyes closed; imaging the urge as a wave that peaks and then fades away; or adding pelvic muscle exercises (*see* below).
4. Record the progress using a voiding chart and provide positive feedback.
5. After the resident becomes continent for 2 consecutive days at the scheduled interval, *increase* the interval by half an hour (e.g., from 1 to 1.5 hours). After continence is achieved at the new interval, extended it again until continence is achieved with voiding intervals of at least 4 hours.

Tips to keep in mind:

- For residents with deficits in locomotion, transfer, or dressing, staff support must be available at the time of the scheduled toileting.
- Once daytime incontinence improves, nighttime leakage improves as well, even though bladder retraining is not implemented at night.
- If a resident is unable to suppress the urge to void, or if urgency occurs too frequently, consider adding a bladder relaxant medication.

PROMPTED VOIDING

With this technique, cognitively impaired residents are prompted to void at intervals short enough to *preempt* leakage; because of their impaired cognition, no attempt is made to restore normal bladder volumes or voiding patterns. Employ positive behavioral reinforcement; avoid negative reinforcement and comments.

Overall, prompted voiding can reduce the frequency of incontinence in most nursing home residents by at least 50%, and restore daytime continence to approximately 25%. Moreover, residents who will respond to prompted voiding can be identified within a few days. They are the residents who, when asked hourly, can appropriately recognize the intermittent need to void and then urinate into a toilet or commode at least half the time. These residents fall into two groups of roughly equal size according to their baseline frequency of incontinence. Those who leak fewer than four times in a 12-hour daytime period will leak on average less than once with prompted voiding; 60% of these patients (or 25% of all incontinent nursing home residents) will actually become dry for 2 or more consecutive days. Fortunately, as the prompting interval is increased to 2 hours, improvement persists in most of these residents. However, for those who leak more than four times during the 12-hour baseline period, the frequency of incontinence will generally decrease by approximately two episodes with hourly prompted voiding, but they still will be wet more than once daily. Unfortunately, increasing the interval in this group attenuates the benefit. Finally, for the 25% of residents who do not respond to prompting at baseline, little benefit is obtained by further prompting. Note that these results were obtained without adjusting fluid balance, knowledge of urodynamic diagnosis, or prescription of appropriate medication. Response rates may be even better if such measures are added, especially for residents who improve but do not become continent with prompted voiding alone.

Even more than with bladder retraining,

success depends on staff motivation. Since normal bladder function is not restored with prompted voiding, continence depends to a major degree on staff input. Such input includes prompting the resident frequently and dependably, escorting the resident to the toilet or commode if necessary, and providing both positive reinforcement and a positive attitude. The time spent with residents may increase, but it will be offset by the reduced time spent coping with incontinent episodes and their sequelae (e.g., skin rashes and breakdown). In addition, much of the time devoted to toileting can be used to address issues that would otherwise be addressed separately, such as assessment of skin integrity, transferring the patient to a chair, and helping with other activities of daily living (ADLs).

Because continued staff vigilance is so crucial, an effective quality assurance program is critical. Residents who do not respond will need either management by containment devices and a checking and changing protocol, or, if clinically appropriate, further evaluation by a specialist to determine the specific type of incontinence.

PROMPTED VOIDING PROCEDURE

The steps to perform prompted voiding are as follows:

- Plan to start the program during a 3-day period when staffing is full and no interruptions are expected (i.e., not during weekends, holidays, illnesses, or trips outside the facility).
- Every 2 hours during the day (not the night), ask whether the resident is wet or dry. Then check for wetness and provide appropriate verbal feedback, positively reinforcing a correct answer and gently correcting an incorrect one. Avoid disparaging intonations and comments.
- Ask the resident if he or she wants to use the toilet, commode, or urinal; eye contact/touching the resident will increase chances

of correct response.

If yes:

o Offer assistance, if necessary.

o If the resident is able to void, record the amount on the voiding record; otherwise, note failure. Provide positive reinforcement for a successful void or for the attempt; spend an extra minute or 2 talking to the resident.

If no:

o Repeat the question once or twice.

o Tell the resident you will be back in an hour and request that voiding be delayed until then.

o If the resident has not voided in past 2 or 3 attempts, repeat the request to use the toilet.

• For those able to void on more than 50% of the occasions that they feel an urge, and whose incontinence has improved with hourly prompting, increase the prompting interval to 2 hours. If success is maintained, continue to increase the interval up to 4 hours.

• For residents whose incontinence does not decrease with hourly prompts for 3 days, continue to check and change absorbent garments on a less frequent but regular basis.

Keep these tips in mind:

o For residents whose incontinence decreases with hourly checks but relapses with increased intervals, consider adjusting fluid excretion (Section II) and prescribing a bladder relaxant medication.

o For nighttime management use either pads or a condom catheter (for men).

Behavioral Treatment to Strengthen Pelvic Muscles (Kegel Exercises)

Several pelvic muscles contribute to continence, and strengthening them can help prevent urine leakage associated with stress maneuvers such as coughing, laughing, straining, or bending over. Several studies have documented success rates of up to 87% (cure plus improvement) in elderly women. However, since maintenance of muscle strength requires regular exertion, pelvic muscle exercises are appropriate only for cognitively intact residents who are committed to continuing them indefinitely.

PELVIC MUSCLE EXERCISES PROCEDURE

The steps to perform pelvic muscle exercises are as follows:

1. Have the resident lie down in a comfortable position in a private area, with legs, buttocks, and abdomen relaxed.

2. Women should imagine trying to prevent urination by tightening the ring of muscles around the vagina, while men should try to tighten the muscles at the base of the penis. Muscles should be contracted slowly and strongly for 3 to 5 seconds. The resident or a staff member should place a hand on the resident's abdomen to ensure that it is not contracting, and ensure that the resident is not tightening leg or buttock muscles.

3. The resident should repeat the contraction/relaxation cycle 10 times; this is called a set. Repeat the sets 3 to 5 times per day.

Keep these tips in mind:

• Coaching a resident with the exercises is often very helpful. Use a clock for accurate timing, and place a hand on the resident's abdomen to ensure relaxation. Abdominal muscle relaxation is particularly important because abdominal muscle contraction exerts pressure on the bladder and may actually push urine out, making the incontinence worse.

• There are several ways to teach the exercises. One way is to instruct the female resident to try to stop the flow when urinating; she should try this only once or twice rather than making it a regular practice. Another way is to insert into the vagina a lubricated foley catheter with the balloon inflated.

When she contracts her pelvic muscles correctly, the catheter should move an inch or so into the vagina. Another way is to prescribe commercially available weighted vaginal cones, which she tries to retain while walking around. These can be used twice a day for 15-minute sessions; once she can retain the lightest cone, she can progress to the next heavier one. Finally, biofeedback programs can help some patients who may otherwise have trouble; these may be available locally for ambulatory patients.

- Continued benefit requires that the exercises be performed daily and indefinitely.
- Once learned, the exercises can be practiced any time, any place, or in any position. It is particularly useful to do them in situations associated with the resident's leakage such as with straining.

After the resident is comfortable with doing the exercises, he or she can practice them in a variety of places and settings in lying, sitting, and standing positions. Encourage the resident to do the exercise when he or she would ordinarily have an incontinence accident, such as when laughing and coughing.

Behavioral Treatment to Improve Bladder Emptying: Voiding Hygiene

This approach is appropriate to improve bladder emptying for any resident whose PVR exceeds 100 mL. Note that these recommendations rely on common sense rather than tested therapies.

AUGMENTED VOIDING TECHNIQUES TO IMPROVE BLADDER EMPTYING

The steps for augmented voiding techniques to improve bladder emptying are as follows:

1. To improve emptying, both men and women should sit to void, with pelvic, leg, and buttock muscles completely relaxed.
2. Do not rush voiding.
3. After voiding has begun, the resident should either strain gently (Valsalva maneuver) or press gently but firmly on the abdomen (Crede maneuver). These maneuvers increase the pressure in the bladder, but they should be done only when urine is flowing.
4. After voiding has stopped, the resident should remain on the toilet and relaxed for at least a minute. He or she should then double-void, i.e., void again using the same technique to empty the bladder further.
5. Encourage the resident to employ this voiding technique for all voids. Continue the program for 7 to 10 days, retraining the resident as necessary, and monitoring adherence and voiding efficacy. If the resident is unable to follow instructions, or if the PVR is unchanged, stop the program.

Medications Used for Urinary Incontinence

Used alone, medications rarely control incontinence. In fact, incontinent residents are more likely to be improved by adjusting or discontinuing a medication than by adding a new one. However, once other issues and offending agents have been addressed and behavioral interventions initiated, medications can be useful. Like all drugs prescribed for the elderly, start with a low dose, increase slowly, and titrate to balance efficacy against side effects. The following sections describe some of the medications that are used to treat urinary incontinence.

Bladder Relaxants

Drugs can be *added* if bladder retraining or prompted voiding is ineffective, or if the interval required is too short to be feasible. Drugs cannot supplant behavioral therapy because they generally do not abolish uninhibited contractions. Studies of less impaired patients demonstrate restoration of continence in up to half of patients and significant improvement in the remainder. There is a lack

Table 27-5. Bladder Relaxant Medications Used to Treat Urge Incontinence[1]

Medication, Class, Name, and Dosage	Comments
Smooth muscle relaxant Flavoxate, 300-800 mg/day (100-200 mg po tid-qid)[2]	Has not proved effective in placebo-controlled trials
Calcium-channel blocker Diltiazem, 90-270 mg/day (30-90 mg po qd-tid) Nifedipine, 30-90 mg/day (10-30 mg po qd-tid)	No controlled trial data; most useful for the resident with another indication for the drug (e.g., hypertension, angina pectoris, or abnormalities of cardiac diastolic relaxation)
Anticholinergic Propantheline, 15-120 mg/day (15-30 mg po tid-5x/day)[3]	Use with particular caution in demented patients and in patients taking other anticholinergic agents
Combination smooth relaxation and anticholinergic Oxybutynin, 5-20 mg/day (2.5-5 mg po tid-qid)[4] Dicyclomine, 30-90 mg/day (10-30 mg po tid)	These medications, which have a rapid onset of action, can be employed prophylactically if incontinence occurs at predictable times; they can also be used continuously
Antidepressants[5] Doxepin, 50-75 mg/day (10-25 mg po qd-tid) Imipramine, 50-100 mg/day (10-25 mg po dq-qid)	May be particularly helpful in women with coexistent stress incontinence; orthostatic hypotension often precludes their use, but a tricyclic antidepressant may be preferred for a depressed incontinent resident without orthostatic hypotension

[1]All drugs should be started at the lowest dose and increased slowly until encountering the maximum benefit or intolerable side effects. All are given in divided doses, except the antidepressants, which may be given as a single daily dose.

[2]Some uncontrolled reports suggest that doses up to 1200 mg/day may be effective with tolerable side effects; efficacy has not been supported by randomized controlled trials at any dose.

[3]Higher doses are occasionally tolerated and effective; should be given in the fasting state.

[4]May also be applied intravesically in residents who can use intermittent catheterization.

[5]May give as a single daily dose of 25-100 mg.

of data about the efficacy and toxicity of drugs in institutionalized residents, and comparative or controlled trials are rare. Since available studies generally show equivalent results among the agents (except for flavoxate, which fares poorly in controlled trials), the decision about which drug to employ is best based on factors unrelated to bladder function.

Many pharmacologic agents are used as bladder relaxants, but most are either anticholinergics or smooth muscle relaxants (most of the latter are calcium-channel antagonists). Table 27-5 lists specific agents and doses. Occasionally, combining low doses of drugs with different mechanisms—such as oxybutynin and imipramine—maximizes efficacy and minimizes side effects.

Regardless of the agent chosen, start with a small dose, monitor for potential side effects, and only increase the dose to achieve the desired effect. Because urinary retention may develop from using any of these drugs, closely monitor the PVR, especially in patients with a high PVR in whom the detrusor is already weak. Retention rarely develops overnight, so such monitoring may be accomplished by daily abdominal palpation and by review of the resident's or staff's impression about urinary output as well as the resident's sense of bladder fullness or incomplete emptying.

In equivocal cases, corroborate the clinical impression by an ultrasound measurement or catheterization. However, inducing urinary retention and using intermittent catheterization may be a viable approach for patients whose incontinence defies other remedies (such as those with DHIC) and for whom intermittent catheterization is feasible.

Because bladder relaxants decrease bladder contractility, they may paradoxically *decrease* functional bladder capacity by increasing PVR proportionately more than total bladder capacity. Thus, subclinical urinary retention may be heralded by attenuation if not reversal of the drug's beneficial effect. In such cases, measure the PVR. Anticholinergic agents also may exacerbate incontinence by causing mouth dryness, which may lead to excess fluid ingestion; substitute another bladder relaxant in such cases. Finally, because of the increased risk of caries from anticholinergic-induced xerostomia, all dentulous patients on anticholinergic drugs should have regular dental care.

ANTICHOLINERGIC MEDICATIONS (INCLUDING TRICYCLIC ANTIDEPRESSANTS)

Anticholinergic medications are prescribed to inhibit cholinergic-mediated bladder contraction, but none of the currently available agents are geared specificically for the bladder. Side effects are common and include visual blurring, nausea, tachycardia, constipation, and dry mouth; delirium and drowsiness occur less frequently. Anticholinergics are contraindicated by pyloric stenosis, intestinal obstruction, and narrow angle glaucoma but not by the more common open-angle glaucoma.

CALCIUM-CHANNEL BLOCKERS

Calcium-channel blockers hinder the influx of calcium into the detrusor, which impedes contraction. However, like anticholinergic agents, they also act on smooth muscle elsewhere in the body. Side effects vary by agent, but include hypotension, fluid retention, and heart block. Since controlled trials of these agents have not been conducted in any population, these drugs are most used appropriately when there is another indication for them, such as angina or hypertension.

AGENTS WITH MIXED ACTIONS

Side effects of these drugs are similar to those of the anticholinergic agents, but they generally cause less confusion. Oxybutynin may cause more mouth dryness than the others but this effect can be helpful for residents who drool.

Alpha-Adrenergic Agonists

Alpha-adrenergic agents increase smooth muscle tone in the bladder neck and proximal urethra, thereby increasing urethral resistance. The best studied agent is sustained-release phenylpropanolamine, administered in divided doses of 25 to 75 mg twice daily. Hypertension is a relative contraindication to its use, but it has been given safely to younger patients whose blood pressure was under adequate control. Although generally well tolerated in younger subjects, the side effects can include anxiety, insomnia, nightmares, agitation, sweating, and cardiac arrhythmias, which may be more common in institutionalized individuals.

Although not traditional alpha-adrenergic agonists, imipramine and other tricyclic antidepressants have an alpha stimulant, as well as anticholinergic properties. Because of this, they have been used to treat women with mixed incontinence although data from controlled studies are not available. In addition to their anticholinergic actions, the side effects of tricyclic antidepressants include nausea, insomnia, weakness, fatigue, and postural hypotension. They have also been linked to an increased risk of hip fracture, so use them cautiously, especially in residents with orthostatic hypotension. Usual doses are 10 to 25 mg orally four times a day; if well tolerated, they also can be given as a single daily dose of 25 to 100 mg.

Alpha Blockers

Alpha blockers decrease the tone of the smooth muscle at the bladder neck and proximal urethra, thereby decreasing bladder outlet resistance. Alpha blockers have not been studied for use in incontinence, but they have proved moderately effective for symptoms of benign prostatic hypertrophy (BPH).

Prazosin is started at 0.5 mg twice a day and increased to 2 mg twice a day as necessary. Terazosin is started at 1 mg at bedtime and increased to 10 mg as needed. Doxazosin is begun at 1 mg at bedtime, and the dose is doubled as needed up to a total dose of 8 mg. The three agents are equally effective; terazosin and doxazosin have a longer half-life than prazosin; they require less frequent dosing, but they are more expensive. The major undesirable side effect of each agent is profound hypotension and syncope, usually following the first dose. Give the first dose or any increased dose at night, when the resident can remain supine for several hours. Other side effects include postural hypotension, nasal stuffiness, and symptomatic hypotension. Use special care for residents with heart disease, especially those with left ventricular hypertrophy, who may be particularly sensitive to preload reduction.

Estrogen

Estrogen is a major growth and trophic factor for most structures in the female pelvis, including the mucosa and submucosal vasculature of the bladder base and the urethra, smooth and striated muscle of the urethra and pelvic floor, and the surrounding ligaments. Restoring normal levels of circulating estrogen strengthens many tissues, returns mucosal surfaces to a more normal state, and supports growth in the vagina of beneficial flora, such as lactobacilli. Estrogen may have beneficial effects outside the urinary tract as well.

Estrogen deficiency may result in or exacerbate urge and stress incontinence. Therefore, estrogen replacement therapy is suggested for all incontinent women who have signs of inadequate estrogen effect and no contraindication to estrogen use. The side effects include breast tenderness, hot flashes, sweating, and vaginal bleeding on withdrawal of estrogen. Contraindications include known or suspected cancer of the uterus, breast, and cervix. Because of the high prevalence of breast cancer, a manual breast examination is a minimum requirement before initiating therapy; a baseline mammogram is recommended as well.

Orally administered estrogen is usually the best tolerated therapy. It can be given as conjugated equine estrogen (Premarin) in a daily dose of 0.3 to 1.25 mg, but more than 0.6 mg is rarely needed. One approach is to administer it daily for 1 or 2 months, and then taper it by eliminating one pill per week each month. In some residents, estrogen can be stopped completely, while in others it may need to be maintained at a very low dose (0.625 mg twice a week) for an indefinite period. If such women still have a uterus, add a progestational agent. Vaginal creams can be used but they are expensive and messy, and they can be embarrassing for elderly women.

Prostate Involutional Agents

Recently, finasteride (Proscar) became available, and similar agents will soon follow. Finasteride, 5 mg/day, competitively inhibits the enzyme that produces the specific form of testosterone that is active in the prostate. Finasteride has not been used for incontinence, but it is theoretically beneficial for men in whom obstruction from BPH is causing DO. Do not use it in men for urinary retention. Despite its benefits, finasteride has some drawbacks: it is expensive; most men experience no benefit; the benefit is moderate and delayed for 3 to 12 months in those men who do benefit; it has not yet been studied in frail elderly men; and, because discontinuation of the drug results in prostate regrowth and symptom recurrence, it must be continued for life.

The side effects include impotence, decreased libido, and decreased ejaculate volume. Sensitivity to the drug is the only contraindication. Female staff members must be careful when handling the drug, since even small quantities can cause fetal deformity in pregnant women carrying a male fetus. Finasteride suppresses PSA production, which reduces the accuracy of PSA as an indicator of prostate cancer, but the usefulness of PSA screening or monitoring of frail elderly men is not yet established.

Cholinergic Medication

Like other agents in this category, bethanechol stimulates cholinergic receptors in bladder smooth muscle, which potentially increases bladder contractility. Unfortunately, these agents have *not* proved effective in published trials, but they may be helpful when used to counteract the anticholinergic effects of another indicated agent, such as an antidepressant that cannot be discontinued or substituted for a less anticholinergic drug.

The side effects include abdominal cramps, diarrhea, nausea, vomiting, bronchial constriction, sweating, salivation, flushing, hypotension and cardiac arrest; atropine is the antidote. Contraindications include obstruction of the gastrointestinal or urinary tract, hyperthyroidism, peptic ulcer disease, latent or active asthma, seizure disorder, bradycardia, vasomotor instability, atrioventricular conduction defects, and hypotension. Bethanechol is given orally, 10 to 50 mg two to four times per day.

Catheters

A catheter is indicated when other measures fail to control incontinence adequately, when precise knowledge of urinary output is crucial (e.g., in pulmonary edema), when a pressure ulcer will not heal in the presence of urine, and when comfort measures require one in the terminally ill patient. Condom catheters are useful for men in whom urinary retention has been excluded, while intermittent or indwelling catheters are useful for men with otherwise untreatable urinary retention with symptoms of hydronephrosis, and for patients of either gender in whom an external catheter is not feasible. An external catheter has recently been devised for institutionalized women but has not yet been widely tested or marketed.

Condom Catheters

Condom catheters are external collection devices made of latex, vinyl, or silicone. They are connected via a tube to an external bag and secured to the penis with a built-in adhesive, an external strap, or a strap with double-sided adhesive. Because they tend to dislodge easily, they are often secured too tightly. Avoid this practice when they are used, and use them for the minimum time possible (e.g., at night only). Other guidelines for indwelling catheters apply, such as the need to keep the drainage bag in a dependent position, to avoid kinking or clamping of the tubing, and to keep the bag clean by daily rinsing in antiseptic solution (*see* the section on indwelling catheter for more information). Also check the penis at least daily, and promptly address any problem. However, even when used carefully, condom catheters cause frequent complications, including urethral obstruction (when they kink), UTI, mechanical friction, contact dermatitis (from the condom or adhesive), and penile maceration and ischemia. Because they cannot decompress an overdistended bladder, condom catheters are contraindicated for men with urinary retention.

Intermittent Catheterization

Intermittent catheterization (IC) consists of inserting and removing a catheter to drain the bladder on a regular schedule, usually several times daily. Consider IC for residents in whom incomplete bladder emptying contributes to or causes incontinence. Because its complication rate is lower than that associated with an indwelling catheter, IC is preferable when feasible. Studies of IC suggest that age alone is not a barrier, but there are few and limited studies of institutionalized elderly available.

The success of IC rests on selecting an appropriate schedule. For a resident whose PVR is 500 mL and whose incontinence occurs only at night when decreased voiding frequency causes urine production to exceed the bladder's reduced functional capacity, a single catheterization at bedtime may be sufficient to restore continence. For another resident, who may be able to use a urinal throughout the night but be unable to get to the bathroom while at activities during the day, IC once after breakfast may restore continence and independence. However, for residents with overflow incontinence, IC may be required every 3 to 8 hours, depending on the volume of urine production. Develop an appropriate schedule by examining the voiding record and scheduling catheterization before the usual time of leakage.

It is appropriate to teach self-catheterization to cognitively intact residents, but the staff must be available and willing to perform the procedure for the remainder. IC can be performed using the clean technique, when multiple caregivers are involved. However, owing to the high prevalence of virulent bacteria in nursing home settings, it may be prudent to use a sterile procedure despite its increased cost.

The side effects of IC include urethritis, UTI, urethral stricture formation, and epididymitis. IC is relatively contraindicated for residents at particular risk for the complications of transient bacteremia; such patients include those with joint or cardiac valve prostheses, or immunosuppression.

Indwelling Catheter

In many, if not most, residents with an indwelling (Foley) catheter, the reason for its placement is usually obscure. Because urinary retention owing to either detrusor areflexia or inoperable urethral obstruction affects fewer than 10% of nursing home residents, caregivers should question the continued need for such a catheter, which is often appropriately placed during hospitalization for an acute illness but never removed. Occasionally, a resident or family member expresses a preference for a catheter, but agree to this only after the resi-

Table 27-6. Removing an Indwelling Urethral Catheter.[1]

1. Correct reversible causes or urinary retention: fecal impaction; pelvic/perineal pain; and use of anticholinergic, alpha-adrenergic agonist, or calcium-channel blocker medications. If an anticholinergic antidepressant/antipsychotic agent cannot be discontinued, consider switching to one with less or no anticholinergic side effects, or consider adding bethanechol. Addition of an alpha adrenoreceptor antagonist may be helpful, but this is unproven in women.

2. Treat delirium, depression, atrophic vaginitis, or UTI, if present.
3. Record urinary output at intervals of 6 to 8 hours for 2 days to establish a pattern of baseline urine excretion.
4. Remove the catheter at a time that permits accurate recording of uring output and allows for postvoiding recatheterization; clamping the catheter before removal is not necessary and can be dangerous.
Reinsert the catheter *only*
   o After the resident voids, to determine PVR volume
   o After the expected bladder *volume* (based on urine output)—not the time since the catheter was removed—exceeds a preset limit (e.g., 600 to 800 mL)
   o If the resident is uncomfortable and unable to void despite ensured privacy and maneuvers performed to encourage voiding (e.g., running water, tapping suprapubic area, or stroking inner thigh)
5. If the resident voids and the PVR volume is:
   o Greater than 400 mL, reinsert the catheter and evaluate further, if appropriate.[2]
   o Less than 100 to 400 mL, watch for delayed retention and evaluate further, if appropriate.[2]
   o Less than 100 mL, watch for delayed retention.
If the resident is unable to void, refer for evaluation if appropriate.[2] If not, the resident requires permanent catheterization.

[1]*Modified from* Resnick NM: Incontinence. In Beck JC, ed: *Geriatric Review Syllabus.* American Geriatrics Society, 1991; 141-154.

[2]Further evaluation is appropriate when the resident and physician feel that if a surgically correctable condition were found (e.g., urethral obstruction), an operation would be preferable to chronic catheterization or the other options described in the text.

dent and caregivers fully understand the risks. Table 27-6 provides the guidelines for removing a catheter.

For the resident in whom an indwelling catheter is appropriate, guidelines for catheter care are detailed in Table 27-7. However, even with the best of care, catheter complications are numerous, and include chronic colonization with urinary pathogens, increased incidence of UTI and urosepsis, bladder spasms, and frequent blockage. Less frequent problems include erosive hypospadias, urethral stricture, hemorrhagic cystitis, increased formation of bladder stones, cancer, and erosion of the bladder neck resulting in loss of the internal sphincter. Another complication is the urethral trauma that results from self-removal of a catheter while the balloon is still inflated, as well as the complications associated with the restraining devices subsequently used to prevent recurrence.

Table 27-7. Principles of Indwelling Catheter Care.[1]

Maintain a sterile, closed-gravity drainage system:
*   Secure the catheter to the upper thigh or lower abdomen to avoid urethral irritation and contamination. Rotate the site of attachment every few days.
*   Empty the bag every 8 hours.
*   Do not routinely irrigate the catheter.
*   Do not clamp or kink the drainage tubing, and keep the urine collection bag below bladder level at all times.
*   Avoid frequent cleaning of the urethral meatus; washing with soap and water once daily is sufficient; periurethral application or microbial creams is ineffective.

If leaking around the catheter (bypassing) occurs in the absence of obstruction, it is likely due to a bladder spasm, which can be minimized by using the smallest balloon that will keep the catheter in place and by treating with a bladder relaxant medication if necessary.

Infection prophylaxis (e.g., with mandelamine or antibiotics), as well as treating asymptomatic bacteriuria, is fruitless and usually leads to the emergence of resistant organisms.

Surveillance cultures are unnecessary and potentially misleading since bacteriuria is universal, frequently changing, and often polymicrobial.

If symptomatic UTI develops, change the catheter before obtaining a culture specimen (cultures obtained through the old catheter may reflect organisms colonizing encrustations rather than the infecting organism). Pending culture results, antibiotic treatment should include coverage for common uropathogens as well as uncommon ones such as *Providencia stuartii* and *Morgana morganii*.

If catheter obstruction occurs frequently, and urine cultures reveal *P. Stuartii* or *Proteus mirabilis*, antibiotic treatment may reduce the frequency of obstruction but induces emergence of resistant organisms. In the absence of such urea-splitting organisms, consider urine acidification if urine output is normal (at low output, acidification may increase blockage due to uric acid crystals). If frequent blockage persists, consider using a silicon catheter.

In the absence of obstruction and symptomatic UTI, there is no consensus on the best time to change the catheter. Some residents form material that frequently clogs the lumen; change their catheters often to reduce such obstruction. Other residents can use the same catheter for years, but it is customary to change it every 1 to 2 months. For residents who are difficult to catheterize, change the catheter less frequently if it remains patent and free of complications.

1*Adapted from* Resnick NM: Voiding dysfunction and urinary incontinence. In Beck JC, ed: *Geriatric Review Syllabus*. American Geriatrics Society. 1991; 144-154.

Absorbent Undergarments and Pads

Absorbent pads and undergarments are appropriately used during the evaluation of incontinence and initiation of treatment, as well as when incontinence proves refractory to other measures. The wide array of available products permits incontinence to be managed in an acceptable manner and skin integrity to be maintained. Available items include disposable underwear inserts, inserts for specially designed and reusable briefs, disposable diaperlike undergarments, and absorbable bed sheets. Many are gender-specific, and some are designed to deal with fecal incontinence as well. In addition, products vary in their absorbency, bulk, and cost. The best results are obtained when selection is tailored to the resident's condition, since one size does not fit all. Help for Incontinent People (HIP, PO Box 544, Union, South Carolina 29379) publishes a helpful catalog of available pads and undergarments.

There are several factors to consider when choosing a product, including the resident's gender, mobility, mentation, manual dexterity, ability to change the garment, type of incontinence, frequency and amount of urine lost, whether normal voiding is still possible, and whether fecal incontinence is also present. Whichever product is chosen, check it on a scheduled program and change it as necessary to prevent skin breakdown.

Prevention of Symptomatic Urinary Tract Infections

Symptomatic UTIs are a common source of morbidity and mortality among nursing home residents, but their frequency can be reduced in many residents and abolished in some. The first step is to identify and address the reversible factors, including atrophic vaginitis and incomplete bladder emptying. For residents who continue to have frequent *symptomatic* UTIs but *do not use an indwelling* catheter, UTI prophylaxis can be achieved using either an antiinfective agent such as methenamine or an antibiotic given in low dose. However, use of the latter can result in selection of resistant organisms and may result in more serious infections.

Methenamine (Mandelamine) is contraindicated in dehydration, renal insufficiency, and hepatic insufficiency; side effects include headache, rash, nausea, vomiting, diarrhea, abdominal cramps, hematuria, dysuria, bladder irritation, and elevation of serum transaminases. The dose of methenamine hippurate (Hiprex) is 1 g twice a day; the dose of methamine mandelate (Mandelamine) is 0.5 to 1 g four times a day. Since both drugs require acid catalysis to be converted to their active form, both must be given with sufficient ascorbic acid to acidify the urine (generally, at least 500 mg–1 g ascorbic acid four times a day). For the low-dose antibiotic regimen, administer the antibiotic at half the usual dose, and swtich the agent every month.

For residents using intermittent catheterization who suffer from recurrent symptomatic infections, bacteriuria also may be reduced through instillation of various solutions, including neomycin and polymyxin. For residents who *do use an indwelling catheter*, antibiotic prophylaxis is fruitless since bacteriuria is not abolished, symptomatic UTI and urosepsis are not reduced, and growth of more resistant organisms is encouraged. Moreover, antiinfective agents such as methenamine are ineffective even in the presence of acid urine since, in the presence of an indwelling catheter, they are in contact with bladder mucosa for too brief a time.

CASE EXAMPLE

An 84-year-old woman was admitted to the nursing home following hospitalization for a hip fracture, which had been complicated by confusion. Previously living at home, she has had type 2 diabetes mellitus for 20 years as well as hypertension. Her initial Minimum Data Set assessment suggested the need for further evaluation using the Resident Assessment Protocols for Delirium, Mood, Incontinence, and Rehabilitation. Care plans were initiated for ADL and Mood. Both the Delirium and Incontinence chapters suggested checking for a UTI: when tests disclosed 10⁵ *Escherichia coli* and hyperglycemia of 350, sulfamethoxazole/trimethoprim was started twice a day, and small doses of insulin were substituted temporarily for her oral hypoglycemic agent until the UTI—and its exacerbation of her diabetes—subsided. The suggested medication review identified several drugs that might be variously contributing to delirium and incontinence: two benzodiazepines (one used for sleep and one for agitation), a narcotic analgesic for pain, both a loop diuretic and an alpha-adrenergic antagonist for hypertension, and an anticholinergic antipsychotic agent. Each drug was eliminated. A thiazide diuretic, (acetaminophen), and a calcium-channel blocker were substituted for the necessary agents while the benzodiazepines and the antipsychotic, prescribed for her acute illness in the hospital, were discontinued without substitution. Within a week, the UTI, delirium, and excess urine output from poorly controlled diabetes had all been identified and treated, and five potentially contributing medications had been discontinued.

Since her incontinence persisted, albeit improved, in the second week, a nurse performed a digital rectal examination, which disclosed fecal impaction. Following disimpaction, several enemas, and adding fiber to her diet, incontinence improved still further. By now, efforts to restore her ADLs had begun to succeed, so that she could transfer with the help of one person, and sit for several hours each day.

In the third week an examination by her primary care physician excluded obvious underlying neurologic problems, but disclosed atrophic vaginitis. Since her breast examination was normal and she had no personal history of breast or endometrial cancer, oral estrogen was started. By the end of the third week, delirium had cleared, the UTI had resolved, the benzodiazepines (and other medications) had been eliminated from her body, her bowels were moving regularly, her mood had improved, her diabetes was controlled without insulin, and she could walk short distances with a walker and an assistant.

However, since the voiding record documented incontinence three times a day, further evaluation was undertaken to determine the cause. Her nurse coordinated the stress test and PVR determination for a time that she usually was able to void. The bladder stress test—performed just before voiding while she stood at her bedside—was negative. Immediately following the void, catheterization disclosed 200 mL of clear, amber residual urine. Thus she fit into incontinence group 2 (for women), with the most likely diagnosis being DHIC. Since her acute illness–associated confusion had resolved, bladder retraining was initiated. A month later, she could wait 3 to 4 hours between voids, and she became consistently continent.

28
Bowel Disorders

Danielle Harari, MD
Pauline Belleville-Taylor, RN, MS, CS
Steven Littlehale, MS, RN, C, CS

Constipation is a common complaint among elderly nursing home residents. Laxatives are administered frequently although they are often not required. Severe constipation can have serious consequences if left untreated. Fecal incontinence is often secondary to constipation and generally responds to treatment. However, evaluation may reveal other, less remediable causes. This chapter discusses the patterns and causes of constipation and fecal incontinence, how to identify residents who require intervention, and how to develop individualized treatment plans based on these findings.

OVERVIEW

Constipation is defined as passing two or fewer bowel movements per week and/or straining more than one in four times when having a bowel movement. Elderly residents often have misperceptions of a normal bowel pattern, and many complain of constipation without fitting this criteria. As a result, laxatives may be prescribed unnecessarily.

Excessive laxative use can cause abdominal bloating and cramps, electrolyte distur-

bances, watery stools, fecal incontinence, diarrhea, and eventually lower bowel dysmotility (altered motility) resulting in true clinical constipation. In turn, untreated true clinical constipation can cause fecal impaction with bowel obstruction, abdominal discomfort, anorexia, and incontinence of feces and urine.

Fecal incontinence is defined as the loss of stool per rectum at inappropriate times, and is often a secondary effect of constipation. Fecal incontinence can increase the risk of development of pressure ulcers and can cause considerable psychological distress to residents and their families.

Patterns of Constipation

There are four patterns of constipation that are found in infirm elderly nursing home residents:

- *Slow transit constipation,* when residents report two or fewer bowel movements per week. Fecal retention is seen in the colon (mainly distally) with a plain abdominal radiograph. This retention is often due to secondary causes such as physical immobility and medications (e.g., antidepressants and neuroleptics with anticholinergic properties, calcium channel blockers, iron supplements, narcotics).

- *Difficulty with rectal emptying* (rectal dyschezia), when residents often report chronic straining, and when the colon is empty of stool but the rectum is full. This difficulty may be due to ignoring the original urge to move the bowels, as in cases of dementia and depression.

- *Fecal impaction with symptoms of colonic obstruction,* when residents present with abdominal pain and distention, vomiting, fever, and with distended bowel and fluid levels seen on a plain abdominal radiograph. This is often associated with acute illness (e.g., systemic infection, acute stroke, myocardial infarction) and dehydration.

- *Cathartic colon, with a distended, noncontracting colon* seen on barium enema. This is often secondary to the prolonged use of stimulant laxatives or constipating drugs such as neuroleptics with anticholinergic properties.

Patterns of Fecal Incontinence

The four patterns of fecal incontinence found in elderly nursing home residents are as follows:

- *Weakened external sphincter,* which causes the continence mechanism to be overwhelmed by soft stool or diarrhea. This is often due to local nerve damage from prolonged straining at stool and/or vaginal delivery (therefore, this is more common in older women), or in some cases to spinal cord dysfunction. An age-related decline in muscle strength may also be a factor.

- *Fecal soiling secondary to fecal impaction,* which is commonly caused by rectal dyschezia with impaction even though the defecation mechanism remains intact.

- *Anorectal pathology,* which damages the anal sphincters so that they cannot be controlled voluntarily. This may be due to rec-

tal prolapse, tumor, or anal surgery.

- *Dementia-related incontinence* (neurogenic disinhibited rectum), resulting from the external sphincter no longer being inhibited by the brain, so the rectum is emptied whenever it is full, usually after a meal (due to the gastrocolic reflex).

Causes of Constipation and Fecal Incontinence

Constipation is the most common cause of fecal incontinence, with either or both conditions often having more than one underlying cause. Typical causative factors include:

- *Mechanical conditions.* Tumor, rectal prolapse, painful hemorrhoids, gut surgery.

- *Medications.* Excessive use of laxatives; polypharmacy (e.g., antidepressants and neuroleptics with anticholinergic properties, calcium-channel blockers, iron supplements, narcotics, diuretics, aluminum antacids).

- *Impaired cognition.* Dementia, depression, poor motivation.

- *Immobility or lack of exercise.* Affects bowel mobility as well as toileting abilities.

- *Other factors.* Acute illness, dehydration, Parkinson's disease, spinal cord problems, hypothyroidism.

IDENTIFYING THE RESIDENT REQUIRING A CARE PLAN

To identify residents requiring a constipation/fecal incontinence care plan, first obtain a history of the problem to confirm that the resident requires a care plan. Ask the following questions:

- Is the constipation or fecal incontinence new?

- Is there a history of laxative use, long-term history of intermittent constipation or diarrhea (irritable bowel syndrome), difficult vaginal deliveries, prolonged straining, or anorectal surgery?

- Was a therapeutic care plan previously implemented? If so, what worked? What did not work?

- When were curative approaches last attempted?
- Were all of the current reversible causes previously addressed?

Consider a constipation/fecal incontinence care plan for any resident who complains of, or is observed to have, any of the following conditions:

- Constipation
- Straining at stool
- Fecal soiling or fecal incontinence
- Unexplained abdominal discomfort
- Vomiting

Further assessment of the resident should include a history of the problem, a physical evaluation, and a laboratory evaluation.

Physical Evaluation

The next step in constipation/fecal incontinence care planning is a physical evaluation, which should include the following assessment steps:

- Maintain and continue a stool diary for at least 14 days to confirm constipation or diarrhea and to establish current bowel pattern.
- Observe fecal incontinence or soiling, straining, and stool characteristics (i.e., consistency, color, blood, mucus).
- Assess for the presence of abdominal pain and distention or rectal pain on defecation.
- Evaluate and remove any physical barriers to toilet access.
- Conduct a digital rectal examination to check for the presence of perianal fecal soiling, fecal impaction of the rectal ampula, hemorrhoids, anal fissure, rectal prolapse, or tumor. If a rectal lesion is found, it must be evaluated. Otherwise, proceed to the next section.
- Conduct a mental state examination (i.e., mood, cognition) to assess the level of cognitive impairment.

Treat any identified problems at any point

in the evaluation process.

Laboratory Evaluation

Laboratory evaluation is done when weight loss, fatigue, pallor, dehydration, fever, lethargy, or delirium occur. In the presence of constipation or fecal incontinence, evaluate and treat any systemic symptoms as appropriate. The following list describes the specific laboratory tests and criteria:

- *Plain abdominal radiography* to assess the extent and distribution of constipation and dilation of the bowel. Perform radiography:
  - o In high-risk residents (with a previous history of impaction and/or one or more risk factors for constipation—*see* the section on causes of constipation and fecal impaction) to look for fecal impaction
  - o When there are signs of a high impaction (abdominal distention, fevers, delirium)
  - o When constipation is refractory to treatment
  - o When diarrhea lasts more than 3 days, or less if vomiting or abdominal distention are present
- *Stool culture, including Clostridium difficile,* to look for an infective cause of diarrhea in:
  - o A resident recently on antibiotic therapy
  - o A resident with diarrhea lasting longer than 3 days
- *White blood cell count.* An elevated white blood cell count may indicate fecal impaction, and/or bacterial enteritis.
- *Stool guaiac* (from an evacuated sample) to check for gastrointestinal bleeding and the presence of internal or external hemorrhoids.
- *Thyroid function tests* to check for hypothyroidism, which can cause constipation or hyperthyroidism resulting in weight loss and diarrhea.
- Perform the laboratory tests listed in Table 28-1 when any of the following are present:
  - o A new onset of constipation

Table 28-1. Laboratory tests for constipation/fecal incontinence

Test	Results
Serum biochemistry	Elevated blood urea nitrogen/creatinine ratio (>25) is indicative of dehydration, either causing constipation or resulting from diarrhea
Calcium	High serum calcium (>10.5 mmol/L) is indicative of hypercalcemia causing constipation
Complete blood count iron studies	Iron deficiency anemia may be indicative of tumor, bowel ischemia, or diverticulitis
Sigmoidoscopy	To check for colitis, presence of tumor

- o Constipation that has not responded to treatment
- o Diarrhea that has lasted for more than 3 days
- o Any other physical or mental symptoms outside the gut (e.g., mental status change, change in ability to ambulate)
- o Bloody diarrhea
- *Barium enema or colonoscopy* (depending on clinical decisions) to look for a tumor, ischemic bowel disease, inflammatory bowel disease, or cathartic colon when:
  - o Diarrhea is of recent onset and persistent
  - o Constipation is refractory to treatment in the absence of other risk factors
  - o There are systemic symptoms (e.g., weight loss)
  - o The presence of iron deficiency anemia not attributed to other causes
- *Anorectal pressure studies* when there is persistent fecal incontinence in the absence of severe dementia.

DEVELOPING THE CARE PLAN

In many residents, constipation and/or fecal incontinence have one or more potentially reversible causes. To identify and treat reversible causes, follow these suggested guidelines:

- Treat all potentially reversible causes simultaneously.
- Follow the progress of therapy though a stool diary of direct observation of the resident's stool output. The diary may be maintained by the resident or staff, as appropriate. If constipation resolves during the course of care, consider discontinuing any ongoing laxative or enema treatment or change to "as needed" therapy.
- If constipation (as assessed by abdominal radiograph) or fecal incontinence persists after all reversible causes are treated, consider further medical assessment (e.g., barium enema, anorectal pressure studies).

To determine an appropriate plan of care for the individual resident, follow these steps:

- Step 1: For the resident who complains of constipation or in whom constipation is not confirmed:
  - *For the resident who complains of constipation*: Determine the resident's bowel pattern by reviewing results of the stool diary (2 weeks minimum), nursing observation notes (3 days minimum and continue for 2 weeks total), rectal examination, and plain abdominal radiography, when appropriate.
  - *If constipation is not confirmed*: Educate the resident (and family as appropriate) about normal bowel frequency in the elderly. This means more than two bowel movements a week, and less than three bowel movements a day. Encourage evacuation without straining. Frequency will be determined by the resident's bowel pattern (established by the stool

diary). Discontinue use of laxatives or enemas.

o *If constipation is confirmed or the resident has fecal incontinence,* proceed to step 2.

- Step 2: If the resident is constipated or has fecal incontinence:

o Review for and treat potentially reversible causes as described in the following section.

o If constipation or fecal incontinence persists following treatment, or reversible causes are not found, proceed to step 3.

- Step 3: Review for serious conditions that cause constipation or fecal incontinence:

o Review the section on care planning for serious conditions requiring review of constipation or fecal incontinence.

o If constipation or fecal incontinence still persists, proceed to step 4.

- Step 4: Develop a treatment plan for persistent constipation or fecal incontinence (i.e., other causes do not exist or have been treated):

o Review the section on care planning for persistent constipation.

o Review the section on care planning for persistent fecal incontinence.

CARE PLAN FOR REVERSIBLE CAUSES OF CONSTIPATION AND FECAL INCONTINENCE

The following sections describe care plans for the reversible causes of constipation and fecal incontinence, the conditions that inhibit rectal evacuation, and the conditions that cause increased stool production.

Conditions that Slow Transit Through the Colon and Rectum

Start treatment when the resident has symptoms of constipation and plain abdominal radiography shows fecal retention in the colon. The following subsections describe conditions that have constipation as a symptom and the methodologies for them.

Immobility

Encourage daily activity within the limits of the functional disabilities. An upright posture alone (in immobile residents) can stimulate gut motility.

Dehydration

Encourage a minimum daily fluid intake of 1500 mL unless medical restrictions apply (*see* Chapter 24, Dehydration, for more information). Increase the minimum daily fluid intake to 2 L during the summer or when additional losses are noted (e.g., polyuria associated with diabetes mellitus or vomiting). Diuretics may precipitate dehydration. When poor fluid intake is associated with acute illness, consider subcutaneous or intravenous hydration. Fecal impaction can develop up to 6 weeks following an episode of dehydration.

Low-Fiber Diet

Increased dietary fiber is recommended for residents who are mobile and able to drink at least 1500 mL of fluid a day. Mix bran with apple sauce to make it more palatable. Residents may complain of bloating and flatulence for the first 2 to 3 weeks of bran intake, but these symptoms should resolve with regular intake. Bran is especially useful in residents with constipation and diverticulosis (seen on a barium enema). However, too much bulk in the diet of immobile residents can promote fecal impaction due to the inability to propel the colonic contents downward. A dietitian should consult with the resident to discuss food preferences and suggest high-fiber alternatives. If residents have low iron or calcium levels, cook their bran. Fruit and vegetables are also high in fiber.

Medication Prescription Pattern

Review the following medications for any possible constipating effects:

- Antihistamines (e.g., Benadryl). Avoid regular use or as a nighttime sedative.

- Antidepressants (e.g., amitriptyline, nortriptyline). Use antidepressants that have less anticholinergic properties.
- Antipsychotics (e.g., Haldol, Mellaril). Decrease use, or use antipsychotics with fewer anticholinergic properties.
- Narcotics (e.g., codeine, morphine, Dilaudid, Darvon). If nonnarcotic analgesics do not provide sufficient pain relief, ensure increased fluid intake and consider a laxative regimen to prevent fecal impaction (*see* the section on care planning for persistent constipation).
- Calcium-channel blockers (e.g., verapamil, nifedipine, nimodipine, nicardipine, diltiazem). Verapamil is the most constipating. Consider a laxative regimen to prevent fecal impaction.
- Antispasmodics (e.g., Donnatal, Bentyl). These drugs are of little benefit to residents with irritable bowel syndrome and may increase abdominal cramps by causing constipation.
- Antidiarrheals (e.g., loperamide, kaolin, morphine, bismuth). These drugs may cause functional obstruction of the bowel and fecal impaction in residents. Avoid using them for more than 48 hours (for exceptions, *see* the section on care planning for persistent fecal incontinence).
- Disopyramide (Norpace).
- Ferrous sulfate and gluconate. Ensure an increased fluid intake and a laxative regimen to prevent impaction if the assessment shows persistent constipation. Stop the laxative therapy after iron supplementation is discontinued.
- Antacids (e.g., aluminum hydroxide, calcium carbonate). Reduce the dosage or administer an alternative, such as sucralfate.

PARKINSON'S DISEASE

Constipation is the most common complaint of residents with Parkinson's disease. Ensure a good fluid intake. Constipation should also improve by using medications such as Sinemet. However, anticholinergic drugs (e.g., Benztropine) can worsen constipation even if they are used occasionally.

Hypercalcemia

This condition is indicated by elevated serum calcium (greater than 10.5 mg/dL). Determine the cause and treat accordingly. Hyperparathyroidism and metastatic cancer are some of the more common causes of hypercalcemia.

Hypokalemia

This condition is indicated by lowered serum potassium (less than 3.5 mg/dL). Review the sources of potassium loss (e.g., urine); treat the condition or remove the cause of potassium loss. Add a potassium supplement to the diet if needed. Intestinal transit time should return to normal when laboratory levels are within normal limits.

Hypothyroidism

Residents may complain of constipation as a presenting symptom. Intestinal transit time should return to normal when laboratory levels are within normal limits on thyroxine replacement (i.e., Synthroid).

Diabetes Mellitus

Intestinal transit may be slowed throughout the gut, secondary to damage to the autonomic nervous system. In the presence of dehydration and acute illness, constipation may be severe. Good fluid intake is essential with control of blood sugar for prevention. Diabetic patients may also have fecal incontinence at night due to an overgrowth of bacteria in the slowed-down gut.

Long-Term Laxative Use

Long-term use (i.e., 10 or more years of daily use) of stimulant laxatives such as senna, bisacodyl, cascara, or castor oil may damage the nerves supplying the lower gut and result in slower transit. Discontinue all stimulant laxatives and start an alternative laxative and enema regimen if constipation persists.

Limited Mobility/Limited Use of Hands

These conditions may affect the resident's access to the bathroom and his or her ability to use the toilet.

Lack of Toilet Access/Privacy

Fear of being interrupted (e.g., by using shared bathrooms) may inhibit defecation and lead to rectal impaction.

Conditions that Inhibit Rectal Evacuation

Start treatment when the resident has symptoms of constipation, particularly straining during bowel movements and the digital rectal examination reveals the presence of stool (in the absence of fecal loading of the colon on plain abdominal radiography). The following subsections describe conditions that have inhibited rectal evacuation as a symptom and the treatment methodologies for them.

Dementia

Residents with dementia ignore or are unable to communicate the urge to defecate due to cognitive impairment. Encourage daily toileting 30 minutes after breakfast to take advantage of the colon emptying reflex that occurs in response to eating.

Depression

Distinguish between the morbid preoccupation with bowels as a symptom of depression and true constipation. Antidepressant drugs may cause constipation, even though the resident's motivation may improve.

Neurologic and Muscular Causes

Weakness of the external sphincter (especially in elderly women) in association with weakness of the abdominal muscles may cause prolonged straining during bowel movements. Elevation of the legs onto a footstool during defecation may make evacuation easier by allowing more efficient use of the abdominal muscles during the Valsalva maneuver.

Medication Prescription Pattern

Medications that cause sedation (e.g., antidepressants, antipsychotics, benzodiazepines, antihistamines) may reduce the sensation of a need to defecate, the motivation to go to the bathroom, or the ability to toilet independently. Reduce the dosages of these medications to promote defecation.

Anorectal Disease

Review anorectal diseases for the following possibly inhibiting effects:
- Painful anal conditions (e.g., hemorrhoids, anal fissure). Treat with anesthetic gel along with specific therapies (e.g., Anusol HC cream or suppositories).
- Anorectal cancer, which may cause bleeding and obstruction.

Conditions that Cause Increased Stool Production

Start treatment when the resident has loose stool or diarrhea associated with incontinence. The following subsections describe conditions that cause increased stool production resulting in incontinence and the treatment methodologies for them.

Gastroenteritis

Viral gastroenteritis occurs sporadically in nursing homes, but usually does not cause constitutional malaise or diarrhea lasting more than 48 hours. Treat by giving additional fluids. Use antidiarrheal medications sparingly (i.e., not more than two doses a day). To treat more severe cases, *see* the next section.

Fecal Impaction

Hard, retained stool irritates the gut mucosa, causing it to overproduce mucus, which may result in fecal staining or incontinence. Treatment of impaction should resolve the fecal leakage. The treatment for impaction is discussed in the section on care planning for persistent constipation.

Excessive Laxative Use

Excessive laxative use is defined as regular use in the absence of constipation. Residents may be overmedicated with laxatives, with resultant looseness of stool and incontinence. Discontinue laxative therapy if there is no impaction and start regular bowel reviews, which should consist of a weekly stool inquiry by the staff or the maintenance of a stool chart for residents with poor memory or impaired communication skills.

Medication Prescription Pattern

Review the following medications for possible loose stool or diarrhea-producing side effects:

- Antacids (e.g., magnesium hydroxide, magnesium sulfate, sodium sulfate, citrate-containing antacids).
- Digoxin and theophylline. Check drug levels for toxicity.
- Broad-spectrum antibiotics. Due to bacterial overgrowth, perform a culture stool for *C. difficile*.

Tube Feedings

For liquid diet supplements, such as Ensure, the recommended treatment is to dilute feedings or to change the rate of feeding.

Malabsorption

Malabsorption occurs with diabetes mellitus and postgastrectomy syndrome. An overgrowth of bacteria in the gut secondary to the slowing of intestinal transit causes diarrhea that is often associated with incontinence. The first line of treatment is to use Reglan. The second line of treatment for severe diarrhea or fecal incontinence is to use limited courses of erythromycin (or other broad-spectrum antibiotic).

Lactose Intolerance

Eliminate foods containing lactose from the diet. If the diarrhea stops (and there is a probable diagnosis), put lactose back into the diet. If the diarrhea starts again, the diagnosis is confirmed, and treatment should be referred to an endocrinologist. This condition is caused by a deficiency of the digestive enzyme disaccharidase. The recommended treatment is to remove all lactose-containing products from the resident's diet.

Thyrotoxicosis

An elevated T4 or T3. Refer the resident to an endocrinologist for further investigation of thyroid function.

Uremia

Elevated blood urea nitrogen levels (uremia). Refer the resident to a nephrologist.

CARE PLAN FOR SERIOUS CONDITIONS REQUIRING REVIEW OF CONSTIPATION OR FECAL INCONTINENCE

After treating these reversible conditions, the clinician needs to check for the presence of serious conditions that cause or accompany constipation or fecal incontinence. The following subsections describe these conditions.

Bacterial Diarrhea

This condition is suspected in the presence of fecal incontinence associated with fever and systemic illness, blood or mucus in the feces, abdominal pain, and watery stools lasting longer than 48 hours. Send feces for culture and antibiotic sensitivities. The treatment will depend on the culture results.

Colitis (Ischemic or Inflammatory)

Suspect colitis in the presence of abdominal or rectal pain, bloody stools, and low serum albumin. The diagnosis is made by sigmoidoscopy and biopsy. Treatment is guided by the gastroenterologist.

Cancer of the Colon, Rectum, or Anus

Suspect cancer in the presence of weight loss and anemia. The diagnosis is made by barium enema and colonoscopy. Refer the resident to a gastrointestinal surgeon for treatment.

Intestinal Obstruction Secondary to Impaction or Other Cause

Suspect this condition if abdominal distention, diminished bowel sounds, and feculent vomiting are present. An abdominal radiograph will show obstruction. Do not give laxatives in the presence of obstruction.

Urinary Retention

Bladder outflow can be obstructed by a fecal impaction with the possible complication of hydronephrosis and renal failure. This condition may also be present in some residents with urinary incontinence (overflow). The diagnosis is made by checking a postvoid residual (PVR) and renal ultrasound if the PVR is greater than 100 mL (*see* Chapter 27, Urinary Incontinence, for more information). Treat the impaction to resolve the urinary retention. If not, *see* the section on urinary problems in Chapter 27.

Rectal Prolapse

If the prolapse cannot be reduced or is associated with chronic fecal incontinence, obtain a surgical opinion.

Care Plan for Persistent Constipation

In care planning for persistent constipation, there are two typical situations, which are discussed in the following subsections.

Persistent Constipation Due to Slow Transit

The stool diary and nursing observation will confirm constipation, and an abdominal radiograph will show fecal retention in the colon. Laxative doses may be titrated upward to achieve regular comfortable evacuation. To treat slow-transit constipation:

1. Exercise, increase fluid intake, and institute a regular toilet habit with attempted defecation daily (30 minutes after eating breakfast).
2. Add prunes to the diet (they contain the natural laxative phenolphthalein). Increase fiber in ambulatory residents.
3. Use a bulk laxative (e.g., Citrucel, Metamucil) for residents who are ambulatory and able to drink good amounts. Use regularly if needed.
4. Use Sorbitol (15 to 30 mL) at night for less mobile residents. The dose may be titrated against bowel movements, with a maximum dosage of 30 mL four times a day. Use regularly if needed.
5. If constipation persists and impaction has been ruled out, add one to three tablets of senna (Senokot) at night until evacuation. Discontinue after 7 days, and then use as required for recurrent constipation.
6. If constipation persists and a radiograph of kidney, ureters, and bladder (KUB) shows fecal impaction, discontinue laxatives until there are no clinical or radiographic signs of obstruction.
7. Give mineral oil retention enemas daily for 3 days, followed 1 hour later by tap water enemas. When signs of obstruction due to impaction resolve, return to steps 1 through 4.
8. If a KUB shows persistent constipation, give Golytely, 1/2 L/day for 3 days with additional fluids.
9. Return to steps 1 through 4 for a maintenance regimen.

Persistent Constipation Due to Rectal Dyschezia

In less mobile residents, or in residents with several predisposing causes for persistent constipation, a combination of recommendations from the previous subsection and this one may be required. To treat rectal dyschezia, use the following steps. If abdominal radiography shows fecal loading, combine these steps with the slow-transit care plan recommendations.

1. Exercise, increase fluid intake, and institute a regular toilet habit within 30 minutes after eating breakfast.
2. Elevate the legs during defecation. If straining persists and more than 2 days pass without a bowel movement, consider the following steps, as appropriate.
3. Manually evacuate the rectum if stool is hard.
4. Follow steps 1 and 2. Administer a bisacodyl suppository before breakfast on alternative days if impaction persists.
5. Administer fleet enemas, or if serum creatinine is 1.0 or more (i.e., there is a risk of hyperphosphatemia), administer tapwater enemas. Use intermittently, except in residents who have chronic difficulties with recurrent impaction who will need triweekly tap water enemas.
6. If stool is hard, give a bulk laxative every day or sorbitol, 15 mL, at bedtime. Colace may cause fecal soiling and is ineffective as a laxative in the elderly.

Care Plan for Persistent Fecal Incontinence

Assess all residents with fecal incontinence for constipation and impaction. When constipation and impaction are confirmed, *see* the procedures in the previous two subsections.

This care plan applies to residents with persistent fecal incontinence that occurs in the absence of acute diarrhea. (To assess and treat diarrhea, *see* the care planning sections for the reversible and serious conditions of constipation and fecal impaction.)

In care planning for persistent fecal incontinence, two situations are typical:

- Persistent fecal incontinence is due to causes other than dementia-related neurogenic disinhibited rectum. Typically, this incontinence occurs several times daily. To treat incontinence other than that caused by dementia-related neurogenic disinhibited rectum:
  o Perform pelvic floor exercises to improve sphincter control. If incontinence persists, refer to a surgeon for possible surgery to repair sphincter mechanism (postanal repair) or rectal prolapse; or medical treatment with biofeedback (training residents to contract the sphincter voluntarily by watching an electrical response to the muscle contraction).
  o If incontinence persists following treatment or the surgical option is ruled out, clean and change the undergarments regularly and perform perineal hygiene.
- Persistent fecal incontinence is due to dementia-related neurogenic disinhibited rectum. Typically, incontinence occurs once a day, after breakfast or other meal. To treat incontinence caused by dementia-related neurogenic disinhibited rectum:
  o Seat the resident on the toilet following breakfast or a hot drink in the morning.
  o If the incontinence persists, give bismuth, 15 to 30 mL, every morning to prevent peristalsis and consequent bowel movement during the day, and give sorbitol, 30 mL at night and/or a bisacodyl suppository before breakfast three times a week.
  o Give bismuth 15 to 30 mL every day and two to three enemas a week (phosphate or tap water, depending on renal function).

CASE EXAMPLE

Mrs. P., an 88 year-old-woman, was recently admitted to the nursing home for long-term care. During the initial assessment, the nurse noted a 10-year history of oral stimulant laxative use (phenolphthalein and bisacodyl tablets). Mrs. P. also reported straining at stool, stating that it was important for her to have a bowel movement daily, although this did not usually occur.

The nurse auscultated active bowel sounds and palpated a supple, nontender, nondistended abdomen. The rectal examination revealed a moderate amount of hard guaiac-negative stool and a small external hemorrhoid. Her underpants were not stained with feces. The examination was otherwise benign. To obtain a complete baseline profile, a care plan was developed that included a stool diary, dietary intake history, close monitoring for abdominal pain, and pain upon defecation. Pharmaceutical interventions were not prescribed.

During Mrs. P.'s first month of residence, the nurse was able to get a baseline of her bowel function. She was unable to pass adequate amounts of stool, and when she did, the feces was hard. She experienced considerable straining during defecation. Enemas were necessary for her to empty her bowels successfully. At one point, Mrs. P. did not move her bowels for several days, and an obstruction was suspected. It became clear that she was chronically constipated. Plain abdominal radiography revealed the presence of feces throughout the colon, but no impaction or other obstruction was visible.

The clinicians decided that a barium enema was required for further assessment. It disclosed a distended, noncontracting colon, which was determined to be the result of prolonged use of oral stimulant laxatives. Accordingly, Mrs. P.'s care plan was revised as fol-lows:

- *Education*. Bowel functioning in the elderly was reviewed. Attention was given to the issue of past ineffective interventions. Mrs. P. agreed that a better solution was necessary. The importance of diet, hydration, and exercise was also reviewed.
- *Diet*. Mrs. P. was placed on an increased dietary fiber diet. She was told that she may feel bloated and experience increased flatulence initially, but that these symptoms would resolve within several weeks.
- *Hydration*. Mrs. P. was encouraged to drink 1500 mL of fluid each day, and 2 L a day during the hot months of the year.
- *Mobility*. Mrs. P. was encouraged to increase ambulation. She was independent in mobility, but the newness of the nursing home had proved overwhelming, so she had generally remained in her room. The staff assisted her in establishing friendships with other residents. With their company she was more inclined to move throughout her environment.

These interventions were successful. Mrs. P. was moving her bowels every third day and passing adequate amounts of formed stool. However, she was still experiencing discomfort during defecation and complained about frequency. Digital examination revealed an empty rectum. It was also noted that her external hemorrhoid was not inflamed. After discussion with Mrs. P., the clinician revised her care plan as follows:

- *Education*. Since Mrs. P. was requesting daily suppositories, the previous interventions were reviewed, along with a restatement about normal bowel functioning in the elderly. Mrs. P. agreed to further dietary modifications, as well as minimal pharmacologic assistance, and was also reminded to let the nursing staff know if her hemorrhoid became sore or painful.

- *Diet*. Prunes were added to Mrs. P.'s diet (two servings daily). This was easily instituted, as she enjoyed eating prunes.
- *Bulk laxative*. Metamucil was given daily since the clinicians were assured that an adequate amount of fluid was being consumed. The importance of this was reviewed again with Mrs. P.
- *Senna (Senokot) as needed*. Three tablets at night were given if Mrs. P. did not move her bowels within 48 hours. Repeated dosing would be reviewed by the nurse and physician.

At 6 weeks into her residency, Mrs. P. was moving her bowels painlessly every other day. She and the clinicians were satisfied with the current regimen, which the nursing staff continued to monitor closely.

29
ADL
Rehabilitation

John N. Morris, PhD
Maria Fiatarone, MD
Pauline Belleville-Taylor, RN, MS, CS
Marie Eckler, RN, MS, CS, CRRN

Helping a resident achieve optional involvement in self-care requires that the nursing staff proceed through a series of evaluative steps. Following these steps, the nursing staff must:

- *Identify opportunities to institute nursing-based rehabilitation and exercise programs*
- *Recognize the reversible causes of functional decline*
- *Target residents for one of three established programs, depending on the appropriate intensity level*
- *Develop and implement specific rehabilitation strategies within the selected program*

OVERVIEW

All residents of nursing facilities are at risk of physical decline. Most have comorbid illnesses or are subject to a variety of other factors that can impact self-sufficiency negatively. For example, cognitive deficits may limit the resident's initiative for self-care or limit their understanding of the necessary tasks involved in completing the activities of daily living (ADLs). Physical and neurologic illnesses may impact on physical factors important to self-care (e.g., stamina, muscle tone, balance, and bone strength). The side effects of medications and other treatments also contribute to a needless loss of self-sufficiency. As a consequence of many possibly adverse influences, a resident's potential for maximum functionality is often underestimated by family, staff, and the resident. In this regard, all residents are candidates for nursing-based rehabilitative care that is focused on both maintaining and expanding self-involvement in their ADLs. In addition, most residents are candidates for a regular program of exercise therapy to improve the physical factors necessary for optimal involvement in self-care.

Background Clinical Review

Gather a background clinical review by identifying the opportunity for rehabilitation, and identify the reversible physical conditions that predispose to functional decline.

Identifying Opportunities for Rehabilitation

While all residents are candidates for some type of supportive or functional enhancement programs, the review described in Table 29-1 helps identify those particular residents who can benefit from an intensive program of nursing rehabilitation—i.e., a program designed to respond to the resident's decline or to take advantage of the resident's residual strengths. Intensive rehabilitation will require frequent care plan updates (usually monthly or quarterly), weekly documentation of progress, extensive communication with the resident and family, and systematic titration of care as progress (or further decline) is noted. While reviewing the items in Table 29-1, consider the following:

- Can newly gained ADL skills be better supported by staff and family?
- Can the resident's functional decline be prevented, slowed, or reversed?
- Have steps been taken to enhance function or reverse decline?
- Can barriers to self-care be eliminated or modified?
- Given the available staffing resources in the facility, are there additional opportunities to enhance the resident's function by employing task segmentation, exercise therapy, or other options?

Reversible Physical Conditions Predisposing to Functional Decline

Functional decline is not an inevitable associate of aging. Rather, it is usually associated with acute or chronic illness, adverse effects of care (e.g., medications, restraints) or physical inactivity. Table 29-2 lists some common conditions associated with functional impairment. Some of these conditions can be improved or resolved with appropriate treatment, which will improve ADL performance and maximize self-care functions in old age. The list is not exhaustive; it can be supplemented with other conditions from your own clinical experience. When a complicating condition is present:

- Select the best treatment for the condition
- Treat the condition

- Determine the results of the treatment
- Adjust the treatment plan according to the results
- Monitor for emerging indicators of improved ADL status

The objective is to treat the underlying conditions, then look for opportunities to focus nursing rehabilitation or exercise therapy in areas where new (or returning) ADL capabilities are noted. For example, a nurse assistant may notice that a resident recovering from a stroke begins to pick up a face cloth and attempt to use it. In an environment in which rehabilitation is valued, staff will encourage this resurgence of independent functioning—licensed nurses will be notified, further monitoring and assessment of abilities will occur, and the rehabilitative plan of care will be altered with resident and family input.

Nursing-Based Rehabilitative Care: Achieving Maximum Function in ADLs

Before creating a care plan that will assist a resident in maintaining current function, retaining newly learned skills, or developing greater self-sufficiency, strength, and stamina, it is necessary to identify the resident's current abilities, performance, and strengths. Correctly targeting residents for the most appropriate rehabilitative care program can greatly increase their chances of success. This section describes the three major rehabilitative groups of residents, which are based on levels of cognitive and ADL performance as determined by the resident's most recent Minimum Data Set (MDS) assessment. These groups are:
- A maintenance group
- A rehabilitation watch group
- An intensive rehabilitation group

Each resident in the facility can be assigned to one of these three rehabilitative groups, evaluated and treated for reversible causes of ADL impairment, and targeted for specific nursing strategies.

Table 29-1. **Identifying Opportunities for Nursing Rehabilitation or Exercise Therapy Programming**

Greater self-sufficiency or capacity for self-care

Has the resident become more self-sufficient in one or more ADLs?

Are these new skills consistently encouraged and supported by staff and family?

Can the resident benefit from such consistent input?

Has the resident recovered from an acute illness that temporarily restricted ADL performance?

Has the resident regained former skills in particular ADLs?

Has the resident responded to a new or altered medication regimen?

Is the resident motivated to become more self-sufficient?

Do staff or family believe that the resident has the potential to become more self-sufficient?

Recent decline or risk for decline in ADL function

Has the resident's performance in one or more ADLs declined?

Does the resident have a condition that increases the risk of decline?

Has the resident experienced a recent transient, self-limited health event (e.g., flu, urinary tract infection)? Is the resident slow to recover?

Has the resident recently experienced a serious health event (e.g., syncope [fainting], stroke, myocardial infarction, congestive heart failure, hip fracture, delirium), or major behavioral change (e.g., severe social withdrawal, aggressive behavior)?

Do some ADLs appear to be particularly vulnerable to decline? For example:

Has the resident become less proficient in particular ADL tasks (e.g., donning clothes in correct order, getting to the toilet on time)?

Does the staff believe that decline can be prevented, slowed or reversed?

Environmental risks to optimum self-care

Are there environmental barriers to self-sufficiency (e.g., heavy bathroom doors, high beds, long distance to bathroom, low toilets, high clothes hangers, glare)? Can modifications be made?

Does the resident lack adaptive devices or equipment necessary for greater involvement in self-care?

Would the resident be more self-sufficient using a brace, orthopedic footwear, walker, long-handled brush, raised toilet seat, built-up utensil, plate guard, or other aid?

Would the resident be better able to participate in a rehabilitation program if hearing or visual appliances were available and regularly used?

If adaptive devices are available, is each device in good operating condition and being used appropriately and consistently?

Has mobility been restricted by the recent introduction of new equipment (e.g., wheelchair, physical restraints)?

Programmatic risks to optimum self-care

Poor communication among interdisciplinary caregivers. For example:

Is communication (both verbal and demonstrative) between therapists and nursing staff (including nurse assistants) adequate for promoting continuity of newly learned skills?

Do nursing assistants caring for the resident know and understand how to implement the care plan?

Lack of training. For example:

Can nursing assistants be better prepared to encourage ADL involvement through task segmentation, rehabilitative care, and exercise therapies?

Has access to occupational therapist (OT), physical therapist (PT), or other rehabilitation specialists been inappropriately restricted?

Is more time required to determine the effectiveness of current rehabilitative/exercise therapy program?

Can better outcomes be expected if staff were more consistent in carrying out nursing rehabilitation activities, if the care plan was more specific, or if the staffing model were more conducive to consistency and continuity (e.g., permanent staff assignments)?

Table 29-2. Reversible Factors Predisposing to ADL Decline

Condition	Comment
Weight loss or dehydration	These problems can reoccur and often go undetected. After an etiology is identified, they can usually be stabilized and possibly reversed. ADL improvement should be noted.
Delirium associated with an acute illness (e.g., infection, CHF)	A decrease in ADL function is often the first sign of acute cognitive deterioration. Any rapid change in ADL performance should prompt an evaluation for delirium and its underlying cause (e.g., infection, adverse medication effect).
Recent decline in ability to understand others or make self understood by others	Impaired communication may be the result of a transitory, reversible condition, such as delirium, cerumen accumulation (ear wax), infections, or depression, or may be attributable to a change in staff assigned to work with the resident, decreased opportunity to interact with an overworked staff, or a change in resident room assignment. The cause may also be related to more permanent, chronic declines in other areas (e.g., change in hearing, Alzheimer's disease, aphasia). At a minimum, the plan of care must ensure that maximum use is made of existing communication skills. Guard against inducing excess disability based on faulty assumptions about the resident's inability to follow instructions or provide information.
Restraint use	If there is a legitimate therapeutic reason to use restraints (e.g., IV hydration), use the least restrictive means and keep the usage brief (both in time per day and total days per week). If there is no legitimate therapeutic reason to use restraints, do not use them. If restraints are in use, evaluate ways to remove or strictly limit their use. Restraints will induce ADL dependency.
Mood distress (e.g., depression, anxiety), problem behavior, withdrawal, apathy, refusal of care by others	Residents who experience mood or behavioral disturbances become less self-sufficient in ADLs. Likewise, declining ADL function can precipitate mood or behavioral distress. When either is present, determine the underlying cause.
Onset of more restricted use of leg, trunk; recent deteriorating balance, stamina, or weakness	When present, determine whether there is a treatable etiology (e.g., medication effect, problem in using a new brace), and treat accordingly. If the problem is of recent origin, refer to a therapeutic professional (OT, PT, or other) for evaluation.
Presence of unstable health condition that makes resident's cognitive, ADL, or behavior status fluctuating, precarious, or deteriorating	When followed for 6 months, the majority of residents who are classified as unstable (at least 60% and potentially many more) respond to treatment and their health status becomes stable. The immediate task is to identify the contributing causal factors and implement an appropriate treatment plan as quickly as possible. Examples of common causal conditions include infections (e.g., pneumonia, flu), multiple falls, CHF, hip fractures, psychiatric conditions (e.g., hallucination, delusions, paranoia), and inappropriate use of psychoactive medications.

CHF—congestive heart failure; IV—intravenous

THE MAINTENANCE GROUP

The maintenance group, comprising about 10% of the residents in a typical facility, includes residents who have few, if any, residual cognitive skills, and who require intensive help with ADLs. Because these residents have difficulty learning new skills, they are candidates for a limited nursing rehabilitation program aimed at preventing the adverse effects of immobility (e.g., pressure ulcers, contractures, pain, isolation, incontinence). This program includes range of motion (ROM) exercises, turning/repositioning, and transferring. The targeting criteria are no ability to make decisions (scored as 3 on the MDS Cognitive Skills item), and dependent (scored as 4 on the Eating item).

Approach to Nursing-Based Rehabilitative Care for Maintenance Group Residents

The objective of care for maintenance group residents is to maintain a regular pattern of physical mobility. To meet this objective:

- Nursing rehabilitative efforts are limited to instituting an active, repetitive program of daily ROM exercises, repositioning, and transferring. Mobilize the resident on a regular schedule and provide an opportunity for engagement in the process to the fullest extent possible. The recommended minimal frequency is:
  - o ROM exercises twice a day
  - o Turning or repositioning every 2 hours while in bed or in a chair
  - o Transferring at least twice per shift on and off a chair, and six to eight times per day on and off the toilet or commode
- When appropriate, encourage the resident to participate actively in performing these tasks (see the suggestions for encouragement in Table 29-3). To decrease stress, engage residents in tasks in which they will be successful. More specifically:
  - o Verbal encouragement may take the form of talking the resident through the activity, soothing the resident to prevent an accident during mobility (e.g., "I'm right here. You're okay"), or providing a simple verbal cue (e.g., "Sit down. Hold on.").
  - o Give the resident enough opportunity to complete the activity (or part of the activity) alone.
  - o Physical encouragement or prompting may include the staff providing hands-on initiation of a movement (e.g., elbow flexion and extension ROM exercise) followed by the resident adoption of that movement. The staff may need to demonstrate the movement while providing an additional verbal cue for the resident to continue the activity (e.g., "Now it's your turn to do this.").
- Provide guidance to families who visit frequently and wish to be involved in the resident's personal care. Include tips to ease resident involvement, e.g., how to do ROM exercises. Note that this rehabilitation group is not discussed further in this chapter. They are not candidates for the more extensive nursing rehabilitation program or the exercise therapy program.

The Rehabilitation Watch Group

The rehabilitation watch group, comprising about 10% of the residents in a typical facility, are fully (or largely) self-sufficient in ADLs. Because these residents are highly involved in self-care, rehabilitation plans for some may be limited to monitoring to ensure that any emerging problems do not go unnoticed. For others, the staff will be providing verbal encouragement to ensure that ADLs are performed in a way that maximizes self-sufficiency. In some instances, residents in this group will also require non-weight-bearing physical assistance (e.g., a light-elbow touch guard while walking long distances). The targeting criteria are:

- MDS ADL Performance scores in the 0 to 2 range, indicating that the resident is neither totally dependent nor receiving extensive assistance in any ADL area except possibly bathing
- Some ability to make decisions (scored as 0

Table 29-3. Encouragement Procedures and Examples

Procedure	Encourage Involvement	Reassure/Compliment
Ambulation	Encourage the resident to walk to the dining room, or to walk for longer distances for one or all meals. Coax the resident to walk to the bathroom	"You walked a lot farther today than you did last week." "Don't worry, I won't let you fall." "I know you are trying."
ROM and turning	Encourage the resident to do upper extremity ROM exercises after a meal. Coax the resident to participate in turning in bed	"Today you were able to get your right arm a lot further back than before."
Transfer	Encourage the resident to transfer out of a chair and walk to a planned activity	"You got yourself into the bed a lot better than you did yesterday."
Meals	Schedule enough time for the resident to eat Encourage the resident to take the first bite or two, then give him or her the opportunity to consume the rest of the food on own initiative Encourage the resident to chew food before swallowing	"You are doing a great job eating that pudding by yourself." "Please put your apron on. It's time for lunch."
Dressing	Encourage the resident to take off an item of clothing alone Encourage the resident to raise arms as you take the shirt off.	"You are getting much better with those buttons. You used to have a very hard time with that."

to 2 on the MDS Cognitive Skills item) or a score of 3 on the MDS Cognitive Skills item and a score of 0 to 3 (nondependent) on the MDS Eating item

Approach to Nursing-Based Rehabilitative Care for Rehabilitation Watch Group Residents

The objectives of care for the rehabilitation watch group are to:

• Actively encourage residents to conduct ADLs independently

• Monitor for the evidence of ADL decline

To meet these guidelines, follow these strategies:

• Encourage resident involvement
• Monitor the resident for signs of decline
• Involve the family in monitoring the resident

Encourage Resident Involvement.

This strategy applies to residents in the rehabilitative watch group who are scored as 1 (supervision) or 2 (limited assistance) on one or more MDS ADL items. About 20% of the residents in this group will require active encouragement to maintain current ADL self-sufficiency patterns, usually in the areas of dressing, grooming, or ambulation). Table 29-3 provides some encouragement procedures (verbal and nonverbal) and examples that will help motivate performance and reduce distractions.

Monitoring.

While many of these residents are self-sufficient in all ADL areas, they are still at risk of decline. Research has shown their ADL decline rates to be comparable to the experience of all other residents. In most instances, however, a decline will be limited to one or just a few areas (e.g., a recent inability to complete part of the dressing activity, a recent tendency to leave some food or fluid at meals, or a recent lack of attentiveness to personal grooming). The first sign of decline is often a new need for staff to provide cues or limited non-weight-bearing support in dressing or locomotion.

To prevent decline, the plan of care should call for at least weekly monitoring by licensed staff for:
- Indications of slower performance in any ADL
- A failure to fully complete ADLs as usual (e.g., grooming, dressing)
- Emerging patterns of greater staff assistance with specific ADLs

This group will also benefit from the preventive exercise therapy program described later in this chapter.

Family Involvement.

Families can play an important role in monitoring the resident for functional decline by reporting their observations and concerns to the nursing staff. Additionally, provide interested families with how-to strategies to support the resident's skills in self-care. For example, show the family how to cue the resident to transfer or use a walker.

The Intensive Rehabilitation Group

The intensive rehabilitation group, comprising about 80% of the residents in a typical nursing facility, includes those who have at least some residual cognitive ability. Residents in this group are candidates for a complete nursing-based rehabilitative care program. The targeting criteria are:
- Scores of 3 or 4 (extensive assistance or dependent) in one or more of the MDS ADL performance areas—excluding bathing where arbitrary facility rules may insist on staff involvement
- Some level of residual cognitive ability, indicating some ability to make decisions—scored as 0 to 2 on the Cognitive Skills item—or a score of 3 on the Cognitive Skills item and a score of 0 to 3 (nondependent) on the Eating item

Approach to Nursing-Based Rehabilitative Care for Intensive Rehabilitation Group Residents

The objectives of care for the intensive rehabilitation group are to:
- Prevent needless decline in ADL involvement
- Sustain recent gains in ADL self-performance
- Expand resident involvement in specific ADL subtasks
- Reverse any recent decline in ADL involvement
- Introduce adaptive devices or environmental modifications to enhance resident involvement in ADLs

For residents in this group, nursing-based rehabilitative care should be a consistent daily activity on all shifts with an emphasis on maintaining patterns of resident involvement in ADLs, and, when possible, extending this involvement (in a stepwise fashion) into new

ADL subtasks. Program intensity will vary (*see* the section on background clinical review) among residents as well as among ADLs for the same resident. For example, some residents will require a nursing rehabilitation program that consists of standby assistance to monitor self-performance. Others will require consistent application of verbal or physical encouragement during ADLs. Others will require a more vigorous, formalized intervention that should be specified in the care plan, carefully implemented, and thoughtfully reassessed at scheduled intervals.

The following sections describe how to select the ADL areas within which nursing-based rehabilitation care will be focused, followed by descriptions of the different strategies available to accomplish this objective. More specifically, this includes:

- Environmental modifications
- Encouraging the resident to perform up to capabilities
- Training the resident in ADL self-care tasks, either during the course of normal performance of an ADL or during specially scheduled supplemental training sessions

Selected ADLs on Which to Focus

Begin by carefully evaluating the resident's current involvement in ADLs. Use the Task Segmentation Protocol (TSP) (*see* Figure A-1 in Appendix A) during the admission and annual assessments. The TSP provides a framework to describe the resident's current involvement in the physical and intellectual subtasks required of activities. TSP assessment areas for each ADL include:

•   Whether the resident understands how to use objects (if needed) to perform the ADL

•   Whether the resident is aware of the need to carry out the ADL

•   A detailed specification of the resident's involvement in the subtask of the ADL task

•   Equipment used to enhance ADL performance

•   Specific types of encouragement and limit-setting procedures that are frequently successful

Limit the TSP review to ADLs in which the resident receives supervision or hands-on support. Exclude from the review any ADL in which the resident is either completely independent or fully dependent on others.

The TSP review helps staff to identify ADL subtasks that can be performed by the resident, as well as others that might eventually be performed by the resident following exposure to a more consistent rehabilitation program. Using the dressing activity as an example, the following description of a resident's abilities could be construed from the TSP review:

- The resident knows how to use clothing, e.g., socks go on feet
- The resident is aware of the need to dress before leaving own room
- The staff currently select and obtain clothes the resident will wear
- The resident dresses upper body but requires help in dressing lower body; is independent for all snaps, ties, zippers, and belts once clothes are on lower body
- The resident puts on clothes in correct order
- The resident depends on the staff to put on shoes and socks
- The resident removes clothes independently, but may undress inappropriately in the middle of the day—particularly if tired; staff must monitor to make sure that this does not occur

The TSP profile, which should be done for each resident at least once a year, enables staff to define the scope of the resident's need for nursing assistance and rehabilitative care. For the resident, this includes the staff's assistance in setup and dressing the lower body, as well as monitoring and encouraging the resident to remain dressed during the day.

Use the TSP profile to determine whether there have been improvements or declines since the last full assessment. If at the time of the annual follow-up the resident is less self-sufficient, and no remedial steps have been taken under the existing plan of care, the need to evaluate the available options is strongly indicated. Or, if the resident's self-care status has stabilized or improved within the past year, the staff should determine whether a still higher level of independence is possible. More specifically, review the subtasks of an activity. Is there an area in which increased self-sufficiency could be sought? For example, in the previous case profile, is it possible for the resident to become more self-sufficient in dressing the lower body or putting on shoes or socks? Have the underlying causes of dysfunction been addressed (e.g., strength training to improve lower extremity weakness)? Has the resident been provided with assistive devices (i.e., a reacher or sock-puller) or adapted shoes to enhance independence? Are there reasons to believe that such improvement is possible, or are there other ADL areas in which progress might be achieved, given more important limited staff resources? Does the resident have the motivation to become more independent?

Strategies for Interaction

The staff should identify the best strategies to interact with the resident, and incorporate these strategies into the rehabilitative care plan. Identify these interactive strategies (or communication techniques) by setting up a few clinical situations with the residents and assessing their responses. The staff will find that these clinical situations are activities that are already a part of their daily routine. The situations or questions are arranged in the following hierarchical order, which must be maintained:

1. Is the resident's functional impairment a result of a sequencing problem? Does the resident perform tasks in the wrong order (i.e., put on shoes after tying them, put a bra on outside the shirt, try to drink from a milk carton before opening it)? Does the resident get distracted by the preparation of items required in the activity (i.e., laying out other items, cutting foods)? If the answer is yes, adjust for these deficits. Put all items in the proper order as they will be needed. With dressing, put clothing into a pile with the first item to be put on the top and the last item on the bottom. With eating, arrange the prepared foods in the order they are to be eaten. If sequencing is not a problem, go to the next question.

2. Is the resident able to maintain attention or comprehend verbal communication? Does the resident react to constant stimulus? If attention is a problem, this resident will be able to perform best in an environment in which the stimuli are acknowledged and controlled. This means that televisions, radios, and excess noise are eliminated when the resident needs to focus on a task. Excess visual stimuli are also minimized (i.e., extra or dirty clothing is not left around, the privacy curtain is drawn, and clutter is removed). If these strategies are not appropriate, go to the next question.

3. Is the resident able to follow one-step commands? Can the resident perform a simple task within physical limits? If you ask the resident to "pick up your sock," does he or she? If yes, use verbal prompts to assist the resident to complete the ADL tasks. Follow the recommendations for controlling the environment, and give the resident one task at a time to complete. This resident cannot be told to get dressed but can perform all the subtasks required to dress. If these strategies are not appropriate, go to the next question.

4. Is the resident able to start the desired activity if handed a familiar object? If handed a shirt, can the resident put it on? If handed a cup, can the resident start drinking? This resident does not respond well to verbal prompts but can initiate activities. Caregivers should maximize this strength and rely primarily on these nonverbal cues to assist the resident. It is possible that the resident may start the desired activity when the staff use the physical prompt, but then stop it before the activity is completed. If this is the case, restart the activity with another physical prompt and allow the resident to continue. For example, you hand a cup to a resident who starts to take a few sips and then returns the cup to the table. After a short period of time, if the resident does not resume drinking, the caregiver may need to put the resident's hand around the cup and move it in the direction of the mouth. The resident will take over the activity and continue the movement. Use verbal cues only to strengthen the nonverbal prompt. If these strategies are not appropriate, go to the next question.

5. Is the resident able to imitate? Face the resident and make eye contact. Begin a simple, familiar activity that is within the resident's physical capabilities. Can the resident mimic your actions? If yes, rely on modeling and gesturing as the primary strategy for interacting with the resident. Use verbal cues only to strengthen the nonverbal prompt. If these strategies are not appropriate, go to the next question.

6. Is the resident able to continue an activity within functional ability once the task is physically started? This is different from physical prompting in that the support is more than just handing the object to the resident. Start the activity (i.e., pulling up pants, guiding the resident's hands through the motion). Over time, allow the resident to assume more of the activity by reducing the amount of support provided (i.e., guide the pants up to the middle of the calves, then the knees, then the thighs, each time allowing the resident to finish the activity).

These communication techniques can be applied to all residents and with all ADLs.

Environmental Modifications

To facilitate resident engagement in ADLs, follow these recommended strategies:

- Structure the schedule of ADLs to minimize distractions to the resident and lessen possible negative reactions as follows:
  o Toilet the resident just before a formal training program session.
  o Begin the program at a time of day when the resident is not drained by other activities, when the resident is feeling best (e.g., after pain medications have started to take effect), or when the resident in a good frame of mind (e.g., after a morning phone conversation with a daughter).
- Physical modifications in unit space
  o Change room assignments, e.g., assign the resident to a room that is closer to the nursing station for better monitoring; separate the resident from the negative impact of a distressing roommate.
  o Rearrange the furniture. Locate appliances in proximity to necessary resources (e.g., the bathroom).
  o Ensure that necessary prostheses and appliances are available, being used, and in good working order. Instruct the staff in the care, cleaning, application, removal, and proper use by the resident of braces, splints, crutches, walkers, and other devices, and monitor his or her performance. Emphasize to nurse assistants and residents the importance of regular use of hearing aids, glasses, and any other appliances that enhance communication, and instruct them to notify

Table 29-4. Examples of Limiting Procedures

Type of Procedure	Adjust Unit Routines to Resident's Needs, Preferences and Strengths	Reorient to Help Overcome Resident's Limited Ability to Make a Good Decision
Ambulation	Take the resident for a walk when he or she is awake and restless during the night Be prepared to offer an individually scheduled walking program Have volunteers or family be with resident as he or she slowly walks or wheels to activity Monitor a fearful resident's reaction to walking in corridors with others	*"Remember, you need your walker when you walk to the bathroom."* *"It is time for lunch. Why don't you start walking to the dining room now?"*
ROM and turning	When the resident is noisy and restless during the night, perform gentle ROM exercises while verbally reassuring the resident	*"Remember, you need to exercise your left hand as well as the right one."* *"Why don't you try doing your leg exercises now while I am here."*
Transfer	Help the resident out of bed and into a chair first thing in the morning to prevent agitation	*"Remember, you need to lock the wheelchair before you get out of it."* *"It's time to go to the birthday party now. Make sure your wheelchair is all set up before I help you get into it."*
Meals	Seat the resident at a small dining table for two if the regular, larger groups are overstimulating and inhibiting to feeding Offer one food at a time to focus attention on the task at hand Arrange tray delivery so that those requiring more time receive trays first	*"Remember, use the fork with the big handle to eat."* *"Don't swallow your food yet, you need to chew."* *"I'll see that your tray is delivered first so that you will have a longer time to eat."*
Dressing	Even though the resident may not always succeed, give the opportunity to take off clothing items when partial independence has been achieved Assist the resident to dress if he or she awakens and wishes to start the day earlier than the other residents	*"Remember, you need to take off your shirt first."* *"Please don't get undressed until you get to your room."* *"You cannot go into the dining room until you are dressed."* *"Why don't you take off your robe now? I'm going to help you get in the tub."*

PT, OT, nursing, or other responsible professional immediately when an appliance or device needs repair.

o Keep the family appraised of the resident's status, progress, and needs for particular types of clothing, shoes, glasses, and other related information. Make specific suggestions about items the family might provide for rehabilitation (e.g., skirts with elastic waist bands, sneakers with Velcro closures; front-zipped dresses).

o Encourage direct care staff (and family when possible) to consistently promote resident involvement in scheduled rehabilitation and exercise programming.

o Initiate an ongoing communication program (posters, flyers, and other media) to generate enthusiasm for the nursing rehabilitation therapy program. The purpose is to create a rehabilitation-oriented environment and philosophy.

o Ensure that licensed nursing staff have been trained to provide instructions to nonlicensed staff on how to complete specific rehabilitation activities when necessary. Schedule an OT or PT consult or inservice on procedures to be followed if the resident is to be involved in ambulation, feeding, dressing, or other procedure.

Table 29-4 provides some examples of limit setting and restructuring procedures (verbal and nonverbal) to use as part of daily resident care in selected ADL areas. They will help motivate performance and reduce problematic distractions.

Encouraging the Resident to
Perform up to Capabilities

Verbal and nonverbal encouragement of a resident's involvement in ADLs is a tenet of good nursing care. When encouragement is lacking or inconsistent, the result frequently is that resident (and family) are confused about the staff's expectations. Such encouragement is especially important for residents who are cognitively impaired. Some will require constant reminders to be engaged in ADLs—e.g., to dress self or to go to activities when scheduled. Others will require less intensive follow-up—typically, cueing or verbal reinforcement—since their decisions will be appropriate most of the time. Whatever the case-specific circumstances, for encouragement to be an effective rehabilitation tool, the following steps are recommended:

• Document in the care plan any encouragement procedures that have worked with the resident in the past.

• Try new procedures—draw on successful experiences with other residents while trying to develop a plan to maximally involve a resident in the ADL activities.

• Train all direct care staff in the use of these procedures.

• Monitor to ensure that the indicated encouragement procedures are applied consistently.

• Inform the resident's family of your plan.

• For staff who do not appear to be following the plan, explain why the plan has been prescribed. Provide specific examples of how the staff have been acting, and provide guidance on how they should conduct themselves.

Refer to Table 29-3 for examples of verbal and nonverbal encouragement procedures for key ADLs.

Training the Resident in ADL Self-Care Tasks

Nursing-based rehabilitative training to improve resident involvement in an ADLs can be either indirect or direct. In *indirect training* the staff work in one activity area hoping that some other ADL functions will be positively reinforced, because the resident is motivated to toilet, incorporate a program to stimulate ambulation when going to the toilet.

In *direct training* the staff's sole training focus is to increase the resident's involvement in a particular ADL area with the resident receiving a specific demonstration on how to complete an activity. This instruction might be verbal without examples or may involve assisted repetitive movement through an activity or part of an activity (e.g., staff physically guide the resident through an ROM exercise or hold the resident's hand and spoon as the first few bites of food are taken).

However the program is focused—indirect or direct rehabilitation—the following recommendations apply.

The scope of the formal rehabilitation program is as follows:
- Schedule a time when the resident will try to do one ADL task (or specific subtasks within that ADL) that has not been accomplished before. The staff should observe this trial situation.
- Start small and go slow as the resident retrains muscles and joints, gains strength, learns an activity pattern, and achieves a sense of confidence in his or her abilities.
- Start with one session per day, 3 days per week. If the resident shows improvement, extend to a maximum of two sessions per day, 5 (or 7) days a week.
- Limit the program duration to 10 to 30 minutes per session, or as appropriate to the resident's normal attention span.
- Extend the time (up to 30 minutes maximum) for residents who demonstrate increased tolerance, interest, and improvements.

The ongoing review is as follows:
- After the nursing staff has organized the resident's care schedule, conduct a weekly review of the resident's performance patterns. How has the performance varied? How can it be improved? What should be the continuing role of direct care staff to ensure that needed ADLs are carried out (with resident input whenever possible)?
- Are there indications that the resident may be overextending his or her ability or experiencing complications (e.g., pain, fatigue, falls, fear)?
- Are there any acute processes that require temporary modification of the training goal?
- A well-conceived program requires continued monitoring for achievement of major milestones. Look at issues of self-initiation, endurance, extent of activity carried out, and reduction of symptoms associated with a sedentary life style (e.g., cramping, pressure ulcers, shortness of breath, restless legs, dehydration, weight loss, depression).
- Where progress is noted, modify expectations (as appropriate) about the resident's and staff's roles in ADL performance.
- Validate progress (or lack of) with the resident.
- When there are signs of recovery from comorbid illness, does the resident become more motivated to self-sufficiency in a specific ADL area?
- For residents who do not achieve the treatment goal that has been set, do not stop rehabilitation prematurely. Rather, consider alternative strategies, such as re-evaluating the goal, extending the time period, setting a more appropriate goal, or reducing the intensity of the training program. A legitimate treatment goal can be to maintain current levels of resident involvement.

The following lists provide examples of indirect rehabilitation procedures—those in which ADL rehabilitation in one area is designed to be linked to the resident's performance of activities in other areas.

Locomotion ADL Focus Area.
Examples of indirect rehabilitation procedures for the locomotion ADL focus area are as follows:

- **Toileting.** *Within functional limits, encourage the resident to walk to and from the bathroom.*
  - o Do not assume the need to transfer the resident with a wheelchair.
  - o Give the resident the option of walking to the bathroom (even with staff physical supports). For, example, place a walker in close proximity to the resident and say, "Let's go for a walk now."
  - o Start the activity on the day shift. If the resident responds positively, extend the program into the evening shift.
  - o If the resident walks to the bathroom on the day and evening shifts, do not rely on a bedside commode or urinal on the night shift. Going to the bathroom not only represents a form of exercise, it also facilitates adequate elimination, and avoids the need to change soiled linens and bedclothes. Say to the resident, for example, "It is good to exercise your leg muscles by standing and walking each time you have to go to the bathroom."
  - o On return from the bathroom, encourage the resident to walk to a pleasurable activity on or off the unit. Say, for example, "Now that you have gone to the bathroom, let's walk to the activity room for the music program."

- **Eating.** *Encourage more independent residents to walk back and forth to the dining room for meals.*
  - o Unless medically contraindicated, the resident should not eat in bed. Have the resident get out of bed and go for meals.
  - o If the resident walks to the midday meal, encourage him or her to walk to supper and breakfast as well.
  - o A nurse assistant can cue, supervise, or provide light touch guard while accompanying a resident walking to the dining area.
  - o Have a dining walking group with one

staff leader. This makes good use of scarce staff resources.
  - o Encourage walking to an area where a pleasurable activity is being held (e.g., birthday or holiday party, tea, wine and cheese party). Encourage the resident to join others in going to the event.

- **Bathing.** *Encourage, cue, supervise, or assist the resident in walking to and from the bathtub or shower.*
  - o Residents can undress and dress in the shower room as an adjunct to the ambulation activity.
  - o Encourage the resident who is reliant on a wheelchair (but able to walk) to use the wheelchair as a walker. Shower supplies can be transported on the seat.

- **Activities.** *Encourage the resident to walk to and from scheduled activities.* For example, say, "I know you are planning to go to ceramics. I'll get your walker so I can help you practice walking, like you did yesterday."
  - o For residents who can be left on their own, or observed from the "corner of my eye," start them to the activity earlier than other residents to avoid the rush.
  - o Provide seats for resting in major facility corridors. Tell the resident that it is okay to stop and rest or sit down on the trip to and from an activity.
  - o Recreational activities can incorporate leg exercises, moving around the room, walking, dance movements, aerobics, and strength training.
  - o Pacing and wandering can become positive activities if a safe pacing area is available (*see* Chapter 30, Activities Programming, for more information).
  - o Suggest that the family may enjoy walking with the resident on the unit grounds.
  - o Ensure that the family is informed of the resident's ambulation program when taking the resident home for a holiday or

other events.

ROM and Turning ADL Focus Area

Examples of indirect rehabilitation procedures for the range of motion and turning ADL focus area are as follows:

- **Toileting**
  - o After the resident has finished using the toilet (commode, bedpan, or urinal), encourage ROM exercises. For example, say, "Now that you have finished washing your hands, this is a good time to do your arm exercises."

- **Eating**
  - o Cue the bedbound resident to turn and position for supper. Remind the resident to do some upper extremity ROM exercises.
  - o While sitting in a chair waiting for a meal, residents can do active ROM exercises of their lower extremities.

- **Bathing**
  - o Spastic muscles become more relaxed in warm water, making it easier and more comfortable to do ROM exercises. For example, say, "After you are out of the tub and dry and warm, I'll help you with your leg exercises, or, "Why don't you brush your hair while I am cleaning the tub?"

- **Activities**
  - o Encourage the resident to do ROM exercises before starting an activity session while waiting for other residents to gather.
  - o Provide a rubber ball to squeeze, or suggest tapping feet to music.
  - o The activity itself can be an opportunity to do ROM exercises (e.g., crocheting, crafts).

Transfer ADL Focus Area

Examples of indirect rehabilitation procedures for the transfer ADL focus area are as follows:

- **Toileting**
  - o Encourage the resident to transfer on and off the toilet or commode. For example, say, "I'll help you get out of bed so that you can walk to the bathroom."
  - o Have any needed transfer devices available, clean, and ready to use.

- **Eating**
  - o Encourage the resident to transfer into a wheelchair to go to the dining room for lunch, and transfer to a dining chair for eating.

- **Bathing**
  - o Encourage the resident to transfer from bed to shower chair or wheelchair to bath, and so on. Many residents become fearful of such transfers. Provide adequate time and reassurance for a successful transfer.

- **Activities**
  - o If interested in going to an activity, offer to help in transfer from a chair to a standing position, or from bed to a wheelchair, and so on. Say, for example, "Time for your art history class now. I'll help you get up using the sliding board that you tried yesterday."
  - o Work on helping the resident achieve independence with the subtask of locking brakes and positioning the wheelchair for a safe transfer.

Eating ADL Focus Area

Examples of indirect rehabilitation procedures for the eating ADL focus area are as follows:

- **Ambulating**
  - o For the resident who would like a snack or a cup of tea, improve stamina by encouraging him or her to walk with you to the kitchen to prepare the item.

- **Dressing/Grooming**
  - o Have the resident perform activities involving the use of fingers, hands, and

arms, as well as eye/hand coordination (e.g., bringing an object such as a washcloth or lipstick to the face).

- Activities
  o Encourage or help the resident prepare a snack at an activity or participate in a cooking group.
  o Support the social aspects of eating. Encourage social exchanges among table mates.
  o For the resident who needs supervision and reminders to repeat the chewing and swallowing tasks until the meal is completed, teach the family how to help in this activity.

Dressing ADL Focus Area. Examples of indirect rehabilitation procedures for the dressing ADL focus area are as follows:

- Toileting
  o Encourage the resident to adjust clothing when using the bathroom. Say, for example, "Now that I have helped you into the bathroom, how about helping to pull down your pants so they won't be soiled."
- Eating
  o Encourage the resident to place a protective apron over clothing. For example, say, "Now that it's time for lunch, why don't you protect your new dress with this apron?" or, "Here is your sweater before you go into the dining room."
- Ambulating
  Encourage the resident to get dressed before ambulating to a favorite activity. Say, for example, "How about wearing your new suit jacket to the concert?"
- Activities
  o Encourage the resident to get dressed before attending an activity or to get undressed after an evening activity.
  o Appraise the family of the dressing program. Let them know how they can help

or participate in the implementation of the care plan (e.g., the resident needs assistance by removing socks and shoes in the evening).

The following lists provide examples of the more direct rehabilitation in targeted ADL area.

Ambulation

Examples of direct rehabilitation in the ambulation area are as follows:

- Demonstrate physical movement using a transfer belt. Provide light touch guard rather than weight-bearing support.
- Specify a walking distance (e.g., an entire corridor, 10 feet around the room).
- Specify the nature of the walking activities (e.g., an inclined ramp, stairs).
- Walk the residents to specific destinations (e.g., to the dining room for meals or off the unit with a staff member who is doing an errand in another part of the facility).
- Recruit family to participate in the care plan if they are routinely at the facility when walking activities are scheduled (e.g., an afternoon walk to the next unit or to the vending machine area, or outdoors).

ROM and Turning

Examples of direct rehabilitation in the ROM and turning area are as follows:

- For residents who are unable to participate in the activity, the nurse assistant should do passive ROM exercises.
- For residents who can perform part of the ROM exercises, the nurse assistant should help with active-assistive ROM.
- For the residents who are capable of doing the ROM exercises alone, the nurse assistant may only need to provide cueing or supervision.
- If the resident is cognitively intact but physically impaired (including sensitivity to touch), train the resident on the importance of changing position and performing activi-

ties at a set interval.

- Include families in the ROM exercises. If the care plan includes ROM exercises in the evening, and the family members always visit at that time, the staff may suggest that the family members help in the activity.

Transfer

Examples of direct rehabilitation in the transfer area are as follows:

- Demonstrate the proper transfer technique (e.g., how to bear weight) and train the resident accordingly.
- Instruct the resident on how to use the arms of a chair to rise.
- Help the resident perceive the right spot and time to sit down.

Meals

Examples of direct rehabilitation in the meals area are as follows:

- Give supplemental nourishment, monitor for full consumption, and remind the resident to continue eating until finished.
- Explain the importance of eating the food provided.
- Try foods that the resident is known to prefer.
- Try foods that can be consumed without utensils.
- Experiment with extending the time allocated for completing the meal.
- Encourage the use of adaptive appliances and retrain the resident, as appropriate.
- Enhance social graces and appropriate eating behavior by providing verbal cues to help the resident understand what is expected.

Dressing

Examples of direct rehabilitation in the dressing area are as follows:

- Lay out the clothes and test whether the resident can be taught to dress through a progressively less intrusive cueing program.

- Experiment with different types of simple instructions.
- When attempting to move the resident into performances of a new dressing subtask, repeat the demonstration of the new task segments.
- Set a time limit within which the resident should dress (or undress).
- Present clothing, selection, and dressing skills in a group session, followed up with individual family and resident sessions. Group and individual sessions can be led by a nurse, OT, or specially trained nurse assistant.

EXERCISE THERAPY PROGRAMS FOR REHABILITATION AND INTENSIVE REHABILITATION WATCH GROUP

A resident's ability to perform the complete series of tasks comprising the ADLs depends on physiologic competence, neuropsychological function, and various social factors. For residents whose ADL dependency is due at least in part to physiologic impairments that can be improved by exercise therapy, the goal of care is to:

- Prevent further decline or improve the resident's capacity to perform ADLs
- Reverse the deconditioning due to chronically low levels of physical activity
- Educate the resident and family that preservation of exercise capacity and maintenance of ADL performance are closely related
- Address the specific remediable decrements in physical capacity attributable to chronic diseases and medications

The introduction of exercise in various forms throughout the day can affect ADL impairment on several levels. Directly, it can reverse some of the muscle weakness, inflexibility, poor balance, and lack of endurance that contribute to physical dysfunction. Indirectly, it can improve a resident's affect, motivation, and self-efficacy, which increases the willingness to participate in other efforts to sustain or improve functional status. Therefore, exercise is an important tool to achieve the goals of the nursing-based rehabilitative care plans.

Assessments

Before the nursing staff increases a resident's level of physical activity, the medical staff should assess residents for stability in acute and chronic medical conditions, and make recommendations for an appropriate activity level. Uncontrolled cardiovascular or metabolic disease, certain kinds of very severe heart disease, and unstable or newly fractured skeletal sites are major medical contraindications to the introduction of increased exercise levels.

Specific examples include malignant arrhythmias, unstable angina, enlarging aortic aneurysm, pulmonary edema, phlebitis, myocarditis, severe aortic stenosis, pneumonia or influenza, hyperglycemia, dehydration, fever, foot ulcers, dislocation of shoulder, or new vertebral compression fracture. However, most residents will have chronic, stable medical conditions accompanied by low levels of activity that make them likely candidates for an exercise therapy program.

Need for Referral

In some cases, it may not be clear from the resident's record whether the level of control of a chronic condition is sufficient to allow the introduction of exercise. In these situations, seek clarification from the appropriate physician or therapist before beginning. Likewise, if a new symptom or exacerbation of an underlying illness arises after the introduction of exercise, seek a referral before continuing. However, it is not necessary to obtain written permission from the physician for every resident about any contraindications, since the exercises involve simple extensions of physical activities that are already performed throughout the day. Barriers to participation will be created in the minds of both nursing staff and residents if increased exercise is seen as a medical prescription rather than as part of the normal, expected daily routine.

Incorporating Exercise Therapy into Nursing Activities

Simple opportunities to exercise present themselves continually throughout the day, and can be incorporated in nursing activities without radically restructuring the workday. For example, calling residents to meals 10 minutes earlier may allow those with impaired mobility to walk to the dining room rather than be dependent on a wheelchair. Many residents spend hours lining the hallways in chairs. Encourage them by using posters or verbal cues to walk or perform seated calisthenics. Strengthening exercises can enliven the sedentary hours with therapeutic exercise without the need for an organized class. Ropes attached to pulleys on the wall of the nursing unit can be used to exercise the upper extremities while sitting. Whatever the activity opportunity, the message to residents should be that active participation is expected and encouraged by the staff.

Targeting Residents for Types of Exercise Therapy

It is likely that every resident will have some degree of deficit in endurance capacity (cardiovascular fitness), muscle strength, balance, and flexibility, due to the combination of deconditioning, aging, chronic diseases, and medications. Therefore, every resident within the intensive rehabilitation and rehabilitation watch groups is a potential candidate for nursing-based exercise therapy, with the exceptions previously noted about specific uncontrolled or untreatable medical conditions.

Some residents, because of their particular

combination of diseases, will benefit from specific types of exercise in the initial stages of therapy. For example, a resident whose mobility is impaired because of painful osteoarthritis of the knees will have deficits in endurance, strength, balance, and flexibility, yet be unable to endure weight-bearing activities such as standing and walking. In such cases, seated or supine strengthening exercises for the quadriceps and hamstrings are recommended as a prerequisite to other forms of exercise in that they will stabilize the joint and allow pain-free weight bearing. This approach is in direct contrast to the usual tactics of providing analgesics, an assistive device, and the advice to walk as much as can be tolerated.

In other cases, use assistive devices to increase mobility in residents whose deficit is due primarily to imbalance. Also, balance training techniques can be practiced safely under nursing supervision, often resulting in safer ambulation with and without assistive devices. Endurance training, progressing from supine to seated to ambulatory activities, is appropriate for a resident recovering from a period of bedrest or hospitalization.

Whatever the case-specific circumstances, it is important to identify the site of the major deficit in order to target residents for specific interventions. Apply the following guidelines to identify the site of major deficit:

- Ask the resident to rise from a chair and walk down the hallway using his or her usual assistive device, and closely observe for these actions:
  o If the resident has great difficulty getting out of a chair, this is due primarily to upper or lower extremity pain or weakness, and *strengthening exercises* are indicated.
  o If the resident rises quickly and easily but is unsteady in standing balance, uses an assistive device for balance, stumbles,

or has a staggering gait, *balance exercises* are indicated.
  o If the resident rises steadily and easily, but tires, develops claudication or becomes short of breath in a very short distance, *endurance exercises* are indicated.

These patterns are not mutually exclusive. Often they occur in combination, and many residents will need all three types of exercises. The classification is useful primarily as a framework to establish an appropriate progression of exercise activities. When in doubt, start with strength and balance, and add endurance later. This is contrary to the usual practice of starting with ambulation (endurance), which may put residents with muscle weakness and balance impairment in danger of falls.

How to Carry Out Exercise Therapy

Consider nursing-directed exercise therapy as a natural component of the ordinary activities of the unit, and not something reserved for a few special cases. The goal is to maintain an adequate level of physical fitness to maximize ADL independence by using various combinations of the three basic kinds of exercise:

- Endurance training (aerobic exercise)
- Resistance training (strengthening exercise)
- Balance and flexibility training. In the following list, each ADL is paired with the physiologic requirements that are predominantly involved in the activity. Prioritize the resident's needs accordingly.

ADL Exercise	Capacity Required
Bed mobility	Flexibility, strength
Locomotion and transfers	Strength, balance, endurance
Dressing	Flexibility, strength
Toileting	Strength, balance
Personal hygiene	Flexibility, endurance
Eating	Strength, endurance

Address each of the indicated physiologic requirements through formal or informal exercise programming. The following ideas, outlined for endurance, resistance, balance, and flexibility training, can be implemented with a minimum of time, expense, and supervision, so their potential range of application is wide.

Endurance Training

Endurance training involves moving the major large muscle groups, which are moved hundreds or thousands of times against little or no resistance in order to improve cardiovascular efficiency. Examples include walking, biking, swimming, and dancing. Obviously, walking is the most immediately available and feasible mode of training for most residents. It is an overlearned activity, requires no extra equipment, and can be carried out in the corridors of any unit at any time of the day or night.

As with any kind of exercise, programming for endurance involves the following considerations:

• Frequency: For sustained benefit, endurance activities should take place at least 3 days per week, up to a 7-day-per-week cycle, as appropriate.

• Duration: Each exercise session should increase gradually from 1 to 5 minutes for very deconditioned residents, up to at least 20-30 minutes of sustained activity for conditioned residents when possible.

• Intensity: Intensity refers to the cardiovascular and pulmonary work required to supply enough oxygen to the exercising muscles. In younger individuals, it is normally measured as the relative rises in pulse and blood pressure. However, many elderly residents have diseases or medications that affect the normal heart rate or blood pressure response to exercise, so it is more appropriate in the nursing home setting to use perceived exertion to monitor the correct level of intensity. The activity should

optimally be at a level between fairly light and somewhat hard, as shown here on the Borg Scale of Perceived Exertion:

6	
7	Very, very light
8	
9	Very light
10	
11	Fairly light
12	
14	
15	Hard
16	
17	Very hard
18	
19	Very, very hard
20	

For residents who cannot understand or read a large posted version of the rating scale, keep the level of intensity below that which produces dyspnea, i.e., the resident should be able to converse while engaging in the activity. The workload required to produce this level of exertion will be unique to each individual and will change as conditioning occurs.

• Progression: Progression refers to the changing of the increase in intensity, duration, or frequency of the exercise that is made by staff in response to the improved cardiovascular fitness of the resident. A target of frequency at least 3 days per week with a duration of at least 20 minutes per session should be observed before increasing intensity. Increase the intensity of walking by altering the speed or grade of ascent, or by having the body support more weight during exercise. With frail individuals, however, it is not appropriate in most cases to progress by increasing speed since this may result in falls secondary to imbalance. However, increase the weight being supported by exercising in a standing as opposed to a seated position, or by using both arms and legs in unison on a rower or cycle. Grade can be increased by walking up a ramp or a staircase with railings if one is available that can be supervised during use.

- Other issues: Successful implementation of an endurance program requires proper footwear and clothing, foot care, appropriate use of assistive devices, timing in relation to meals and medications that may cause postural hypotension, administration of pain medications to increase mobility, optimal correction of vision, and family support and encouragement during visiting hours.

Resistance Training

Resistance training refers to activities in which the muscles are used to produce an unusual amount of force to move or resist an object just a few times in order to increase muscle strength. It differs from endurance training in that the muscle is overloaded and the number of contractions (or repetitions) needed to achieve a training effect is very small by comparison. Examples include weight lifting (i.e., dynamic resistance training) and pushing against an immovable object (i.e., static or isometric training). Lifting something more closely approximates real-life ADL needs, and is preferred, but in many cases the lack of equipment in the nursing home dictates the use of static or isometric strengthening exercises. However, the advantage of this mode of training, in addition to no need for equipment, is that there is little chance of injuring joints or aggravating arthritis since there is no movement of the joints.

The following general recommendations apply to all forms of resistance training:

- Frequency: Resistance training activities should take place 3 days per week for maximum benefit, although twice a week still provides substantial benefit.
- Duration: Duration will vary with the number of strengthening exercises prescribed.

In general, about 3 to 5 minutes for each muscle group exercised is all that is needed. This will involve approximately 10 slow repetitions (one set), a rest period of 1 to 2 minutes, and then another set of 10 repetitions. Slow means that the repetitions should take approximately 6 to 9 seconds to complete. If not done slowly, the muscle will not be stressed, and momentum and gravity will do all the work. For residents who are too weak to complete 10 repetitions of a particular exercise in the beginning, gradually increase the number of repetitions until the whole set can be done. Then increase the intensity of the resistance.

- Intensity: Intensity refers to the difficulty of the task or the heaviness of the load lifted, relative to the maximal strength of the individual. In order for a training effect to occur, the task must involve exertion between 50% and 80% of the capacity of a particular muscle group. For example, if someone can lift a maximum of 10 pounds with his or her biceps, he or she needs to lift 5 to 8 pounds initially during training to improve strength. In many cases the resident's maximum capacity at the outset will not be known. Use the Borg Scale to determine the relative effort involved. Strengthening exercises should aim for a level of "Somewhat hard" to "Hard" (13 to 15) on the scale.
- Progression: Progression refers to the increase in intensity of the exercise in response to the improved muscular strength of the resident. Unlike endurance training, modify only the intensity; the frequency (3 days per week) and duration (two sets of 10 repetitions) should be held constant. The reason for this is that a muscle is made stronger by resisting heavier loads, not by resisting light loads more times. Therefore, after the target duration for each exercise has been reached, progress by increasing the load. The load can be increased in many ways. For example, if pushing against an immov-

able object such as a wall or bed, the resident may start by resisting moderately and progress to pushing as hard as possible during each repetition. If strengthening the quadriceps (knee extensor) muscle, the resident may start by tensing the muscle at the front of the thigh (as though trying to lock the kneecap) while in bed, advance to extending the lower leg against gravity while seated, and finally to standing up from a chair without using the arms to assist. In this progression, more and more of the body weight is used as resistance as the muscle becomes capable of resisting a heavier load. The following examples are ways to train other muscle groups. Both static and dynamic techniques are described.

o *Dorsiflexors* of the ankle (muscles at the front of the calf): While seated in a chair facing the bed, hook the front of the shoes under the bed. Pull the toes upward as hard as possible and hold in that position for 6 seconds.

o *Plantarflexors* of the ankle (muscles at the back of the calf): While standing and holding onto a railing, lift the body so that it is supported by the toes, then slowly lower back to the ground. To progress, place a sturdy book under the feet so that the heels are hanging below the level of the forefoot. Lift the body until it is supported by just the toes and hold, and then slowly lower back to the starting position. Enhance balance and strength by toe walking along the length of the hall while holding onto the railing.

o *Triceps* (muscle at the back of the upper arm): While seated in a chair or wheelchair with the brakes locked, lean forward slightly at the waist. Push down on the arms of the chair, attempting to lift the buttocks off the seat. Even if the body cannot be lifted initially, trying to lift it is a beneficial isometric (static) exercise.

o *Biceps* (muscle at the front of the upper arm): While standing with the back against a wall and holding onto a walker or cane with both hands, bend the elbows to bring the walker or cane as close to the shoulders as possible and hold. Slowly lower the walker back to the floor, keeping the back against the wall at all times. Progress by lifting heavier objects. For example, add a walker bag filled with progressively heavier objects, such as fruit, cans, and books.

o *Shoulders, triceps*: After a cane or walker is brought to the shoulders as in the previous exercise, continue to raise it straight up over the head as high as possible. Hold it in this position and then slowly lower it back to the starting position.

Balance Training

Balance training consists of activities whose purpose is to improve static and dynamic balance by stimulating the central and peripheral balance system. In static balance training, the goal is to extend the base of support gradually and decrease proprioceptive input while maintaining an upright posture. For example, standing with the feet apart and eyes open, train the resident to stand on one foot gradually with the eyes closed. In dynamic balance training, the goal is to train the reflexes and musculoskeletal response necessary to resist disturbances of the environment or the body mass. Examples include leaning as far as possible in all directions without moving the feet, tandem (heel to toe) walking, and stepping over obstacles. In general, balance training can be accomplished by manipulating the body weight and simple, easily obtainable props. The following general programming considerations are the same as for the other forms of exercise:

• *Frequency*: Practice balance exercises at least 1 day per week, up to a 7-day-per-week cycle, as appropriate.

- *Duration*: Five to 10 minutes is required, depending on the number of different exercises practiced. Usually, each movement is practiced five times during one session.
- *Intensity*: Intensity refers to the difficulty of the maneuvers chosen. For safety reasons (i.e., prevention of falls) begin with activities that stress the balance system only mildly. Intensity will be regulated by:
  - o The narrowness of the base of support (e.g., feet apart versus feet together stance)
  - o The sensory cues allowed (e.g., eyes open versus eyes closed; hard linoleum floor versus soft foam pad to stand on)
  - o Environmental manipulation (e.g., height of the steps to climb up or size of the obstacle to step over)
  - o The degree of displacement of body mass (e.g., amount of lean attempted, extent of position transfer required as in transferring from standing to bed or chair versus standing on the floor)
- Progression: Progression must be competency-based, and will involve moving to a more complex task. Residents must be able to demonstrate that they can perform the task safely and repeatedly without spotting (i.e., observation by the staff) of any kind before the next level is prescribed. Progression can also mean application of the newly mastered balance task to ADL and mobility activities during the course of the day. For example, if a resident can rise safely from a seated to standing position, encourage the resident to do this independently every time he or she transfers during the day, rather than relying on assistance from the nursing staff to speed things along. The following examples are progressively more difficult tasks presented in their approximate order of difficulty:
  - o Static balance training. Hold each position for as long as possible, up to 30 seconds:

- Stand holding an assistive device
- Stand without an assistive device
- Stand with feet side by side
- Stand with feet in tandem position (heel to toe)
- Stand on one foot

For safety, practice all these positions with the resident standing 12 inches in front of a wall, with a staff member spotting from the side. After these positions are mastered, ask the resident to repeat the sequence with his or her eyes closed. Finally, a more compliant surface can be added: Proceed from linoleum to carpet to a foam mattress pad in order to decrease proprioceptive input and increase task difficulty. Flat-soled shoes should be worn during these exercises; bare feet are also acceptable.

- o Dynamic balance training. Repeat each task five times or as tolerated. Practice one task from each category during a session.
- o Transfers
  - Transfer from bed or chair to standing position
  - Transfer from bed or chair without using arms to assist
  - Transfer from standing to supine position on floor and back
- o Ambulation
  - Tandem walk for 20 feet using a railing or assistive device
  - Tandem walk for 20 feet without an assistive device or railing
  - Climb up and down steps or staircase using a handrail
  - Climb up and down steps or staircase without using a handrail
  - Step over progressively larger obstacles (shoe, box, book, stacked books)
- o Leans
- o Lean as far as possible to the front, back, and each side while in seated position
- o Lean as far as possible to the front, back, and each side while in standing position

o Lean as far as possible to the front, back, and each side while standing holding a 5-pound ball or weight in outstretched hands

Flexibility Training

The purpose of flexibility training is to increase tissue elasticity and allow greater ROM across the joints. To accomplish this, slowly stretch the targeted areas and hold the stretch in the maximally attained position for a sustained time. Stretching is never done ballistically by bouncing or jarring the joints, which may cause tears or strains. The proper method is to move as far as possible toward the desired position, then completely relax the stretched muscles, stretch a little further, and then hold that position as long as possible, with a goal of 30-60 seconds.

Do not perform stretching with cold muscles. Stretching is best accomplished after an endurance exercise, such as walking as part of the cool-down routine, or after a warm bath.

The following general recommendations apply to all forms of flexibility training:
- Frequency: One to 7 days per week
- Duration: One minute per stretch; five to 10 stretches of major muscle groups such as quadriceps, hamstrings, shoulders, plantar flexors, hip flexors, lower back, and abdomen. There are thousands of opportunities during the day to perform stretching exercising. For example, when drying the back with a towel, instruct the resident to hold the towel diagonally behind the back, and alternate extending the upper arm as fully as possible. Dressing provides another opportunity. While putting on shoes, flex the hip up as far as possible toward the chest and hold this position while fastening shoes. Use the hours spent lining the hallways in chairs. While seated, the toes can be flexed and held up, the knees can be extended to stretch hamstrings, and the arms can be lifted straight over the head. It is important to prac-

tice proper durations for each stretch: one stretch held for 60 seconds is very effective; bouncing into position but not holding it more than a second or two is not effective, even if done many times.
- Intensity. The intensity of stretching routines is generally maintained by always stretching to the limits attainable without producing pain. There is never a need to go beyond this threshold to achieve increased flexibility.
- Progression. As flexibility increases, hold the stretch in its maximum position for longer durations, until a 60-second hold can be achieved. At the same time, the amount of the stretch will gradually be increased as the tissue elasticity improves.

Care Plan Documentation

If exercise is to be taken seriously as an integral part of the nursing care plan, it must be documented like other therapeutic interventions. The easiest way to document the success of an exercise program is to outline the mode, frequency, duration, intensity, and progression of the categories of exercise previously described. When no progression is observed over time, it is likely that the principles are not being followed, or that the resident is not compliant with the recommendations. In the latter instance, find creative ways to enhance exercise adoption and adherence, including more staff and family participation, fitness groups, awards ceremonies, and posting of graphs of progress in common areas. This will also allow the physician to correlate any positive or negative changes in underlying conditions, with the actual exercise participation rate.

Monitoring Resident Response to the Program

The best way to measure resident response to the program is to re-evaluate ADL capacity as the specific physiologic deficit is addressed through the training program. If the program has been adhered to, physiologic benefit should result unless there is intercurrent illness, progression of disease, or injury. The resident can keep logs to monitor adherence rates, if possible, or they can be kept by the staff and family if needed. This feedback will enhance compliance and visibility of the program on the unit.

Equipment and Environmental Modifications

The environment on the nursing unit should be safe and inviting for the kind of exercise programming described here. Hallways that are uncluttered with wheelchairs and carts provide a good walking path. An even better adaptation is to mark off a route like a real track, with markers indicating the distance traveled, motivational posters and exercise tips along the way, arrows painted on the floor, and provision for rest stops and railings. Routes for more advanced or supervised residents might include ramps, stairs, and areas to practice tandem walking for balance. Good lighting is always essential to prevent falls.

The ambiance of the nursing unit is key to the success of such programming. If the visual message conveyed is that residents are expected to lie down or line the hallways in chairs for most of the day between meals, that is what will happen. However, if some chairs are replaced by exercise bikes or strength-training devices, or a track is clearly designated around the unit, or logs of distances walked each day are posted in the dining room, the expectations of the residents and their families will likely be quite different. Hopefully, nursing home design in the future will not assume sedentariness as it often does now, but instead the architectural plans will include provisions for a wide range of ADL-enhancing exercise options.

30
Activities Programming

Nancy Mace, MA
Ruth Perschbacher, RMT-BC, ACC
Heike Tuplin, CTRS, ACC
Michael Westerman, CTRS
Jane Carlson
Gail Schober, RN

Activities are important in the lives of nursing home residents. They are a source of pleasure and provide opportunities for positive engagement. They can invoke smiles, rekindle meaningful roles, lessen a dysphoric mood, strengthen self-identity, and alter physiology.

A resident's physical and psychosocial well-being can benefit directly from daily participation in activities. Most cognitively intact residents are able to set their own schedule and choose activities that are interesting to them. For these individuals, a wide array of activities are possible—depending on their needs and preferences. An effective activities program provides opportunities to exercise individual initiative, interactive social skills, and self-control, whether in individual or small group settings.

For the diverse spectrum of cognitively impaired residents, however, it is staff and family who must play a central role in specifying daily routines and activity options. As a resident's decision-making ability declines and consistent communication becomes more problematic, staff and family collaboration be-

comes increasingly important. Since the resident's preferences continue to have meaning and must be respected, strategies will be required to ensure the match between resident response and the desired outcome.

With the cognitively impaired, individual attention or small group settings are usually appropriate, but some larger group activities may also be warranted. In designing programs, success depends upon correctly perceiving the needs and responses of the resident involved. Although some general principles apply, be prepared to be surprised by the adaptive ability and activity preferences of the cognitively impaired population in your facility.

Because activities are so important to quality of life, a planned program of daily activities is an essential element of total care. To formulate an activities care plan, the staff should know the resident's present history (i.e., medical history, physical or mental deficits, emotional and social strengths, sources of enjoyment) and past history (who the person used to be and how the past may be relevant to the present). For example, residents with ap-

parently low cognition for whom listening to opera was once an important part of their lives might respond to recordings in ways that could not have been predicted.

OVERVIEW

Activities are a basic part of human life, and they are required no matter where a person resides. In the nursing home, some residents will spend long hours in both passive and active pursuits that are meaningful, enjoyable, and ultimately in line with their own preferences and choices. Many will be able to decide what they can and cannot do, focusing on activities that have meaning to them. Other residents, however, because of diminished capabilities and changed situations, must work with and depend on staff and family to ensure that their preferred activities are recognized and available in an institutional setting.

If this is the approach taken in better nursing homes, it is also true that many residents are in facilities where activity involvement is severely constrained. In such instances, the challenge to activity directors is to start programmatic improvement so that the activity needs of residents are recognized to be a vital component of total care and an important, integrating force for positive adaptation.

Entering and living in a nursing home inevitably involves losses—including health (due to accompanying illness), home and privacy, family involvement in familiar surroundings, pets, and the possessions of a lifetime. Other losses, too, can be keenly felt and severely disabling to the resident, including the loss of independence, identity, friendships, security, dignity, mastery and control, success, pleasure, and self-esteem. The purpose of activity therapy in the nursing home setting is to sustain and strengthen the affective aspects of normal life, i.e., the stuff of life's daily experience, involving the emotions, feelings, and sense of social and physical identity.

These activities are not a one-time therapy given after the morning meal like a daily dose of a medication. Do not consider them to be simple diversions that help ensure that residents do not disrupt the health care team. Rather, activities must be seen as a central, driving force in the resident's daily life and plan of care. By building on the resident's sense of independence, identity, and dignity, and enabling the resident to create and nurture friendships and achieve mastery, success, and pleasure, activities therapy gives greater meaning and satisfaction to what the resident does all day—before and after formal activities sessions as well as during what appears to be more independently motivated and controlled times of the day. A good activity program identifies quality of life areas that have been lost to the resident, and finds ways to restore them.

Risk-Taking, Autonomy, and Control

For an activities program to be successful, it must resolve the inevitable philosophical tension in the nursing home setting between risk-taking, autonomy, and control. It is not uncommon for the rights and responsibilities of the facility, the resident, and the resident's family to be in conflict. For example, in formulating an individualized activities care plan, how much risk should the resident (or the family, if the resident is not competent to participate in these decisions) be encouraged or willing to accept? Some residents—or their families, or the nursing facility itself—will place a high value on preserving independence, and opt for high-risk activities such as continuing to walk in the garden even though the resident is prone to falls. Others will take a low-risk position, such as not venturing or restraining the resident from venturing out of the room for fear of falling, which increases dependency. Such decision-making is invariably complex, involving issues of autonomy, i.e., the legal right of the resident to do what he or she wishes as long as others are not placed at risk or harmed.

Assessment

If a resident finds an activity meaningful, include it in the resident's total activity program. These activities may include:

- *Unstructured activities*, such as family visits, socializing with other residents and staff, watching television, and other related activities
- *Structured activities,* such as large and small group programs and one-on-one visits from activity staff

In all cases, carefully consider the resident's individual needs, particularly those of residents who are more impaired and less able to articulate these preferences and choices.

Assume a situation to be problematic when:

- The resident prefers more or different activity pursuits than those in which he or she is presently engaged.
- The resident has little involvement in activities and shows signs of distress. This is a concern with residents who are bedfast, whose communication and cognitive abilities exceed their physical skills, or who have communication and cognitive impairments.
- The more unusual situation when a resident has become overly involved in activities, is awake all or most of the time, and is at risk for overexertion. In this case, a psychiatric consult is recommended.

The activities assessment for these residents will rely and build on the medical, nursing, and rehabilitation therapy evaluations that are included in the resident's file. The Health Care Financing Administration-mandated Minimum Data Set (MDS) documentation of resident attributes will provide useful information on the resident's past activity interests, level of current activity involvement and preferences, and whether the resident prefers more or different activities. Be sure also to include input from nurse assistants, who can often provide crucial insight into the resident's likes and dislikes.

Medical assessment information provides insight into how much and what kind of things the resident can do comfortably, the medical limitations and sensory capacities (vision, hearing, smell, taste, touch), and any medications that might impair function. Nursing assessment items provide information on the resident's special needs (e.g., for a catheter or support in the wheelchair) or behavioral patterns and risks (e.g., wandering). Other valuable information pertains to language skills, range of motion, use of limbs, potential for recovery, function, and psychosocial status.

Cognitive assessment items focus on memory and decision-making ability, including an evaluation of whether cognitive function varies over time—for better or for worse. Changing involvement in activities can be a key indicator of altered cognitive status. Cognitive function itself will vary greatly between individuals, even on a nursing unit comprised of a supposedly homogeneous population. One resident may be unable to name an object but still remember how to use it. Another may be unable to sit still. Another may be apathetic. The ability to plan, remember a goal, do overlearned motor skills, select among objects, initiate or stop behaviors, ignore distractions, do things in sequence, or tolerate stress is never consistent among individuals, and all of these factors directly affect their ability to perform activities.

Perform an assessment of the resident's mental health status. Many nursing home residents are depressed, while others will have various psychological problems. The facility should make the best use of available mental health resources, with the activities staff consulting with the psychologist or psychiatrist to design individualized activities for the resident that will support the therapist's interventions. Most mental health professionals are eager to participate in joint care planning exercises.

Mental health problems require special approaches. The resident who complains incessantly is suffering. The resident who is depressed will not cheer upon request or upon being moved bodily to a picnic. With such residents, it is best to introduce an activity in small, easy steps. Providing specialized activities for residents in mental distress, enabling them to achieve dignity, control, and self-esteem, is more likely to mute their difficult behavior than punishment or rewards.

The following list provides the positive attributes that can be used by activities planners to construct a meaningful program for the individual resident:

- How well can the person get about? Walk independently? Need a wheelchair? Slow? Need assistance? What help is needed for the person to find his or her way about the unit?
- How well can the resident's toileting needs be met? Independent? Need assistance? Able to locate toilet?
- How much assistance will the resident need to get ready for activities? Independent? Reminders?
- Will the person need encouragement to participate?
- What physical abilities does the resident retain? How can the function be supported? What motor skills remain?
- What is the resident's mood? Shy? Depressed? Irritable? Amiable?
- Afraid of failure? Discouraged? Retains sense of humor? Under what circumstances?
- How much of a resident's customary activity can he or she still do? Read? Cook? Shop? Sing? Play piano? Tell a joke? What can be done to enable a resident to continue to enjoy activities that were important earlier in life?
- What social skills remain? Smiling, laughing, staying focused? Responds to social cues? Is socially appropriate? Will talk about others (gossip)? Who does the resident still recognize? How small a group is needed to bring the resident out?

- What cognitive functions does the resident have? Sensory functions? Ability to understand? Ability to stay focused? Memory, logic, abstraction, understands quantities, able to put things in proper sequence, able to make choices, able to plan, initiate? Can the resident follow one- or two-step commands? How long is attention span?
- What behaviors can be channeled into meaningful activity? Repetitious activities? Physically active tasks?

Careplanners who learn more about a resident are better able to restore positive, effective feelings and enrich the resident's daily life. In researching the resident's personal history, ask about:

- Occupations, travels, hobbies, interests, daily activities (e.g., she liked to mow the lawn, he enjoyed washing or drying the dishes)
- Family and professional roles, ethnic background, pets, the old neighborhood, etc. Learn about the resident's family relationships, feuds, roles (e.g., controlling mother, stern father, dominating brother), any unfulfilled goals (if the resident had any)

For example, a resident badly crippled by strokes may be able to achieve her goal of learning how to use a computer, and gain great satisfaction from showing people how "a crippled old lady" has learned modern technology. Or, a resident now crippled with arthritis who may have once loved to quilt, may be able to quilt again using an adapted cutting tool and fabric adhesives provided by the activities therapist.

Consider, too, the impact of the environment on the resident's ability to participate in activities. Is there enough light? Too much glare or noise? Too many distractions? Uncomfortable chairs? Tables too high for stooped bodies? Unpleasant smells? Residents enjoy outings. To plan them, assess various modes of transportation, the walking surface, weather, availability of hand rails, noise, light, and other environmental factors. Adapt environments when possible to allow fuller resident participation in outings.

Developing and Implementing the Activities Care Plan

The purpose of activities is to build on or restore the resident's sense of independence, identity, dignity, friendship, mastery and control, success, pleasure and self esteem. These are the same objectives that drive the resident's overall care plan (i.e., activities of daily living [ADLs], rest, and therapies), so the activities personnel must be an integral part of the caregiving staff. For example, if a resident cannot exercise any decision-making, control, or independence about dressing, the goal of activities must be to restore these experiences for the resident, however briefly.

Long periods of idle time are not therapeutic for any individual. For all residents, including those with dementia, boredom can lead to restless activity, apathy, and a further weakening of identity and self-esteem. Boredom can also lead to depression or surly, unpleasant behavior. A resident's day must include scheduled rest periods, but there should not be periods of unscheduled idleness lasting more than 1 hour. Fill that time with planned activities. These may be slow-paced and simple (e.g., watching television or observing groups) or more energetic (e.g., singing, exercising), as appropriate. To consider an activity therapeutic, the resident must be actively involved in it. Someone who is near the television but not involved in watching a program is not engaged in that activity.

Activities may range from individual or one-on-one interactions to large group programs such as sing-alongs or church services. The duration of activities depends on many factors. Cognitively intact residents who are involved in group planning of a fund raiser may be actively engaged for 2 hours; a wine and cheese night may last even longer. However,

a cognitively impaired group may be able to tolerate as little as 5 minutes or as much as 45 minutes of involvement in any one type of activity. Even within supposedly homogeneous groups, individual tolerances vary and must be accommodated. Never force a resident to attend or to stay in an activity either verbally or by using restraints.

A key element in activities care planning is to build on the resident's remaining strengths while making no demands on his or her disabilities, since any demand on disabilities confirms the resident's experience of lost independence or low self-esteem. In a group activity in which residents with dementia are making soup, one person can use chopping skills, another can peel vegetables, another can pour in the water, another can hold the bowl, another can taste, and another can sit and criticize, which in this case represents a positive participation since the resident may be reliving an old role and so recapturing some self-esteem.

Setting Care Plan Goals

Matching the resident's assessed activity preferences to the array of program options offered by the nursing home is key to developing effective treatment approaches. For example, an oriented resident who prefers more or different activities may be lacking activity options that adequately challenge his or her cognitive potential, interests, and levels of function. Therefore, develop the initial care plan for individual, small, or large group activity programs that match the resident's functioning and interest levels if current programs do not do so. Offer program alternatives designed to meet individualized goals and outcomes.

Goals for an Activity Pursuit Program

Address the following central goals in an activity program (or parts of the program):
• Facilitate self-expression

- Facilitate social interaction with other residents, staff, or family
- Reduce agitated and disruptive behaviors
- Facilitate involvement in a productive activity
- Make use of leisure time and find gratification in activity pursuits
- Increase sensory and tactile stimulations
- Provide the appropriate cognitive challenges and opportunities to make decisions
- Take more responsibility for setting a schedule, building greater self-direction and control over what the resident does during the day

The following list provides 12 guidelines for therapeutic activities that are responsive to the prior goals:

- The activity must have an obvious purpose and meaning for the resident.
- The activity must offer a reasonable chance of success.
- The activity must reestablish old roles.
- The activity must confirm dignity. It must never be perceived by the residents as childish or inappropriate to social status.
- The activity must provide pleasure.
- The activity must not reinforce inadequacy or add to anxiety.
- The activity must be individualized.
- The activity must be voluntary.
- The activity must capitalize on the resident's remaining abilities.
- The activity must break down tasks into steps.
- The activity must meet basic human needs for identity, mastery, and self-esteem.
- The activity must encourage social interchange.

PROBLEMS, OBSTACLES, AND CHALLENGES

Sometimes an activity professional's day can seem to go from one crisis to another like this: residents refuse to participate; staff do not seem to support activities, and there is no space, time, or budget to accomplish one's responsibilities. In addition, the behavior of people with dementia can disrupt the best planned activity.

This section discusses how to react to those realities. The wise activity professional will:

- Build a support network outside the facility
- Build alliances within the facility and network with them
- Use a problem-solving approach and be creative and flexible
- Learn to recognize which problems can be solved and which cannot—and learn to tell the difference.

Activity directors often encounter residents who do not participate. A common problem is refusal to do any activity that may reflect an unmet need. For example, Mrs. Jones refused to participate in any activity. She required a wheelchair and was generally unpleasant and uncooperative. Staff assumed that she was just too difficult to place in an activity. They said she "has to take a positive attitude unless she wants to be miserable here." The activity professional spent time building Mrs. Jones' trust and eventually learned that Mrs. Jones was depressed by the idea of ball toss, exercise, discussing Ann Landers, and crafts. All she really wanted to do before she died was to go fishing. This was not possible and Mrs. Jones was seen by staff as needing to face reality. They said, "she needs to recognize that she is in a wheelchair and lives in a nursing home now."

In fact, facilities have taken multiply impaired, and even confused, residents fishing with no accidents. Volunteers can augment staff and safety can be ensured by carefully planning the activity. The barrier is often not the resident but the facility's ability and willingness to provide activities that residents may enjoy.

Refusal often occurs when the resident does not see the point of an activity, cannot remember the goal, or does not share the goal. Problems often arise around childish activities or crafts.

Depression

Depression is a major factor in a resident's refusal to participate in activities. Depression is rampant in nursing homes. It is often unrecognized and untreated, and the resources are not always in place to address the problem. The situation is gradually improving, however, as discussed in Chapter 13, Depression.

Activities alone may not be enough to treat depression, but activities that help self-esteem and social interaction are an important part of the treatment plan. Begin with small steps. Look outside the usual list of activities. Ask the resident to identify one small thing that will truly make him or her feel useful.

Residents with depression may have very little energy and may have difficulty concentrating on a task. Plan for this; you may not be able to change it until the depression lifts. Do not try to cheer people up or reassure them that they can do more than they say they can. This can make them feel misunderstood and become more depressed. Pressuring or coaxing a resident to participate may also make things worse.

Embarrassment

Embarrassment may cause residents to be reluctant to participate because of unsightly ostomy bags, loss of hair due to chemotherapy, loss of limbs, or fear of incontinence. Contact the voluntary associations for help with these problems and advice on how to locate and pay for wigs, attractive garments, and other items to improve self-esteem. Involve the resident in this process from the beginning and include this step in a care plan.

Severe Physical Impairment

Severe physical impairment, such as when residents are severely crippled by stroke or arthritis, may be impediments that staff are unprepared to deal with. Contact the voluntary associations for information on how to plan adapted activities. Ask for information

such as asking for a good film, a local consultant, or similar recommendation. Also consider obtaining an occupational or physical therapy consult. These specialists have extensive resources for adaptive devices that can be modified for activities. They also know how to position and support people so that they can participate.

Fatigue or Pain

Fatigue or pain can cause residents to refuse activities. Fatigue is genuine, so do not consider it malingering. Getting active may not relieve fatigue. When associated with illness or depression, fatigue can be crippling. Work with the resident to identify one small thing he or she really wants to do (e.g., write to her son, go to church, listen to religious music) or that will make him or her feel useful. Avoid activities that seem pointless to the resident. Involve the resident in planning and chart this as therapeutic time.

Pain is also genuine, even when the resident's report seems more severe than it appears. Much pain is overlooked, especially in residents with dementia, which can result in restlessness and irritability. (*See* Chapter 10, Cognitive Loss, for more information.) Aggressive pain management improves quality of life and supports function. Prevent pain to the extent possible, and time medications so that residents will not have to wait for them. Obtain a physical therapy consult when positioning or movement is contributing to pain. Arrange for the residents to receive their pain medication so that it will be at peak effectiveness when they join an activity group.

Impairments in Vision and Hearing

Impairments in vision and hearing are common and require that:
- The sensory loss be supported by environmental interventions such as improved lighting, the absence of glare, and the absence of background noise.
- The use of adaptive devices.

- Adapted activities (e.g., large-print books, playing cards, and computer screens; talking books).

Make sure that adapted activities are adult in character. Giving a visually impaired person a children's puzzle as a substitute for a complex jigsaw puzzle may lower the person's self-esteem. A new activity such as gardening might be more rewarding for the resident. For example, as an old man, artist Paul Matisse could no longer paint. Instead, he began to cut large shapes out of brightly colored paper, creating some of his most beautiful and moving work. Consult the voluntary associations for more help and information.

Cognitive and Behavioral Deficits

Cognitive and behavioral deficits can impede involvement in activities. Sometimes the behavior of people with dementia is disruptive to group activities. Try to provide separate activities for these people.

It is easy to blame residents whose behavior (e.g., being manipulative, controlling, rude, or demanding) excludes them from groups ("she has to stop insulting the others if she is going to be in the groups"). However, by the time a person reaches a nursing home many of these behaviors are unlikely to change. Powerful, but hidden, emotional pressures support their continuance. Further, when people enter a nursing home, they experience many losses. Many are in great distress—experiencing physical and mental anguish and difficulties adapting to the new environment. Activities provide the opportunity to restore some positive feelings, especially in people whose behavior reflects their suffering. (Do not overlook the other residents. They, too, are facing aging, losses, and death and are in need of feeling good about themselves.)

Fear for Privacy or Safety

Residents often refuse to participate in activities because they need to protect their room from wandering residents; they are fearful of noisy, agitated residents; or their escort is late, careless, or leaves them sitting in the hall. These are legitimate concerns. It is the responsibility of the facility to ensure a resident's privacy and safety of possessions and to employ competent staff.

The problems that arise between cognitively intact but often frail residents and people with dementia are best met by separating these residents. The staff will also appreciate this. A facility may choose separate living areas, parallel programming, hours during which the confused residents are off the unit (day care in the nursing home), and so forth.

Taking the First Step to Overcome Obstacles

Many problems in nursing homes arise from the lack of internal communication or the different goals of different staff. Periodic team meetings to discuss a resident is an excellent first step to begin change. By discussing a resident together, it may become evident for the first time to the staff that they are almost meeting a resident's needs. With simple changes the staff will be able to affect the resident's quality of life. All that may be needed is better transport coordination, pain management timed to allow for the resident's best performance during scheduled activities, or ensuring that a resident goes to activities with an empty bladder and a clean incontinence pad.

Problem-based charting with positive notations will ensure that regulatory requirements are met, will set staff goals, and will identify successes. Consider the following examples:

"Mrs. Jones is despondent over the changes in her life and has one goal before she dies. The team has decided to help the daughter and a volunteer take Mrs. Jones fishing. The activity director will teach the daughter ...."

"Evelyn cannot comfortably leave her room. She has asked to have visitors in her room. A tea party with the following activities has been planned in her room with five other residents."

"Mable will not participate in exercise classes. The group is noisy and the confusion is too stressful for Mable. She and four other ladies will be offered special programming by the activity aide."

"So much of George's self-esteem revolves around being needed, that he will be asked, as a therapeutic activity, to sweep the corridors. This will not alter the facility's normal provision of janitorial services."

The Second Step to Overcome Obstacles

As a second step, engage residents as much as possible in solving problems and chart this time as a one-to-one activity with the goal of providing increased control for the resident. The amount of activities accomplished will rise and leave the staff with a paper trail documenting the resident's needs and the staff's ability within current constraints to deliver the necessary programming.

There will often be little time and resources to provide care for a very impaired person. The staff may not make big changes. However, making one small positive change for a resident is often enough to make a big difference.

Staff members may not think that their facility has the resources discussed here. For example, it might be 6 months before the physical therapist can see a resident, and Medicare will not pay for it because the resident is not in a rehabilitation program, or there may be no psychiatrist who can see the depressed residents. The lack of resources is a major problem for long-term care facilities across the nation. Often the activity professional will have only a limited ability to change conditions.

Do not use this fact as an excuse for inactivity, however. For example, consider having the physical or occupational therapist conduct meetings for the staff on the units, giving general advice on how staff and the nurses can apply this knowledge to residents. Consider having someone on staff attend seminars on depression and then work with physicians to improve conditions. Also consider whether

any of the voluntary associations have valuable information for the care and comfort of residents with the illness they represent. These associations may also have educational materials or be willing to do seminars for the staff. These resources will vary from region to region, but they are worth contacting for help.

Many homes will have family members and others who are willing to act as volunteers. Volunteers can work in nursing homes, but volunteerism requires a talented, dedicated person to recruit, train, and retain them. Consider these people as an option for special activities that a resident wishes (e.g., playing chess, going fishing, talking about some esoteric interest).

Other Ideas to Overcome Obstacles

Some facilities will be able to match their own nonclinical staff with "buddies" for some individual time, or a local philanthropic organization may agree to purchase a few pretty garments or adaptive devices. Be open to whatever options might be out there.

However, after the activity professional has done all that can be done, there may still be major obstacles to the type of program being designed. Among these noteworthy obstacles are the severity of the resident's multiple illnesses, public policy, lack of funds and professional resources, a destructive physical environment, the value others place on activity therapy, and poor management. A major problem for some activity professionals is the limited control over the mix of residents to be served. Staff may face frail, cognitively intact residents and people with a range of cognitive deficits, including the severely impaired, all in one group. Cognitively well residents may resent the confused residents, and with so much going on, many of the confused residents will become agitated. A very needlessly limited range of activities will limit the chance that any activity will meet any resident's needs.

A similar problem is the requirement to individualize care when staffing levels for activities are too low to even meet with each resident individually or when resources are not available to enable care. Lack of adequate staffing often means that the activity director can only serve large groups, even though many residents can only benefit from small groups. The activity director is often caught in the middle of this debate.

These can be troubling situations. Unless the activity professional can find a crack in the system in which to begin to make changes (or has been given a mandate to make changes), this person must accept the limits to what can be accomplished. When these situations exist in an atmosphere where change is unlikely, the activity professional will not be able to meet goals.

The operative word is the *potential* for change. For example, can the activity professional find funding to break one group a day into two groups? Gain assistance in recruiting volunteers? Have some aides cross-trained as activity aides? Arrange for people with dementia to spend a few hours each day in separate programming? Gain a team approach so that other staff help to learn what residents prefer as activities? If the activity professional can begin to make a change, then the residents will have help in being cared for.

Servicing Different Populations

A nursing home can provide care for many different types of populations. Some residents are transient, entering acutely ill from the hospital and leaving as soon as they recover. Often delirious and frequently immobile, they may require only simple, solitary activities for a short time span in addition to intensive nursing care. For them, education regarding adapting activities once they return home is often a valuable approach. Other residents are permanent, intending to live at the home for the remainder of their lives. They may be cognitively intact, have a wide range of physi-

cal or psychological deficits, or (in the rare case) be comatose with very little ability to interact with their environment.

Task Breakdown and Assessment of Complexity

Adapt all activities to fit the retained abilities of residents. The following list describes the process of task breakdown for individualized activities:

- In advance
  - o Identify a task.
  - o Write out each step.
  - o Check whether any steps were missed.
  - o Mark the steps the resident can do.
  - o Mark the steps the staff will do.
  - o Before starting the task, ask:
    - Is the resident rested and calm?
    - Is this a calm environment?
    - Was enough time allowed to very slowly move the resident?
    - Am I treating the resident as a friend?
    - Am I using touch, affection, appropriate humor?
- Carry out the task.
  - o Identify both visually (show it to the resident) and verbally (name it) the first item to be used.
  - o Say what is to be done with it. Use clues that do not involve language (point, start the resident's arm in motion).
  - o Be patient. Many residents move very slowly.
  - o Give positive feedback ("That's right. That looks good.")
  - o Repeat for each step.
- After the task is complete, review the plan.
  - o Mark the places where the resident had trouble.
  - o Divide this step into simpler ones.
  - o Are there any steps the staff did that the resident might be able to do?
  - o Does the environment need to be changed?
- Try out the modified tasks. If there are still problems, get suggestions from the family

and coworkers.
- The following list describes the task breakdown for group activities:
- In advance
  o Identify a task.
  o Write out each step.
  o Note which resident can do each step (remember that actively watching is participation).
  o Indicate which steps the staff will do.
  o Consider the group environment:
    - Are the residents rested and calm?
    - Is this a calm environment?
    - Has the staff allowed enough time for people to complete the tasks slowly?
    - Will the atmosphere encourage pleasure and friendship?
    - Does this task meet the requirements for appropriate activities?
- Carry out the task.
  o Get each resident started on his or her task in sequence.
  o Provide verbal and nonverbal cues.
  o Allow plenty of time.
  o Make positive comments.
- After the task is completed, review the success of the plan. Note which residents were successful or unsuccessful at tasks, and which might be able to do other tasks.

Apply these techniques for residents with cognitive, physical, or sensory disabilities. When changes occur in a resident's status, review the breakdowns and simplify the tasks, as appropriate. When residents improve, fewer task breakdowns will be required. In many instances, steps can be done for the resident in advance, often before the one-on-one activity begins or the group assembles. For example, have tools laid out, be sure project components are precut, and so on. The resident may then participate in as many tasks or task steps as ability will allow. Some residents will enjoy helping with this preparation.

Activity Options for Cognitively Intact Residents

While some individuals demand and enjoy traditional pursuits (e.g., bingo, sing-alongs), others find they have no interest. Some can be coaxed to participate while others will flatly refuse. Activities that fail to meet affective needs can reinforce negative feelings that one's life is void of meaning or interest.

Activities for cognitively intact residents should encourage independence and try to capitalize on old lifestyles and personalities. Accomplishing this objective can be a challenge to nursing home management, which is also responsible for ensuring safety, economy, and efficiency of operation.

A few innovative programs allow cognitively intact residents significant autonomy in major aspects of nursing home life, with assistance—but minimal control—from staff. The following examples are drawn from facilities throughout the United States:
- Residents can plan, set up, stock, and staff a gift shop.
- Residents can publish an inhouse newspaper, which they write, edit, and distribute. The staff may assist in photocopying.
- On determining the need for a VCR for the commons room, residents can plan a fund raiser and select a model (after visits to the home from several dealers).
- Residents can organize a pub night.
- Resident councils can play a role in addressing real-life problems, such as what to do about confused people who wander into their rooms.
- Residents can have good ideas about how to draw the community (including their old friends) into the home. Pub night is a good time to invite guests. Residents can plan a small restaurant, to which they can invite friends and pay for the meal by having the bill put on their account.
- If the nursing home provides a child-care area for its staff, residents can provide much

of the child care, to the enrichment of both generations. Other ways can also be found to link children and residents, e.g., a program to "adopt" a handicapped child who visits several times a week.

- Some residents will welcome the opportunity to learn a skill they have always wanted to learn (e.g., quilting, painting, weaving, silk painting). The tools can be adapted to support arthritic hands or vision disabilities. Silk painting is a failure-free activity—it is impossible to create something that is not lovely. For unsure, depressed, or negative people, it provides instant rewards.
- Residents may choose to personalize their rooms or paint murals in the halls. Be sure to get permission from the local fire marshall and facility administrative staff as appropriate.
- Residents can engage in handicap-modified sports, which can be organized and conducted facility-wide as a Senior Olympics.

If some of these activities seem too ambitious, try scaled down versions or trials with small groups. Consult with the occupational therapist for further suggestions.

For able residents who disdain commonplace activities, find out what they want or what bothers them about the activities program, and encourage them to take a leadership role in planning for change. The planning exercise is itself a valuable activity, although predictably it will take time for residents to become certain of themselves and establish their own peer hierarchy.

ACTIVITY OPTIONS FOR RESIDENTS WITH DEMENTIA

The magnitude of cognitive loss will vary for residents with dementia, and this variability usually correlates with the resident's interest and involvement in activities. For many of the more impaired residents, low-key, calm, and quiet activities with obvious meaning and purpose are enough to occupy them throughout the day. Such activities can help reduce problem behaviors and improve the quality of life. Agitated residents with dementia will benefit from a more lively, stimulating activity program. The following list shows some successful activities for residents with dementia.

- Social activities:
  - Holidays; parties; coffee groups; discussing gossip columns; controversial discussions (morals of youth, politics, religion); retelling war stories (men); bingo.
- Religious activities:
  - Men will often set up the chairs. Be sure the symbols (crosses, the Jewish candlestick, flowers) are present.
- Music, dance:
  - If a piano is available, some people will play it independently. Dancing is popular, and it is enjoyed by watchers as well as participants.
- Outdoor activities/outings:
  - Sightseeing; walking; raking; sitting; "riding along" short distances on the bus; picking flowers; sweeping walks.
- Facility bus:
  - For men; looking under the hood; discussing tires; wiping it down.
- Activities using large movements:
  - Bowling; shuffleboard; sweeping; raking.
- Activities that give immediate feedback:
  - Preparing food; grooming; tasting the food; weeding.
- Personal care:
  - Hair; nails; dressing; pedicure. (Looking good and care of clothing are also important to many men.)
- Domestic chores:
  - Food preparation; sweeping; folding; wiping up; dusting.
- Visits from children and pets
- Activities that use old overlearned motor skills or repetitive, rhythmic tasks:
  - Sanding; rocking; scrubbing potatoes; brushing lint.
- Activities that help sustain family ties:

o A memory album with pictures and notes; a letter that the family writes during a visit; talking about the family visit and when they will return.

- Activities that use old memories:
  o Discussing antiques; old Valentines; rummaging through drawers for things that interest or belong to the resident; a purse with one's own belongings.

The following list describes activities to avoid for people with dementia, but they meet the previous warning that staff may be surprised by the interest and capacity of the demented resident:

- Tasks that require decisions involving several steps:
  o Crafts that require decisions about which to select, what step is next.
- Tasks that are new to the resident:
  o Using modeling clay; finger paints; listening to rock and roll; crafts the resident does not usually do.
- Tasks that convey a childish message:
  o Childish games; puzzles that use children's supplies (crayons, laces).
- Tasks that depend on lost skills:
  o Commonly relying on verbal language (discussion groups), fine motor skills (paper folding), judgment.
- Tasks with unpredictable elements
- Tasks that require abstract thought, math, or visualization
- Tasks that Encourage Tuning Out:

Tasks that the resident cannot follow, understand, or see.

The following list shows activities that may be more appropriate to male residents with dementia:

- Yardwork, including repetitive, simple tasks (e.g., picking up leaves or trash).
- Looking under the hood of a car, discussing whether "it will run again."
- Stacking things (e.g., newspapers, plastic chairs, light pieces of firewood).
- Have an old carburetor steam cleaned and then set it out for the men to take apart.

- Give the men a set of keys so they can "work on the locks."
- Filing, sanding, and simple painting of wood pieces to be sold at a bazaar. Sanding is a failure-free, repetitive, easy skill that is likely to have been done in earlier years, and it has meaning to most men.
- Have someone bring in sports equipment to look at. Adopt bowling, shuffleboard, shooting baskets, or other simple indoor sports. Do not plan to play by the rules.
- Provide and use a pool table (do not promote rules, just shoot the balls). Since pool cues are dangerous, use shortened sticks or only use one cue and maintain control of it, or have the men just roll the balls without using the cues.
- Men like to admire and hold babies and pets. Remember these types of activities are not limited to women.
- Visit a horse or use large pictures of horses to talk about racing, horse breeding, or farm work.
- Use old pictures to talk about the war and war experiences. Before trying this, find out from the family if the resident is upset by talk of the war. Ask families to bring in war medals for sharing in the discussions.
- Go through auto magazines or gun magazines.
- Read *Sports Illustrated* together.
- Take lots of walks.
- Handle or watch model trains.
- Use model trains, ships, horses, or airplanes to stimulate discussion. Let residents touch the models. Ask hobbyists to visit with their models.
- Get antique items (a store owner may bring them in). Look for tools, pieces of harness, or other items that men may have used.

Simplify activities by using the task breakdown methodologies previously described. By making activities accessible to confused people and eliminating steps that are stressful, the possibility of discouragement or angry outbursts is minimized.

Individualize interventions—even if staff resources are limited. Plan activities so that residents participate at their own skill and attention level. Do not assume that all the participants in a group will enjoy the same activity. If some become restless, irritable, or tuned out, reassess the goals and guidelines and repeat the task breakdown and complexity analysis.

Group size has a significant impact on participation. Many residents with dementia are able to pay attention or participate only when involved in very small group situations. If a resident is disruptive or does not participate, try a smaller group. Residents with dementia will rarely be able to benefit from independent, unsupervised activities. Review the resident's ADLs. These activities may be made more therapeutic and meaningful for the resident without increased staffing.

Avoid idle time as much as possible. Repeat successful activities since residents with dementia are often reassured by routine and the expectation that events will occur at the same time every day. In addition to regular events, plan others that are new, and some that are occasional (e.g., religious services). Even when an activity is apparently successful, review its efficacy since both residents and their capacity to participate change, sometimes for the better. For example, if a resident has recovered from an acute illness, he or she may be ready for more challenging tasks.

Encourage residents with dementia to participate in activities you know they like, while avoiding forced compliance. People with dementia often lose their ability to initiate movement. They may not understand what is being suggested or may be unable to get started. Try to assess whether a resident's refusal to participate represents a genuine dislike for the activity or is based on misunderstanding and the inability to initiate. Use the resident's responses throughout the day as a guide.

Residents with dementia also often lose their ability to stop an action; they will do the same thing over and over. Take advantage of this in planning activities. There is no reason why a resident cannot wipe the same table over and over, or sweep the same side of the hall repeatedly.

Residents with dementia are highly vulnerable to stressors such as not feeling well, noise, confusion, large groups, poor light, glare, patronizing staff, upsets from family visits, misunderstanding of what is going on, fearing that one will make a fool of one's self, and so on. If they become restless, irritable, or withdrawn, look carefully for stressful triggers. However, do not be reluctant to try adventurous things. Positive stimulation is not a stressor. Small groups of these residents have been successfully taken swimming and to shopping malls and restaurants. Such events enrich total affective experience, but require full staffing (perhaps involving family members as volunteers) and careful planning for every contingency.

Schedule the day's activities to match natural biorhythms. Plan activities when the residents are awake and alert. For example, a walk after lunch may be less successful than resting and listening to music. Ideally, offer activities during the second shift up to the normal bedtime.

Do not be surprised if residents with dementia become upset after a pleasant activity period, since they may have become disoriented. When moving a group from room to room, tell them what is going on. When they are brought back to the unit, reorient them (e.g., "Its almost dinner time," or "Here is your nursing assistant coming to meet you.")

Environmental Settings

Residents with dementia are extremely sensitive to the setting or ambience of the activity, which can often convey messages about the appropriateness of various behaviors. For example, a neuropsychologist was using blocks to carry out psychometric testing with residents. All went well until the nursing assistants began placing bibs on everyone in preparation for lunch. Suddenly, the residents began putting the blocks in their mouths. The bibs changed the message, implying that the residents were babies and were now permitted to do baby things. Does the activity setting convey dignity or institutionalization? Adultness or childness? Well roles or sickness roles? The following list describes some ideas on appropriate environmental settings:

- Put a tablecloth on the table and serve tea or coffee in cups. Help one of the residents pass the cookies.
- Invite a child to join you for children's games such as "Doing the Hokey Pokey" or parachute-tosses.
- Have a few people fold their own clothes. Use a laundry hamper. Discuss what needs mending, what's pretty, and so forth. Quickly resort them before storing.
- Wash and style a resident's hair.
- Have higher-functioning, cognitively impaired residents make aprons out of pretty fabric, and use them instead of bibs.

Social Interaction

Residents with dementia have few opportunities for social interchange, so facilitate this to the extent possible. Even arguing between two residents may be considered a meaningful interaction. Seat people together if they show signs of interacting and set up social situations (e.g., having coffee). People will sometimes help each other spontaneously. However, do not automatically seat a high-functioning resident where that person can help a lower-functioning resident. This can be exploitative, and is often done in nursing homes when there is not enough staff. The high-functioning residents have their own needs. However, if an assessment of the higher-functioning resident identifies a need or willingness to help others, consider building on the tendency. For example, an oriented resident may enjoy volunteering as a music therapy assistant or book reader with a small

group of dementia residents. If this was part of the resident's customary routine before entering the nursing home, this may become his or her most important and valued activity during the day. Document the reasons for using a resident as a volunteer.

TYPES OF ACTIVITIES TO CONSIDER

This section describes activity options that are often successful in the nursing home setting. In specifying these activity options, include a definitive statement of goals in the resident's care plan and also provide an environment in which the resident's decision-making capability is stimulated. The facility's activity program must be responsive to the needs of all residents, show support for the decision-making process of the cognitively impaired, and provide an interesting set of options for the cognitively intact.

Exercise

Exercise is essential for all residents. However, as cognitive status declines, the challenge is to find creative ways to motivate residents and develop stimulating physical programs. Generally, it is possible to incorporate direct exercise programs as well as any indirect program that promotes exercise (*see* Chapter 29, ADL Rehabilitation, for more information). For example, consider direct exercises such as chair calisthenics, walking, swimming, stretching, bed exercises, transfer exercises, and range-of-motion exercises, or indirect exercises that incorporate resident mobility or muscle exercise such as singing or gardening.

Some residents will not see the point to activities such as parachute toss and ball toss, or will regard them as childish or demeaning. Whenever an activity appears to be damaging to a resident's self-esteem, need for mastery, or personal dignity, discontinue it immediately. However, first determine whether such an activity will be accepted if the purpose behind the use of a piece of equipment is explained beforehand. In each activity option, consider special adaptations and modifications for specific types of population (e.g., residents with dementia).

Games

Residents will have a history of involvement in many types of games—puzzles, bowling, cards, bingo, and so forth. Use this past experience as the basis for specifying activity pursuit options. For example, for cognitively intact people who have enjoyed bingo in the past, this is an excellent activity that supports friendship and encourages continued cognitive mastery. Allow residents to set up the game, call the numbers, and perform other related tasks as their capability permits. Schedule the games at a convenient time.

For cognitively impaired people, particularly if they have played bingo in the past, relaxed, "no-rules" bingo can be rewarding. Awarding prizes to all participants, regardless of whether they actually won, may ensure lots of success and laughter. At the same time, avoid trivializing the experience, which can be counterproductive.

Some residents may find bingo demeaning. Coaxing or requiring these individuals to participate is damaging to self-esteem and subversive of autonomy, so avoid forcing them to participate. Likewise, do not force residents who lack the hearing, fine motor skills, or vision necessary to play bingo.

Discussions and Reminiscence

Group discussion sessions are enjoyable to many residents, but they may place undue demands on those with impaired hearing or communication skills, in which case one-on-one reminiscence activities may be more successful. In a reminiscence activity, use picture albums, home movies, slides, newspaper clippings, or any objects to bring back memories of people, places, and times that were important to the resident's life as an entry to reminiscence about family members or the old neighborhood. When more general discussion

sessions are possible, use small groups and nonstressful settings and rely on topics that are appropriate to the residents' language skills. For example, residents with dementia who cannot express themselves verbally may still enjoy demonstrating the use of an antique tool. However, some persons with dementia will not be able to enjoy discussions or reminiscence activities in any form.

Music

Most residents retain an ability to respond to music, but the form of enjoyment will vary from resident to resident. For example, residents (with or without family) can listen to favorite music or softly sing together. If the activities staff is not sure of a favorite type of music, try tunes popular during the resident's teenage years or early 20s, sing-along music, religious music from a resident's church or synagogue, or relevant ethnic music.

Try to combine music and movement. For example, for residents who retain some range of motion in their extremities (including those who are chairbound), the following programmatic approach may be useful:

- Begin by greeting each resident
- Motivate the group by singing and clapping in rhythm to the song
- Dance with each resident, trying to incorporate as full a range of arm movements (up-and-down, in-and-out, side-to-side) as possible
- Encourage each resident to touch head, shoulders, waist, knees
- Using theraband elastic, have three residents at a time do in-and-out, up-and-down arm movements while holding the band
- Conclude by applauding the group and thanking everyone with a handshake

Crafts

Crafts are the mainstay of many activity programs in the nursing home, and many active residents enjoy them. However, for residents with cognitive impairments such as dementia, crafts may be unfamiliar and too complex and demanding of fine motor skills, vision, and so on. In addition, many elderly people of the present generation value only work-related activities.

Holidays

Holidays offer a change of pace to the daily routine and provide residents with new activities to do. They also provide a sense of continuity with lifelong values and customary activities. Celebrating holidays can include old recipes that were favorites of the resident, music, old ethnic costumes on display, or objects such as pictures that were brought in by family members. Ask families to send all residents on the unit cards or pictures related to the particular holiday. Consider planning a celebration activity, including food and a social hour, with some family members assisting or participating. However, recognize that for some older people holidays will carry only unhappy memories, or are pleasurable only if there are children around. Therefore, some residents may prefer a low key approach to holidays. A sensitive awareness of individual feelings is the best guide.

Toys

Using children's toys (e.g., stuffed animals, trains, coloring books) may provide comfort, success, and a sense of engagement for very impaired elderly people. Conversely, they may persuade the resident that he or she is "in a second childhood" and has nothing worthwhile to contribute in life. In determining whether toy-play is appropriate in the individual instance, ask whether the presence of such items subtly change staff's behavior toward the resident, so that they treat the resident like a child, even slightly. If so, role-playing inservices may be warranted, or the activity avoided altogether. Even very impaired persons, who may not register the stuffed toy as childish, can read subtle, patronizing body language.

Task-Focused Activities

All elders will have performed a variety of valued tasks during their adult years. To identify these tasks, review links to role activities on the job, in the home, with the family, in the church, with friends, or in the community. There are many ways to use this information to design an individually meaningful activity program. For example, a small group may plan and carry out a display depicting these common religious, education, or occupational experiences.

The following subsections describe programs that will be useful for some resident groups—hobby shop, gardening, and domestic chores.

Hobby Shop

Bring together small groups of residents to work on a common project or on related projects in a group environment. For more cognitively impaired residents, start with simpler exercises (e.g., sanding a piece of wood or hammering nails into a piece of wood for a purpose). Prepare the staff to reinforce and maintain schedules, provide guidance and encouragement, praise success, and reminisce about the past. When setting up physical space, ensure that there is enough space between residents to allow working without contact or conflict.

Gardening

Raised flower beds allow for easy access, but a large flower pot set on an inverted flower pot will also work. Fill flower beds or pots with soil and allow enough drainage so that the residents can water the plants as often as they wish without damaging the flowers. Consider planting herbs for their fragrance, tomatoes, and fast-growing summer squash. Watching these plants grow is a weekly activity. When ripe, picking them and cooking them becomes another activity. Individual residents may have their own plots, window boxes, or potted plants.

Domestic Chores

Domestic chores are the core of what most people have done since retirement and what most women have always done. They are old, well-learned tasks, primarily involving gross motor skills. They are often desirably repetitive and provide opportunities to rekindle old roles, achieve success, and get needed physical exercise. They are status-appropriate, have purpose and meaning, and do not create anxiety or embarrassment. Although some cognitively intact residents may not wish to do any more housework, these activities often work well with cognitively impaired residents.

In the United States, state and federal regulations protect residents from exploitation by nursing homes that would require them to work. Documenting the therapeutic rationale for the activity before starting it is usually enough to meet federal regulatory requirements.

The following domestic chores are often spontaneous activities for individuals or small groups. Be sure they remain meaningful. One confused resident pointed out, "they give me these towels to fold to keep me busy."

- Wiping tables
- Washing dishes (they will later be returned to the dishwasher)
- Putting laundry into and out of washer and dryer
- Folding laundry
- Sweeping
- Dusting
- Helping to make one's bed
- Straightening one's room
- Sorting one dresser drawer
- Polishing
- Stacking chairs (lightweight plastic)

- Moving tables (be alert to the possibility of falls)
- Outdoor domestic work, as appropriate, includes:
- Raking leaves
- Trimming grass
- Planting flower beds
- Hanging clothes on an old fashioned clothesline, and taking them in (whether they need it our not)
- Pushing a wheelbarrow
- Pushing an old manual lawn mower

For many people these kinds of activities form the core of the day. After selecting the tasks, reduce them to manageable steps and justify their therapeutic intent so they can be easily encouraged and monitored by nursing staff.

Wandering Hallway

This program is designed for the subgroup of residents who wander, or have a short attention span, and are unable to tolerate more structured group activities (e.g., they become disruptive). This program only works if it is led by a staff person or family member. The program takes place in a hallway where residents can wander and move about at will. On the walls at various stations are task-oriented activities, which can be manipulated by the residents as they walk. Stations may include tactile aprons, magazine racks, drawers with clothing, activity boards, and brooms. Place a park bench along one wall, perhaps with a painting of a street sign from the residents' "old neighborhoods" positioned nearby. Depending on the residents, the program can run from a few minutes to about half an hour in length.

Pets and Children

Pets make wonderful therapists in the nursing home setting. They have the capacity to reach severely ill, withdrawn, depressed, or impaired residents. There are several ways to involve animals: ask an animal shelter to bring in pets as visitors; ask community volunteers or staff to bring in pets; or start an institutional pet on the unit program. Select animals that have an even temperament and are friendly. Birds and fish can also add interest. If you use birds, select little finches, which breed easily. The chirping of baby birds adds life to an entire facility.

Children are almost always welcomed by residents, especially very impaired residents who typically love to watch babies at play. Some facilities provide day care for their staff. With supervision, residents can provide rocking, feeding, and playing. Also, nursery and elementary schools can visit, and middle school and high school students can pair up with residents for friendship.

Volunteers

Volunteers are extremely helpful in working with the elderly, especially with residents with dementia, but never consider them "free labor" for a facility that is understaffed. Assign a staff person to supervise the volunteer program and be responsible for recruiting, training, and onsite support. Some facilities successfully engage noncaregiving employees as volunteers. They are excused from their regular duties for 30 minutes a day to spend with a "special friend." Such volunteers need prior training, and need to be matched carefully to residents. For example, in one facility the handyman stopped by regularly to visit a confused resident. The two of them sorted through a toolbox and talked about the tools the resident had once used.

Evaluating the Activity Program

Staff often feel that they are too busy to conduct a formal program evaluation. This failure to evaluate a program is a failure to grow. In addition, since very little has been tested about good activity care in nursing

homes, particularly for residents with dementia, even simple findings will find an interested readership and be welcomed by professional journals.

Evaluations should be prospective. Plan before, not after, for what to learn and how to achieve it. Ask:

- Are there activities that residents are asking for?
- Are there activities that cannot be done due to economic, space, or other barriers? What can be done instead?
- What impact (more smiles, less behavior problems) are the activities having on the people with dementia?
- Do schedules need modification?
- How well do innovations work? What characteristics work best?
- What positive things do the staff have to say?
- What negative things do the staff have to say?

CASE EXAMPLE

In many nursing homes, activities are an afterthought, something to be done only "if there's time" when the "more important" caregiving tasks of the day are completed. The connection between increased resident dependency, problem behaviors, and lack of meaningful activities is frequently unrecognized.

This case example describes how nursing and recreation therapy staff of one cognitively impaired unit got together and conducted a systematic modification of the activities program, with beneficial results for residents and caregivers.

As a first step toward achieving interdisciplinary cooperation between nursing and activities staff, a series of educational sessions was given by the recreation therapist and nurse manager to nurses and nursing assistants on the 7 to 3 and 3 to 11 shifts. The night shift staff were provided updates. In the sessions, the theories about recreation therapy and their application to cognitively impaired residents were discussed. Nursing staff responded positively, indicating they had gained a better understanding of the importance of activity care planning in improving residents' affect, behavior, and quality of life. As part of this orientation, the hobbies of nursing assistants were identified, and the nursing assistants were encouraged to use these skills in the groups they ran with residents.

The program devised by the interdisciplinary team on the unit involved activities planning for days, evenings, and weekends. One group convenes at 10 AM on Tuesdays and Thursdays, and is run jointly by a recreation therapist and a nurse who has received additional training in occupational therapy and recreation therapy. The size of the group varies, but generally compromises no more than six residents who are less cognitively impaired than others on the unit and exhibit a need to be useful and complete a project. They collate material, separate papers, staple items, and work together toward a common goal. Two-step tasks are possible with this group, rather than one-step tasks, which is usually the objective with less cognitively intact residents. Staff refer to the group members as "workers," and as they lead the residents into the room they tell them they will "be doing a job for us." When the group finishes, they receive a snack and many thanks for a job well done.

The evening group was designed as an intervention to decrease agitated behavior, which was noted to occur immediately after the evening meal. As nurses prepared to eat their dinner and nursing assistants collected trays and began to put a few residents to bed, other residents would voice concern over "What should I do?" and some tried to leave the unit to "go home." With the assistance of the recreation therapist, the nurses now run a group that meets five evenings a week at 6:15 PM. Various guest activities, such as listening to soft music tapes or having a tea party to reminisce are offered. Since implementation, the mood of the unit after dinner is more mellow, and residents are going to bed later, sleeping better, and are more available for family visits in the evening.

The weekend group was developed to fill a gap in recreational programming. Residents were fighting and falling more frequently on Saturdays and Sundays, and staff attributed this to a lack of activities. Educational sessions were held with the weekend shifts to discuss the principles of recreational therapy and to reaffirm the need of the residents to be actively engaged in positive situations. Two-person teams of nursing assistants run the weekend groups. Activities include exercise, bowling, listening to music, and playing musical instruments. In addition to the benefit to the residents, including less need for intervention and direction by caregiving staff throughout the day, the self-esteem of the nursing assistants involved in the program has increased significantly.

While no programs are currently being held during the night, unit staff are planning for a varied initiative—the availability of warm milk, cake or cookies, opportunities for quiet conversations, and televisions and talking books with individual head phones.

31
Restraint Reduction

Carter Catlett Williams, MSW, ACSW
Sarah Greene Burger, RN, MPH
Katharine Murphy, RN, MS

People who live in nursing homes have the right to make choices about their treatments, and to be free of physical restraints except as indicated for the medical treatment with which they concur and only for temporary periods of time. Focus care plan discussions on the resident, who knows what it feels like to be tied down. As reported by virtually all who have had such an experience, being restrained is one of degradation, humiliation, punishment, fear, anxiety, and pain. Residents may spend not only months but years of their lives in nursing homes. If physical restraint is practiced, then residents are constantly at risk of being tied down. It becomes a matter of civil rights as well as maintenance and/or enhancement of function.

Broadly defined, a physical restraint is any device that cannot easily be removed that restricts voluntary movement or access to one's body. Included are any manual method or physical or mechanical device, material, or equipment that results in such a restriction by being attached to or adjacent to the resident's body.

Examples of physical restraints include leg, arm, wrist, trunk, waist, and crotch devices consisting of straps, belts, vests, or sheets of any material, whether or not they are considered postural supports; as well as gerichairs, hand mitts, pelvic rollbars, and halters; and full bedside rails and split rails that have only a small opening midway. Additionally, locked wheelchairs, reclining chairs, and tables placed in front of the resident are considered physical restraints if they prohibit mobility.

OVERVIEW

In the 11 years before the passage of the nursing home reform law (OBRA 1987), the use of physical restraint rose nationwide by almost 60%, from 25% to 41% of all residents.

In the past, four reasons were commonly given by caregivers for restraint use:

- To prevent falls
- To achieve proper trunk position
- To control residents who were agitated and confused
- To prevent interference with medical treatment

In addition, there was the mistaken belief that restraints were necessary in order to avoid legal liability over resident falls.

There is now evidence that restraints offer no guarantee against falls, often increase agitation, and are not effective or comfortable as trunk positioners. Restraints can only be justified for brief periods of time in connection with monitored medical treatment to which the resident has agreed, or because of some immediate emergency situation.

Adverse Effects of Restraint Use

Restraint use has destructive effects both physically and emotionally. Physical hazards include the loss of muscle mass, contractures, loss of mobility and balance, skin breakdown, increased constipation, incontinence, falls, loss of appetite, abnormal biochemical and physiologic changes related to immobility and the stress of being tied down, and an increased risk of death. Additionally, residents who are restrained are at risk of receiving inadequate medical evaluations because it is difficult and time-consuming for physicians to examine people when they are tied to beds or chairs. Emotional and psychological hazards include withdrawal; feelings of isolation, shame, and depression; agitation (screaming, struggling to untie the restraint, pleading with passersby, hitting, biting); verbal abuse; broken spirit; decreased social interaction; greater dependency; and loss of coping abilities.

The practice of restraining people also has negative effects on staff from both clinical practice and personal perspectives. First, used as a panacea for managing difficult situations, restraint use eliminates the necessary search for the underlying causes of residents' problems, removes the possibilities for creative interdisciplinary team and family problem-solving, and fails to use the knowledge of the nursing assistant. Second, having to tie another person down can be stressful to the caregiver, particularly if the resident pleads to be left free. The person who applies the restraint may thereafter avoid the resident. Restraints are obstacles to communication with residents and to knowing them as individuals.

The sight of a relative tied down to bed or chair has a depersonalizing and distancing effect on families and friends. In society at large, restraint use has the effect of devaluing older people. You are not your own person when you are tied down by others.

As to the legal situation, a thorough research of court cases reveals that there have been no successful lawsuits against nursing homes based only on the failure to place a restraint on a resident. When plaintiffs' suits have been successful there were always one or more other failures on the part of the facility, such as faulty assessment, inadequate monitoring of the resident's condition, or lack of timeliness in responding to a resident leaving the facility. The conclusion is that the burden of proof now rests on the facility to show that no less restrictive approach to the resident's needs can be discovered.

In some European countries there are facilities with little or no use of physical restraints. In the first few years following OBRA 1987, we started to see many nursing homes in the United States begin to move toward restraint-free care and many have already achieved it. Unfortunately, there are many facilities that continue to restrain residents and manufacturers who continue to invent and market devices that severely restrict mobility.

THE OPPORTUNITIES FOR RESTRAINT-FREE CARE

First, eliminating the habit of using restraints calls for the staff to establish human, caring relationships with residents, and to think creatively about care needs, causal factors, and constructive intervention plans. Second, restraint-free care has a distinct order of operational priorities. Third, restraint-free care is not something accomplished once and for all, but is an ongoing process, not only with each resident, but facility-wide. A successful program requires flexible schedules and routines, and the habitual use of individualized strategies for supporting residents.

Thinking About Caring for Residents

To facilitate restraint elimination, it is important to know each resident as a *person*. Try to learn something about each person's earlier years, particularly what and who is most important to each individual, what that person is most proud of, most disappointed or angry about, and how each has coped with life's problems. What does this person laugh about? What does this person enjoy doing? What is upsetting to this person? The answers to these questions will be discovered over a period of time, and in the process will help build a relationship that is the foundation for all caregiving work.

Above all, find out what makes a good day for this person, and then incorporate these factors into the resident's daily routines. Ask the person for information on what has meaning for him or her. For those who cannot communicate verbally, learn gradually through observation and from friends and family what particular sources of satisfaction, even joy, have been (and are still) of importance.

A Different Order of Priorities: Individualized Care

For the resident to have as familiar and satisfying a daily life as possible, care must be individualized. Responding to personal preferences will result in a more tranquil, less hectic unit. Residents should determine their own times of getting up and going to bed, times and location for eating breakfast, napping, going outdoors, and should choose times and kinds of snacks and drinks they prefer between meals. By developing this flexibility, the staff will put less pressure on residents and will have more opportunity to use their talents and energies in ways that are creative and appreciated. Also note that the schedules for taking people to the bathroom should not be determined by the time when most staff are available, but rather by the individual resident's bowel and bladder elimination patterns and needs.

Just as customizing familiar daily routines will contribute to resident well-being, familiar and homelike physical surroundings help people have a sense of continuity in their lives. Connections with the past are strengthened and people have a sense of being in control of their own space if they have their own belongings (e.g., furniture, photographs, mementos, artwork, pillows) around them. Home furnishings in dining and day rooms also add ease and comfort. Such environments may enhance feelings of wellness and reduce feelings of despair that accompany a more institutional-like atmosphere.

The time spent in learning residents' preferences and habits will be more than compensated for by the removal of many of the difficulties that occur in connection with trying to get people to do things that are unfamiliar, uncongenial, and uncomfortable to them. Time will be gained, too, by reducing the number of accidents that have to be cleaned up because people cannot go to the bathroom on someone else's schedule.

To help build relationships and rapport, it is necessary to adopt a primary nursing model of care. In this type of staffing model both licensed and nonlicensed nursing staff are assigned to care for a particular group of residents permanently. By working together for long periods of time, residents and staff build relationships, come to know each others' habits, and reach mutually agreed on ways of doing things. This often results in saving time for all concerned as well as greater satisfaction for residents and staff.

Restraint-Free Care is an Ongoing Process

Restraint-free care begins by building relationships and getting to know each individual resident. Concurrently, assessment is taking place, a plan of care is agreed on with the resident, and the outcomes are monitored and reevaluated with the resident. This cycle continues as an ongoing process as the resident changes over time. Assessment and care planning as they relate to restraint elimination are discussed in more detail later in this chapter.

As residents come to be seen as people with the right to make choices about how they lead their daily lives and what risks they choose to take, the facility administration will need to develop flexibility. Philosophy, policies, and procedures, as well as the role of residents in the facility, should be seen as living, growing things, not laws, habits, and attitudes set in stone.

OBRA 1987 Regulations and Guidelines Support Individual Care

Both the overall rehabilitative thrust of OBRA 1987 and many specific sections of the law and regulations support the development of care plans that are individualized to the residents' specific needs. The individualized approach is spelled out in the law's requirement that "a nursing facility must provide services and activities to attain or maintain the highest practicable physical, mental, and psychosocial well-being of each resident in accordance with a written plan of care which describes the medical, nursing, and psychosocial needs of the resident and how such needs will be met..."

Regulations for this section of the law on quality of life state that "The facility must promote care for residents in a manner and in an environment that maintains or enhances each resident's dignity and respect in full recognition of his or her individuality." Again, the resident has the right to "make choices about aspects of his or her life in the facility that are significant to the resident."

In the Interpretive Guidelines for the same section, it is stated that "reasonable accommodations of individual needs and preferences" means adaptations of the facilities' physical environment and staff behaviors to assist residents in maintaining independent functioning, dignity, well-being and self determination."

PREVENTING RESTRAINT USE

Restraint-free care falls into two categories: preventing restraint use and discontinuing restraints (see the next section).

Preventing restraint use depends on the following factors:

- A facility-wide policy that expects and supports a philosophy of individualized care without a reliance on restraint use
- Prohibits the use of restraints for residents who are admitted to the facility unrestrained, except in life-saving situations to which the resident agrees
- In-depth assessment and care planning, taking into account the needs and preferences that are significant to the resident

Preventing restraint use differs from prevention of other adverse outcomes (e.g., pressure ulcers), in that standards of care are just now evolving. Facilities have limited experience in preventing restraint use. Preventive practices must often be defined on an individual basis. Good outcomes require vigilance, a commitment to minimizing restraint use, and a consistency in applying preventive measures. The staff must think creatively, drawing on individual experiences to eventually create consistent preventive guidelines in this area.

IDENTIFYING RESIDENTS IN NEED OF ATTENTION

The four general categories of people who are at risk for being restrained are those who:

- Fall easily or are at risk of falling
- Slip out of chairs or have trouble maintaining trunk control
- Become agitated, confused, and wander
- Need life-sustaining medical treatment (e.g., intravenous fluids or medications)

The staff who know that restraints are not an option (except in narrowly prescribed temporary circumstances) are immediately free to be creative in solving problems in other ways. How does this work? The following sections discuss some methods to solve these problems.

The Resident Who Falls Easily or is at Risk of Falls

Why does this resident fall so easily? Careful, systematic assessment to determine the reason for the fall is in order (*see* Chapter 18, Falls, for more information). After identifying the cause:

- Take measures to remove the cause (e.g., drugs causing sedation or hypotension)
- Change the circumstances that contribute to falls (e.g., inappropriate shoes, bed too high)
- Enhance independent functioning (e.g., muscle strengthening and gait training)
- Deal with sensory impairment (e.g., provide eyeglasses or hearing aids)
- Remove a frail or defenseless resident from an environment in which others may push or harm the resident
- Institute a scheduled toileting program based on the person's bowel and bladder elimination patterns

If a resident continues to fall despite treatment of the underlying causes, consider how to prevent injury in this individual during a fall. The plan is to make the environment as safe as possible to reduce the risk of injury.

Discuss with the resident and family the risk of injuries associated with both falling and restraint use. Help them to determine which risks and benefits are preferred. Resident involvement in care planning is particularly important in finding agreeable solutions to minimize risks. If the staff make a decision to protect the resident from falls in ways that do not take account of individual needs and preferences, then the resident will feel powerless and probably will not follow the plan. For example, a woman who has worn high heels all her life may reject safer, flat shoes or sneak-

ers as undignified. She may perceive the risk of falling while dressing the way she wants as preferable to a life without that choice. Try to achieve a compromise, such as suggesting that the resident purchase a medium height, wider heeled, nonskid shoe to reduce her fall risk while remaining fashionable.

The Resident Who Slips Out of Chairs

Determine why this resident slips out of chairs so easily. Sometimes the cause can be found and removed. For example, a resident may be weak from a recent infection, or bored because of a lack of activities that are relevant to the resident. However, if the cause cannot be removed, then the staff must devise safe seating.

Creativity is the key to preventing residents from slipping out of chairs. In the past, a new 100-bed nursing home would open with 120 resident chairs exactly alike for each room. Yet each resident has different needs. The chairs in each person's home are different, so why should it not be the same in the nursing home? Once the person's size, shape, and unique needs are known, then specialized seating can be arranged. Another common but inappropriate practice in the nursing home is to keep residents in wheelchairs all day. Wheelchairs are generally very uncomfortable and not very supportive. Except in unusual circumstances where necessary, only use wheelchairs for mobility and use other types of chairs for sitting. Whatever chairs are used, they must be specifically fitted.

Take the resident's style of life into account (e.g., active or inactive, seated most of the day or alternating between bed and chair). What is comfortable for this particular resident? How can a chair be retrofitted to fit the resident's needs? Who can help? A therapist? The maintenance department? Nursing? Does the resident agree with the plan and is he or she comfortable with the final seating arrangement(s)? Has the seriously demented resident been observed carefully for comfort? Has the family been consulted?

The Resident Who Wanders, or Becomes Agitated or Confused

Why is this person feeling restless and agitated? Often, the underlying cause is some form of dementia. Comprehensive resident assessment, such as the minimum data set, holds many pieces of information that will shed light on the resident who wanders and becomes restless. A person who is demented, without reliable recent memory, usually depends on old habits or customary daily routines. Past work life may also be another clue to finding out why a resident is restless. For instance, a housewife may become restless every day around the time her children or husband would have come home. She was used to watching out and providing for them. Likewise, a night owl is not going to take kindly to being put into bed at 8 PM or getting up at 6 AM. The nursing home must adapt to meet that resident's customary daily routine in order to prevent or alleviate behavioral symptoms.

A resident with sudden agitation or confusion may have an infection, drug reaction, or other underlying condition that needs treatment. Sometimes agitation leads to aggressive behavioral symptoms, which pose a threat to others. Remembering that all behavioral symptoms have meaning is very important in finding the cause and meeting the unmet need.

In all these situations, including the resident in the care planning process is very important. If a resident is unable to participate, then include a surrogate, such as a family member. Often, the resident or family member provides the clue to addressing behavioral symptoms successfully without restraints.

The basic thrust of care for many residents is to keep them involved in meaningful activities. Chapters 15 and 30, Psychosocial Well-Being and Activities Programming, respec-

tively, both have informative suggestions to consider. For example, relevant activity options should be available on the day and evening shifts. Consider varying activities -- sometimes a resident may wish to rest and be alone, and at other times may wish to be in the action. Anticipating these needs can ensure that the resident does not wander or risk falling by seeking these activities without assistance. For residents who do wander, modifying the environment, moving the resident to a safer environment, or using one of the electronic monitoring devices now on the market may ease the problem.

Emergency Life-Sustaining Treatment

Look for the cause of the emergency. A common cause is delirium, a life-threatening disorder manifested by confusion and behavioral symptoms such as agitation and hallucinations. In order to complete a medical evaluation, including laboratory tests, and provide appropriate treatment (e.g., intravenous fluids and antibiotics), physical restraints are sometimes necessary to prevent the resident from pulling out tubes. If necessary, they should be used for only a very short time under close staff monitoring.

When the cause of the emergency is the expected result of a terminal illness, then the cause, usually dehydration, must be assessed within the context of the resident's advanced directives. If intravenous rehydration is chosen, restraints may be necessary temporarily. Life-saving treatment of someone who is terminally ill must be done in the context of that resident's wishes. If comfort care is the choice, then provide that within the context of that resident's lifelong experience.

INTERVENTION TO REMOVE RESTRAINTS

Previous studies indicate that for the majority of restrained residents, the staff can no longer recall the initial reason restraints were initiated. For most of these residents, there no longer is an indication and restraints can be removed readily. For others, the challenge is to find an alternative way of caring for the resident. The same processes of assessment and care planning are used. A resident who has been restrained has already suffered negative consequences and often needs restorative care. Many residents will have to be prepared for this new freedom. Inform the family, discuss with the resident and staff what is to happen, and institute the necessary rehabilitative plans. Such plans may include:

• Instituting a toileting program
• Instituting muscle strengthening exercises or a supervised walking program
• Informing direct care and licensed staff of the need to maintain a systematic monitoring program during the weeks following program implementation
• Having a planned program to redirect or reorient a resident who becomes agitated
• Evaluating the need for feeding tubes
• Providing mobility or transfer assist devices
• Training the staff in how to approach the resident (e.g., from the front) to avoid hitting or other disruptive episodes
• Asking families or other companions to increase their presence on the unit

Determine the Circumstances
Related to Restraint Use

The first step in determining how to eliminate restraint use and provide alternative methods of care is to evaluate the circumstances in which restraint is used. Ask the following questions:

• Why is the resident restrained? Has the resident wandered into unsafe areas or into others' rooms uninvited? Does he or she have a history of injurious falls? Do staff feel they have been unable to provide adequate supervision if the resident has an unsteady gait? Most importantly, can staff still identify why the restraints are in use, or are they just carried forward based on pre-

cedence?

• What types of restraints are used? Trunk and chair restraints are the most common types of restraints used on elders in nursing homes. For multiply-impaired persons, often more than one type is used at a time, having the effect of doubly restricting mobility.

• During what times of day is each type of restraint used? Determine whether different types are used at different times of the day. For example, the resident may be restricted in a chair with a locked lap board during the day, and a vest restraint at night. Be sure to find out if the resident is restrained on shifts other than your own. It is not uncommon to find that the resident who is restraint-free during the day is being tied down at night. Other caregivers may have already found ways to remove restraints successfully when the resident is in their care. Learn from their examples.

• Where is the resident restrained (e.g., in a bed, in a chair, in the hallway)? Each location has its drawbacks and adverse effects on residents. The resident restrained in bed may experience a more fearful reaction to restraint such as abandonment by caregivers, or the possibility of being trapped in the event of a fire, and subsequently have difficult evening and nighttime behavioral symptoms of distress (e.g., calling out or agitation). The resident who is publicly restrained may feel more shame and humiliation and be reluctant to be involved in social activities.

• How long is the resident restrained at a time? Are restraints used intermittently? Intermittent use can increase the risk for falls because the residents become deconditioned while restrained and then, when not restrained, attempt ambulation. Are restraints used most of the time, necessitating that the resident receive physical rehabilitation to restore muscle strength and ambulatory capacity during the restraint removal process?

- Under what circumstances is the resident restrained (e.g., when left alone, after family leave, when not involved in a structured activity, when eating)? If the circumstances can be determined, often an activity or social contact with the staff can be substituted for the restraint.
- Who suggested the resident be restrained (e.g., staff who feel stress and do not know alternatives; family who are fearful their relative will sustain injury)? Sometimes educating the person who suggested restraints about risks and alternatives can help reduce their concerns.

Since physical restraints often increase agitation, restrained residents may also be receiving psychotropic drugs to treat agitation; therefore, the procedures discussed in Chapter 14, Psychotropic Drugs, are also useful. Once physical restraints are eliminated, psychotropic drugs may also be reduced or eliminated.

Intervention Strategies

Interventions that eliminate the need for physical restraint use include:

- Meeting basic needs for food, toileting, and sleep according to each resident's customary daily routine (i.e., individualizing care).
- Individualizing seating in wheelchairs, lounge chairs, and dining room chairs. If the resident is capable of rising but the chair impedes this activity because it is too high, too low, or too soft, seek alternatives or have the staff ask regularly if the resident needs help in rising. For residents requiring trunk control or support of a limb, use nonrestraining wedges, positioning pillows, antislipping material (such as Dycem) on a chair seat, one-sided bars on beds, wheelchair inserts, back supports, antitipping devices for wheelchairs, self-release devices for chairs or wheelchairs, or beds that are lower to the floor.

- Creating a homelike environment with the sights, sounds, and smells of home.
- Taking into consideration a person's past interests. Provide interest baskets of safe objects, (e.g., magazines, photographs) for those with a dementing illness.
- Assigning staff to the same residents to promote a more complete knowledge of each person, as well as continuity in care, and to enable staff to bond with residents and become their advocates.
- Training staff to support and comfort residents who have cognitive impairment. For example, if a resident appears frightened by the institutional bath, then try giving a thorough sponge bath as a substitution.
- Providing safe outdoor space with interesting things to explore such as a statue, garden benches to sit on, tables to sit at, and people to watch.
- Using patience and good humor in responding to residents, especially those who are demented. These may be the only things left they can respond to. Be sensitive. Remember that some residents may misinterpret jokes as personal insult.

32
Advance Directives

Myles Sheehan, MD
Terri Fried, MD
Katharine Murphy, RN, MS
David A. Levine, PhD

Advance directives allow an individual to prepare for the time when he or she can no longer make health care decisions. A written advance directive allows a resident's previously expressed wishes and values to guide treatment choices at a time when the resident cannot participate in the decision-making process.

Depending on applicable state law, an advance directive may take the form of:

- *A living will or medical directive, in which the individual specifies therapies that he or she would or would not accept as treatment for specific medical conditions*

- *A health care proxy or durable power of attorney for health care, in which the individual designates a surrogate decision maker in the event that he or she is unable to make decisions.*

- *A combination of both, in which the individual makes specific choices regarding therapy as well as designating a surrogate decision maker*

Under current federal law, the Patient Self-Determination Act of 1991 states that anyone admitted to a skilled nursing facility who receives Medicare or Medicaid funding must also be given information about the state's laws regarding advance directives. Federal law does not require all individuals to execute an advance directive. However, it does mandate that nursing homes ask whether new residents have advance directives and provide all persons admitted to the facility the opportunity to create such directives. Nursing homes must provide residents with the following information:

- *A statement of the individuals' rights under state law (whether statutory or as recognized by the courts of the state) to make decisions regarding their medical care, including the right to accept or refuse medical treatment and the right to formulate advance directives*

- *A statement describing the nursing home's written policies about implementing individuals' rights under state law*

In addition, as a further requirement to participate in Medicare and Medicaid programs, nursing homes must agree to:

- *Document in the medical record of each resident whether or not the individual has executed an advance directive*

- *Not condition the provision of care or otherwise discriminate against a resident based on whether or not he or she has executed an advance directive*

- *Ensure the institution's compliance with re-*

quirements of state law, whether statutory or as recognized by the courts of the state, regarding advance directives

• *Provide, individually or with others, education for the staff and the community on issues concerning advance directives*

This chapter is not intended to serve as legal advice to the resident, the resident's family, or the nursing home. The usual caveat about legal matters applies; if you have a specific legal problem or question, seek the advice of competent legal counsel. Note, however, that in most cases in the United States an attorney is not required to draft a comprehensive and binding advance directive. Many states with health care proxy or similar laws provide simple forms and instructions on request. In other countries, this process will vary considerably—some countries have no provisions for advance directives.

OVERVIEW

The creation of advance directives provides an opportunity to improve care and promote communication between physicians, other health care workers, residents, and their families. Advance directives are an attempt to preserve individuals' choices about their health care in the event that they cannot participate in the decision-making process. Given the nature of communication and the ability of individuals to misunderstand each other, advance directives will never be perfect. However, in long-term care settings, advance directives provide guidance to the facility staff about treatment decisions when residents can no longer express themselves; provide families with written documentation of a relative's wishes; and minimize conflict among family members and between the staff and families by clarifying the resident's wishes.

Formulating advance directives requires thoughtful planning. Physicians and other health care professionals often object because discussing advance directives may be upset-

ting to residents. However, the majority of elderly persons are willing and eager to discuss advance directives, and these discussions usually result in feelings of increased control and relief. From the perspective of the primary caregivers, two separate issues are involved in promoting the creation of advance directives for nursing home residents. They are:

• Process—what is the nursing home's internal procedure for ensuring that advance directives are properly created?

• Content—What are the resident's values, beliefs, and preferences regarding the future course of treatment?

The following sections discuss these issues.

INTERNAL PROCEDURE FOR CREATING ADVANCE DIRECTIVES

To ensure compliance with federal regulations, all nursing homes in the United States should have a policy regarding advance directives. More important than statutory compliance is a policy that encourages effective communication between residents and care providers. This type of communication is not always easy. Discussing matters of life and death is not easy. The staff must be open to the variety of strong feelings and potential for conflict that may arise in these discussions.

Advance directives are not a cure for every ethical problem that arises in the nursing home, but rather a chance for residents to make their own health care decisions. If that goal is reached, then the nursing facility has made great progress in respecting the wishes of its residents.

The topics frequently covered in advance directives—limiting medical therapy; instituting, withholding, or withdrawing some treatments; allowing residents to die without transfer to a hospital— overlap with several ethical concerns that arise in chronic care. Advance directives should be created in the context of institutional policies regarding management of serious ethical questions and conflicts. If a nursing home has not considered these issues or does not have an ethics committee, the federal requirement provides an opportunity to address these issues.

Institutions must identify the types of treatment they consider obligatory parts of basic care. Most nursing homes identify emotional support, religious support, skin care, turning, positioning, grooming, and oral feeding as obligatory care. Other facilities may have specific types of care, such as using tubes, which they consider obligatory. Residents should be notified of these restrictions before admission. The intent in mandating advance directives is to respect the wishes of the individuals entering health care facilities. These facilities must be clear about their restrictions on resident choice.

Most advance directives describe the type of care and therapy that a resident would or would not want, should an illness prevent the resident from making his or her own decisions. However, not all persons wish to limit their medical therapy in an advance directive. For example, a resident may request resuscitation in the event of cardiac arrest or the use of a feeding tube if he or she is unable to eat and drink normally.

Other residents will be unwilling or unable to create an advance directive. A comatose resident or one with advanced dementia is incapable of expressing his or her wishes. In such situations, care decisions are usually made by consulting with relatives, and are decisions based on both the resident's previous expressions and the traditional ethical principles of preserving life while avoiding burdensome and useless treatments. Obviously, there may be conflict between staff and family members regarding the benefits and burdens of treatment and defining what constitutes a useless therapy. Ethical guidelines provide a framework for decision making but will not solve each dilemma to the everyone's satisfaction.

In considering the formulation of advance directives and the limiting of medical therapy, nursing homes must distinguish between orders that prohibit resuscitation only (Do Not Resuscitate or DNR orders) and those with other treatment limitations. The objective of a DNR order is highly specific: If a resident is found pulseless or without respirations, then cardiopulmonary resuscitation will not be started. It is important that the meaning of DNR orders is clear to nursing home staff members. A DNR decision need not mean that other aspects of care are limited. For example, a resident may wish to have a DNR order but may also want aggressive medical treatment and hospitalization in the event of serious illness. For residents who request limitations of treatment beyond DNR, their treatments must be individualized to reflect their wishes.

The formulation of advance directives requires attention to a number of details which are addressed in the following subsections.

Asking the Resident

Facilities must devise a procedure that establishes the existence of an advance directive document, and the creation of such a document, if the resident wishes so. Depending on the size of the nursing home, it may be the responsibility of the administrator, admitting social worker, or nurse to provide this mandated information about advance directives and the individual's rights under state law to accept or refuse medical treatment. It is good practice to have the physician caring for the resident review the contents of the advance directive and discuss them with the resident.

Determining the Type of Advance Directive to Use

The specific type of advance directive that is used is dependent on state laws. In some states only a health care proxy is formally recognized; others allow for the formulation of living wills and the appointment of durable power of attorney for health care decisions. Facilities should develop a policy describing how to handle out-of-state documents. At a minimum, these documents should be respected as important expressions of an individual's wishes. Determining the exact status of these documents is also dependent upon state laws.

Facility Policies for Specific Therapies

Some facilities may have policies about specific therapies, especially feeding tubes, DNR (Do Not Resuscitate) orders, and Do Not Hospitalize (DNH) orders. Nursing homes and other facilities should have guidelines about providing, withholding, and withdrawing specific therapies. For example, if a facility will not allow the withholding and withdrawal of feeding tubes, residents must be made aware of this before admission. It is wise for facilities to develop policies about resuscitation, hospitalization, and other treatments (e.g., antibiotics, oxygen use, protocols for terminal care, etc.) to maintain consistency in the care of residents. The existence of these policies can often limit conflict in crisis situations.

For facilities with a particular philosophy of care (e.g., nursing homes with religious affiliations), developing these policies in conjunction with advance directive policies can ensure that residents are aware of the approach to health care in the facility, and that residents are able to express their wishes about therapy within that context. These policies also give residents and their families the opportunity to seek another facility if these regulations conflict with their wishes.

Advance Directive for Cognitively Impaired Residents

There are no steadfast rules for the development of advance directives for residents with dementia. Severely demented individuals lack the capacity for such decisions. Some degree of cognitive impairment, however, does not mean that an individual's requests for therapy are not valid. Many residents with dementing illnesses can express a clear preference about specific therapies, which shows both an awareness of the choice involved and the consequences.

For example, a resident with moderately severe Alzheimer's disease may be confused and disoriented, yet when questioned will consistently reject aggressive attempts to prolong life. Document these preferences along with information that gives evidence of their consistency and the resident's recognition of the consequences. Ask family members and friends to verify that the resident's wishes are consistent with his or her long-held beliefs. Other residents, who are unable to specify treatment choices, can name a surrogate decision maker.

Determining the true desires of residents with cognitive impairment can be aided by a supportive family, who can confirm that the residents' statements conform to past expressions or long-held beliefs. Conversely, families in conflict or strained relationships may make a difficult situation even worse. In cases in which there is family conflict about the resident's wishes, legal guardian proceedings may be necessary..

In situations in which a resident with cognitive impairment requests or rejects treatment, and this decision conflicts with previous expressions, proceedings can be difficult. Again, a supportive family may be able to clarify the situation. However, in some cases, the staff will be in the difficult situation of balancing the desire and obligation to comply with the resident's desires versus the concerns that the resident does not understand the implication of the decision. There are no set rules to follow in these circumstances. However, the staff should note the consistency and clarity of the resident's current desires; the ability of the resident to articulate the consequences if the requests are followed; the place of the resident's desires within the total medical condition; and the severity of the resident's cognitive impairment.

Chart Placement for Advance Directives and Resident Transfers

Place the advance directives in the patient chart so that they are readily accessible in an emergency. This provides guidance to temporary or "on-call" health care workers. For residents who are transferred to the acute care hospital, develop a mechanism so that the resident's previously expressed wishes are readily available to the hospital. Many nursing homes consistently refer residents to only one or two hospitals, and communication between the facilities about these transfers ensures that advance directives will be respected. In some states, after residents are transfered to a new facility, the advance directives are reviewed at the receiving facility and the residents or their proxies are asked if they agree with the document's contents.

Residents Who Are Unable to Decide or Who Do Not Want an Advance Directive

Residents are not required to have an advance directive regarding their health care. Residents who do not want an advance directive should have this noted in their chart. However, preferences about resident's health care decisions should be determined in the event of serious illness. Ask these residents about resuscitation, hospitalization, and individuals to be consulted, should they become unable to make decisions. Document the wishes of the resident.

At the time of admission to long term care facilities some residents will be unable to make decisions regarding their health care. The facility should try to determine if the resident created an advance directive (e.g., ask family members, check with the primary physician, request a review of the hospital chart). In the absence of any directive, treatment decisions can be made in concert with the resident's closest family members or through legal guardianship procedures.

When Advance Directives Take Effect

The timing in which an advance directive takes effect depends on applicable state law. The presence of a directive does not mean that the physician immediately turns to surrogates without determining whether or not the resident can make decisions. Generally speaking, when the resident is no longer able to communicate or make decisions, the provisions of the advance directive or the surrogate decision maker are to be honored. However, if the resident recovers and demonstrates an awareness of the situation, decision-making power returns to the resident.

Family Disagreements with Advance Directives

Ethically, the facility staff must recognize that their first responsibility is to the residents. Residents who refuse therapy should not receive such treatment when they are unable to object. When faced with angry relatives, the staff may be concerned with the possibility of civil liability. In developing advance directive procedures, seek the opinion of legal counsel on how best to protect the wishes of the residents and limit the facility's potential for liability.

Staff Objections to Advance Directives

The facility staff is not obliged to honor advance directive wishes that are illegal. For example, an advance directive cannot compel a physician or nurse to participate in active euthanasia. Often, ethical objections to care decisions can also be a problem. In devising an advance directive policy, institutions should consider conscientious objection to decisions by the staff and allow for individuals to withdraw from the care of a resident. In smaller nursing homes, this may create staffing problems, so it is important that facilities be clear on their philosophy of care.

When to Review Advance Directives

Because values and treatment preferences may change with time and health, the staff should speak with residents about their wishes on a regular basis (at least once a year) and/or when there has been a major change in their physical condition or functional status (e.g., after hospitalization).

DETERMINING THE CONTENT OF ADVANCE DIRECTIVES

Advance directives reflect the wishes of residents in proportion to the time and care spent by the staff in speaking with residents. Whether creating an advance directive or reviewing the content of an advance directive brought to the facility, a conversation with the resident about medical care preferences should take place directly after admission. Considering the time that residents spend in nursing homes compared with that in acute care hospitals, the staff of nursing homes should adopt a high standard in determining the preferences of their residents. This may well require communication between various staff—physicians, nurses, aides, social workers, and others—to obtain the complete picture. A team approach to care can facilitate this process, including discussion of advance directives as a part of team meetings.

It is impossible to provide a detailed script for a conversation between the staff and a resident here. However, the following points can serve as suggestions for these conversations. With experience, individual staff members will develop their own questions, recognize pitfalls in discussion, and devise their own approach to asking residents about care preferences. In discussing advance directives with residents, the staff will always have their own preferences and values. Some ethicists urge the staff to be value neutral; others object that value neutrality is impossible in every situation. Ideally, an awareness of preferences and values will help the staff recognize ways in which they may bias the conversation unfairly.

Introduce the Topic of Advance Directives

Both the staff's anxiety about the discussion and the resident's concerns can be eased by sensitive and careful introduction to the topic of advance directives. The meanings of "sensitive" and "careful" depends heavily on the staff's personality and the resident's condition, but here are some general guidelines. Begin with an open-ended statement such as, "Many of my patients are concerned about what would happen to them if they suffered from an accident or a serious illness. Have you ever thought about that? Can we talk about your treatment preferences if that ever happened to you?"

Resident Values and Advance Directives

Asking residents about things in life that are important to them provides a context in which to discuss specific therapies. It gives residents the chance to articulate important values and provides the staff with insight into the people for whom they are caring. For example, ask, "There are a number of therapies available that we use to maintain life and restore function. Sometimes they are successful and sometimes they are not. Help me to understand what is more important to you–every day of life or other personal goals?"

Discuss the Goals and Options of Specific Therapies

Discussing the resident's values leads to consideration of the benefits and burdens of different therapies. A distinction must be made between short-term trials of aggressive treatment and prolonged, open-ended therapy. Be alert to the resident's fears and misconceptions that are masquerading as genuine desires. Residents may be so predetermined to avoid prolonged treatment when there is little hope of recovery that they never consider the possibility of a brief period of treatment in reversible situations. A resident may say, "Just let me die, I don't want any tubes." However, the resident may agree to mechanical ventilation and intensive care for a short period in a reversible illness such as pulmonary edema.

Residents may accept or reject therapy, depending on their underlying medical condition. For example, a resident with Parkinson's disease may want a feeding tube placed if severe dysphagia developed in relation to the Parkinson's disease, but would reject tube feedings in the case of severe dementia.

Situations can also occur in which residents desire aggressive and intensive therapies that have little likelihood of achieving success. Although respect and sensitivity are called for, as well as avoiding an ageist attitude that could reject potentially life-saving treatments because the resident is old, the staff can point out what they consider unreasonable therapy. Determining what constitutes 'unreasonable therapy' can be quite arbitrary, and the staff must be aware of their own biases. Recommendations to residents, either for or against specific treatments, should be based on clinical experience and literature.

Residents who arrive at a nursing home with complete advance directives should review their options. Many residents will arrive at the nursing home with a living will calling for "extraordinary care" and "quality of life," which are terms that are difficult to apply in specific situations and emergencies. Conversely, some directives may contain very detailed instructions about the use of some therapies. However, documents such as these may cause difficulties when the clinical situation does not match that of the document. In both situations, a discussion with the staff can provide insight into the wishes of the resident. In some instances, the resident may even wish to dictate a new directive.

Specific therapies that should be considered include, at a minimum, resuscitation, artificial feeding, hydration, and mechanical ventilation. Therapies such as dialysis and surgery should also be considered. Discussing care issues about a terminal illness is especially important for elderly residents in long-term care settings. Residents should discuss their preferences about hospitalization or a hospice approach to care.

Surrogate Decision Makers and Advance Directives

Some states allow residents to designate a surrogate decision maker. Often, advance directives that outline specific treatment options are limited by unanticipated situations and ambiguity in the document. The appointment of a surrogate decision maker, or someone who will speak for the resident if he or she cannot, helps to overcome these limitations. Depending on the jurisdiction, the surrogate decision maker can be termed a *health care proxy* or be empowered with *durable power of attorney* for health care decisions.

The purpose of a surrogate is to determine what the resident would want in a given situation. To maximize the effectiveness of this type of designation, the nursing home should encourage a discussion regarding the resident's wishes with the resident, surrogate, and staff. Without such a discussion, proxies will not be adequately informed to make decisions and may impose their preferences rather than those of the resident. The nursing home should have the necessary information to contact the surrogate in case of an emergency.

Review the Resident's Wishes

Because of the importance of advance directives in the determination of the resident's care in life and death situations, these directives should be revised at the time of discussion to ensure they express the resident's wishes. Staff caregivers may suggest that the resident take time and consider the discussion before formally agreeing. The resident may also wish to speak with others about the directive and obtain the advice of relatives, friends, legal counsel, and clergy.

CASE EXAMPLES

The following case examples describe two advance directive scenarios.

CASE EXAMPLE 1

The laws governing advance directives vary from state to state, so this case describes a hypothetical admission in the state of Massachusetts. The law here specifies the appointment of an individual as health care proxy rather than the formulation of a living will.

Mrs. C. was an 87-year-old woman admitted to the nursing home after a 2-week admission to the local community hospital for the repair of a hip fracture. Mrs. C. had suffered two strokes in the past with a mild residual left-sided weakness. She had previously lived in a small apartment where she received considerable assistance from her daughter. A son, estranged from the family, lived in a distant state. On admission to the nursing home, the nurse asked Mrs. C. about any advance directives. Mrs. C. had no such document but expressed interest in further information. She was given a copy of the informational packet provided by the nursing home to all new admissions, which contained a description of the Massachusetts Health Care Proxy law as well as information about her rights and responsibilities as a resident. The nurse explained that Mrs. C. would be examined by her new physician at the nursing home and that she could discuss her wishes with the doctor as well as ask the nurse any questions.

After performing a physical examination, the doctor reviewed his findings with Mrs. C. The nurse on the floor confirmed the physician's impression that Mrs. C. was mildly forgetful but aware of her environment and her decisions. The physician asked Mrs. C. if she had considered appointing anyone as her proxy for health care decisions. She responded that she would like to name her daughter as her proxy. The doctor also inquired as to Mrs. C.'s values and her thoughts about specific treatments. Mrs. C. responded that she had a strong religious faith and that she was not particularly afraid of dying. She did not want any effort made to restart her heart, but agreed with the doctor that she would be willing to undertake a brief period of intensive treatment if there was a reasonable hope of recovery. She wanted "the machines shut off" if she did not get better quickly.

In the event she was unable to eat normally, Mrs. C. felt that she would want a feeding tube if she could interact with her family. The physician contacted Mrs. C.'s daughter who agreed to be her mother's proxy and confirmed that her mother's statements about her care were consistent with previous comments. The physician assisted Mrs. C. in completing the Health Care Proxy form, and recorded in the chart Mrs. C.'s preferences about specific treatments. Per nursing home policy, a copy of the Health Care Proxy form was placed in a specially marked portion of the chart and a copy sent to the local hospital for inclusion in Mrs. C.'s record. Mrs. C. did well for the next 18 months at the nursing home. At a yearly review she reiterated her desires not to be resuscitated but to receive aggressive short-term therapy for reversible illness.

One evening, Mrs. C. was found unresponsive after dinner. She was transported to the hospital. A neurologic examination suggested a large stroke. Mrs. C.'s daughter was contacted and told of the poor prognosis. She agreed with a plan of intravenous fluids and supportive therapy, but she did not wish her mother intubated in the event of respiratory arrest. She asked that a priest be called to attend to her mother and stated she would notify her brother and come to the hospital.

Mrs. C.'s condition remained unchanged over the next 48 hours. A high fever was then noted with a chest radiograph suggesting aspiration pneumonia. Mrs. C.'s son arrived and appeared greatly distressed at the situation. He argued with his sister, who had agreed to the use of antibiotics for the pneumonia, but again refused the option of mechanical ventilation. The son spoke with the attending physician and demanded his mother be transferred to the intensive care unit, intubated, and given all available therapies. He threatened legal action against the physician and hospital should the doctor refuse. Mrs. C.'s physician reviewed with the son her conversations with his mother, showed him the Health Care Proxy, and expressed her sorrow over Mrs. C.'s illness but informed the son that she would not go against the decisions of his sister or Mrs. C.'s previous wishes. Mrs. C. died the next day in the company of her daughter and grandchildren.

CASE EXAMPLE 2

Mr. S. is an 87-year-old man with multiinfarct dementia, who was admitted to the nursing home after being hospitalized for pneumonia. He had lived alone for 5 years after his wife's death, and because of an inability to care for himself, moved to the home of his daughter and son-in-law and their three young children because he was unable to care for himself. He lived at their home for 2 years before hospitalization. At the time of the hospital admission, Mr. S. required assistance with bathing, dressing, and toileting, and was frequently incontinent.

Mr. S. was transferred to the nursing home from the hospital because his care had become too much for his family to manage. He was weak and frail as a consequence of his pneumonia, required assistance with eating, and the dementia had progressed to the stage that he was disoriented, often agitated, and

he sometimes wandered. On admission to the nursing home, the admitting physician found Mr. S. unaware of his surroundings; grossly confused as to the year, month, and date; and asking for his wife. The physician asked Mr. S. about his care in the hospital and whether he would want to be resuscitated. He responded, "Take care of me. Do everything." Further questioning did not clarify what Mr. S. meant by this.

The physician, nurse, and social worker received little new information from Mr. S. in the next few days of his stay. He frequently yelled, "Take care of me." When asked specific questions about his preferences, he would answer, "Do everything!" The staff held a team meeting with Mr. S.'s two daughters. The physician expressed his impression that Mr. S. was unaware of the meaning of his statements and asked the impressions of Mr. S.'s daughters. The daughter with whom Mr. S. had lived related that Mrs. S. had died after several heart attacks and a long struggle in the intensive care unit. After his wife's death, Mr. S. had frequently expressed to his daughter and son-in-law that he wished to die peacefully; did not desire any sort of intensive care; would not want to have cardiopulmonary resuscitation or be put on a ventilator; and desired only treatments that were simple. The other daughter agreed with her sister's recollections.

The physician said that he would place a DNR order in the chart on the basis of this conversation. He and the other members of the team stated that Mr. S. would receive attentive care and that everything would be done to ensure his comfort. The daughters agreed with this plan and asked to be informed of any changes in their father's condition.

SUMMARY

The case of Mrs. C. demonstrates a relatively straightforward example of a resident articulating her desires and appointing a health care proxy. It shows the physician's responsibility to respect the wishes of the patient, and not succumb to threats by family members. Specific points to note in the case include:

- The physician's involvement in the formulation of advance directives allowed her to provide appropriate care at the end of Mrs. C.'s life, despite a difficult family situation
- Mild cognitive impairment need not mean lack of clarity in the resident's conveyance of her wishes for care
- The sharing of the health care proxy form with the local hospital will facilitate care in the event of an emergency
- A yearly review of advance directives is advised
- The importance of having a family member appointed as proxy, who insisted that the resident's wishes be respected

The case of Mr. S. is less clear. His response, "Take care of me! Do everything!" could mean that he should be a full code and receive aggressive treatment. In the example, the physi-cian and staff were concerned about the meaning of Mr. S.'s response given his dementia. Appropriately, they consulted with family members, and the physician submitted a DNR order on the basis of this conversation. If the family had been at odds with one another or less clear about Mr. S.'s previously expressed wishes, then the nursing home staff should consider their next move carefully, and suggest that the family try to resolve their differences. If that was impractical or impossible, then other avenues could have been explored, including legal guardianship for Mr. S. The major point of this case is the care that must be taken to balance the values of preserving life, respecting a person's wishes, and providing appropriate care. Cases in which the staff and family believe a resident's preferences for care are inappropriate must be approached with great caution. In such circumstances, involving an ethics committee can be invaluable to the situation.

33
Terminal Care

Linda H. Kilburn, MSSS
Katharine M. Murphy, RN, MS
Kate Kelley, RN, MPH

Terminal care in the nursing home setting is that provided to residents who have a limited prognosis and for whom the goals of treatment shift from curative to palliative outcomes. In terminal care, the focus becomes maximization of the quality of remaining life, rather than the prolongation of life. Formal hospice programs in the United States initially were focused primarily on the care of patients with cancer diagnoses. Hospice care is now available to nursing home residents under the Medicare Hospice Benefit. To be eligible for this benefit, the resident must be terminally ill (regardless of diagnosis), with a prognosis of 6 months or less. However, this time limitation may be less applicable to persons with AIDS (see Chapter 5, AIDS, for more information) and residents with noncancer diagnoses, i.e., those whose disease progression may have significant variations, but whose terminal disease progression must nevertheless be affirmed by their physicians.

Caring for the terminally ill involves considering and addressing a wide variety of physiological, psychological, social, and spiritual needs in addition to administrative issues. The scope of care of terminally ill nursing home residents has been further expanded by the development of hospice-specific third-party benefit and licensure regulations and by demands related to the care of persons with AIDS. (See Chapter 5, AIDS, and the section on Community Hospice Services in the Nursing Home, in this chapter, for more information.)

This chapter addresses direct resident care and support concerns and identifies key administrative issues to be considered when adapting the nursing home environment to special resident care needs, applicable federal regulations, and relevant administrative and staff concerns.

OVERVIEW

In the nursing home, death is common and often expected. However, caring for dying residents in the nursing home is less common because a relatively large percentage of terminally ill residents are transferred to acute care hospitals at the end of life. Among frail elderly nursing home residents, death is often preceded by an extended period of immobility, incontinence, mental deterioration, and the inability to communicate. However, because satisfactory prognostic indicators have heretofore been lacking among persons with multiple interacting physical and mental illnesses, it has often been difficult to determine the appropriateness of continued life-sustaining interventions (e.g., tube feedings, antibiotics, mechanical ventilation). Residents are often transferred to the acute care hospital setting when an emergency arises.

Unnecessary and burdensome tests and treatments can result from lack of communication among residents, families, and interdisciplinary staff about the following issues:
• Resident's prognosis
• Values regarding the quality of life
• Objectives of care
• Resident's wishes for life prolongation and improved quality of life through symptom control

Nursing homes are appropriate facilities for providing the intensive, noninvasive nursing care needed by dying residents. At some point, any multiply impaired, terminally ill resident may benefit from receiving a palliative approach to care, so explore this option with the resident, family, and staff. The overall objectives of a palliative approach include:
• Promoting comfort and quality of remaining life through symptom control, providing interventions with a low resident burden and high benefit, and withholding treatments of unproven value
• Promoting as much functional autonomy as possible
• Maximizing the resident's role in decision-making by informing the resident (or surrogate) about the condition and treatment alternatives in terms he or she can understand and seeking his or her input into the process; this means keeping the resident as alert as possible while simultaneously securing maximum physical comfort
• Facilitating open communication between the resident, family, and interdisciplinary caregivers
• Educating the resident and family about care techniques and encouraging family involve-

ment in resident care and support
• Fostering a homelike environment that is conducive to resident comfort and well-being

IDENTIFYING RESIDENTS WHO MAY BENEFIT FROM PALLIATIVE CARE

In a study using longitudinal nursing home resident assessment (i.e., Minimum Data Set) data, approximately 15% of the sample had died at 6-month follow-up. However, only 1.1% of the residents had been diagnosed by their physicians as being terminally ill at the beginning of the 6-month study period.

This section describes how to identify residents who may be approaching the end of life by reviewing common functional markers of terminal conditions rather than disease diagnoses. This review should prompt further discussion to determine whether the resident has reached a transition point at which an explicit palliative/hospice approach to care would provide a greater benefit to the resident's quality of life than the current approach.

Assessment and decision-making about care of the terminally ill requires interdisciplinary teamwork and ongoing, open communication with the resident and family. There are no firm rules; the process involves a high degree of uncertainty, and necessitates flexibility and creativity. It is imperative that nurse assistants, who will be providing the majority of direct resident care, be involved in the process and understand the meaning of a shift in care focus. Those involved need the chance to share information and insights, discuss options and goals, ask questions, and take time to think and consult with others as necessary. At times it is helpful to have the facility chaplain or social worker join the team to facilitate problem-solving.

This section also highlights key resident, service, and resource variables to use in evaluating whether a shift in care focus (i.e., palliative) is warranted and appropriate. It also prompts clinicians to think about what to do to create an environment that is conducive to offering quality palliative care (e.g., staff education, links to community hospice). The issues to consider are described in the following sections.

Resident Evaluation

Perform the following resident evaluation:

- End-stage disease: Is the resident in the late stage of a chronic disease for which no cure is possible and intercurrent acute illnesses (e.g., aspiration pneumonia) or acute manifestations of the problem (e.g., congestive heart failure) are highly probable?
- Recurrent near-death episodes: Has the resident been at the point of death several times in the past year and recovered with treatment? Since recovery, what is the resident's quality of life (e.g., ability to communicate, level of socialization, mood, physical function)?
- Severe dementia: Is the resident in the late stage of a dementing illness, i.e., totally dependent on others for personal care and nourishment, unable to make decisions, noncommunicative, physically contracted, incontinent, and asleep much of time?

Consider the resident's potential reaction to treatment. Does the resident understand the disease process or need for tests, treatment, or transfer to another location for care? Anticipate the resident's response to treatment or hospitalization based on previous reactions to acute illness and relocation.

- Severe dysphagia: Does the resident have swallowing difficulty that inhibits adequate nutrition, hydration, and enjoyment? Is the problem acute with hope for recovery, or is the prognosis for restoration of oral feeding poor? (*See* Chapter 26, Feeding Tubes, for more assessment information.)
- Verbal expressions of being ready to die (or that death is approaching): Does a chronically debilitated resident make statements such as "I've had enough;" "I'm ready to join (deceased);" "I wish God would take me."? Are these comments manifestations of a treatable depression or do they reflect true readiness in frail, chronically ill resident? (*See* Chapter 13, Depression, for more information.)
- Verbal requests to withhold life sustenance such as refusing food or fluids and stopping medications: Are these informed, rational requests or do they reflect hopelessness that may accompany a treatable depression? (*See* Chapter 13, Depression, for more information.)
- Demonstrated resistance to current treatment, medication, or nourishment in a nonverbal resident: Such actions may include spitting out food and medications or repeatedly pulling out a feeding tube. Try to differentiate whether such actions reflect a treatable discomfort or an aversion to the treatment (e.g., bad-tasting drug, sore throat from tube), or if they represent the resident's preference to not be burdened by the treatment.
- Resident's goals and values: What are the resident's goals? Has he or she previously expressed wishes about the type of care to receive at the end of life? Does the resident have personal goals yet to be achieved (e.g., attending a granddaughter's wedding; celebrating the next holiday or birthday)? Is the resident able to do the things that he or she wishes to do? How does the resident perceive the quality of his or her life? The assessment and care approach should take these questions into consideration.
- Timing of death: Would death in the near future be premature for this resident, or would it be appropriate and acceptable? Death is considered premature if treatment may provide the resident with a good quality of remaining life, or if it will buy time for the resident who is not yet prepared to die.

Appropriate timing is a subjective phenomenon based on levels of physical and emotional comfort and goals for the future.

Service Evaluation

Perform the following service evaluation:

- Advanced directives: Are the resident's and family's wishes about more aggressive interventions known or can they be ascertained? Is there a living will or medical power of attorney in place? Has an advanced directive to withhold certain treatments (e.g., Do Not Resuscitate) been developed and recorded in the resident's record? If so, is the directive current? Are there any known disagreements between the resident, family, and caregivers regarding the philosophy of care that need to be addressed?

- Treatment burden: What is the potential level of intrusiveness of possible interventions and what are the implications for the resident's comfort if these interventions are undertaken? Is the anticipated treatment perceived to be more burdensome than the natural disease process itself? Will the treatment be painful (e.g., frequent needle sticks for blood tests, postoperative pain), prolonged, or involve using physical restraints that will undermine the resident's freedom or sense of self? Are uncomfortable side effects common? Limiting treatment may increase the resident's comfort.

- Recurrent hospitalizations: Has the resident had multiple acute hospitalizations in the past year for acute exacerbations of chronic life-threatening illnesses (e.g., CHF, respiratory insufficiency, unstable diabetes, recurrent aspiration pneumonia, dehydration)? Is this pattern likely to continue given the resident's condition?

Facility Resource Evaluation

Perform the following facility resource evaluation:

- Philosophy of care: What is the facility's philosophy of care? Is there an atmosphere of caring and respect for the residents' wishes and preferences? Does the facility make an effort to accommodate unique cultural aspects of death and dying (e.g., bedside vigils, preparation of the body)? Does the facility encourage family involvement in resident assessment, care planning, and caregiving? Is there flexibility to accommodate family needs and preferences at the end of a loved one's life (e.g., rooming-in options)?

- Facility preparedness: Do staff know how to provide palliative care? Do they have a knowledge of symptom control measures or resources (e.g., community hospice services) and make them accessible to residents and families? Have the staff, particularly the nonlicensed direct caregivers, been prepared psychologically and physically to care for dying residents and to attend to their dead bodies?

- Facility resources: Do residents, families, and staff have access to clergy, social workers, and volunteers? Is there respite for primary staff caregivers (caregiving can become physically and emotionally draining)?

- Facility policies: Does the facility have policies and procedures for the following:

  o Helping residents and families prepare advanced directives (e.g., living wills, health care proxies)
  o Formally communicating the news of a death to the residential community
  o Observing death within the residential community (e.g., memorial services, transportation to wakes and funerals, discussion on the unit with the social worker)
  o Informing direct care staff and family of the resident's condition
  o Telling the truth to the residents
  o Notifying families (determining ahead of time when families want to be called, who to call)

CARE PLANNING

Note: The authors of this chapter wish to acknowledge the contributions of the following former members of the Hospice of the Good Shepherd clinical team whose work, "Multidisciplinary Team Manual for the Hospice Patient and Family," served as the foundation for the palliative, psychosocial, and spiritual care portions of this chapter. Principal authors of the initial work included Sheila Flynn Scott, MSN; Sandra Skelly Skinner, RN, MA; Helen Marino Connolly, BSN, MS; Elinor Robinson, MEd; and Kate Leornard, PhD, under the supervision of Linda Kilburn.

Teamwork

The roles of physicians and nursing home staff working with terminally ill residents should be closely interrelated. The physicians ultimately make decisions about the appropriate medical intervention and its intensity and timing, but it is the daily observations of and interactions with the resident by nurses, nursing assistants, and other staff that are important in monitoring and validating current care plan effectiveness, identifying new problems or changes in the resident's condition, and maximizing the resident's comfort. Close contacts and interaction with social workers, volunteers, and the resident's family or significant other may also provide important clues about nonphysical factors that may impact the resident's reaction both to the terminal condition as well as to pain and other symptoms of discomfort.

Family Involvement

If available, family input is crucial in delivering quality care to residents approaching the end of life. However, family members often feel helpless and anxious in medical settings. Staff efforts to welcome the family as important members of the care team can enhance communications on the resident's behalf, avoid misunderstandings or sabotage of care plan intent, and maximize support to the resident. Concrete suggestions about ways in which the family members can help are generally welcomed and can make a major difference in the resident's quality of life. However, families who do not feel welcome or who are not provided opportunities to be concretely involved in care, may tend to visit less frequently or develop adversarial relationships with the caregiving staff.

During the terminal phase of a resident's life, family issues are often highly complex, usually involving multiple generations. The nature of marital, parent-child, and multigenerational relationships may change drastically. Common spousal concerns may include fear of losing a long-term partner, lover, or supporter who may well be the primary sustaining relationship in the resident's life. Fears about "What will happen to me?" and anger at pending desertion (death) are also common.

For adult children, there may be issues related to role reversals as their parent becomes increasingly debilitated and dependent; fears about being able to cope and of the emotional and physical drain; lack of knowledge, fear, and guilt related to the disease process, proposed care interventions, and their own abilities to be involved in the process; and the loss of a sustaining support in their own lives. There may also be financial burdens.

Younger children in the family, although usually taking their cues from adults and therefore reflecting similar fears, may have their own fears exacerbated by being more cut off from the information-sharing and decision-making processes. Their own grieving process can be greatly complicated by family conspiracies of silence and their own self-imposed sense of guilt.

Both residents and family members may need assistance in sorting out their feelings to adapt to changes and stresses arising from the terminal condition. Nursing homes should provide interested families with opportunities to be involved in decision-making and caregiving, teach ways to promote resident comfort, and support their participation at whatever level they feel comfortable. The guidelines for family involvement include the following:

- Support the family at its level of functioning. Recognize and reinforce the strengths of each family member. Encourage questions and tailor information to the individual's level of understanding.
- Teach the family about the disease process, the resident's requirements, and reasonable treatment options for care. Correct misconceptions about illness, the dying process, and death. Promote family participation in decision-making and caregiving at levels appropriate to their capabilities, preferences, and comfort.
- Describe for the family what care will be provided to prevent the misperception and fear that the resident will be abandoned and neglected by staff.
- Anticipate conflicts over treatment regimens. Conflicts between a nursing home resident and his or her family may arise from any number of factors, including differences in religious or spiritual beliefs, differences in understanding or level of acceptance of the resident's prognosis, and fears or lack of understanding about the proposed care plan, its intent, and potential impact. Assist the family in devising a means of negotiating differences. Support the resident and family choices. When in conflict, it is essential to advocate for the resident's preferences, and assist family members in understanding and accepting the resident's choices.
- Identify barriers to or fears of communicating, and address these directly if appropriate and desired. Common emotional barriers might include fears of upsetting the resident or a family member, difficulties with

truthtelling (this can also affect staff), and the desire to protect the resident or family member. Provide alternative opportunities for the resident or family members to vent their concerns if they are unable or unwilling to do so more directly with each other.

- Role playing staff-family interactions is an effective way to ensure positive effective communication. The ways in which questions are framed are important to ensure the type of care the resident wishes to receive. For example, posing the question, "Do you want everything done for your mother?" will elicit a less accurate response than, "Do you think your mother would want to be resuscitated (brought back to life) when she dies?"
- Explore with family members ways they can participate in care; even young children are often eager to help and their aid can be enlisted in simple tasks like carrying a snack, fetching an extra blanket, assisting the resident to drink with a straw, or drawing a picture to decorate the resident's room.
- Assist the family in its effort to reorganize roles, set priorities, and maintain family integrity and functioning. Make referrals for supplemental services if needed or requested.
- Encourage family members to identify, develop, and pursue other supports, interests, and activities to help them cope with the anticipated loss of a loved one.
- Notify family members of imminent death. Provide opportunities for a time of family privacy with the body after death if possible and desired.

General Care of the Terminally Ill Resident

Many problems encountered by the terminally ill are also experienced by the nonterminally ill and are addressed in other chapters in this manual. This section details additional or alternative care plans specific to residents near the end of life.

Nutrition and Hydration

The approach to nutrition and hydration is different for the terminally ill resident than for the nonterminal resident. In the terminal phase, the need and desire for food often decrease. Clinicians should focus on evaluating and alleviating the symptoms that interfere with a resident's desires for food intake. New dietary preferences must be identified and provided when the resident feels hungry or thirsty. Flexibility is crucial in maintaining comfort. Although most institutions are geared toward providing three meals a day as the primary dietary routine, meeting the somewhat different needs of the terminally ill resident need not be cumbersome if the nursing home provides staff and families with sufficient resources for quick preparation on the nursing unit.

Ideally, the equipment can include a refrigerator, blender, toaster, or microwave oven. Juices, custards, puddings, the makings for milkshakes, and other items brought by family members can then be easily stored and quickly prepared. Encourage family members, other visitors, and volunteers to use these facilities to provide nutrition and hydration more readily when the resident is feeling up to eating or drinking.

Consider these nutrition guidelines:
- Consult with a dietitian. Involve the resident in identifying foods and drinks that appeal to him or her. As taste disturbances occur, some items may no longer be palatable. More or different spices and flavorings may need to be added to make food more appetizing. Also, breakfasts are often the resident's best meal. Breakfast foods and snacks provided at other times of day may have an appeal.
- Provide meals and snacks that are high in protein and carbohydrates. Nutritional supplements can be added to food or taken

separately.
- Small, more frequent meals or snacks are more effective than large ones. Terminally ill residents often feel full after only a few bites of food or sips of fluids. It is often more palatable to take frequent small bites or sips than to take large amounts at once.
- Encourage family members or significant others to bring residents' favorite foods and drinks, and to spend time with them during meals. Social interaction can augment the desire to take nourishment. However, caution family members against developing, "the eat a little more" syndrome. Meal and snack times should be pleasant, not a battle, and family members may need support and education about naturally changing needs and desires for food and fluids.
- A glass of wine or beer should be permitted because it might stimulate the appetite.
- Allow enough time for the resident to eat. Reheat food and fluids in the microwave if the resident eats slowly.
- Check for and address any physical problems that may interfere with eating and drinking.

Mouth Care

Maintaining good oral hygiene and avoiding common complications are essential to comfort and well-being. The most common oral problems in the terminally ill include xerostomia (dry mouth), stomatitis (sore mouth), coated tongue, and thrush (candidiasis). Nearly all terminally ill residents experience dry mouth. About 70% of residents with oral cancer will develop thrush.

Oral problems may stem from poor oral hygiene, ill-fitting dentures, drug reactions, mouth breathing, dehydration, radiotherapy, infections, tumors, or disorders of the salivary glands.

It is important to encourage as much resident autonomy as possible in maintaining daily mouth care. However, as the resident's condition deteriorates provide assistance to ensure oral hygiene.

Follow these guidelines for general oral care:

- Brush teeth at least twice a day (if the resident accepts). Note that some residents in end-stage illness who are dependent in oral hygiene find such care disagreeable. Offer oral rinses instead.
- Check dentures for fit and comfort, clean them daily, remove them at night, and seek a dental consult as needed.
- Clean the tongue and teeth every 2 to 3 hours with toothettes (foam stick applicators) to remove debris (the toothette can be dipped in water, sodium bicarbonate, or club soda). Avoid lemon glycerin swabs, which can exacerbate dry mouth.
- Rinse the mouth every 2 to 3 hours with diluted mouthwash. (Mouthwashes with a high alcohol content may cause stinging or drying; carbamide peroxide is available commercially as an 11% gel (Proxigel) or 10% solution (Gly-Oxide).
- Apply vaseline or lip balm to lips. Check for sores.

SYMPTOM CONTROL

In elderly residents with multiple interacting illnesses, the distinction between treatment aimed at improving the quality of life through symptom control and treatment aimed at prolonging life is unclear. Sometimes palliative treatment actually extends life as in the case of giving antibiotics or diuretics to treat underlying causes of severe shortness of breath. Decisions are particularly difficult when the intervention involves hydration because a person can only live a short time without fluid. According to ethical theory, it is helpful to consider two ethical principles when making difficult treatment decisions at the end of life:

- **The principle of "proportionality,"** which specifies the use of only those interventions that can demonstrate a proportionately

greater benefit than burden to the resident. For example:

o If a resident is dehydrated, uncomfortable, and cannot drink water, then intravenous fluids for comfort make sense, since the benefit in this case may outweigh the burden of therapy. However, remember that introducing intravenous hydration often precipitates fluid overload, an additional burden of discomfort in persons close to death.

o If the resident is dying without feeling thirst, and fluids and nutrition merely prolong the dying process, then the interventions are judged to be disproportionate to the outcome and are optional.

- **The principle of "double effect,"** which specifies that one action can have two or more effects, one good and the others bad. For example, one action of using high doses of morphine sulfate to control pain can produce two effects—control of pain and suffering and depressed respirations. The first duty is to control pain and suffering. If the resident is in pain during the last days of life, provide analgesia regardless of the adverse side effects, which by this point have no valid meaning.

In some cases, intervention approaches for pain and other symptom control problems of the terminally ill may differ from those used for similar problems among the nonterminally ill. This section reviews symptom control measures for common sources of discomfort in the terminally ill.

Pain Management

Pain is experienced by more than 75% of terminally ill cancer patients and is also very common in those with other diagnoses (e.g., angina in end-stage cardiac disease, joint pain). It may be caused by an injury, disease progression, treatment interventions, reactions to debilitating disease, positioning, and/or psychological/physiological response to circumstances. It may not always be possible to ascertain the complete causes of pain. *If the resident feels pain, it exists and should be evaluated and treated.*

Common sources of disease-related pain may include tumor infiltration of bone, nerve, hollow viscous, viscera, or soft tissues, muscle spasm, edema, raised intercranial pressure, infection, myopathy, obstruction, or pathological fractures.

Common sources of treatment-related pain may include postoperative pain or adhesions, postradiation fibrosis or necrosis, postchemotherapy necrosis, or peripheral neuropathy. Pain can also be exacerbated by a lack of, insufficient, or inappropriate treatment interventions, including the failure to bring the resident to (and maintain) a sufficient level of analgesic relief.

Common sources of pain associated with debilitating disease include constipation, contractures, pressure ulcers, joint inflammation, or infection. Residents may also experience pain related to other medical conditions (e.g., migraine headaches, musculoskeletal complaints).

The resident's psychological state can also directly cause or exacerbate pain. Common contributing factors may be in response to terminal prognosis and its implications, as well as from such other factors as family or life situation, disagreements between the resident and caregivers about appropriate treatment interventions, or anticipation of pain due to inadequate analgesic regimens.

The cognitively impaired resident may be unable to identify, remember, or communicate the nature and scope of the pain. Instead, the resident may have increased agitation, restlessness, and noisiness, which may or may not be indicative of pain or a specific pain source.

Assessment

Good pain management starts with a thorough assessment that takes into account the combined physiological, psychosocial, and spiritual factors that contribute either to the pain itself or the resident's tolerance of it. Insomnia, fatigue, anxiety, fear, anger, helplessness, boredom, isolation, abandonment, and depression are some of the factors that can decrease the resident's tolerance for pain significantly. Address the following factors to maximize comfort:

- General medical history, including disease progression, diagnostic workups, and treatments.
- Determine pain history, analgesic drug history (e.g., drug names, dosages, frequency, effectiveness, side effects), and alternative methodologies and their efficacy.
- Determine the current pain experience, including location, intensity and severity, quality, degree of radiation and timing, as well as any factors that appear to ameliorate or provoke the pain experience. For residents with communication difficulties, use a body chart to help the resident locate the pain; use simple terms or scales to help the resident describe and rate the pain (e.g., throbbing, stabbing, radiating, intermittent, burning).
- Document factors that ameliorate the pain (or that have done so in the past). Provide cues to help the resident identify these factors. For example, is the pain better with position changes, involvement in an activity, or after medications?
- Identify factors that increase pain. Cue the resident if necessary. For example, is the pain greater at the end of the medication cycle, does it occur when the resident is tired, when the resident has remained in one position for a prolonged period, at night?
- For residents with communication difficulties observe for physical cues related to discomfort (e.g., moaning, grimacing, favoring a body part, agitation) and anticipate the resident's needs. If the resident continues to be highly agitated after inter-

vention to relieve discomfort, reassess the situation

- Assess and document pain and the effectiveness of pain relief measures as an ongoing process. Solicit input from caregivers in contact with the resident on a round-the-clock basis.

Intervention

The goals of treatment should include relief of pain, prevention of recurrence, erasure of the memory of pain, ease of administration of pain relief measures, and keeping the resident as mentally alert as possible. The range of interventions may include:

- Medications
- Relaxation/diversion/distraction (e.g., encourage activity, visitors, use of music or visual stimulation; decorate the room differently with pictures or personal items; reminisce; get the resident out of the room as much as possible)
- Modification of pathological processes by shrinking tumors, treating pneumonia, relieving painful obstructions, and so forth (e.g., palliative radiotherapy is the treatment of choice to treat bone pain that has not responded to antiinflammatory or opioid analgesics)
- Acupuncture/acupressure
- Nerve block
- Cutaneous stimulation
- Being there, including psychosocial and spiritual support and intervention
- Physical exercise (e.g., range of motion exercises, stretching to reduce muscle tension)

The following sections discuss these interventions.

Guidelines for Pharmacologic Analgesia

Remember that the primary goal of palliative care is resident comfort. Some sedation and respiratory depression are preferable to cycles of pain. The guidelines for pharmacologic analgesia are as follows:

- When choosing a medication for pain control, use the analgesic ladder. Mild discomfort calls for mild analgesia. Move to increasingly stronger medications if comfort is not achieved (e.g., aspirin, Tylenol with codeine, percocet, Dilaudid, morphine).
- Be aware of equi-analgesic dosages if switching from one drug to another (Table 33-1). The equi-analgesic dose refers to the relative potency of a single dose of a particular drug compared with a single dose of another drug (often morphine).
- The ideal route of administration should be the least intrusive route that achieves desired pain relief. If possible, avoid intramuscular or subcutaneous injections since they are another source of pain, particularly in cachectic (highly wasted) residents. Residents who are no longer able to take medications orally can achieve good relief with suppository or dermal patch alternatives.
- Evaluate the need for regular versus as-needed administration. Most residents respond best to regular administration. As-needed dosing tends to result in cycles of pain wherein the anticipation of the pain's return not only increases the pain but also highly decreases the resident's overall comfort level. If a resident's pain is continuous (usually in persons with pain secondary to cancer), round-the-clock analgesia is the mode of choice.
- Know the duration of action for the drug of choice, and schedule dosages at the appropriate intervals. Note that these intervals may vary somewhat for individual residents, depending on such factors as body weight, rate of absorbtion, and reaction to drug combinations.
- Give the drug in high enough dosages. Doses that are too low are often the cause of pain control failure, particularly with medications given orally; titrate drugs regularly. Individualize drug dosages, eventually using the lowest possible dosage from

which comfort can be achieved. Consider the resident's body weight, age, past drug and medication history, and the physiological ability to break down and eliminate drugs. Some initial drowsiness will probably occur and it may take several days for this side effect to abate. If drowsiness persists after 2 or 3 days, lower the dosage. It is better to try a higher dosage of one drug than to continually add other drugs or switch to other alternatives.

- Remember that over time, tolerance to a given drug will occur and dosage levels will need to be increased to continue to achieve pain relief.
- Residents near death may become less conscious as part of the normal dying process. If the resident has had a history of pain, do not reduce pain medications at this time since the pain will likely recur. Likewise, do not withhold analgesics if respirations are depressed. Remember, the primary goal of care is to help provide a comfortable death.
- Adjuvant medications should be the rule rather than the exception. For example, Thorazine and Vistaril have some analgesic properties, as do some antidepressants. Other classes of drugs that may be helpful are dextroamphetamines, antianxiety drugs, diuretics (particularly helpful if the resident has shortness of breath or edema), antibiotics, steroids, and sedatives.
- Observe for side effects and treat appropriately with particular attention to bowel function and appetite. Constipation, nausea, and sedation are the most common side effects.

Acupuncture and Acupressure

Acupuncture and acupressure are appropriate methods for pain relief in terminal malignant disease, and may reduce opioid analgesic requirements. However, some of the problems with their use include resident receptivity and lack of access to appropriately skilled practitioners in the nursing home. For persons with difficulty tolerating medications, or for those who express a preference for alternatives (acupuncture and acupressure are used extensively in Eastern societies), it is worth exploring resident access to such practitioners. Studies on acupuncture generally indicate effectiveness in about 60% of the patients. Generally, multiple sessions are needed.

Nerve Blocks

A nerve block is a neurosurgical procedure in which a needle is inserted close to a nerve in order to inject a solution to cause a neural blockade (either temporary or permanent). It is most often used as a mechanism for relieving chronic pain. For the terminally ill, it is generally a procedure of last resort when pain is intractable and when other methods have failed to achieve effective pain relief. Request a neurosurgical consult to ascertain the viability and appropriateness for the presenting pain problem, and to weigh the benefits versus the potential side effects.

Cutaneous Stimulation

Transcutaneous electrical nerve stimulation (TENS) units have been used with some success both for patients with cancer pain as well as for those with some musculoskeletal pains (e.g., cervical spondylosis). It can, however, exacerbate nerve pain and should not be used for this. The units are thought to work in one of two ways: High-frequency TENS (80 to 200 Hz) were developed as the result of the gate theory of pain, in which the stimulation of skin mechanoreceptors is thought to induce presynaptic inhibition of pain transmission. Low-dose TENS (2 to 6 Hz) are thought to release endogenous opioids in the spine and midbrain, similar to acupuncture.

Optimum conditions for the use of TENS include:

- Resident receptivity and cognitive clarity

- Self-adhering 2.5-mm electrodes
- Use of a good contact medium
- A frequency of 4 Hz
- Intensity settings to cause distinct pulsation (not pain)
- Electrodes applied to acupuncture points
- A treatment duration of 15 to 20 minutes (usually daily)

Ideally, try to use a portable unit with a frequency range of 0 to 200 Hz and a minimum of two channels. TENS units have the added advantage of giving residents some control over their pain and may enable the reduction of opioid analgesics. However, it is necessary to engage the assistance of a professional with expertise in assessing TENS appropriateness and facilitating usage and monitoring at the nursing facility.

Controlling Symptoms that Interfere with Eating

The following sections discuss how to control symptoms that interfere with eating.

Nausea and Vomiting

Nausea and vomiting may be caused by the primary disease process, drug side effects, or fecal impaction, or may be a physiological response to pain or anxiety. Consider the following:

- Review the drug regimen for drugs having nausea and vomiting as side effects. Obtain relevant serum drug levels (e.g., digoxin, theophylline). Discontinue or reduce the dosage of the drug as appropriate.
- Check for fecal impaction, particularly if the resident's food and fluid intake is poor or if the resident has been receiving drugs that tend to constipate (e.g., codeine). Relieve the impaction if present (*see* Chapter 28, Bowel Disorders, for more information).
- Ensure the adequacy of pain or anxiety management.
- Administer an antiemetic drug 1 hour be-

fore each meal if the problem is severe. The typical drug of choice is Compazine 5 to 10 mg by mouth.

- Provide salty foods and ice-cold drinks to help control the nausea; suggest keeping crackers and juice readily available at the bedside to stave off nausea.
- Avoid greasy or very sweet foods; they may aggravate nausea.
- Encourage the resident to eat slowly and chew thoroughly, to rest before and after eating, and to eat when he or she feels less nauseated and more hungry.
- Provide smaller, more frequent meals. The smell of food may aggravate nausea and the resident may do better eating when the routine food carts are not present on the unit.

Dry Mouth

A large percentage of residents suffer from dry mouth due to dehydration, thrush (candidiasis), the effects of anticholinergic drugs, diuretics, or morphine. Suggested care plans include:

- Provide mouth care every 2 hours.
- Review the drug regimen and stop unnecessary drugs or, alternatively, use those with the least anticholinergic side effects.
- Evaluate for candidiasis by thoroughly inspecting the oral cavity and throat. *Candida* infections typically present as white patches or reddened mucous membranes. If present, treat with nystatin suspension, 1 to 2 ml every 6 hours. Swish nystatin around the mouth and do not give the resident any food or fluids for at least 30 minutes afterward. For resistant candidiasis, give one clotrimazole lozenge dissolved slowly in the mouth.
- Moisten the mouth by placing a humidifier in the room, particularly if the resident is mouth breathing. Provide frequent lubrication with ice chips, small sips of liquids, popsicles, sugarless drinks, pineapple chunks, or melon. Stimulate saliva with sour

Table 33-1. Narcotic Analgesics for Severe Pain

Route[a]	Equi-analgesic Dose[b]	Duration (hours)	Plasma Half-Life (hours)	Comments
Morphine				
IM	10	4–6	2–3.5	Standard for comparison; also available in
PO	60	4–7		time-release tablets
Codeine				
IM	130	4–6	3	Transformed into morphine in the body;
PO	200	4–6		useful as an initial pain killer
Oxycodone				
IM	15	—	—	Short-acting pain killer
PO	30			
Heroin[c]				
IM	5	4–5	0.5	Illegal in the United States; comparable to
PO	60	4–5		morphine in analgesic effect, side effects, and influence on mood
Levorphanol (Levo-Dromoran)				
IM	2	4–6	12–16	Good oral potency; requires careful
PO	4	4–7		supervision by a physician because of drug build-up
Hydromorphone (Dilaudid)				
IM	1.5	4–6	2–3	Available in high-potency injectable form for
PO	7.5	4–6		very sick patients and as rectal suppositories
Oxymorphone (Numorphan)				
IM	1	4–6	2–3	Available in parenteral and rectal
PO	10	4–6		suppository forms only
Meperidine (Demerol)				
IM	75	4–5	3–4	Should not be used for patients with renal disease
Methadone (Dodophine)				
IM	10		15–30	Works well when taken orally, but dosage must be carefully monitored by physician

Adapted from Foley KM: The Treatment of Cancer Pain, *N Engl J Med,* 313(2):90, 1985.

[a]IM = intramuscular; PO = oral.
[b]The relative potency of a single dose compared with a single dose of morphine.
[c]Heroin is used in the UK as a potent pain medication that can also be effective in terminal care.

or bitter cough drops, sugarless gum, or use oral bethanecol (e.g., Urecholine), 10 to 20 mg daily for 3 or 4 days, to stimulate saliva and counteract anticholinergic agents.

Sore Mouth and Stomatitis

Sore mouth and stomatitis occur most commonly as a result of candidiasis, loose or ill-fitting dentures, gingivitis, or mouth ulcers. Suggested treatments include:

- Maintain good basic oral hygiene. Seek a dental consult for denture fit problems commonly experienced with terminal residents who have lost weight and oral tissue. Failure to address denture problems can also result in increased mouth soreness and altered self-image.

- Assess for mouth ulcers and, if present, treat with local anesthetic suspensions, particularly before meals. Suggestions include dyclonine (Dyclone) 1% gel, one or two drops orally every 2 to 4 hours, or viscous lidocaine 2% 15 ml orally (swish and swallow) every 3 hours, up to eight doses per day.

- Inspect for and treat candidiasis.

- Inspect for gingivitis, which presents as inflamed, reddened, swollen gums often accompanied by bleeding. If present, treat with metronidazole (e.g., Flagyl).

- Try a soft, bland diet that is less irritating. Avoid highly acidic, spicy, or raw foods. Use a blender to soften foods that may be too hard to eat. Foods taste better if they are cooked first, then blended. Serve food lukewarm, rather than hot.

- Reposition the resident as necessary to make swallowing easier. Encourage the use of straws or cups so that the resident can drink fluids and pureed food.

Coated Tongue

Coated tongue, which presents as a layer of whitish or yellowish material, often causes halitosis and predisposes the resident to oral candidiasis. Treatment options include:

- Effervescent vitamin C tablets placed twice daily on the tongue.

- Fresh pineapple, which contains the proteolytic enzyme ananase. Reduce the potential sting by freezing pineapple slices and dipping them in powdered sugar.

Loss of Taste

The treatment options for the loss of taste include:

- Consult with the dietitian and family to provide more strongly flavored foods. Add bacon bits, sliced almonds, ham strips, or pieces of onion to vegetables for more flavor. Marinate meat, chicken, or fish in sweet fruit juices, sweet wines, Italian dressing, or sweet and sour sauce for more taste. Use stronger seasonings such as basil, oregano, rosemary, thyme, lemon juice, or mint. These seasonings can be left at the bedside or in the unit kitchen for convenience.

- If meats no longer have an appeal, provide chicken, turkey, or fish instead. Eggs, dairy products, and beans can also provide protein substitutes.

- Suggest that the resident rinse the mouth with ginger ale, tea, or club soda before eating.

Diarrhea

The treatment options for diarrhea include:

- Reduce dietary fiber and fat. Encourage liquids between meals rather than with them; encourage fluid intake to replace lost fluids and salts.

- If cramps are a problem, avoid foods or liquids that may cause gas or cramps (e.g., carbonated beverages, beer, beans, cabbage, cauliflower, spicy foods, sweets, chewing gum). Cue the resident to chew with his or her mouth closed to avoid swallowing air, which increases the potential for gas or cramps.

(For more information, *see* Chapter 28,

Bowel Disorders.)

Anorexia and Cachexia

Anorexia is a loss of appetite that occurs as only one of several symptoms of cancer cachexia or other end-stage disease. Cachexia is an overall state of malnutrition and wasting. Signs and symptoms may include:

- Weight loss
- Muscle depletion
- Electrolyte and water disturbances
- Possible decrease in hematocrit/hemoglobin
- Decrease in serum albumin
- Decrease in total iron-binding capacity
- Fatigue
- Decreased mental alertness
- Decreased food intake and an increased metabolic rate
  Cachexia can be caused by:
- A change in central hypothalamic controls
- A change in glucose and/or lipid metabolism that leads to a satiety signal
- Taste disturbances
- Side effects of treatment (e.g., medications, chemotherapy, or radiation therapy)
- Mechanical defects and malabsorption
- Psychological factors (e.g., stress, depression)
- Another problem (e.g., infection, constipation)
  The treatment options for anorexia and cachexia include:
- Provide oral care before meals and as needed. Rinse the mouth with diluted mouthwash or club soda and lemon. Check daily for sores or infection.
- If mouth pain or ulceration is a problem, use a mouthwash consisting of equal parts Benadryl elixir, viscous Xylocaine, and Kaopectate.
- Evaluate all medications for side effects that may contribute to decreased appetite. Ensure that analgesic drugs are properly titrated and that pain is not a contributing factor.

- Oral zinc, 15 mg twice a day, may be helpful in diminishing taste disturbances due to altered metabolism.
- Low-dose steroids or a medrol dose pack may stimulate appetite and improve the resident's sense of well-being.
- If poor intake is related to mechanical problems (e.g., swallowing difficulties), consider evaluation for G-tube placement. Nonoral nutrition is not appropriate for end-stage terminal illness.
- If the problem is malabsorption, consult with a dietitian to consider using supplemental feedings with Vivonex.
- Educate the family about the disease process related to anorexia; help them to deal with their own frustration over the resident's decreasing appetite and to learn other, nonfood means of nurturing the resident (e.g., back rubs, reading aloud).

Dehydration

- Carefully consider the treatment of dehydration in the terminally ill resident. If the resident's prognosis is more extended, the problem that precipitated the dehydration is acute in nature, and the resident cannot tolerate oral rehydration, then parenteral fluid replacement may be appropriate. However, if the source of the problem is recurrent, then the decision to replace fluids should be made by the resident and family at each episode (see Chapter 24, Dehydration, for more information). Suggestions for care with end-stage illness include:
  o In the resident at end-stage illness who is dehydrated because death is imminent, parenteral replacement is usually not appropriate because added fluids may:
  o Increase gastrointestinal fluids, which in turn can cause increased vomiting
  o Increase respiratory secretions, which can exacerbate shortness of breath
  o Increase edema and ascites, which in turn can cause pain and discomfort

o Increase urine output, which will necessitate more frequent resident movement (possibly increasing discomfort)

o Increase urine output, which can lead to urinary retention, particularly in residents receiving anticholinergic medications

- Focus the treatment of dehydration in end-stage illness on comfort and include the following:

o Treat dry or sore mouth, avoiding the use of lemon-glycerine swabs that may contribute to dry mouth.

o Rinse the mouth often with a mouthwash solution diluted to the resident's taste.

o Provide ice chips, hard candy, or small sips of fluid.

o Use antiemetics or antidiarrheal agents to prevent further fluid loss.

o Brush the teeth and tongue with a soft brush or toothette.

Managing Common Respiratory Problems

The following sections describe the symptomatic management of common respiratory problems in the terminally ill.

Shortness of Breath

Shortness of breath (SOB) may be described as air hunger resulting in labored or difficult breathing, sometimes accompanied by pain. Breathing is usually audibly labored and the resident may exhibit signs of nostril dilatation, protrusion of the abdomen and expanded chest, gasping, cyanosis, and distress.

The symptoms are usually related to insufficient oxygenation of blood resulting from disturbances in the lungs, circulatory disturbances, or hemoglobin deficiency. SOB may occur as the result of lymphangitic tumor spread, pleural effusion, bronchial obstruction, treatment modalities (e.g., radiation), or metastatic diseases that restrict diaphragmatic movement (e.g., ascites, abdominal tumor). Other causes may include anemia, edema, acidosis, excessive CO_2 content of blood, lesions of the respiratory center, asthma, emotional excitation, medication side effects, or orthopnea. SOB may also be a subjective feeling in the absence of underlying disease.

The supportive interventions are as follow:

- Elevate the head of the bed or suggest that the resident rest in a reclining chair. Encourage frequent rests between activities. A room vaporizer or table fan sometimes helps. Use postural drainage and percussion when appropriate. This is often not appropriate in residents who are severely cachectic.

- Give oxygen for symptom relief. Maintain flow at 2 liters per minute or less for residents with a history of CO_2 retention. Delivery by nasal cannula is generally effective and more comfortable than by mask.

- If the resident is cognitively capable, teach relaxation or breathing techniques such as pursed lip or diaphragmatic breathing.

- Consider thoracentesis and sclerosis as palliative measures to treat pleural effusions. Likewise, radiation may be appropriate in select cases to reduce tumor size.

Consider the following pharmacological interventions:

- Give morphine sulfate to decrease SOB and to reduce feelings of panic. Morphine sulfate elixir can be given orally or sublingually.

- Try steroids (e.g., prednisone, inhalers).

- Try bronchodilators (by nebulizer).

- Give adivretic if the cause is CHF.

- If dyspnea is anxiety-related, give a low-dose, short-acting antianxiety drug such as lorazepam (Ativan) and observe for relief.

Ineffective Airway Clearance

Some residents experience real or potential threats to respiration that are usually related to partial or complete airway obstruction. Ineffective airway clearance may be caused by the resident's inability to maintain proper position, ineffective cough, pain, viscous secretions, fatigue, weakness, drowsiness, chronic cough, or tumor mass.

The treatment options for ineffective airway clearance include:

- Provide emotional support and reassurance as the experience can be frightening.
- Position the resident for optimal breathing by raising the head of the bed. Proper positioning should prevent slouching and cramping of the thorax and abdomen. The resident may be more comfortable in an adjustable reclining chair.
- Give an antitussive (e.g., suppressants such as codeine or morphine; expectorants such as iodinated glycerol [Organidin]).
- Where appropriate, teach the resident diaphragmatic breathing, and to deep breath and cough. Provide oxygen through a nasal cannula as needed.
- If pain is preventing effective coughing and expectoration, administer pain medications as needed. Keep the oral mucosa moist. Use anesthetic lozenges or gargle if oral discomfort is present.

End-Stage Care

This section describes the signs and symptoms commonly associated with approaching death, and discusses suggestions for care that maximize resident comfort and avoid unnecessary, intrusive interventions. Not all of these conditions will appear in every dying resident nor will they appear simultaneously. Some residents may be free of any of these conditions. It is most important to provide family and nurse assistants with explanations about these signs and symptoms, which can be alarming to the unprepared.

Skin and Mobility

As circulation slows down, the extremities become cool to touch. The underside of the body may become dark in color as blood pools. Use the following guidelines to treat these symptoms:

- Provide extra blankets, socks, and other articles to maintain warmth. Do not use an electric blanket, heating pad, or hot water bottle.
- Turn and reposition the resident at least every 2 hours to prevent skin breakdown and discomfort. Maintain position with pillows, cushioning the areas of bony prominence.
- Provide daily passive range of motion unless the resident has bone pain or fractures.

Cognitive and Sensory Function

As metabolism changes, the resident will spend increasing amounts of time sleeping and may, at times, become difficult to arouse. With changing metabolism and decreased oxygen circulation to the brain, the resident may become increasingly restless (e.g., pulling at bed linens) and have visual hallucinations. The resident may become increasingly confused about time, place, and the identities of familiar people. Clarity of vision and hearing also decrease slightly. To address these concerns:

- Educate the family and staff about expected changes in levels of alertness and orientation as death approaches. Encourage them to communicate with the resident even if the resident does not respond; hearing often remains intact. Instruct the family and staff to touch and hold the resident if possible.
- Plan communications for times when the resident seems more alert. Talk calmly and assuredly so as not to frighten or further confuse. Reorient the resident by frequent reminders of the time of day, who you are, and what you are doing.
- Keep a soft light on in the resident's room.

Respiratory Function

During sleep, the resident will experience changes in breathing patterns and periodic apnea for up to 30 seconds or more (Cheyne-Stokes respiration). This symptom is indicative of decreased circulation and buildup of body waste products. Oral secretions are likely to become more profuse and to accumulate in the back of the throat, producing a gurgling sound (death rattle). Death rattle usually results from a decrease in fluid intake and the inability to cough up normal saliva production. To treat these symptoms:

- Elevate the head of the bed to 20 to 30 degrees.
- Consider giving two to four transdermal scopolamine patches every 48 hours to reduce secretions. This may cause more confusion but the benefits of comfort usually outweigh this effect unless the resident becomes highly agitated. Use tonsil suction only as a last resort since it is quite invasive.
- Educate the family and staff that these respiratory changes are common and not always troublesome to the resident. The staff will need to educate the family about the causes of respiratory changes.

Elimination

Urinary or fecal incontinence may occur or worsen as death becomes imminent. In addition, the frequency and amount of output is normally diminished at this stage. To assist in elimination:

- Consider an indwelling catheter for incontinent residents for whom bed and clothing changes are painful or disruptive, for residents who have skin irritations or stage III or IV pressure ulcers, or for residents with urinary retention. Expect urine output to decrease as fluid intake decreases. However, periodically check to make sure the catheter tubing is not blocked by sediment. Use syringe irrigation with normal saline.
- For men, consider applying a condom catheter if no urinary retention is present.

PSYCHOSOCIAL CARE OF THE TERMINALLY ILL

Interdisciplinary staff should anticipate, assess, and plan for the unique psychosocial needs of terminally ill residents, as well as the family and significant others who may be involved in the resident's care and support. In addition, staff may need to coordinate services with social workers and hospice volunteers from other agencies (e.g., hospital discharge planners, community hospice staff). For residents cared for under hospice-specific benefit programs (*see* the guidelines in the section on community hospice services in the nursing home), make efforts to coordinate services carefully in order to avoid service overlap.

The diagnosis of a terminal condition has implications for both the resident and the family. Individualized care plans will be more effective if both perspectives are taken into account. It is also possible that a resident and family have longstanding psychosocial problems not related to the resident's terminal condition, or that the resident and family have a more pathological reaction to the circumstances surrounding the terminal diagnosis. In these cases, clinical staff may benefit from consultation with a mental health professional to develop an effective and responsive care plan.

General Principles of Care

The general principles of psychosocial care of the terminally ill are as follow:

- Establish trusting relationships with the resident and family so that they feel comfortable expressing their feelings, preferences, needs, and wishes. Anticipate that they will have feelings of loss, anger, and concern, and encourage them to verbalize them.
- Provide accurate information to the resident and/or family regarding:
  o Typical emotional responses in this type of situation
  o Reality testing of their expectations
  o Additional services that may be available and how to gain access to them
- Encourage communication among and between:

o Staff caregivers and the resident and family
o Resident and family
o Family members
o Other involved supports (e.g., religious affiliation) if applicable
• Educate members of the interdisciplinary team (including nurse assistants) about family functioning and current coping mechanisms.

Anxiety

For the cognitively intact resident, the diagnosis of terminal disease raises a number of issues for both the resident and family. Anxiety may be manifested in many ways: physical tension, hyperactivity, worrying, fears, difficulty in concentrating, insomnia, somatic symptoms such as shortness of breath or nausea), impatience, inability to relax, and irritability.

Mentally compromised residents often experience anxiety but are less likely to verbalize their distress and fears. Anxieties are more likely to be manifested in reaction to physical discomfort, rather than to the knowledge and fears of the terminal condition. Therefore, the staff should focus assessment on the physiological cues suggestive of anxiety:

• Assess and treat potential underlying physical causes of anxiety (e.g., pain, shortness of breath).
• Facilitate relaxation through physical exercise, relaxation techniques, visualization, meditation, and leisure and social activities as appropriate considering the resident's level of cognitive function.
• Problem-solve with the resident or family. Explore options for further relief, including counseling and antianxiety medication.
• Additionally, for the cognitively impaired resident, provide ongoing reassurance and as much structure as possible, to increase the resident's sense of safety and control.

Grief and Bereavement

Grief and bereavement include the resident's or family's sadness over the resident's impending death (anticipatory grief), as well as the adjustment to the death itself. The actual period of grieving varies considerably for each individual, but it is not uncommon for the postdeath bereavement period to last several years.

Persons experiencing grief may have both physical and emotional responses. Physical responses may include sleep disturbances, eating disturbances, smoking or substance abuse, changes in appearance, and a host of psychosomatic disorders. Emotional responses may include the need to tell the story of the terminal illness, expressions of loss and sadness, anger, guilt, denial, confusion, decreased coping skills, and possible suicidal ideation. Responses may be heightened by the stresses inherent in changing roles and responsibilities and financial pressures. Also note that among residents with significant cognitive impairment, grief responses are more likely to be in response to physiological decline, rather than cognitive understanding of losses.

The majority of nursing home staff are more likely to be involved with residents and families dealing with anticipatory grief, as most nursing homes do not provide formal postdeath bereavement services. However, staff involved with those going through anticipatory grief may be able to identify those family members who may be at greater risk for difficulties following the resident's death. In these cases, make the appropriate referrals at or near the time of the resident's death. Contact from the nursing home's social service department after the resident's death can also help to encourage referral follow-up.

Sadness and depression are common responses to losses and grief, and are a normal response to the diagnosis of terminal disease and all its implications. Because depression is a normal and expected response to terminal illness, caregivers need to understand that it is neither possible nor appropriate to relieve all the symptoms. Depression is part of the normal grieving process; therefore, it is an important role of caregivers to offer opportunities for the resident and family members to vent their grief.

An essential part of bereavement assessment is ascertaining whether the problems identified are representative of a normal grief response or are more pathological in nature. The scope of grief responses varies considerably from individual to individual, and the line between a normal grieving response and a more pathological one is generally only a matter of degree. If the problems are more pathological, then referrals for other counseling, medical and supportive services may need to be made. (*See* Chapter 13, Depression, for more information.) Some of the indicators for a more pathological response, or, at a minimum, a response that may need outside intervention, might include one or more of the following criteria:

- Repeated suicidal ideation
- Inability to carry out the most basic of activities of daily living and self-maintenance
- Prolonged self-imposed isolation
- Increase in alcohol or other substance abuse
- Prolonged sleep or eating disturbance
- Profound depression

Care Planning

Follow these guidelines to help cope with grief and bereavement:

- Listen. Provide opportunities for the resident to do a life review without judgment. Provide opportunities for the resident to identify sources of satisfaction and regrets about his or her life. Provide opportunities to express feelings of loss.
- Facilitate resident and family articulation of their feelings about impending death and loss. Encourage them to discuss past experiences with death and loss that

may impact on the nature of their reaction to the current loss.
- Educate the family about the grieving process and normal grief responses. Validate each person's experience of grief. Caution them on the use of sedatives and tranquilizers that may prevent and delay emotional expressions of loss.
- Encourage and facilitate family members' support of one another. Encourage participation in social activities in areas of interest to the bereaved; encourage reinvolvement in old and new networks and social systems. Refer for additional support and intervention services as needed and as appropriate.
- Make the appropriate referral if additional professional assistance is needed (e.g., psychiatric or social support and intervention).

SPIRITUAL CARE OF THE TERMINALLY ILL

Spiritual assessment, care planning, and intervention are among the most varied and least developed areas of terminal care in the nursing home setting. While some nursing homes may have chaplaincy programs, the vast majority do not use the services of community clergy to meet residents' spiritual needs. For many residents and their families, the diagnosis of terminal disease and the process of coming to terms with its realities commonly raise spiritual concerns, even if the resident or family has not been particularly active in organized religion.

While referrals to local clergy may be appropriate, it is also possible that nursing staff, social workers, and other staff who are good listeners and sounding boards may offer residents and their families important opportunities to explore their more spiritually oriented concerns. It is not necessary to have a divinity degree to do this effectively. It is also important that staff identifying spiritual concerns convey them to the interdisciplinary team and chaplain. Such concerns may well influence their receptivity to and compliance with the nonspiritual aspects of care. From the perspective of caregiving staff and administration, the death of a resident may also raise both spiritual and grieving concerns for other residents, particularly those close to the dying resident.

Religious or spiritual concerns are those that may arise out of a given philosophy or set of beliefs and related practices that govern a person's understanding of the meaning of life and death, and the person's relationship to the larger world in which he or she exists. This set of beliefs and related practices may or may not recognize higher powers or authority. The resident's beliefs are also likely to have defined and influenced the manner in which he or she has lived or how the resident currently evaluates the manner in which he or she has lived. Beliefs and practices may not only affect day-to-day existence, but may also affect the resident's decision-making, particularly as it relates to treatment options.

Spiritual concerns may or may not be an issue for a given nursing home resident. The challenge for caregivers is to identify the level of importance a given belief system may hold for an individual, family, or significant other, and to assist them in dealing with religious or spiritual concerns (either directly or through referral), and to understand how belief systems may affect their understanding of and receptivity to the disease process, care planning, and various treatment options.

Common Spiritual Concerns of the Terminally Ill

It is impossible to define the full range of spiritual issues that may arise as concerns for the terminally ill person and the family, but there are some common themes that have been identified:

* **Adjusting to feelings of alienation** from the religious or spiritual community.
* **Difficulties finding meaning in suffering**

or approaching death. For some residents in the nursing home, the dying process can be prolonged. Death may be preceded by an extended period of increasing debilitation, discomfort, and diminished quality of life. A common question that may be raised by the resident during this period is, "Why do I go on living?" Anger at God, caregivers, and life in general is not uncommon.

* **Adjusting to the need for reconciliation with God, others, and self.** It is common for the terminally ill to conduct a life review process in which relationships, accomplishments, and regrets are identified and evaluated. This process can occur over a fairly extended period of time and residents are likely to discuss these types of concerns with any staff member, including housekeeping and support personnel, with whom they feel comfortable. Unfinished business is likely to be identified.
* **Lack of or diminished religious or spiritual ritual or symbols.**
* **Holding beliefs opposed by family, peers, and health care professionals.**
* **Concerns related to continuing to live or wanting to die.**

Spiritual Assessment

Follow these guidelines to obtain a spiritual assessment:

* **Does the resident practice a specific religion or spiritual belief system?** What is the resident's current level of involvement? Even if there is not a formal affiliation with a given spiritual or religious community, it is essential that staff try to identify habits, customs, values, or beliefs the resident holds or practices, and to understand how these beliefs and practices may affect the resident's attitudes about life, health, and illness, pain, dying, and death.
* **What is the religious or spiritual orientation of the resident's family or signifi-**

cant other? Family religion or other spiritual orientation and involvement may be important, particularly if their beliefs and practices differ significantly from those of the resident. If the family's persuasion differs from that of the resident, it is important to ascertain how and if these differences are reflected in such areas as reaction to the terminal diagnosis, receptivity to prescribed care interventions, or disagreements between the resident and family in key decision-making.

- **Does the resident have contact with a particular clergyperson or spiritual counselor?** If not, would the resident wish to do so, and if so does the resident have a particular person in mind or want assistance in contacting someone?
- **Are there specific spiritual rituals or practices** in which the resident would like to participate but feels limited due to his or her condition?
- **Are there particular spiritual issues** that the resident wishes to discuss or resolve? (*See* the sample problem list in the sections to follow.)
- **What are the resident's and family members' expected religious, spiritual, or cultural practices or restrictions related to dying and death** (including discussion of death or actions to be taken or avoided at the time of death)?
- **What are the resident's or family's desires related to funeral planning?**

Care Planning

The following care planning guideline assumes the resident's desire and consent to reestablish religious or spiritual ties:

- **To facilitate resident adjustment to feelings of alienation from the religious or spiritual community,** contact former clergy or spiritual advisor to request renewed involvement. If there are no prior contacts in the community, seek a new contact of the appropriate religious persuasion. Maintain

periodic contacts with the spiritual advisor or clergy as part of the approach to care. Make arrangements with a family member, clergy member, or volunteer to tape religious services or programs if desired. Request that church and synagogue bulletins and newsletters be sent to the resident. Arrange for contacts by representatives of the resident's church lay ministry, community outreach, and friendly visitor programs.

- **To assist the resident to find meaning in suffering or approaching death,** encourage the resident and family to verbalize questions. Encourage the staff (including volunteers) to listen without offering judgment or answers. Explore the resident's issue of anger with God (or other supreme being). Explore the resident's and family's views on the meaning of hope and life after death. Use written resources if appropriate (e.g., read *When Bad Things Happen to Good People* by Harold S. Kushner [New York, 1981, Avon Books]). Talk with the resident about any unfinished business or unmet goals that may still be of concern. If it is possible to aid the resident in completing such a goal or task, facilitate this. If not, aid the resident in exploring feelings of regret in not being able to do so. The resident who hangs on in a lingering death may need permission to go. Say, for example, "It's OK that you haven't done this; you don't need to worry about it any more."
- **To help the resident adjust to the need for reconciliation with God, self, and/or others,** assist him or her in defining life goals and measuring feelings of success or failure in meeting those goals. Encourage the resident's search for meaning in his or her life (e.g., roles, accomplishments, relationship to others). Discuss feelings of guilt and resentment for unfulfilled or unmet goals. Assist the resident in accomplishing any remaining goals and tasks that are realistic within

istic within the confines of the illness, increasing disability, and family or peer constellation.

- **To assist a resident who lacks religious or spiritual ritual or symbols,** encourage the search for symbols that express a life story. For example, go through a family photo album, the family Bible, a personal recipe book, a diary, or other text; or, alternatively, aid the resident in creating such a legacy. Encourage participation in familiar rituals that give comfort or life meaning. Encourage the staff and volunteers to pray with the resident if appropriate and if the staff or volunteer is comfortable with this. Assist the resident and family to prepare for funeral rituals either directly or through referral. Enlist the aid of clergy, spiritual advisors, or lay representatives to assist in rituals as desired by the resident (e.g., taking communion, last rites, and other rituals).

- **If the resident's beliefs are opposed by family, peers, and/or health care professionals,** assist the staff to support the resident's beliefs, even if the beliefs conflict with personal values (and within the limits of standard medical practice). Educate the resident to the consequences of holding to the beliefs (e.g., refusal of analgesia or blood transfusions) and implications for effectiveness of care intervention. Encourage the resident to seek information and discuss the perceived belief system restrictions with others in the resident's religious group. Included in the discussion should be staff clarifications of the implications of decisions for the promotion or nonpromotion of resident comfort. The resident's perceptions about restrictions, or alternatively, the interpretations of the restrictions may not be accurate. Clarifications may help to avoid denying the resident access to such comfort measures as effective pain medication. Assist the resident, peers, and family members to share

feelings about differences in beliefs and concerns about the implications of those beliefs for each other. Help differing members acknowledge their mutual caring, even if their beliefs differ. Often differences are motivated by caring, even though they may not be perceived as such.

The authors wish to thank Rev. Jack M. Maxwell, PhD, for his review and comment of this section.

ADMINISTRATIVE ISSUES: DEALING WITH DYING AND DEATH IN THE NURSING HOME SETTING

Nursing home administrators and clinical supervisory staff can deal most effectively with death and dying in the facility by attempting to understand the issues from not only the perspectives of terminally ill residents and their families but also those of other residents and caregiving staff.

Other Residents

Many nursing home residents develop friendships and strong ties with other residents with whom they have regular contact. The terminal illness and subsequent death of a fellow resident not only raise fears of one's own mortality but may also result in strong feelings of grief and bereavement. Suggestions for helping other residents cope with the dying and death of fellow residents include:

- Individual contacts by staff with affected residents (friends, roommates of the dying/deceased) to offer them opportunities to discuss their feelings about the death and its implications for themselves.

- Facility recognition of the death. For example, the deceased may be acknowledged at facility religious services, at a residents' meeting, or within a facility newsletter. Family, staff, and other residents often benefit from participating in memorial services by relating personal anecdotes of their relationship with the deceased resident. Failure to acknowledge deaths diminishes the importance of the death and its impact on those left behind.

Staff Caregivers

Staff personal attitudes about death and dying can affect their desire to be involved in the care of the terminally ill, to be effective listeners, and to be appropriately sensitive to the wide variety of physical, emotional, and spiritual issues relevant to care of the terminally ill. Staff with many fears about their own mortality or those with previously negative and unresolved experiences with death and dying (either personal or professional) may be highly ineffective as caregivers. In addition, the attitude that "there's nothing more we can do," which is a far too pervasive attitude among caregivers today, may have a highly detrimental effect on staff attention to the details of care and the kind of reassurances critically important to a terminally ill resident's comfort.

The cognitively impaired terminally ill resident may also be in need of even greater attention, reassurance, and structuring. Staff who have cared for a given resident over an extended period of time may also experience major grief at the resident's death. Suggestions for administrative and supervisory personnel to improve the effectiveness of caregiving staff in care of the terminally ill include:

- Careful monitoring of staff involved in caring for terminal residents to identify caregivers who seem to have particular difficulties in dealing with death and dying, or who seem to be avoiding their terminal residents.
- Explore with staff their personal past experiences with death and dying and identify any experiences that may be affecting their attitudes negatively. Help them to resolve these issues or, at a minimum, separate their past experiences from their current responsibilities.

- Conduct group discussions with staff, including nurse assistants to identify culturally diverse perspectives of dying and death. Every culture has unique perceptions, beliefs, and values (e.g., silence about dying) that caregivers bring to the bedside. Unless they are acknowledged and addressed openly, such mores can greatly affect the care provided to an individual who holds beliefs different from those of caregivers.
- Provide specific training on such things as palliative assessment and care techniques, with a focus on how palliative care techniques and approaches may (and should) differ from approaches for a similar problem in a nonterminal resident. Perform this type of training at all levels, not just for professional staff. The caregivers who have the most contact with residents (i.e., nursing assistants) may benefit the most. Staff may also need assistance in better identifying discomfort, anxiety, depression, and distress in cognitively impaired residents.
- Provide opportunities for staff members closely involved with deceased residents to express their grief. Attending the resident's funeral may be appropriate.

COMMUNITY HOSPICE SERVICES IN THE NURSING HOME

The nursing home industry is a late arrival to the field of hospice care, but its involvement has increased dramatically in the last 10 years. Under the provisions of the Medicare hospice benefit (and, in states where it exists, the Medicaid hospice benefit), a nursing home may function as a care provider in the following four ways:

- As a direct provider of the full range of care, including home care
- As a provider of institutional respite care or short-term acute inpatient care, under contract to a Medicare-certified hospice
- As an institutional alternative to home care
- As a direct provider of lower-level, residen-

collaboration with a Medicare-certified hospice

This section describes terminal care in the nursing home setting under hospice-specific regulations and third-party benefit programs.

Medicare and Medicaid Hospice Benefits

The Medicare and Medicaid hospice benefits are of an array of service options available to eligible recipients. Residents who are terminally ill, with a prognosis of 6 months or less, may elect the hospice benefit with the understanding that they waive all rights to other Medicare benefits except those applying to conditions unrelated to the terminal illness and the services of their attending physician.

The hospice benefit includes coverage for nursing care, medical social services, physician services, counseling services, short-term inpatient care, and respite care; medical appliances and supplies (including drugs and biologicals for palliation and management of symptoms); home health aide and homemaker services; and physical, occupational, and speech therapies. Covered services must be provided by a Medicare-certified hospice that meets the conditions of participation and, where applicable, is state licensed. The type and scope of services to be provided to the resident are determined by the care plan as developed by the interdisciplinary hospice team.

To be covered under the Medicare benefit, hospice services must be "reasonable and necessary for the palliation and management of the terminal illness as well as related conditions." Benefits are allocated in a series of benefit periods. Under current law, the last benefit period can be extended indefinitely, provided that the resident continues to meet all other defined eligibility criteria, including the 6-month prognosis.

The hospice benefit is paid by Medicare on a per-diem basis at one of four levels of care (determined by the hospice team): routine home care, continuous home care, institutional respite care, or general inpatient care. Payment for care provided by a nursing home may be made directly if the nursing home is a comprehensive, certified provider. More often, however, the nursing home functions as a subcontractor under agreement with a Medicare-certified hospice provider.

Some or all of the Medicare hospice regulations may apply to nursing homes, depending on whether the nursing home is a direct provider of care or is delivering some portion of care through contract or collaboration with a Medicare-certified hospice provider. Medicaid regulations, which have Medicare hospice regulations as a starting point, may impose additional requirements under state law.

Structure of Hospice Care in the Nursing Home Setting

Under provisions of the Medicare/Medicaid hospice benefits, there are four ways in which a nursing home may function as a hospice care provider:

- **The nursing home as the direct provider of hospice care.** There are very few nursing homes nationwide that are direct providers of hospice care as per Medicare definitions, since in order to qualify under Medicare a nursing home must also be a provider of home care. If a nursing home wishes to explore the possibility of providing hospice care directly, the National Hospice Organization can provide detailed documentation and technical assistance, including designs for feasibility studies, advice on structuring services and preparing for the Medicare hospice survey, and listings of nursing home-based programs that are currently operational.

- **The nursing home as provider of inpatient care under contract to a Medicare-**

certified provider. Typically, there are two types of contracts. The first is for institutional respite care, i.e., a short-term stay in the nursing home, which is negotiated by the hospice team to provide respite to the terminally ill resident's primary, home-based caregivers. While many nursing homes have such contracts in place, use by hospices is low because of the difficulties inherent in negotiating short-term stays, resident resistance to institutional admission, and the fact that it is usually easier and less disruptive to the resident to provide respite care in the home setting. Since the allowable Medicare rates for respite care are generally low, nursing homes also tend to be disinterested. The second type of contract is for short-term, acute care. However, the great majority of hospices make these arrangements with hospitals, not nursing homes, because nursing homes tend to lack sufficient medical and diagnostic coverage and capabilities to meet resident assessment and care needs. Most of the inpatient stays under these contracts involve diagnostic workup for pain management or other symptom control problems. To obtain sample contract formats contact the National Hospice Organization (*see* the References for more information).

• The nursing home as an institutional alternative to home care. This is the most common form of nursing home involvement in hospice care. The nursing home acts in lieu of the resident's home, at whatever nursing home care level is deemed appropriate by the Medicare-certified hospice team working in coordination with the nursing home staff. The source of per diem payment to the nursing home may be private pay and/or any type of third-party coverage except Medicare. This option has become increasingly popular, since it allows nursing home residents to access additional expertise and services that are available

through the Medicare hospice benefit. Specifically, these include hospice or nursing care, including continuous care for periods of crisis and additional help at the time of resident need; extended psychosocial supports (e.g., social workers and volunteers) for both resident and family; 24-hour access to hospice expertise in care planning and assessment, particularly in areas of pain management and symptom control for end-stage disease; avoidance of unnecessary hospitalizations; and additional supports, education, and collaborative opportunities for nursing home staff. Where the contractual arrangement calls for collaboration between the Medicare-certified hospice team and nursing home staff, certain administrative and interpersonal issues must be addressed:

o Nursing home staff and hospice staff must work together to establish the criteria by which a resident needing hospice care will be identified.

o Nursing home staff (all shifts) must be educated to the specifics of the Medicare hospice benefit, including care plan authorizations, procedures, and documentation.

o Nursing home staff and hospice staff must work together on policies and procedures governing all the particulars of their collaboration, including communication, care plan changes, authorization procedures, and interdisciplinary team meetings. Where possible, adapt the existing policies and procedures of the nursing home. Experience has shown that when such issues are addressed forthrightly, and those involved begin to recognize and value the others' capabilities and contribution to resident and family care, the problems inherent in any insider-outsider collaboration tend to disappear.

o Particularly during the initial stages of the contractual arrangement, nursing home staff and hospice staff—especially the nursing home charge nurse and hospice director of nursing—must be alert to operational problems and intervene promptly to resolve conflicts. Both nursing home and hospice staff must develop the appropriate mechanisms to evaluate the effectiveness of the collaboration, and provide emotional support to staff, as needed, upon the resident's death.

• The nursing home as a provider of lower-level, residential-type care. The alternative residence option, which may or may not involve collaboration with a Medicare-certified hospice, is the fastest growing segment of the hospice industry. It differs from hospice inpatient care (as defined by Medicare and state regulations) in that it is essentially a nonmedical model, providing an alternative home setting and surrogates for the primary, home-based caregiver. It addresses the needs of a large number of terminally ill persons who:

  o Lack a primary caregiver in their home
  o Have a primary caregiver who is limited in caregiving capabilities (e.g., a frail, elderly spouse)
  o Are proceeding through the end stages of life in more expensive inpatient settings (i.e., acute care hospitals) for lack of a viable home-based alternative. In this model, the primary caregiver is a paid nursing home staff member having the approximate caregiving capabilities of a family member at home. Care is supplemented by the professional expertise of a Medicare-certified or licensed hospice or home-care team, or by an interdisciplinary team established by the nursing home for that purpose.

Regulations governing the alternative residence option are just beginning to appear in various states (e.g., Vermont and New Hampshire). Such regulations governing New Hampshire were developed under its Supported Care

guidelines. In addition, there are several demonstration projects underway or being planned through third-party payers, so the possibility exists that a more secure revenue stream will be forthcoming. In the interim, payment for this type of care may be available through channels such as personal care assistance, foster care, sheltered care, supported care, private pay, partial payment through Medicare hospice benefits where the program is part of the hospice's service offerings, and special grant programs (e.g., AIDS funding programs). Nursing homes are logical strategic partners with area home care and hospice teams in the development of alternative residence units.

CASE EXAMPLES

The following case examples describe two terminal care scenarios.

CASE EXAMPLE 1: THE NURSING HOME AS AN ALTERNATIVE TO HOME IN HOSPICE CARE (RESIDENT WITH NONCANCER DIAGNOSIS)

Mrs. C., a 78-year-old woman, was admitted to the nursing home from a local hospital. She had a longstanding history of CHF and chronic obstructive pulmonary disease. In the preceding 2 years, Mrs. C. had been hospitalized many times and had been responding increasingly poorly to therapeutic interventions. During the hospital stay just prior to her nursing home admission, Mrs. C. decided she wanted no further aggressive medical intervention for her life-threatening conditions, including no further hospitalizations, saying she wished to "die in a natural way." Her 85-year-old husband agreed with her decisions, but indicated he was unable to provide sufficient care to maintain her at home.

The option of having nursing home care combined with community hospice services was discussed with Mrs. C. in the hospital, first by her physician and later by a hospice nurse. She understood and agreed to the option, and was discharged to the nursing home, with coordinated care to be provided under the local hospice program.

Upon admission to the nursing home, Mrs. C.'s cardiac and respiratory status were fairly stable. On a regimen of diuretics, oxygen at 2 l/minute, and bronchodilators, Mrs. C. was able to participate in self-care activities, albeit with extensive assistance. She was also able to ambulate a few steps within her room with physical assistance from one person. However, she spent most of her days resting in a recliner at her bedside listening to classical tapes and visiting with relatives.

Within 3 weeks of admission, Mrs. C's condition deteriorated. Her respiratory rate increased to 35 to 40 breaths per minute. Current treatments provided little relief. She spent increasing amounts of time in bed and became extremely fatigued in transfers of any kind. She became anxious and restless with increasing shortness of breath.

The natural inclination of nursing home staff was to encourage Mrs. C. to continue getting out of bed, fearing the adverse effects of decreased function if she did not. A joint meeting of the hospice team, nursing home staff, and Mr. C. was convened to discuss her condition and plans for care. At first, because they were used to transferring residents in Mrs. C.'s condition to an acute care hospital, the nursing home staff expressed concern about providing only palliative care. However, when they understood the nature of Mrs. C's prognosis and accepted that Mrs. C. had been cognitively intact when she made her health care decisions to receive comfort measures only, the staff shifted their orientation to a more palliative mode of care.

The nursing home charge nurse and hospice nurse spoke with Mrs. C.'s physician to discuss her deteriorating condition and associated comfort needs. Morphine elixir, 2 mg sublingually every 3 hours as needed, was prescribed for respiratory rates of 25 to 35

breaths per minute, and 4 mg as needed for rates above 35. The morphine helped relieve Mrs. C.'s respiratory symptoms and improved her feeling of well-being. For 3 days after starting morphine, Mrs. C. was sedate and breathing easier, but was rousable for meals and some interaction. After her system became adjusted to the drug, she became more alert, though she slept more than she did previously.

After a temporary rally due to improved comfort related to morphine, Mrs. C.'s cardiac output deteriorated, leading to increased cyanosis, leg edema, and feelings of chest pressure. She talked openly of "wanting to let go." She slept more and remained in bed. The physician increased her morphine dose to 4 mg every 3 hours for respiration rates up to 30 breaths per minute, 6 mg every 3 hours for respiration rates up to 35 per minute, and 8 mg every 3 hours for respiration rates above 35 per minute. Because she was constantly symptomatic, morphine was ordered to be given around the clock instead of as needed. Additional attention was given to maintain her skin integrity.

The hospice social worker met with Mrs. C. both alone and with her husband. Mrs. C. was able to tell her husband that she had "no unfinished business." A hospice home health aide spent 2 hours with her every evening to assist with personal care, help her sip drinks as tolerated, and make her comfortable for the night. Mrs. C. had refused a hospice volunteer, saying that she was deriving sufficient support and comfort from her family and the hospice and nursing home staffs.

Despite minor adjustments in Mrs. C.'s cardiac medications, her cardiac condition continued to deteriorate. She slept more and began refusing to eat. The facility nurses educated the nursing assistants about not forcing Mrs. C. to eat, explaining that the tendency to decrease food intake was part of the natural process of dying. The hospice nurse instructed all caregivers to check for a gag reflex prior to giving Mrs. C. oral fluids.

Mrs. C. slipped into unconsciousness. She developed increased pulmonary congestion and noisy breathing. The physician prescribed three scopolamine patches transdermally every 3 days to decrease respiratory secretions. This medication was effective within 2 hours. As her respiratory rate fluctuated, she moaned periodically. Because Mrs. C. was unable to swallow, morphine was given subcutaneously and all other medications were discontinued. Fluids were withheld and attention to mouth care was provided. She seemed comfortable and died peacefully. Bereavement follow-up contacts were made with Mr. C. by members of the hospice team.

CASE EXAMPLE 2: THE NURSING HOME AS AN ALTERNATIVE TO HOME IN HOSPICE CARE (RESIDENT WITH A DIAGNOSIS OF CANCER)

Mrs. D., a 74-year-old widow, was diagnosed with rectal cancer with bone and pelvic metastases. She had been a resident of the nursing home for 5 months before receiving community hospice services. She was referred for hospice care by the nursing home at the request of her family. The referral enabled Mrs. D. to remain in the nursing home, for which she paid privately while accessing benefits under the hospice Medicare benefit program, which included additional hands-on and supportive care and assistance in pain management and other symptom control.

At the time of Mrs. D.'s admission to the hospice program, presenting problems included lower back pain radiating down both legs, which had been controlled intermittently, and a nonhealing stage II sacral pressure ulcer. Pain was exacerbated by movement, and the family was concerned that pain management was becoming less effective. Her regimen for pain at the time of hospice admission was acetaminophen (Tylenol), 650 mg orally every 4 hours as needed, hydromorphone (Dilaudid), 4 mg orally every 4 hours as needed, and sustained-release morphine sulfate (MS Contin), 45 mg orally at 8 AM daily and 30 mg orally at 8 PM daily.

Initial assessment by the hospice team confirmed that Mrs. D.'s comfort was inconsistent, with a major worsening of symptoms in the evening. To improve her level of comfort, an indwelling catheter was inserted to eliminate unnecessary, painful transfers. Efforts to increase and regularize the Dilaudid dose not only failed to provide consistent relief, but had the negative side effect of excessive drowsiness. To provide respite from pain, all analgesics were discontinued and replaced by fentanyl (Duragesic) transdermal patches, 50 g every 72 hours. This regimen provided a temporary respite from pain, but 3 days later Mrs. D. again experienced breakthroughs of pain. Therefore, the dosage was increased to 75 g every 72 hours; 3 days later it was increased to 100 g every 72 hours. Comfort was achieved, necessitating no further changes to the pain regimen.

Socially, Mrs. D.'s family had been experiencing interpersonal problems for many years. There were five adult children. Two of her daughters remained in regular contact, participating in some of their mother's personal care. Her sons were estranged from each other and from their mother, which was distressing to Mrs. D. She chose not to try and re-establish links with her sons, although she did manage to express her sadness about the situation. Although it was impossible for her to reverse the family's established pattern of relationships, Mrs. D. was at least able to achieve partial resolution by expressing her grief over the way things had been.

Prior to her mother's admission to the hospice program, one daughter had had numerous conflicts with the nursing home staff. Communications were strained and the daughter was highly critical of the care provided. At the suggestion of the hospice team, two meetings that included family, hospice, and nursing home staff were convened. One meeting was held with day staff, the other with evening staff. In the course of airing the problems that had developed over the previous 5 months, the nursing staff suggested that the family be less accusatory and more helpful in determining the difficulties being experienced by their mother. In turn, the nursing staff agreed to respond more quickly to the family's stated concerns. As a result, the family and staff became more of a team in their efforts on behalf of Mrs. D.

The nursing home staff also came to a greater understanding of the family history behind the emotions being displayed. For example, it became apparent that much of one daughter's criticism of the staff was rooted in her guilt at being unable to care for her mother at home. A hospice social worker began to make regular visits with Mrs. D. and her daughters to explore their concerns, not trying to resolve the long-standing family divisions. In addition, a hospice volunteer was assigned to assist Mrs. D and her daughters with relaxation techniques, enabling the three women to spend some less stressful time together.

Since both resident and family problems appeared to exacerbate in the evening hours, a 3-hour home health aide shift was instituted in the nursing home. The aide was able to respond to Mrs. D.'s needs quickly, as well as to reinforce and support the family's efforts. Additional volunteer time was also added in the evening.

Several days prior to death, Mrs. D. slipped into semicoma, experiencing acute confusion and severe agitation. Thioridazine (Mellaril), 25 mg orally every 6 hours, was then prescribed to reduce her distress. As she was approaching death, for her last 2 days the hospice provided a registered nurse to care for Mrs. D. around the clock to assess the nature of the agitation and the effectiveness of the interventions. This could be provided through the Medicare hospice program because Mrs. D. required skilled nursing care at least every 2 hours. Mrs. D.'s agitation was reduced successfully by the Mellaril and one-to-one care, and she died peacefully.

This case provides an example of effective teamwork between nursing home and hospice staff. The hospice team was able to provide important pain management and symptom control assistance, objectivity in facilitating nursing home staff and family to cope with myriad family problems and miscommunications, and mechanisms for the family to vent their frustrations over a long history of family problems. The ability of the hospice team to supplement nursing staffing coverage at crucial transition points was made possible by the Medicare hospice benefit.

34
Discharge Planning

Sue Nonemaker, RN, MS
Vincent Mor, PhD
Katharine Murphy, RN, MS, C
John N. Morris, PhD

The American Nurses Association defines discharge planning as "that part of the continuity of care process which is designed to prepare the patient or client for the next phase of care and to assist in making any necessary arrangements for that phase of care, whether it be self care."

This chapter focuses on the interdisciplinary processes used to identify and prepare residents for their return to the community. This coordinated process includes a needs assessment to evaluate key medical and functional factors that impact the return to the community, as we'l as subsequent continuing care needs. The assessment serves as the basis for developing a viable strategy to expedite the transition and start the postdischarge plan of care.

OVERVIEW

Advanced age is often characterized by a continuum of change in health status, functional abilities, and social support associated with complex patterns of acute and chronic illness. These changes are usually accompanied by a series of transitions in the type, amount, and location of medical, nursing, and support services.

At any given time, approximately 5% of persons over the 65 years of age reside in nursing homes. However, over a lifetime, it is estimated that 40% or more of older people will receive nursing home care, particularly after an acute hospitalization. Deteriorating health and functional status alone are not determinants of the need for nursing home care. Only one in three elders with disabilities resides in a nursing home; the remainder live in community settings with various types and levels of support. From 15% to 30% of all persons admitted to nursing homes are discharged to the community, usually following a short stay of 4 months or less. After 6 months, discharges are rare. This chapter focuses on ensuring a consistent and thorough review process during the first few months of a resident's stay.

Targeting Residents for Discharge

The focus here is on residents who are identified during their first few months of residency as being candidates for discharge—those for whom nursing homes provide transitional, rehabilitative, or supportive care—as well as residents with similar characteristics, but whom the staff have not traditionally identified as discharge candidates. Some residents will meet the potential discharge profile at admission; others will move into this status as they continue to improve during the first few months of residency.

Unfortunately, a significant number of new residents who fit a potential discharge profile are not discharged. Therefore, the goal of this chapter is to help facility staff target and plan appropriately for all residents with discharge potential. Discharge decisions are influenced by many factors, including resident or family characteristics, staff actions or values, facility characteristics, and the extent of service and housing options in the community. For example, some facilities such as hospital-based skilled nursing facilities (SNFs) specialize in providing short-term, rehabilitative services, and therefore have high turnover rates. Thirty percent of newly admitted Medicare patients go home after short stays (median of 29 days). Another 20% go home within a median of 100 days. Conversely, there are other specially targeted nursing homes in which life-care residential services are provided. These homes require a commitment for lifetime residency; the average length of stay is in years and almost all discharges will be due to death.

At the resident level, functional status weighs heavily as a determinant of discharge potential—focusing on factors such as cognition, activities of daily living (ADLs), and behavioral status. In the few studies that have looked at the role of these factors, discharge is more prevalent among residents who are independent in bed mobility, continent of urine, cognitively intact, and free of problem behaviors (e.g., no wandering or verbal abusiveness).

Sociodemographic characteristics do not appear to play a major role in discharge potential. For example, married individuals tend to enter nursing homes at a much later stage in their disease and functional progression, but their rate of discharge is only slightly lower than that of unmarried individuals.

At the same time, there is little systematic information to help make generalizations regarding the specific selection of individuals who will be discharged successfully to the community. There is not enough information about the characteristics of family or support systems that facilitate discharge from the nursing home.

Changing Role of Nursing Homes Within the US Health Care System

There are numerous reasons why the nature of the discharge planning process may have become more important in recent years. Nursing homes increasingly provide short-term care after hospitalization or illness at home. The nursing home can provide supportive care during recovery from an illness, or temporary respite support for an informal caregiver who provides continuing care in the community. The following factors contribute to this process:

- Reducing the length of hospital stays. Before implementing the Medicare Prospective Payment System for hospitals in 1983, many elderly patients left hospitals without having fully regained their presurgery or preillness status. For some, a short-term stay in a nursing home has now become an integral part of the total program of recuperative care.
- Increasing the complexity of posthospital discharge care needs that may have been resolved before hospital discharge. The case mix of many nursing facilities includes higher percentages of residents who require short-term care that cannot be provided in the community. For these residents, the goal of nursing home care is rehabilitation, restoration of health, and discharge to the community.
- Rise of hospital-based SNFs. As of 1992, 9% of nursing homes certified to participate in Medicare or Medicaid were hospital-based units. Hospital-based SNFs have evolved

increasingly to meet the needs of the high-tech hospital discharge. Such programs provide a variety of services, including intravenous antibiotics, chemotherapy, total parenteral nutrition, enteral tube feedings, and artificial ventilation through a respirator. The care needs of residents in hospital-based SNFs can be divided into two categories:

o Those who need skilled rehabilitative care after acute care procedures, such as a total hip replacement

o Those with complicated nursing or medical conditions who are medically stable but in need of skilled nursing care or monitoring

Additionally, the provision of much skilled care has shifted to community settings. The availability of these services has increased nursing homes' responsibilities to conduct discharge planning and arrange for these community-based follow-up services.

• Changes in social structures/family support systems. Social changes, such as an increased prevalence of households in which both spouses are working, or where children may reside at great distances from the parent, has resulted in an increased need for a period of formal long-term care services after hospitalization. In these cases, elders may not have someone at home to assist them, and nursing homes can provide the short-term care to help them recover their functional resources following an illness or surgical procedure.

Screening Assessment of Discharge Potential

The guidelines for discharge planning are as follows:

• Begin early. Consider the possibility for potential discharge during the preadmission phase by reviewing the resident's application, interviewing the resident and family, and speaking with current formal caregivers.

• During the preadmission phase advise the resident and family to consider not selling the home or giving up an apartment for at least 3 months after admission. Having a home to return to is extremely important.

• Assume that all first-time admissions with a home to return to have the potential to be discharged.

• Remember that a resident who is capable of making decisions has the right to choose where and how to live, unless the rights and interests of others are jeopardized. Present available options to the resident and family and assist them in the decision-making process.

• From admission, all staff who provide care to the resident should be aware of and have input into the discharge planning process. The composition of the team may vary, depending on the needs of the resident and the type and intensity of services to be provided to expedite movement of the resident to another level of care. It is important to include the nurse assistants in this information exchange process since they are probably the most reliable informants about the resident's functional performance in self-care and daily routines.

• Identify a discharge planner to assume responsibility for coordinating the discharge plan, establishing necessary links, making referrals to other disciplines and home care services as needed, and ordering necessary medical equipment. In the nursing home, continuing care planning is usually the responsibility of a registered nurse or social worker, and those individuals often have many other competing demands. Therefore, teamwork is essential. In many facilities the nurse assumes the role of discharge planner. The nurse is in direct contact with the resident and family on a daily basis, and may be best able to conduct an ongoing assessment of the resident's functional status and postdischarge care needs. The social worker then assumes the role of liaison

with the family and community services.
- Individualize the discharge plan, taking into account the resident's unique needs, strengths, values, and goals as well as those of potential family caregivers.

Discharge Planning Process

The following terms refer to aspects of the discharge planning process:
- Screening refers to the process of identifying residents who have potential for discharge from the nursing home (see the section on screening: assessment of discharge potential).
- Needs assessment is the process of evaluating the resident's present and projected medical status and care needs in conjunction with psychological, social, environmental, and financial factors that influence the ability to manage continuing care needs at home. The needs assessment provides the foundation for the development of a postdischarge plan of care (see the section on Needs Assessment).
- The postdischarge plan of care is that portion of the resident's care plan that addresses what the facility is doing to prepare the resident for discharge. It may include teaching the resident and family members how to manage self-care activities after discharge; making referrals to other care providers such as home care, day care, or a hospice; or ordering medical equipment. One aspect of these services is to make arrangements for a home evaluation. The factors to review include safety, the need for adaptive equipment, and the need to make arrangements for food or medical supplies.

Information about the resident's status and care needs, preferences for continuing care, and availability of family and community resources are then used to identify options available to the resident and develop the discharge plan (see the section on developing and implementing a postdischarge plan of care).

Take into account medical stability and the availability of follow-up when planning to discharge. Will the resident require ongoing monitoring of vital signs or weight; administration of oxygen, inhalers, or parenteral medications; periodic clinic visits; or blood tests (e.g., prothrombin times to monitor anticoagulant therapy)? These procedures must be arranged at home if discharge is to be successful.

SCREENING: ASSESSMENT OF DISCHARGE POTENTIAL

There is a need to focus on new admissions. Federal regulations require an evaluation of discharge potential each time a comprehensive assessment is completed. This means that each resident's discharge potential must be evaluated on admission to the facility, when there is significant change in status, and at least annually. Having made that assessment, an item on the Health Care Financing Administration's (HCFA's) Minimum Data Set (MDS) is provided to indicate which residents are candidates for discharge. The focus of this chapter is on new admissions, representing the only group of residents for whom homes have demonstrated an ability to expedite return to the community.

The prognosis for long-stay residents (i.e., 180 days or longer) to be discharged to the community is rather dismal. In part, this may be driven by reimbursement policy, requiring residents to spend down in order to qualify for publicly financed long-term care. After an individual's home and furnishings have been disposed of, it is usually very difficult for a nursing home to assist that individual to return to the community.

Due to interstate variation, have the discharge planning staff investigate the availability of state or local programs that provide community-based services to eligible individuals, and prepare to expedite the unusual discharge of the long-stay resident. Nevertheless, spend the time to ensure the maximum discharge of new admissions during the early months of their stay.

Preadmission Screening

Begin discharge planning in the preadmission period. At that time many elders about to enter a nursing home and some family members will be receptive to considering return to the community. They may still be discussing the need for placement versus other options. An individual may become depressed or resist entering the nursing home, or may take this opportunity to communicate with family in a way that they have avoided in the past.

By effectively engaging the person and the social supports, a foundation is built for strengthening stable family relationships and support networks. At the same time, this transition period is difficult, and many elders and their families will not be open to this type of discussion, particularly when entry to the nursing home is to be immediate. There are many possible disturbing scenarios, so be sensitive when approaching this topic. For example, in some cases the resident will want to return home, but the family will be unwilling to consider this possibility. The complications of such a pattern are many, and involve financial, legal, and ethical issues.

Start to address this issue by talking separately with the resident and his or her family members. Invite both the resident and family members to attend the interdisciplinary team meeting where one of the scheduled topics will be the potential for return to the community. However, for residents capable of making decisions on their own, staff (if not family) must respect and pay careful attention to the wishes of the resident.

During this time, the admissions staff should consider the individual's residential and services pathway immediately before entering the nursing facility. Such consideration may both

benefit residents with the potential for discharge to the community (e.g., the staff and the resident are aware of the need to hold onto the resident's apartment for a period of time), and assist the facility to anticipate and plan for future bed availability (e.g., the staff can track where new residents are coming from).

Admission from another nursing facility and return admission to the facility from an acute hospital are common pathways to admission. Other scenarios are as follows:

- A precipitating medical event (e.g., hip fracture secondary to a fall) that necessitated acute hospitalization followed by a period of rehabilitation.

The majority of admissions to acute hospitals are over 65 years of age. Under the current prospective payment system hospitals tend to discharge patients quicker and sicker in an effort to keep health costs down. On discharge many elders do not need long-term care, but neither are they functionally capable of returning home. Because it may take longer for an older person to recuperate, many elders require a period of functional rehabilitation and health teaching at this transition point. The nursing home can provide services to enable successful transition back to the community.

Additionally, during short hospital stays following a major health event, difficult choices about living arrangements must be made by elders and their families on very short notice. Both parties may be anxious and fearful about the possibility of dependency and choose nursing home placement. Nursing home care can provide residents and families with time to adjust to change and to gain perspective about the realities of care and feasible future options.

- A second pathway to admission involves a long period of deterioration in health, function, or cognition, necessitating ongoing heavy physical assistance and social support from others.

It is common for families to provide elders with an inordinate amount of care before nursing home placement. Placement is usually a last resort when caregivers are no longer able or willing to continue caregiving responsibilities. Their own deteriorating health and competing role responsibilities, as well as assumptions about the elder's future prognosis are major reasons why families suggest a transition to nursing home care. The absence of available caregivers places dependent elders at high risk for long-term institutionalization.

Discharge Targeting Model

Using the data from HCFA's MDS, the team that developed the MDS system has created a model to specify which residents to consider during this review process. This model will identify more residents for discharge than is traditional at most facilities. Some of these residents can be excluded because of disease or complicating functional syndromes that are not referenced in the model. Other residents will exclude themselves from this process: some families or the residents themselves may be adamant in their refusal to return to the community. In other cases, the situation will be less clear-cut, and whenever possible start the discharge review process.

The specific rules for the discharge potential model are shown in Table 34-1. Assign the resident into the Discharge Potential Re-

view Group when four or five of the conditions listed in the table apply. (The items and their category response descriptions come from the HCFA's MDS.)

In the experience of the MDS development team, most new admissions who were discharged at or before 6 months came from among those who had four or five of the conditions listed in Table 34-1. In an analysis of a collection of data from HCFA, discharge rates for this subgroup (which comprised two thirds of new admissions) varied as a function of how the staff judged the discharge potential of each resident. Discharges were highest for the subgroup of residents whose discharges had been seen by staff to be planned in the prior 3-month period (comprising 16% of the previous discharge group): 56% of these residents returned to the community, 14% died, and 30% were still in a nursing home or hospital 6 months after admission.

The discharge experience of those who met the criterion of having four or five of the characteristics listed in Table 34-1 was much less positive when staff felt that the resident would not return to the community in the next 3 months (comprised of 69% of the previous discharge group): only 10% of these residents returned to the community. While many residents seem to have the functional criteria that permit return to the community, staff identify only a subset of these residents under the practice patterns that are operational in many fa-

Table 34-1. Items that Identify the Discharge Potential Review Group

MDS Items	Categories that Suggest Discharge Potential
Cognitive Skills for daily decision making	Independent to moderately impaired
Making self understood	Understands or usually understands
ADL self performance in eating	Independent or supervision
Trunk control problem	None
Lifted (manually, mechanically)	No

cilities. Whether this can be reversed is open to question; using the Discharge Potential Review Group assignment model ensures that many more residents than at the current time will be considered for potential return to the community.

Consider as having discharge potential a first admission to a nursing home in which the resident has four or five of the positive characteristics listed in Table 34-1. As a group, initial stay residents are the most likely to be discharged. Factors such as caregiver availability, medical needs, and patient compliance are additional predictors of discharge planning outcomes of hospitalized patients. Consider the following factors in an expanded review of those who fall into the Potential Discharge Review Group:

• Mood problems
• Behavior problems
• Chronic health complications (e.g., chronic falls)
• Difficulty complying with complicated health routines
• The presence of intensive rehabilitation that might result in significant functional improvement
• Resident motivation for continued improvement
• Resident and family commitment to the resident's return to the community
• Staff belief that the resident can become more self-sufficient

Carefully evaluate the psychosocial factors since an individual may become depressed on admission to a nursing home or try to reconcile goals with what is perceived to be an inevitable long-term nursing home stay.

NEEDS ASSESSMENT

Comprehensive assessments to determine an individual's personal, health, and social care needs and the availability of family and community support are critical to the resident's ultimate rehabilitation and return home.

Link the needs assessment in a meaningful fashion to the postdischarge care environment. For example, a resident to be discharged to live with his daughter and her family will have very different needs than the resident returning home alone. For residents identified as having discharge potential, assess the following areas and use them in conjunction with HCFA's Resident Assessment Instrument data in developing a postdischarge plan of care:

• Resident and significant other's goals and preferences for continuing care.
• Availability of family or other informal (nonpaid) support to assist with self-care activities after discharge.
• Ability to perform Instrumental ADLs, such as meal preparation, medication administration, telephone use, housekeeping, shopping, handling finances, and transportation use.
• Discharge environment, such as living arrangements before admission and whether they are still available to the resident; and barriers that need to be modified to make the environment safer and more accessible.
• Financial resources to cover formal support services, medical equipment, home maintenance, and living expenses in the community.
• Nursing and other care requirements, such as the need for skilled nursing or other therapeutic services; or the need for unskilled, supportive services necessary to meet self-care demands.
• Resident and significant other's health educational needs to learn technical or support skills that must be mastered before discharge; how to recognize and respond to a decline in health or function.
• Need for durable medical equipment or other types of supplies.
• Community services used before nursing home admission that the resident may continue to use after discharge.

- Availability of medical supervision and follow-up.

DEVELOPING AND IMPLEMENTING A POSTDISCHARGE PLAN OF CARE

A well-developed and comprehensive discharge plan will provide needed continuing and follow-up services at the most appropriate level of care. The following needs assessment serves as the basis for developing the plan:

- On admission, encourage the family to remain involved with the resident's care.
- Guide the resident and family through the discharge planning process.
- Ensure that the facility staff and the attending physician agree with the goal of return to the community. At least ensure that all parties are aware of the wishes of the resident.
- Present the resident and family with information about the resident's specific care needs that are expected to continue after discharge. Discuss viable alternatives to meet continuing care needs.
- Implement proscribed formal occupational, physical, and speech therapy programs to help the resident regain lost functional abilities. For residents on the discharge path, use this knowledge to help motivate their success in these programs. This involves setting realistic target dates for progress to be observed, encouraging the resident to complete the scheduled program, and involving family in motivational activities if the resident appears to have plateaued at a low level of functioning.
- Follow the procedures described in Chapter 29, ADL Rehabilitation, to institute either a nursing-based functional rehabilitation or muscle-strengthening activity program. For residents who might have difficulty with key instrumental ADL activities after they are back in the community, consider starting a training program in these

areas. For example, practice dialing the phone, counting money, walking to activities off the unit with only minimal staff monitoring, making the bed, tidying up the room, and putting on appliances (e.g., glasses, hearing aide). If facilities with proper staff oversight are available, give the resident an opportunity to prepare cold and hot foods, use a stove, or go shopping.

- Use regular family conferences and educational programs to provide information, seek input from potential caregivers, and maximize their involvement in discharge planning.
- Prepare residents and families to make informed choices about how the individual's care needs will be met after discharge. By involving the resident and family in the decision-making process, goals are mutually established and will be more realistic and attainable. The degree of satisfaction with a discharge plan is related directly to the level of resident involvement. Residents who are not involved adequately may feel powerless or manipulated, which may result in feelings of anger or noncompliance.
- If the resident will live with family after discharge, suggest that the family take the resident home for a brief visit and progressively longer overnight visits. Ask the family also to give the resident an opportunity to retry certain key activities on these visits, e.g., buying food in a neighborhood market, making change, using appliances in the home. If these activities are tested, the staff must debrief the family on how well they were carried out, e.g., back to old performance levels, some improvement, still a problem.
- Sometimes it is helpful to have a caregiver or family member come in and spend a morning (or day) with the resident. The family member will better understand how the resident has progressed, and the staff can

use the time to teach needed (or new) caregiver skills. This experience can also serve as a reality check for residents or families with unrealistic expectations.

- Respond to questions, clarify options, and assist the resident or family in resolving conflicts.
- Teach the resident and caregiver skills and self-care practices to successfully manage chronic illness or compensate for functional deficits. Instruct on safety factors or needs and suggestions for environmental modifications as follows:
  - o Assess the person's readiness for learning:
    - ¬ Focus on the emotional factors that affect the ability to assimilate material as well as the individual's preexisting knowledge base
    - ¬ Determine the teaching method and level of content based on the resident and family's ability to read and comprehend, visual/hearing function, and any unique factors that relate to the cultural context of the resident and family.
  - o Assess learning needs:
    - ¬ Skills that must be mastered before discharge (e.g., walking with a walker, colostomy care, medication administration, applying a splint)
    - ¬ Information that must be assimilated for health and safety (e.g., recognizing medication side effects, diet)
  - o Provide written take-home instructions for reference. Beware of how the material is presented—are there educational or cultural biases that may preclude effective use of the materials? Instructions must be written in clear, simple language, not medical or nursing jargon.
- Order necessary equipment such as oxygen, raised toilet seat, life-line emergency response system.
- Identify community services or programs to meet resident and family needs, and make referrals for continuing care. Have all prescriptions written to cover 1-month of administration or a quantity to last until the resident's next scheduled physician visit. Make sure the resident has an appointment for a follow-up physician visit once he or she returns to the community. Impress on the family and the resident, that it is important to keep this appointment.

- Provide the resident and the caregiver with written information listing the names, numbers, and other pertinent information, of referring agencies, suppliers, follow-up appointments, and a list of medications.

There may be problems that trouble the family, or factors that prevent the family from accepting the resident's return to the community. Examples might include issues of mood, compliance with medication regimen, wandering, verbal aggressiveness, muscle weakness, or uncertainties about the prognosis and the likely rate of decline. In some instances, information supplied by the staff to family members or a referral to a knowledgeable community agency (e.g., the local chapter of the Alzheimer's Association) may be all that is required.

In all cases, bring the identified problems into the care planning process. These key problems are among the most important targets for the resident's initial care plan.

Also keep in mind the possibility that family either has unrealistic expectations or their description of resident problems may be inaccurate. Relationships between the resident and family members may not have been supportive or close. The staff must be careful not to seem judgmental or authoritarian. Misperceptions or troubled family members may be the key issue to address. Consider family group involvement, referral to outside support agencies, family education by facility staff, or the need to identify other family members (or significant others) who can be recruited to assist the staff and the resident to devise and implement a plan to return the resident to the community.

CASE EXAMPLE

Mrs. M. is a 78-year-old widow who has lived alone for the past 15 years. Her social contacts are limited to her landlord and daughter. Her residence is a second floor walk-up apartment that is accessed by an outside staircase. Mrs. M. has a friendly relationship with her landlord, who lives on the first floor and has limited financial resources and is functionally impaired. As a consequence, the building has become more and more hazardous, and Mrs. M. seldom ventures outside of her apartment.

Mrs. M.'s primary medical problems—high blood pressure, dizziness, unsteady gait, painful arthritis, and recurrent falls—have limited her willingness to leave the apartment. She spends her time watching soap operas, caring for her cat, and talking with her daughter. She has always been a positive person, putting few demands on others.

Her daughter, Amy, who is single, lives 25 miles away in her own four-room apartment. She visits her mother at least every other day, and calls several times each week. She loves her mother and has often thought that Mrs. M. needed a better living arrangement, but they have never discussed living together.

In reality, Mrs. M. is highly dependent on her daughter for both physical help and in making decisions. Mrs. M. has been isolated from others and, while intellectually capable, has made a habit of responding to the wishes of her daughter.

Mrs. M. became a candidate for nursing home residency following her most recent fall. While walking down the stairs to look for her cat, Mrs. M. became unstable and fell down the final three stairs onto a concrete landing. She braced herself with her left hand, hitting the railing with her face and knee as she fell. She broke her wrist, wrenched her knee, and has multiple bruises and cuts on her face and scalp. Her neighbor saw the fall, called for an ambulance, and Mrs. M. spent 4 days in the local hospital. During this time she became very depressed, and refused to bathe, change her clothes, or walk on the floor.

The hospital discharge staff, Mrs. M.'s doctor, and Amy decided that it would be best if Mrs. M. entered a nursing home for further rehabilitation. Amy and her mother also agreed that it would be too dangerous for Mrs. M. to return to her own apartment. At the same time, neither women wanted Mrs. M to stay in the nursing home permanently.

Mrs. M. was admitted to the nursing home. She and her daughter met with the facility social worker. Amy and Mrs. M. decided it would be best for the two women to live together.

Amy lives in a modern building with an elevator. She has enough room in her apartment and is very positive about this decision. Both Amy and Mrs. M. attended the interdisciplinary care planning meeting. The facility staff reviewed the plan of care and discussed Mrs. M.'s progress and discharge plans. The group set a goal for discharge to Amy's apartment in 2 weeks.

The social worker had already started making arrangements to have a home health aide come twice a week and help Mrs. M. take a bath.

The occupational therapist made an appointment to conduct a home evaluation of Amy's apartment in 1 week. After the home evaluation, the social worker planned to order any needed special equipment. She assured Amy and Mrs. M. that any necessary equipment and services would be set up before discharge from the nursing home.

Mrs. M. and Amy were very happy with the plans for discharge. Amy would be able to continue working and still provide a safe and secure environment for her mother. Mrs. M. was glad she had made progress and was able to go to her daughter's home.

BIBLIOGRAPHY

AIDS AND HIV

Allers CT: AIDS and the older adult, *Gerontologist* 30:405-407, 1990.

Benjamin AE and Swan JH: Nursing home care for persons with HIV illnesses, In Generations: AIDS in an aging society, 13(4):63-64, 1989

Crystal S: Persons with AIDS and older people: Common long term care concerns. In Ory MG, Riley MN, Zablotsky D, editors: *AIDS in an aging society*, New York, 1989, Springer Publishing Company.

Fillit H, Fruchtman S, Sell L, and Rosen N: AIDS in the elderly: a case and its implications, *Geriatrics* 44(7):65-68, 70, 1989.

Lusk P: Who's knocking now?, *Gerontol Nursing* 16(6):8-11, 1990.

Martin JP, et al: *AIDS home care and hospice manual*, ed 2, San Francisco, 1990, Visiting Nursing and Hospice of San Francisco.

Whipple B and Scura KW: HIV and the older adult: taking the necessary precautions, *Gerontol Nursing* 15(9):15-19, 1989.

ARTHRITIS

American Nurses Association: *Outcome standards for rheumatology nursing practice*, Kansas City, MO, 1984, American Nurses Association.

Arthritis Health Professionals Section of the Arthritis Foundation: *Self-help for patients with arthritis*, Atlanta, 1980, The Arthritis Foundation.

Bowsher D: Assessment of the chronic pain sufferer, *Surg Rounds Orthop* 70-73, 1989.

Pigg JS: Nursing care of the hospitalized patient with rheumatic disease, In Erhlich GE: *Rehabilitation management of rheumatic conditions*, Baltimore, 1980, Williams & Wilkins.

Schumacher RH, editor: *Primer on rheumatic diseases*, Atlanta, 1988, The Arthritis Foundation.

ACTIVITIES

Murray JM: *Activities, adaptation and aging*, Binghamton, NY, 1990, The Haworth Press, Inc.

Coons DH: Assessment as a basis for intervention. In Coons DH, editor: *Specialized dementia care units*, Baltimore, 1991, Johns Hopkins University Press.

Bell V: Tapping an unlimited resource: building volunteer programs for patients and their families. In Mace NL, editor: *dementia care: patient, family, and community*, Baltimore, 1990, Johns Hopkins University Press

Coons DO: Activities and staff approaches: the impacts on behaviors. In Coons DO, editor: *Specialized dementia care units*, Baltimore, 1991, Johns Hopkins University Press.

Gibbons AC: Popular music preferences of elderly people, *Music Ther* 14(4):180-189, 1977.

Green L: Humor and lighthearted activities. In Coons DO, editor: *Specialized dementia care units*, Baltimore, 1991, Johns Hopkins University Press.

Mace NL: Principles of activity therapy. In Sloane PD and Matthew LJ, editors: *Dementia units in long term care*, Baltimore, 1991, Johns Hopkins University Press.

Mace NL: Therapeutic activities. In Mace NL, editor: *Dementia care: patient, family, and community*, Baltimore, 1990, Johns Hopkins University Press.

Moore B: Growing with gardening: a twelve-month guide for therapy, recreation and education, Chapel Hill, NC, 1989, University of North Carolina Press.

Perschbacher B: Assessment: *the cornerstone of activity programs*, 1993, Venture Publishing.

Reminiscence: finding meaning in memories, Washington, DC, 1989, American Association of Retired Persons.

Weaverdyck SE: Intervention-based neuropsychological assessment. In Mace NL, editor: *Dementia care: patient, family, and community*, Baltimore, 1990, Johns Hopkins University Press.

Zgola Y: *Doing things*, Baltimore, 1987, Johns Hopkins University Press.

ADVANCE DIRECTIVES

Annas GJ: The health care proxy and the living will, *N Engl J Med* 324(17):1210-1213, 1991.

Doukas DJ and McCullough LB: Assessing the values history of the elderly patient regarding critical care and chronic care. In Gallo JJ, Reichel W, and Anderson L, editors: *Handbook of geriatric assessment*, Rockville, MD, 1988, Aspen Systems.

Emanuel L: The health care directive: learning how to draft advance care documents, *J Am Geriatr Soc* 39(12):1221-1228, 1991.

Gamble ER, McDonald PJ, and Lichstein PR: Knowledge, attitudes, and behavior of elderly persons regarding living wills, *Arch Intern Med* 151(2):277-280, 1991.

Lo B, McLeod GA, and Saika G: Patient attitudes to discussing life-sustaining treatment, *Arch Intern Med* 146(8):1613-1615, 1986.

McCloskey E: The patient self-determination act, *Kennedy Inst of Ethics J* 1:163-169, 1991.

Practicing the PSDA, Special Supplement, *Hastings Cent Report*, 21(5):S1-S16, 1991.

Wolf SM et al: Sources of concern about the patient self-determination act, *N Engl J Med* 325:1666-1671, 1991.

AGING AND COMMUNICATION

American Speech-Language and Hearing Association: *Communication problems and behaviors of the older american*, Rockville, MD, 1979, American Speech-Language and Hearing Association (includes booklet and VHS tape).

American Speech-Language and Hearing Association: *Communications disorders and aging*, Rockville, MD, 1985, American Speech-Language and Hearing Association (includes leader's guide and participant's manual).

Beasley D, Davis GA: *Aging: communication processes and disorders*, New York, 1981, Grune and Stratton.

Holland A: *Language disorders in adults: recent advances*, San Diego, 1984, College Hill Press.

Mueller H and Geoffrey V: *Communication disorders in aging: assessment and management*, Washington, DC, 1987, Gallaudet University Press.

Schow R, Christenson J, and Nerbonne M: *Communication disorders of the aged: a guide for health professionals*, Baltimore, 1978, University Park Press.

Shadden B: *Communication behavior and aging*, Baltimore, 1988, Williams and Wilkins.

Shanks S: *Nursing and the management of adult communication disorders*, San Diego, 1983, College Hill Press.

Ulatowska H: *The aging brain*, San Diego, 1985, College Hill Press.

APHASIA

Boone D: *An adult has aphasia*, Austin, TX, 1983, Pro-Ed.

Brady W: *Aphasia: communication and the family*, Austin, TX, 1989, Pro-Ed.

Chapey R: *Language intervention strategies in adult aphasia*, Baltimore, 1986, Williams and Wilkins.

Hooper C and Dunkle R: *The older aphasic person*, Rockville, MD, 1985, Aspen Systems Publishing.

National Stroke Association: *Understanding speech and language problems after stroke*, Englewood, CO, 1992, National Stroke Association.

Sarno MT: *Understanding aphasia: a guide for the family and friends,* ed 11, New York, 1986, New York University Medical Center.

BEHAVIOR

Blazer D and Busse E: *Geriatric psychiatry*, Washington, DC, 1991, American Psychiatric Press.

Fogel BS and Stone AB: Practical pathophysiology in neuropsychiatry: a clinical approach to depression and impulsive behavior in neurologic patients. In Yudofsy SC and Hales RE, editors: *American psychiatric press textbook for neuropsychiatry*, ed 2, Washington , DC, 1992, American Psychiatric Press.

Fogel BS: Beyond neuropolitics. In Light E and Lebowitz BD, editors: *The elderly with chronic mental illness*, New York, 1991, Springer Publishing Company.

Salzman C: *Geriatric psychopharmacology*, ed 2, New York, 1979, Elsevier.

COGNITIVE LOSS/DEMENTIA

Alzheimer's Association, DeBruin J, 1980. 1992 Products Catalogue, 1992. Creative, hands-on science experiences using free and inexpensive materials. Carthage, IL, 1992, Good Apple (includes packages of activities programs).

Alzheimer's Association, Patient and Family Services: *Guide for dignity: goals of specialized Alzheimer/dementia care in residential settings*, ed 1, Chicago, 1992, Alzheimer's Association.

American Psychiatric Association: *Diagnostic and statisical manual of mental disorders, ed 3, revised*, Washington, DC, 1987, American Psychiatric Association.

Brawley E: Alzheimer's disease: designing the physical environment, *Am J Alzheimer's Care Rel Disord Res*, 7(1):1-8, 1992.

Burton J: Programming to meet the needs of the elderly in institutions: part I, *Can J Occup Ther* 49(1):7-10, 1982.

Calkins MP: *Design for dementia*, Baltimore, 1988, National Health Publishing.

Cohen U and Weisman GD: Holding on to home: *designing environments for people with dementia*, Baltimore, 1990, Johns Hopkins University Press.

Coons DO, editor: *Specialized dementia care*,

Baltimore, 1991, Johns Hopkins University Press.

Corder EH et al: Gene dosage of apolipoprotein E type 4 allele and the risk of Alzheimer's disease in late onset families, *Science* 261(5123):921-923, 1993.

Cummings JL and Benson DF: *Dementia: a clinical approach*, Stoneham, MA, 1992, Butterworth-Heinemann.

Davis KL et al: A double-blind, placebo-controlled multicenter study of tacrine for Alzheimer's disease: the Tacrine Collaborative Study Group, *N Engl J Med* 327(18):1253-1259, 1992.

Dowling JR: *Keeping busy, a handbook of activities for persons with dementia*, Baltimore, 1995, Johns Hopkins University Press.

Edelson JS and Lyons WH: *Institutional care of the mentally impaired elderly*, New York, 1985, Van Nostrand Reinhold.

Farlow M et al: A controlled trial of tacrine in Alzheimer's disease: the Tacrine Collaborative Study Group, *JAMA* 268(18):2523-2529, 1992.

Folstein MF, Folstein S, and McHugh PR: Mini-Mental State: a practical method for grading the cognitive state of patients for the clinician, *J Psych Res* 12(3):189-198, 1975.

Gwyther L: *Care of Alzheimer's patients: a manual for nursing home staff*, published jointly by American Health Care Association and Alzheimer's Disease and Related Disorders Association, 1985, Chicago.

Hachinski V et al: Cerebral blood flow in dementia, *Arch Neurol* 32:632-637, 1975.

Hellen CR: *Alzheimer's disease: activity-focused care*, Stoneham, MA, 1992, Andover Medical Publishers.

Hiatt LG: Supportive design for people with memory impairments. In Kalicki A, editor: *Confronting Alzheimer's disease*, Owings Mill, MD, 1987, National Health Publishing/American Association for the Aging.

Jarvik LF and Winograd CH, editors: *Treatments for the Alzheimer patient*, New York, Springer Publishing Company, 1988.

Lutz CW, Fischer L, and Arnold RM: *The erosion of autonomy in long term care*, New York, Oxford University Press, 1992.

Knoll J: Deprenyl Medication: a strategy to modulate the age related decline of the striatal dopaminergic system, *J Am Geriatr Soc* 40(8):839-847, 1992.

Lehane MS: *Science tricks*, New York, 1980, Franklin Watts.

Mace NL, editor: *Dementia care: patient, family, and community*, Baltimore, 1989, Johns Hopkins University Press.

Mace NL: The management of problem behaviors. In Mace NL, editor: *Dementia care: patient, family, and community*, Baltimore, 1989, Johns Hopkins University Press.

Mace NL: Principles of activities for persons with dementia, *Phys Occup Ther Geriat* Vol 5(3) 1987.

Mace NL and Rabins PV: *The 36-hour day: a family guide to caring for persons with Alzheimer's disease, related dementing illnesses, and memory loss in later life,* ed 2, Baltimore, 1981, Johns Hopkins University Press.

Mace NL, Whitehouse PJ, and Smyth KA: *Management of patients with dementia*, In Whitehouse PJ, editor: *Dementia*, Philadelphia, 1993, FA Davis.

Marshall PJ: Vascular dementia. In Whitehouse PJ, editor: *Dementia*, Philadelphia, 1993, FA Davis.

Mayeux R et al: The clinical evaluation of patients with dementia. In Whitehouse PJ, editor: *Dementia*, Philadelphia, 1993, FA Davis.

McKhann et al: Clinical diagnosis of Alzheimer's disease: report of the NINCDS-ADRDA Work Group under the auspices of Department of Health and Human Services Task Force on Alzheimer's Disease, *Neurology* 34:939-944, 1984.

Meggendorfer F: Uber die hereditare disposition zur dementia senilis, *Zeitschrift Neurol Psychiatrie* 101:387-405, 1926.

National Institutes of Health Consensus Conference on Differential Diagnosis of Dementing Diseases, *JAMA* 258(23):3411-3416, 1987.

Poirier J et al: Apolipoprotein E polymorphism and Alzheimer's disease, *Lancet* 342(8873):697-699, 1993.

Rebeck Gwet, Et al: Reduced apolipoprotein epsilon 4 allele frequency in the oldest Alzheimer's patients and cognitively normal individuals, *Neurology,* 44(8):1513-1516, 1994.

Ritter L: Developing a therapeutic activities program in a dementia unit. In Sloan PD and Mathew LJ, editors: *Dementia units in long-term care*, Baltimore, 1991, Johns

Hopkins University Press.

Robinson A, Spencer B, and White L: *Understanding difficult behaviors: some practical suggestions for coping with Alzheimer's disease and related illnesses*, Ypsilanti, MI, 1989, Geriatric Education Center for Michigan, Eastern Michigan University.

Seubert P et al: Isolation and quantification of soluble Alzheimer's beta-peptide from biological fluids, *Nature*, 359:325-327, 1992.

Siu AL: Screening for dementia and investigating its causes, *Ann Intern Med*, 115(2):122-132, 1991.

Sheridan C: *Failure-free activities for Alzheimer's patients: a guidebook for caregivers*, San Francisco, 1987, Cottage Books and San Francisco, 1989, Reminiscence/Elder Press .

Shoji M et al: Production of the Alzheimer amyloid beta protein by normal proteolytic processing, *Science* 258(5079):126-129, 1992.

Sloane PD and Mathew LJ, editors: *Dementia units in long-term care*, Baltimore, 1991, Johns Hopkins University Press.

Somerset Pharmaceuticals package insert for Elderpryl, Tampa, FL, 1995.

Tune LE and Lucas-Blaustein MJ, and Rovner BW: Psychosocial interventions. In Jarvik LF and Winograd CD, editors: *Treatments for the Alzheimer patient: the long haul*, New York, 1988, Springer Publishing Company.

Weaverdyck SE: Intervention-based neuropsychosocial assessment. In Mace NL, editor: *Dementia care: patient, family, and community,* Baltimore, 1989, Johns Hopkins University Press.

Whitehouse PJ, editor: *Dementia*, Philadelphia, 1993, FA Davis.

Zgola JM: Therapeutic activity. In Mace NL, editor: *Dementia care: patient, family, and community,* Baltimore, 1989, Johns Hopkins University Press.

Zgola JM: *Doing things: A guide to programming activities for persons with Alzheimer's disease and related disorders*, Baltimore, 1987, Johns Hopkins University Press.

COMMUNICATION AND FACILITY

Lubinski R: A model for intervention: communication skills, effectiveness and opportunity. In Shadden B: *Communication behavior and aging*, Baltimore, 1988, Williams and Wilkins.

Lubinski R: Environmental considerations for elderly patients. In Lubinski R: *Dementia and communication*, Philadelphia, 1991, B.C. Decker.

Lubinski R, Morrison E, and Rigrodsky S: Perception of spoken communication by elderly chronically ill patients in an institutional setting, *J Speech Hear Disord* 46:405-12, 1981.

DEHYDRATION

Clarkin C: Fluid volume replacement. In Rogers-Seidl, editor: *Geriatric nursing care plans,* St. Louis, 1991, Mosby-Year Book.

Davis KM and Minaker KL: Disorders of fluid and electrolytes balance. In Hazzard W and Anders R, editors: *Principles of geriatric medicine and gerontology,* New York, 1990, McGraw-Hill.

Gaspar PM: What determines how much patients drink, *Geriatr Nurs* 221-228, 1988.

Hirschhorn N and Greenough WB: Progress in oral rehydration therapy, *Sci Am* 264:50-56, 1991.

Hoffman NB: Dehydration in the elderly: insidious and manageable, *Geriatrics* 46(6):35-38, 1991.

Kositzke JA: A question of balance: dehydration in the elderly, *Gerontol Nurs* 16(5):4-11, 1990.

Lavizzo-Mourney RJ: Dehydration in the elderly: A short review, *J Nat Med Assoc* 79(10):1033-1038, 1987.

Lavizzo-Mourney RJ, Johnson J, and Stolley P: Risk factors for dehydration among elderly nursing home residents, *JAGS* 36:213-218, 1988.

Lipschitz S et al: Subcutaneous fluid administration in elderly subjects: validation of an under-used technique, *JAGS,* 39:6-9, 1991.

Phillips PA et al: Reduced thirst after water deprivation in healthy elderly men, *N Engl J Med* 12:753, 1984.

DELIRIUM

Blackburn T and Duna M: Cystocerebral syndrome: acute urinary retention presenting as confusion in elderly patients, *Arch Int Med* 150:2577-2578, 1990.

Gustafson Y et al: Acute confusional states in elderly patients treated for femoral neck fracture, *JAGS* 36:525-530, 1988.

Inouye SK et al: Clarifying confusion: the confusion assessment method, *Ann Intern Med* 113:941-948, 1990 .

Levkoff SE, Besdine RW, and Wetle T: Acute confusional states (delirium) in the hospitalized elderly, *Annu Rev Gerontol Geriatr* 6:1-26, 1986.

Levkoff SE et al: Delirium: the occurrence and persistence of symptoms among elderly hospitalized patients, *Arch Intern Med*, 152:334-340, 1992.

Lipowski ZJ: Delirium in the elderly patient, *N Engl J Med* 320(9):575-581, 1989.

Liptzin B et al: An empirical study of diagnostic criteria for celirium, *Am J Psychiatry* 148(4):454-457, 1991.

Morris RK et al: Delusions in newly admitted residents of nursing homes, *Am J Psychiatry* 147(3):299-302, 1990.

Rabins PV: Psychosocial issues and management: aspects of delirium, *Int Psychogeriatr* 3(2):319-324, 1991.

Schor JD et al: Risk factors for delirium in hospitalized elderly, *JAMA* 267(6):827-831, 1992.

Sullivan N and Fogel B: Could this be delirium?, *Am J Nurs* pp 1359-1363, 1986.

Williams MA: Delirium/acute confusional states: evaluation devices in nursing, *Int Psychogeriatr* 3(2):301-308, 1991.

DEMENTIA AND COMMUNICATION

Bayles K and Kazniak A: *Communication and cognition in normal aging and dementia,* Austin, TX, 1987, Pro-Ed.

Cummings J and Benson D: *Dementia: a clinical approach,* London, 1983, Butterworth.

Lubinski R: *Dementia and communication,*

Philadelphia, 1991, BC Decker.

DISCHARGE PLANNING
Weaver F and Burdi M: Developing a model of discharge planning based on patient characteristics, *J Aging Health* 4(3):440-452, August 1992.

DYSARTHRIA
Darley F, Aronson A, and Brown J: *Motor speech disorders*, Philadelphia, 1975, W.B. Saunders.

FALLS
Granek E et al: Medications and diagnoses in relation to falls in a long-term care facility, *J Am Geriatr Soc* 35:503-511, 1987.

Lipsitz LA et al: Causes and correlates of recurrent falls in ambulatory frail elderly, *J Gerontol* 46(4):114-122, 1991

Lipsitz LA et al: Syncope in institutionalized elderly: the impact of multiple pathological conditions and situational stress, *J Chronic Dis* 39:619-630, 1986.

Robbins AS et al: Predictors of falls among elderly people, *Arch Intern Med* 149:1628-1633, 1989.

Tinetti ME: Factors associated with serious injury during falls by ambulatory nursing home residents, *J Am Geriatr Soc* 35:644-648, 1987.

Tinetti ME and Speechley JF: Prevention of falls among the elderly, *N Engl J Med* 320:1055-1059, 1989.

Tinetti ME, Williams TF, and Mayewski R: Falls risk index for elderly patients based on number of chronic disabilities, *Am J Med* 80:429-434, 1986.

FEEDING TUBES
Edes TE: Diarrhea in tube-fed patients: feeding formula not necessarily the cause, *Am J Med* 88:91-93, 1990.

Harris JA and Benedict FG: *A biometric study of basal metabolism in man*, Washington, DC, 1919, Carnegie Institute of Washington.

Long CL et al: Metabolic response to injury and illness: estimation of energy and protein needs from indirect calorimetry and nitrogen balance, *JPEN* 3:452, 1979.

Morley J et al: Geriatric rounds: nutrition and the elderly, *J Am Geriatr Soc* 34:823-832, 1986.

Nelson RC and Franzi LR: Nutrition and aging, *Med Clin North Am* 73(6):1531-1550, 1989.

Silver AJ: The changing role of tube feeding, *Long-Term Care Forum* 2(2):2-4, 1992.

Taylor CA et al: Predictors of outcome after percutaneous endoscopic gastrostomy: a community Study, *Mayo Clin Proc* 67:1042-1049.

Wilmore DW and Van Woert JH: Enteral and parenteral nutrition in hospital patients. *Sci Am* 1992.

FOOT CARE
Gudas CJ: Common foot problems in the elderly. In Catkins E, Ford AB, and Katz PR, editors: *Practice of geriatrics*, Philadelphia, 1992, WB Saunders.

Helfand AE: Foot health for the elderly patient. In Reichel W, editor: *Clinical aspects of aging*, Baltimore, 1979, Williams and Wilkins.

Jahss MH: Geriatric aspects of the foot and ankle. In Rossman I, editor: *Clinical Geriatrics*, Philadelphia, 1979, JB Lippincott.

Annual Review of Gerontology and Geriatrics, *Podiatry for the geriatric patient*, Vol 4 Chapter 8, 1984.

HEARING LOSS

Armbruster J and Miller MH: *How to get the most out of your hearing aid*, Washington, DC, 1981, Alexander Graham Bell.

Hull R: *Hearing impairment among aging persons*, Lincoln, NE, 1977, Cliffs Speech and Hearing Serios-Professional Educators Publications, Inc.

Laufner B: *Have you heard? Hearing loss and aging*, Washington, DC, 1984, American Association of Retired Persons.

Maurer J and Rupp R: *Hearing and the aging: tactics for intervention*, New York, 1979, Grune and Stratton.

Weinstein B and Amsel L: Hearing loss and senile dementia in the institutionalized elderly, *Clin Gerontol*, 4:3-15, 1986.

HIP FRACTURE

Baker PA, Evans OM, and Lee C: Treadmill gait retraining following neck-of-femur, *Arch Phys Med Rehab* 71:649-652, 1991.

Bonar SK et al: Factors associated with short- versus long-term skilled nursing facility placement among community living hip fracture patients, *JAGS* 38(10):1139-1144, 1990.

Cornell CN: Management of fractures in patients with osteoporosis, *Orthop Clin North Am* 21(1):125-130, 1990.

Jette AM et al: Functional recovery after hip fracture, *Arch Phys Med Rehab* 58:735-740, 1987.

Kumar VN and Redford JB: Rehabilitation of hip fractures in the elderly, *Am Fam Phys* 29:173-180, 1984.

Labelle LW, Colwill JC, and Swanson AB: Bateman bipolar hip arthroplasty for femoral neck fractures, *Clin Orthop Rel Res* 251:20-25, 1990.

Mossey JM et al: Determinants of recovery 12 months after hip fracture, *Am J Public Health* 79(3):279-286, 1989.

INFECTION

Irvine PW, Van Buren N, and Crossley K: Causes for hospitalization of nursing home patients: the role of infection, *J Am Geriatr Soc* 32:103, 1984.

Kurtz D and Chow AW: Infected pressure and diabetic ulcers. *Clin Geriatr Med* 8(4):835, 1992.

Maginer J et al: Prevalence and characteristics of nursing-home acquired infections in the aged, *J Am Geriatr Soc* 39:1071, 1991.

Verghese A and Berk SL, editors: *Infections in nursing homes and long-term care facilities*, Basel, Switzerland, 1990, Karger Publishers.

Warren JW: The catheter and urinary tract infection, *Med Clin North Am* 75:481, 1991.

Yoshikawa TT: Treatment of nursing home-acquired pneumonia, *J Am Geriatr Soc* 39:1040, 1991.

LARYNGECTOMY

Keith R and Darley F: *Laryngectomy Rehabilitation,* ed 2, San Diego, 1986, College Hill Press.

Salmon S: *Alaryngeal speech for clinicians by clinicians,* Austin, TX, 1991, Pro-Ed.

Shanks J: Current strategies for rehabilitation of the laryngectomized patient. In *Seminars in speech and language vol* 7, New York, 1986, Theime.

Weinberg B: Speech rehabilitation of the laryngectomized patient: advances and issues. In Costello J and Holland A, editors: *Speech and language disorders,* San Diego, 1986, College Hill Press.

DEPRESSION

Hall RCW, editor: *Psychiatric presentations of medical illness-symptomatic disorders,* New York, 1980, SB Medical and Scientific Book.

Heston LL et al: Inadequate treatment of depressed nursing home elderly, *JAGS* 40:1117-1122, 1992.

Jenike MA: *Geriatric psychiatry and psychopharmacology,* St. Louis, 1989, Mosby-Year Book.

Kramer-Ginsberg E et al: Hypochondriasis in the elderly depressed, *JAGS* 37:507-510, 1989.

Levinson AJ and Hall RCW, editors: *Neuropsychiatric manifestations of physical disease in the elderly,* New York, 1981, Raven Press.

Mackenzie TB, Robiner WN, and Knopman DS: Differences between patient and family assessments of depression in Alzheimer's disease, *Am J Psychiatry* 146(9):1174-1178, 1989.

NIH Consensus Development Panel on Depression in Later Life: Diagnosis and treatment of depression in late life, *JAMA* 26(8):1018-1024, 1992.

Parmelee PA, Katz IR, and Lawson MP: Incidence of depression in long-term care settings, *J Gerontol* 47:M189-M196, 1992.

Parmelee PA, Katz IR, and Lawson MP: Depression and mortality among institutionalized aged, *J Gerontol* 47:3-10, 1992.

Rovner BW et al: Depression and mortality in nursing homes, *JAMA* 265(8):993-996, 1991.

Salzman C: *Clinical geriatric pharmacology.* Baltimore, 1992, Williams and Wilkins.

NUTRITION

Blackburn GL et al: Nutrition and metabolic assessment of the hospitalized patient, *JPEN* 1:11, 1977.

Fischback F: *Manual of laboratory and diagnostic tests,* ed 4, Philadelphia, 1992, JB Lippincott.

Nutrition interventions manual for professionals caring for older Americans, The Nutrition Screening Initiative, Washington, DC 1992.

Pagano KD and Pagana TJ: *Mosby's diagnostic and laboratory test reference,* St. Louis, 1992, Mosby-Year Book.

ORAL CARE

American Heart Association Guidelines, December 1990.

Gordon SR and Jahnigen DW: Oral assessment of the dentulous elderly patient, *JAGS*

34:276-282, 1986.

Gordon SR and Jahnigen DW: Oral assessment of the edentulous elderly patient, *JAGS* 31(12):797-800, 1992.

PARKINSON'S DISEASE

Cummings JL: Depression and Parkinson's disease, *Am J Psychiatry* 149:443-454, 1992.

Hughes AJ et al: Accuracy of clinical diagnosis of idiopathic Parkinson's disease: a clinicopathological study of IDO cases, *J Neurol Neurosurg Psychiatry* 55:181-184, 1992.

Goetz AA and Stebbins GT: Risk factors for nursing home placement in advanced Parkinson's diease, *Neurology* 43-2227-2229, 1993.

Huber SJ, Shuttleworth EC, and Freidenberg DC: Neuropsychological differences between the dementias of Alzheimer's and Parkinson's diseases, *Arch Ne* 46:1287-1291, 1989.

Koller WC et al: Falls and Parkinson's disease, *Clin Neuropharmacol* 12:98-105, 1989.

Koller WC, Silver DE, and Lieberman A: An algorithm for the management of Parkinson's Disease, *Neurology* 44 (suppl 10):57-552, 1993.

Larsen JP: Parkinson's disease as community health problem: study in Norwegian nursing homes, *BMJ* 303:741-743, September 1991.

Levi S et al: Increased energy expenditure in Parkinson's disease, *BMJ* 301:1256-1257, 1990.

MacMahon DG, Overstall PW, and Marshall T: Simplification of the initiation of bromocriptine in elderly patients with advanced Parkinson's disease, *Age Aging* 20:146-151, 1991.

Parkinson's Study Group: Effect of deptemyl on the progression of disability in early Parkinson's disease, *N Engl J Med* 321(20):1364-1371, November 1989.

POLYPHARMACY

Avorn J and Gurwitz JH: Principles of geriatric pharmacy. In Cassel CK et al, editors: *Geriatric Medicine,* ed 2, New York, 1990, Springer-Verlag.

Avorn J et al: A randomized trial of a program to reduce the use of psychoactive drugs in nursing homes, *N Engl J Med* 327:168-173, 1992.

Beers MH et al: Psychoactive medication use in intermediate-care facility residents, *JAMA* 260:3016-3020, 1988.

Beers MH et al: Explicit criteria for determining inappropriate medication use in nursing home residents, *Arch Intern Med* 151:1825-1832, 1991.

Beers MH et al: Inappropriate medication prescribing in skilled-nursing facilities, *Ann Intern Med* 117:684-689, 1992.

Bradley JD et al: Comparison of an antiinflammatory dose of ibuprofen, an analgesic dose of ibuprofen and acetaminophen in the treatment of patients with osteoarthritis of the knee, *N Engl J Med* 325:87-91, 1991.

Everitt DE and Avorn J: Systemic effects of medications used to treat glaucoma, *Ann Intern Med* 112:120-125, 1990.

Greenblatt DJ, Sellars EM, and Shader RI: Drug

disposition in old age, *N Engl J Med* 306:1081-1088, 1982.

Greenblatt DJ et al: Sensitivity to triazolam in the elderly, *N Engl J Med* 324:1691-1698, 1991.

Griffin MR, Ray WA, and Schaffner W: Nonsteroidal antiinflammatory drug use and death from peptic ulcer in elderly persons, *Ann Intern Med* 109:359-363, 1988.

Gurwitz JH, Soumerai SB, and Avorn J: Improving medication prescribing and utilization in the nursing home, *J Am Geriatr Soc* 38:542-552, 1990.

Gurwitz JH and Avorn J: The ambiguous relation between aging and adverse drug reactions,
Ann Inter Med 114:956-966, 1991.

Gurwitz JH et al: Aging and the anticoagulant response to warfarin, *Ann Intern Med* 116:901-904, 1992.

Gurwitz JH et al: Nonsteroidal antiinflammatory drug-associated azotemia in the very old, *JAMA* 264:471-475, 1990.

Heston LL et al: Inadequate treatment of depressed nursing home elderly, *J Am Geriatr Soc* 40:1117-1122, 1992.

Monane M: Insomnia in the elderly, *J Clin Psych* 53(suppl 6):23-28, 1992.

Montamat SC, Cusack BJ, and Vestal RE: Management of drug therapy in the elderly, *N Engl J Med* 321:303-309, 1989.

Ray WA et al: Psychotropic drug use and the risk of hip fracture, *N Engl J Med* 316:363-369, 1987.

Ray WA et al: Reducing antipsychotic drug use in nursing homes: a controlled trial provider education, *Arch Intern Med* 153:713-721, 1993.

Reidenberg MM et al: Relationship between diazepam dose, plasma level, age, and central nervous system depression, *Clin Pharmacol Ther* 23:371-374, 1978.

Salzman C: *Clinical geriatric psychopharmacology,* ed 2, Baltimore, 1992, Williams & Wilkins.

PRESSURE ULCER
Allman RM: Pressure ulcers among the elderly, *N Engl J Med* 320:850-853, 1989.

Bergstrom N and Braden BA: Prospective study of pressure sore risk among institutionalized elderly, *J Am Geriatr Soc* 40:747-758, 1992.

Bergstrom N et al: Treatment of pressure ulcers. *Clinical Practice Guideline, No. 15,* Rockville, MD, US Department of Health and Human Services, Public Health Service, Agency for Health Care Policy and Research. AHCPR publication number 95-0652, December 1994.

Brandeis GH, Morris JN, Nash DJ and Lipsitz LA: The epidemiology and natural history of pressure ulcers in elderly nursing home residents, *JAMA* 264(22):2905-2909, 1990.
Cooper DM: Pressure ulcers, *Nurs Clin North Am* 22(6), 475-492, 1987.

Krasner D, editor: *Chronic wound care: A clinical source book for health care professionals*, King of Prussia, PA, 1990, Health Management Publications.

Maklebust J and Sieggreen M: *Pressure ulcers: guideline for prevention and nursing management*, West Dundea, IL, 1991, S-N Publications.

Melcher RE, Longe RL, and Gelbart AO: Pressure sores in the elderly, *Postgrad Med* 83(1):299-308, 1988.

National Pressure Ulcer Advisory Board: Pressure ulcers prevalence, cost and risk assessment. Consensus Development Conference Statement, *Decubitis* 2(2):24-28, 1989.

Panel for the Prediction and Prevention of Pressure Ulcers in Adults: *Pressure ulcers in adults: prediction and prevention*, Clinical Practice Guideline Number 3, AHCPR Publication

No. 92-0047, Rockville, MD, Aging for Health Care Policy Center, Public Health Service, US Department of Health and Human Services, May 1992.

Spector W, Capp MC, Tucker RJ: Factors associated with presence of decubitis ulcers at admission to nursing homes, *Gerontologist* 18(6):830-834, 1988.

Standards Committee of the International Association for Enterostomal Therapy: *Standards of care, dermal wounds: pressure sores*, Irvine, CA, 1987, International Association for Enterostomal Therapy.

PSYCHOTROPIC DRUGS

Birren J, Sloane RB, and Cohen GD, editors: *Handbook of mental health and aging,*, ed 2, San Diego, 1992, Academic Press.

Devanand DP et al: The Columbia University Scale for Psychopathology in Alzheimer's Disease, *Arch Neurol* 49:371-376, 1992.

DeVane CL: *Fundamentals of monitoring psychoactive drug therapy*, Baltimore, 1990,

Williams and Wilkins.

Hamilton M: A rating scale for depression, *J Neurol Neurosurg Psychiatry* 23:56-62, 1960.

Hamilton M: The assessment of anxiety states by rating, *Br J Med Psychol* 32:50-55, 1959.

Lohr JB et al: Treatment of disordered behavior. In Salzman C, editor: *Clinical geriatric psychopharmacology,* ed 2, Baltimore, 1992, Williams and Wilkins.

Overall J and Gorman DR: The brief psychiatric rating scale, *Psychol Rep* 10:799-812, 1962.

Ray, WA et al: The nursing home behavior problem scale, *J Gerontol Med Sci* 47:9-16, 1992.

Salzman C and Nevis-Olesen J: Psychopharmacologic treatment. In Salzman C, editor: *Clinical geriatric psychopharmacology,* ed 2, Baltimore, 1992, Williams and Wilkins.

Spitzer R, Endicott J, and Robins E: Research diagnostic criteria, *Arch Gen Psychiatry*, 35:773-782, 1978.

Stoudemire A et al: Psychopharmacology in the medical patient. In Stoudemire A and Fogel BS, editors: *Psychiatric care of the medical patient*, New York, 1993, Oxford University Press.

Stoudemire A and Fogel BS: Psychopharmacology in the medically ill. In Stoudemire A and Fogel BS, editors: *Principles of Medical Psychiatry*, Orlando, 1987, Grune & Stratton, Inc.

Stoudemire A, Fogel BS, and Gulley LR: Psychopharmacology in the medically ill: An update. In Stoudemire A and Fogel BS, editors: *Medical psychiatric practice, vol 1*, Washington, DC, 1991, American Psychiatric Press, Inc.

Yesavage JA et al: Development and validation of a geriatric depression screening scale: a preliminary report, *J Psychiatr Res* 17:37-49, 1983.

Yudofsky SC et al: The overt aggression scale for the objective rating of verbal and physical aggression, *Am J Psychiatry* 143:35-39, 1986.

Zung WWK: A rating instrument for anxiety disorders, *Psychosomatics* 12:371-379, 1971.

PULMONARY REHABILITATION

Anonymous, Diagnostic techniques, *Clin Chest Med* 8(1), 1-175, 1987.

Durstine JL et al, editors: *Resource manual for guidelines for exercise testing and prescription: American College of Sports Medicine,* Philadelphia, 1993, Lea and Febiger.

Ferguson GT and Chernak RM: Management of chronic obstructive pulmonary disease, *N Engl J Med* 328(14):1017-1022, 1993.

Kacmarek RM, Dimas S, and Mack CW: *The essentials of respiratory therapy*, Chicago, 1982, Year Book Medical.

Make BJ, editor: Cardiac/pulmonary rehabilitation, *Semin Respir Care* 14(2), 1993.

Nocturnal Oxygen Therapy Trial Group: Continuous or nocturnal oxygen therapy in hypoxemic chronic obstructions lung disease, *Ann Intern Med* 93:391-398, 1980.

Paine R and Make BJ: Pulmonary rehabilitation for the elderly, *Clin Geriatr Med* 2(2):313-335, 1986.

Shapiro BA, Harrison RH, and Trout CA: *Clinical application of respiratory care*, Chicago, 1981, Year Book Medical.

Tockman MS: Aging of the respiratory system. In Hazzard et al, editors: *Principles of geriatric medicine and gerontology*, New York, 1990, McGraw-Hill.

RESTRAINT-RREE CARE

Kapp MR: Nursing home restraints and legal liability: merging the standard of care and industry Practice, *J Legal Med* 13:1-32, 1992.

The Kendal Corporation: *Untie the elderly: resource manual*, Kennett Square, PA, 1991, The Kendal Corporation.

May MI et al: *Managing institutional long-term care for the elderly*, Rockville, MD, 1991, Aspen Publishing Systems.

Rader J: A comprehensive staff approach to problem wandering, *Gerontologist* 17:756-760, 1987.

Werner P et al: Physical restraints and agitation in nursing home residents, *JAGS* 37:1122-1126, 1989.

SLEEP DISORDERS

Ancoli-Israel S: Epidemiology of sleep disorders. In Roth T, editor: *Clinics in geriatric medicine*, Philadelphia, 1989, WB Saunders Company.

Ancoli-Israel S et al: Sleep apnea in female patients in a nursing home: increased risk of mortality, *Chest* 96(5):1054-1058, 1989.

Ancoli-Israel S and Kripke DF: Now I lay me down to sleep: the problem of sleep fragmentation in elderly and demented residents of nursing homes, *Bull Clin Neurosci* 54:127-132, 1989.

Ancoli-Israel S et al: Sleep fragmentation in patients from a nursing home, *J Gerontol* 44:M18-M21, 1989.

Bliwise DL et al: Sleep and sundowning in nursing home patients with dementia, *Psychiatry Res* 48(3):277-292, 1993.

Campbell SS et al: Exposure to light in healthy elderly subjects and Alzheimer's patients, *Physiol Behav* 42:141-144, 1988.

Clapin-French E: Sleep patterns of aged persons in long-term care facilities, *J Adv Nurs* 11:57-66, 1966.

Cohen D et al: Sleep disturbances in the institutionalized aged, *J Am Geriatr Soc* 31:79-82, 1983.

Cohen-Mansfield J and Marx MS: The relationship between sleep disturbances and agitation in a Nursing Home, *J Aging Health* 2:42-57, 1990

Evans LK: Sundown syndrome in institutionalized elderly, *JAGS* 35:101-108, 1987.

Gillick MR and Serrel NA: Adverse consequences of hospitalization in the elderly, *Soc Sci Med* 16:1033-1038, 1982.

Jacobs D et al: 24-Hour sleep/wake patterns in a nursing home population, *Psychol Aging* 4(3):352-356, 1989.

Mendelson WB: *The use and misuse of sleeping pills*, New York, Plenum Publishing Co., 1980.

Miles L and Dement WC: Sleep and aging, *Sleep* 3:119-120, 1980

Pollack CP and Perlick D: Sleep problems and institutionalization of the elderly, *Sleep*
Res 16:407, 1987.

Regestein QR and Morris J: Daily sleep patterns observed among institutionalized elderly, *J Am Geriatr Soc* 35:767-772, 1987.

Sanford, JRA: Tolerance of debility in elderly dependents by supporters at home: its significance for hospital practice, *BMJ* 3:471-473, 1975.

Spielman AJ, Saskin P, and Thorpy MJ: Treatment of chronic insomnia by restriction of time in bed, *Sleep* 10:45-56, 1987.

STROKE

Albert MD and Helm-Estabrooks N: Diagnosis and treatment of aphasia: parts 1 and 2, *JAMA* 259 (7 and 8):1043-1047 and 1205-1210, 1988.

Damasio AR: Aphasia, *N Engl J Med* 326:531-539, 1992.

DeLisa JA and Gans BM: *Rehabilitation medicine*, Philadelphia, 1993, JB Lippincott Company.

Folstein MF, Folstein SE, and McHugh PR: Mini-mental state: a practical method for grading the cognitive state of patients for the clinician, *J Psychiatry Res* 12:189-198, 1975.

Hamilton M: A rating scale for depression, *J Neuro Neurol Psychiatry* 23:56-62, 1960.

Mahoney FI and Barthel DW: Functional evaluation: The Barthel Index, *MD State Med J* 14(2):61-65, 1965.

Perry J and Keenan MAE: Rehabilitation of the neurologically disabled patient. In Aminoff MJ, editor: *Neurology and General Medicine*, New York, 1989, Churchill

Livingstone.

Zung W: A self rating depression scale, *Arch Gen Psychiatry*, 12:63-70, 1965.

TECHNOLOGICAL AIDS FOR THE ELDERLY
American Speech-Language and Hearing Association Series:
Augmentative Communication for the Medical Community
Augmentative Communication for the General Public
Augmentative Communication for Consumers
Rockville, MD, 1986, American Speech-Language and Hearing Association

American Speech-Language and Hearing Association: *Assistive listening devices and systems*, Rockville, MD, 1986, American Speech-Language and Hearing Association.

American Speech-Language and Hearing Association: *Breaking the silence barrier*, Rockville, MD, 1985, American Speech-Language and Hearing Association.

TERMINAL CARE
Billings JA: *Outpatient management of advanced cancer: symptom control, support and hospice in the home*, Philadelphia, 1985, JB Lippincott Company.

Boulder County Hospice: *Signs and symptoms of approaching death*, Boulder, CO, 1983.

Center for Thanatology Research. Publishes a comprehensive bibliography serving the educational and research needs of the international thanatology community in the study and care of the aged, dying, and the bereaved. 391 Atlantic Avenue, Brooklyn, NY 11217, 212-858-3026.

Code of Federal Regulations, #42 Parts 400 to 429. Public Health, revised October 1986 (describes the hospice-specific Medicare regulations.

Kaye P: *Notes on symptom control in hospice and palliative care*, Essex, CT, 1991, Hospice Education Institute.

Kilburn L: *Hospice operations manual: a comprehensive guide to organizational development, management, care planning, regulatory compliance, and financial services*, Arlington, VA, 1988, National Hospice Organization (describes the methodologies to prepare for Medicare Certification compliance).

Magno JB: Hospice care: an overview, *Henry Ford Hosp Med J*, 39(2):72-73, 1991.

Magno JB: Management of terminal illness: The hospice concept of care, *Henry Ford Hosp Med J* 39(2):74-76, 1991.

National Hospice Organization. Publishes a large number of hospice-specific items including a national directory of existing programs, information on various aspects of hospice operations, sample contract formats, and other related information, and maintains an updated listing of hospice-related legislation. They also distribute an extensive amount of audiovisual materials and maintain current bibliographical lists. For more information, contact: National Hospice Organization, 1901 N. Moore St, Suite 901, Arlington, VA 22209, 703-243-5900 fax 703-525-5762

Portenoy RK, editor: *J Pain Symptom Manage*, New York, Elsevier Science Publishing Co. For subscription information, call: 212-633-3950 or fax 212-633-3990

Scott SF: The philosophy of hospice nursing.

In Skinner SS, et al, editors: *Multidisciplinary team manual for the hospice patient and family,* Waban, MA, 1984 (unpublished), Hospice of the Good Shepherd.

Skinner SS, O'Connor T, Pollack V, et al: *Multidisciplinary team manual for the hospice patient and family,* Waban, MA, 1984 (unpublished), Hospice of the Good Shepherd.

US Department of Health and Human Services, Health Care Financing Administration: *Medicare hospice manual,* US Department of Commerce, National Technical Information Services, HCFA Publications 21 to T27, January 1992 (for more information, write to NTIS, US Department of Commerce, Springfield, VA, 703-487-4630).

Volicer L et al: Ethical issues in the treatment of advanced Alzheimer's dementia: hospice approach. In *Clinical management of Alzheimer's disease,* Rockville, MD, Aspen Systems Publishing, 1988.

URINARY INCONTINENCE

Resnick NM and Baumann MM: Urinary incontinence and indwelling catheter. In Morris JN and Hawes C editors: *Minimum Data Set and resident assessment instruments,* Boston, 1991, Eliot Press.

Resnick NM and Ouslander JG, editors: NIH consensus development conference proceedings, *J Am Geriat Soc* 38:263-387, 1990.

Resnick NM, Yalla SV, and Laurino E: The pathophysiology and clinical correlates of established urinary incontinence in frail elderly, *N Engl J Med* 320:1-7, 1989.

Resnick NM and Yalla SV: Evaluation and medical management of urinary incontinence. In Walsh PC, Retik AB, Starney TA, and Vaughn, Jr ED, editors: *Campbell's urology,* ed 6, 1992.

Urinary Incontinence Guideline Panel: Urinary incontinence in adults: clinical practice guideline. AHCPR Publication No. 92-0038, Rockville, MD, Agency for Health Care Policy and Research, Public Health Service, US Department of Health and Human Services, 1992.

VISION

Faye EE, editor: *Clinical low vision,* Boston, 1984, Little Brown.

Faye EE and Stuen CS, editors: *The aging eye and low vision: a study for physicians,* New York, 1992, The Lighthouse, Inc.

Genensky S et al: *Visual environmental adaptive problems of the partially sighted,* Santa Monica, CA, 1979, Center for the Partially Sighted.

Lighthouse low vision catalog, ed 7, New York, 1992, Lighthouse Low Vision Products.

Pavan-Langston D and Dunkel E: *Handbook of ocular drug therapy and ocular side effects of systemic drugs,* Boston, 1991, Little Brown.

Rosenbloom A and Morgan M, editors: *Vision and aging: general and clinical perspectives,* New York, 1986, Professional Press Books.

VITAL SIGNS

Bates B: *A guide to physical examination and history taking,* Philadelphia, 1987, JB Lippincott Company.

Kirkendall W et al: Recommendations for human blood pressure determination by sphygmomanometers, AHA Committee Report, in News from the American Heart Association, *JAMA* 2:1146A-115A, 1980.

McFadden JP et al: Raised respiratory rate in elderly patients: A valuable physical sign, *BMJ* 284:626-627, 1982.

Messerli FH, Ventura HO, and Amodeo C: Osler's maneuver and pseudohypertension, *N Engl J Med* 312:1548-1551, 1985.

Nelson WP and Egbert AM: How to ensure blood pressure—accurately, *Primary Cardiol* 14-26, 1984.

O'Brien ET and O'Malley K: ABC of blood pressure management, *BMJ* 982-983, 1979.

Stoneking HT et al: Blood pressure measurements in the nursing home: are they accurate?, *Gerontologist* 32:536-540, 1992.

RESOURCE GROUPS TO CONTACT FOR MORE INFORMATION ON COMMUNICATION OF THE ELDERLY

Academy of Neurologic Communication Disorders
Dept. of Speech and Hearing Sciences
University of Arizona
Tuscon, AZ   85721

Alexander Graham Bell Association for the Deaf
3417 Volta Place NW
Washington, DC 20007

American Academy of Otolaryngology
1101 Vermont Avenue NW Suite 302
Washington, DC 20005

American Speech-Language and Hearing Association (ASHA)
10801 Rockville Pike

Rockville, MD   20852

National Aphasia Association
P.O. Box 1887
Murray Hill Station
New York, NY   10156

National Association of Activity Professionals,
1225 I St NW, Suite 300,
Washington, DC 20005.

National Association of the Deaf
814 Thayer Avenue
Silver Spring, MD   20910

National Center on Technology and Aging
University Center on Aging
University of Massachusetts Medical Center
55 Lake Avenue North
Worcester, MA   01655

National Hearing Aid Society
2713 Ontario Road NW
Washington, DC   20009

National Hearing Association
1010 Jorie Blvd.
Oak Brook, IL   60521

National Information Center on Deafness
4848 Battery Lane Suite 100
Gallaudet College Kendall Green
800 Florida Avenue NE
Washington, DC 20002

National Institute for Neurological Disorders and Stroke
Public Information Office
DHHS/NIH
9000 Rockville Pike, Building 31
Bethesda, MD   20892

National Institute on Deafness and Other Communication Disorders (NIDCD)
Information Inquiry

Building 31 Room 1 B62
9000 Rockville Pike
Bethesda, MD 20892

Resources for Rehabilitation
33 Bedford St Suite 19A
Lexington, MA 02173

Self Help Group for Hard of Hearing People,
   Inc. (SHHH)
7800 Wisconsin Avenue
Bethesda, MD 20814

Stroke Club International
805 12th St.
Galveston, TX 77550

FILMS

American Speech-Language and Hearing Association: *An inservice training program on the communication needs of older persons*, American Speech-Language and Hearing Association, 10801 Rockville Pike, Rockville, MD 20852, 1987.

American Speech-Language and Hearing Association: *Communications disorders and aging*, American Speech-Language and Hearing Association, 10801 Rockville Pike, Rockville, MD 20852, 1987.

Audiovisual Catalogue 1989-1990, The House Ear Institute, 256 S. Lake St., Los Angeles, CA 90057 (as an example, they carry *Hearing Aids in Adults: Current Concepts*).

Designing the physical environment for persons with dementia, Terra Nova Films, Inc., 9849 S. Winchester Ave, Chicago, IL 60643, 1987.

Helping people with dementia in activities of daily living, Terra Nova Films, Inc., 9849 S. Winchester Ave, Chicago, IL 60643, 1987.

Nevlund G and Jones R: *Experiencing aphasia: an inservice model demonstrating aspects of aphasia*, Tuscon, AZ, Communication Skill Builders.

Shadden B, Raiford C, and Shadden H: *Coping with communication disorders in aging*, Tigard, OR, 1983, CC. Publication.

ASSOCIATIONS

For information on the nearest Alzheimer's Association chapters, call 1-800-272-3900

Glossary

abulia

A loss of the ability or a reduced capacity to exhibit initiative or to make decisions.

acetaminophen

An analgesic and antipyretic drug used in many nonprescription pain relievers. It has no antiinflammatory properties.

acid-fast bacillus (AFB)

A type of bacillus that resists decolorizing by acid after accepting a stain; examples include Mycobacterium tuberculosis and M. leprae.

Acquired immunodeficiency syndrome (AIDS)

A disease involving a defect in cell-mediated immunity that has a long incubation period, follows a protracted and debilitating course, is manifested by various opportunistic infections, and has a poor prognosis. AIDS was found originally in homosexual men and intravenous drug users but now occurs increasingly among female sex partners of bisexual men and children of those with the disease.

Observations: A resident is characterized as having AIDS if he or she has contracted HIV and exhibits one or more of 23 specific signs or symptoms, including various types of pneumonia, cancer, and fungal and parasitic infections. AIDS is also determined by the level of the resident's T4 lymphocytes, indicating the efficiency of the person's immune system. If that number drops below 200 to 500/mm3, compared with a normal level of 1000 lymphocytes/mm3, the person may be identified as having AIDS. The causative agent is a retrovirus, identified as HIV, transmitted through sexual contact or exposure to contaminated blood or other body fluids of infected residents, including breast milk. Initial symptoms include extreme fatigue, intermittent fever, night sweats, chills, lymphadenopathy, enlarged spleen, anorexia and consequent weight loss, severe diarrhea, apathy, and depression. As the disease progresses, there is a general failure to thrive, anergy, and any number and kind of recurring opportunistic infections may appear, most commonly Pneumocystis carinii pneumonia, meningitis, or encephalitis caused by aspergillosis, candidiasis, crytococcosis, cytomegalovirus, toxoplasmosis, or herpes simplex. Most residents with the disorder are susceptible to malignant neoplasms, especially Kaposi's sarcoma,

Burkitt's lymphoma, and non-Hodgkin's lymphoma, which cause as well as result from immunodeficiency.

ACTH (adrenocorticotropic hormone)

See adrenocorticotropic hormone.

actinic keratoses

A slowly developing, localized thickening of the outer layers of the skin as a result of chronic, prolonged exposure to the sun. Treatment of this potentially malignant lesion includes surgical excision, cryotherapy, and topical chemotherapy. Also called senile keratosis, senile wart, solar keratosis.

activities of daily living (ADL)

Activities usually performed in the course of a normal day in a person's life, such as eating, toileting, dressing, washing, or brushing the teeth. The ability to perform ADLs may be compromised by a variety of causes, including chronic illnesses and accidents. The limitation imposed may be temporary or permanent; rehabilitation may involve relearning the skills or learning new ways to accomplish an activity. Health care professionals have significant roles in helping a person to maintain or regain his or her ability to perform the necessary ADLs, thus remaining independent to the greatest degree possible. An ADL checklist is often used before discharge from a hospital. If any ADLs cannot be performed adequately, arrangements are made with an outside agency, such as a visiting nurse service, or with family members to provide the necessary assistance. Follow-up with physical therapy or other health care professionals such as occupational therapy on an outpatient basis may be useful in maintaining or increasing the resident's ability to perform the ADLs.

adipsia

Absence of thirst.

ADL (activities of daily living)

See activities of daily living.

adrenocorticotropic hormone (ACTH)

A hormone of the anterior pituitary gland that stimulates the growth of the adrenal cortex and the secretion of corticosteroids. ACTH secretion, regulated by corticotropin releasing factor from the hypothalamus, increases in response to a low level of circulating cortisol and to stress, fever, acute hypoglycemia, and major surgery. Under normal conditions there is a diurnal rhythm in ACTH secretion with an increase beginning after the first few hours of sleep and reaching a peak at the time a person awakens. ACTH stimulates the formation of cyclic adenosine monophosphate (cAMP), which is thought to activate the enzyme system that catalyzes the conversion of cholesterol to pregnenolone, the precursor of all steroidal hormones. A purified preparation of ACTH in gelatin is used widely in the treatment of rheumatoid arthritis, acquired hemolytic anemia, intractable allergic states, various dermatologic diseases, and many other disorders. Normal findings range from 15 to 100 pg/ml or 10 to 80 ng/L (AM) to less than 50 pg/ml or 50 ng/L (PM). Also called adrenocorticotrophic hormone, corticotropin.

advance directives

The means by which an individual prepares for the time when he or she can no longer make his or her own health-care decisions. See also written advance directive.

AFB (acid-fast bacillus)

See acid-fast bacillus.

agonist

1. A contracting muscle whose contraction is opposed by another muscle. 2. A drug or other substance having a specific cellular affinity that produces a predictable response.

AIDS (acquired immunodeficiency syndrome)

See acquired immunodeficiency syndrome.

akathisia

A pathologic condition characterized by restlessness and agitation, such as an inability to sit still.

allopurinol

A xanthine oxidase inhibitor.

Indications: It is prescribed in the treatment of gout and other hyperuricemic conditions.

Alzheimer's disease

Presenile dementia, characterized by confusion, memory failure, disorientation, restlessness, agnosia, speech disturbances, inability to carry out purposeful movements, and hallucinosis. The patient may become hypomanic, refuse food, and lose sphincter control without focal impairment. The disease usually begins in later middle life with slight defects in memory and behavior, and occurs with equal frequency in men and women. Typical pathologic features are miliary plaques in the cortex and fibrillary degeneration within pyramidal ganglion cells. Treatment can only be palliative. Nursing care is concerned primarily with preventing injury, promoting activity, promoting sleep, and preventing agitation and violence.

amaurosis fugax

Transient episodic blindness due to decreased flow to the retina.

amyotrophic lateral sclerosis

A degenerative disease of the motor neurons that is characterized by weakness and atrophy of the muscles of the hands, forearms, and legs, spreading to involve most of the body and face. It results from degeneration of the motor neurons of the anterior horns and corticospinal tracts, beginning in middle age

and progressing rapidly, causing death within 2 to 5 years. There is no known treatment.

anhidrosis

An abnormal condition characterized by inadequate perspiration.

anomia

A form of aphasia caused by a lesion in the temporal lobe of the brain. It is characterized by the inability to name objects.

anthropometric measurements

The science of measuring the human body with regard to height, weight, and size of component parts, including measurement of skinfolds, to study and compare the relative proportions under normal and abnormal conditions.

anticholinergic

1. Of or pertaining to a blockade of acetylcholine receptors that results in the inhibition of the transmission of parasympathetic nerve impulses. 2. An anticholinergic that functions by competing with the neurotransmitter acetylcholine for its receptor sites at synaptic junctions. Anticholinergic drugs reduce spasms of smooth muscle in the bladder, bronchi, and intestine; relax the iris sphincter; decrease gastric, bronchial, and salivary secretions; decrease perspiration; and accelerate impulse conduction through the myocardium by blocking vagal impulses. Many anticholinergic agents reduce parkinsonian symptoms; atropine in large doses stimulates the central nervous system and in small doses acts as a depressant. Among numerous cholinergic blocking agents are anisotropine methylbromide, belladonna, glycopyrrolate, hyoscyamine sulfate, methixene hydrochloride, and scopolamine. Various members of the group are used to treat spastic disorders of the gastrointestinal tract, to reduce salivary and bronchial secretions preoperatively, or to dilate the pupil.

antiemetic

1. Of or pertaining to a substance or procedure that prevents or alleviates nausea and vomiting. 2. An antiemetic drug or agent. Belladonna derivatives, bromides, barbiturates and other sedatives, and substances that protect the stomach lining, such as lime water or mild gastric astringents, have weak antiemetic properties. Chlorpromazine and other phenothiazines are sometimes effective antiemetic agents. In motion sickness scopolamine and antihistamines provide relief. Marijuana may alleviate the nausea induced by certain antineoplastic drugs in cancer patients.

antiinflammatory

1. Of or pertaining to a substance or procedure that counteracts or reduces inflammation. 2. An antiinflammatory drug or agent. Betamethasone, prednisolone, prednisone, and other synthetic glucocorticoids are used extensively in treating inflammation. The basis of the antiinflammatory effect of salicylates and nonsteroidal antiinflammatory agents, such as phenylbutazone and indomethacin, appears to involve inhibition of prostaglandin biosynthesis.

aphasia

An abnormal neurologic condition in which language function is defective or absent owing to injury to certain areas of the cerebral cortex. The deficiency may be sensory or receptive, in which language is not understood, or expressive or motor, in which words cannot be formed or expressed. Sensory aphasia may be complete or partial, affecting specific language functions, as in dyslexia or alexia. Expressive aphasia may be complete, as in dysphasia, in which speech is impaired, or as in agraphia, in which writing is affected, or it may be partial, diminishing either or both functions. Most commonly, the condition is a mixture of incomplete expressive and receptive aphasia. It may occur after severe head trauma, prolonged hypoxia, or cardiovascular accident. It is sometimes transient, as when the swelling in the brain that follows a stroke or injury subsides and language returns.

apraxia

An impairment in the ability to perform purposeful acts or to manipulate objects. Ideational apraxia is characterized by impairment caused by a loss of the perception of the use of an object. Motor apraxia is characterized by an inability to use an object or perform a task without any loss of perception of the use of the object or the goal of the task. Amnestic apraxia is characterized by an inability to perform the function because of an inability to remember the command to perform it. Apraxia of speech is an articulatory disorder caused by brain damage that results in an inability to program the position of speech muscles and the sequence of muscle movements necessary to produce understandable speech.

atelectasis

An abnormal condition characterized by the collapse of lung tissue, preventing the respiratory exchange of carbon dioxide and oxygen. Symptoms may include diminished breath sounds, a mediastinal shift toward the side of the collapse, fever, and increasing dyspnea. The condition may be caused by obstruction of the major airways and bronchioles, by pressure on the lung from fluid or air in the pleural space, or by pressure from a tumor outside the lung. As the remaining portions of the lung eventually hyperinflate, oxygen saturation of the blood is often nearly normal. Loss of functional lung tissue may secondarily cause increased heart rate, blood pressure, and respiratory rate. The retained secretions are rich in nutrients for the growth of bacteria, a condition often leading to stasis pneumonia in critically ill patients.

Babinski's reflex

Dorsiflexion of the big toe with extension and fanning of the other toes elicited by firmly stroking the lateral aspect of the sole of the foot. The reflex is normal in newborn infants and abnormal in children and adults, in whom it may indicate a lesion in the pyramidal tract.

bacteremia

The presence of bacteria in the blood. Undocumented bacteremias occur frequently and usually abate spontaneously. Bacteremia is demonstrated by blood culture. Antibiotic treatment, if given, is specific for the organism found and appropriate to the locus of infection.

bacteriuria

The presence of bacteria in the urine. The presence of more than 100,000 pathogenic bacteria per milliliter of urine is usually considered significant and diagnostic of a urinary tract infection.

basal cell carcinoma

A malignant epithelial cell tumor that begins as a papule and enlarges peripherally, developing a central crater that erodes, crusts, and bleeds. Metastasis is rare, but local invasion destroys underlying and adjacent tissue. In 90 % of cases the lesion is seen between the hairline and the upper lip. The primary cause of the cancer is excessive exposure to the sun or to x-rays. Treatment is eradication of the lesion, often by electrodesiccation of the lesion or cryotherapy. Also called basal cell epithelioma, basaloma, basiloma, carcinoma basocellulare, hair matrix carcinoma.

blepharitis

An inflammatory condition of the lash follicles and meibomian glands of the eyelids, characterized by swelling, redness, and crusts of dried mucus on the lids. Ulcerative blepharitis is caused by bacterial infection. Nonulcerative blepharitis may be caused by psoriasis, seborrhea, or an allergic response.

Bouchard's node

An abnormal cartilaginous or bony enlargement of a proximal interphalangeal joint of a finger, usually occurring in degenerative diseases of the joints. Compare Heberden's node.

bradykinesia

An abnormal condition characterized by slowness of all voluntary movement and speech, such as caused by parkinsonism, other extrapyramidal disorders, or certain tranquilizers.

Broca's area

An area involved in speech production that is situated on the inferior frontal gyrus of the brain. See also aphasia.

CDC (Centers for Disease Control)

See Centers for Disease Control.

cellulitis

A diffuse, acute infection of the skin and subcutaneous tissue that is characterized most commonly by local heat, redness, pain, and swelling, and occasionally by fever, malaise, chills, and headache. Abscess and tissue destruction usually follow if antibiotics are not taken. The infection is more likely to develop in the presence of damaged skin, poor circulation, or diabetes mellitus. In addition to appropriate antibiotics, treatment includes warm soaks, elevation, and avoidance of pressure to the affected areas.

Centers for Disease Control (CDC)

A federal agency of the US government that provides facilities and services for the investigation, identification, prevention, and control of disease. It is concerned with all aspects of the epidemiology and laboratory diagnosis of disease. Immunization programs, quarantine regulations and programs, laboratory standards, and community surveillance for disease are among the activities of the CDC, which is located in Atlanta. Many state and local health workers and scientists receive training in specific techniques there. Originally named the Communicable Disease Center, it was concerned only with communicable diseases; today its interests include environmental health, smoking, malnutrition, poisoning, and issues in occupational health. It's name was changed again in 1992 when 'and Prevention" was added.

central nervous system

One of the two main divisions of the nervous system of the body, consisting of the brain and spinal cord. The central nervous system processes information to and from the peripheral nervous system and is the main network of coordination and control for the entire body. The brain controls many functions and sensations, such as sleep, sexual activity, muscular movement, hunger, thirst, memory, and the emotions. The spinal cord extends various types of nerve fibers from the brain and acts as a switching and relay terminal for the peripheral nervous system. The 12 pairs of cranial nerves emerge directly from the brain. Sensory and motor nerves of the peripheral system leave the spinal cord separately between the vertebrae but unite to form 31 pairs of spinal nerves containing sensory and motor fibers. The neuroglia is comprised of more than 10 billion cells. The neurons and the neuroglia form the soft, jellylike substance of the brain, which is supported and protected by the skull. The brain and the spinal cord are composed of gray matter which contains primarily nerve cells and associated processes and white matter which consists of bundles of predominantly myelinated nerve fibers.

cerebral vascular accident (CVA)

An abnormal condition of the blood vessels of the brain characterized by an embolus, thrombus, or cerebrovascular hemorrhage, resulting in ischemia of the brain tissues normally perfused by the damaged vessels. The sequelae of a CVA depend on the location and extent of ischemia. Paralysis, weakness, sensory change, speech defect, aphasia, or death may occur. Symptoms remit somewhat after the first few days as brain swelling subsides.

chalazion

A small, localized swelling of the eyelid resulting from obstruction and retained secretions of the meibomian glands. It is a nonmalignant condition that often requires surgery for correction.

chickenpox

An acute, highly contagious viral disease caused by a herpes virus, varicella zoster virus. It occurs primarily in young children and is characterized by crops of pruritic vesicular eruptions on the skin. The disease is transmitted by direct contact with skin lesions, or more commonly, by droplets spread from the respiratory tracts of infected persons, usually in the prodromal period or the early stages of the rash. The vesicular fluid and the scabs are infectious until entirely dry. Indirect transmission through uninfected persons or objects is rare. The diagnosis is usually made by physical examination and by the characteristic appearance of the disease. The virus may be identified by culture of the vesicle fluid. Also called varicella.

chronic obstructive pulmonary disease (COPD)

A progressive and irreversible condition characterized by the diminished inspiratory and expiratory capacity of the lungs. Persons with COPD complain of dyspnea with physical exertion, difficulty in inhaling or exhaling deeply, and sometimes a chronic cough. The condition includes chronic bronchitis, pulmonary emphysema, asthma, or chronic bronchiectasis and is aggravated by cigarette smoking and air pollution.

circadian rhythm

A pattern based on a 24-hour cycle, especially the repetition of certain physiologic phenomena, such as sleeping and eating.

claudication

Cramplike pains in the calves caused by poor circulation of the blood to the leg muscles. The condition is commonly associated with atherosclerosis. Intermittent claudication is a form of the disorder that is manifested only at certain times, usually after an extended period of walking, and is relieved by rest.

clonus

An abnormal pattern of neuromuscular activity, characterized by rapidly alternating involuntary contraction and relaxation of skeletal muscle.

closed reduction of fractures

The manual reduction of a fracture without incision.

computed tomography (CT)

A radiographic technique that produces a film representing a detailed cross section of tissue structure. The procedure is painless, noninvasive, and requires no special preparation. CT employs a narrowly collimated beam of x-rays that rotates in a continuous 360 motion around the patient to image the body in cross-sectional slices. An array of detectors, positioned at several angles, records those x-rays that pass through the body. The image is created by computer using multiple attenuation readings taken around the periphery of the body part. The computer calculates tissue absorption, displays a printout of the numeric

values, and produces a visualization of the tissues that demonstrates the densities of the various structures. Tumor masses, infarctions, bone displacement, and accumulations of fluid may be detected. Formerly called computerized axial tomography.

conduction aphasia

A dissociative speech phenomenon in which there is no difficulty in comprehending words seen or heard and in which there is no dysarthria, yet the patient has problems in self-expression. The patient may substitute words similar in sound or meaning for the correct ones but is unable to repeat from dictation, to spell, or to read aloud. The patient is alert and aware of the deficit. A common cause is an embolus in a branch of the middle cerebral artery. The caregiver should try to reduce tension and frustration in the patient, encourage socialization, find the best means of communication for the patient, use simple language and direct questions requiring simple answers, and help the family to understand the problem and to deal with it.

congestive heart failure

An abnormal condition that reflects impaired cardiac pumping, caused by myocardial infarction, ischemic heart disease, or cardiomyopathy. Failure of the ventricle to eject blood efficiently results in volume overload, chamber dilatation, and elevated intracardiac pressure. Retrograde transmission of increased hydrostatic pressure from the left heart causes pulmonary congestion; elevated right heart pressure causes systemic venous congestion and peripheral edema.

contracture

An abnormal, usually permanent condition of a joint, characterized by flexion and fixation and caused by atrophy and shortening of muscle fibers or by loss of the normal elasticity of the skin, such as from the formation of extensive scar tissue over a joint.

crystal-induced arthritis

Acute arthritis due to the release of crystalline material into the joint space. Crystal material usually consists of sodium urate (gout), calcium pytophosphate (pseudogout), or hydroxyapatite.

CT (computed tomography)

See computed tomography.

CVA

See cerebral vascular accident.

dementia

A progressive, organic mental disorder characterized by chronic personality disintegration, confusion, disorientation, stupor, deterioration of intellectual capacity and function, and impairment of control of memory, judgment, and impulses. Dementia caused by drug intoxication, hyperthyroidism, pernicious anemia, paresis, subdural hematoma, benign brain tumor, hydrocephalus, insulin shock, and tumor of islet cells of the pancreas can be reversed by treating the condition; Alzheimer's disease, Pick's disease, Huntington's disease, and traumatic injuries to the brain are not amenable to treatment. Types of dementia include Alzheimer's disease, dementia paralytica, Pick's disease, secondary dementia, senile dementia, and toxic dementia.

depression

1. A depressed area, hollow, or fossa; downward or inward displacement. 2. A decrease of vital functional activity. 3. A mood disturbance characterized by feelings of sadness, despair, and discouragement resulting from and normally proportionate to some personal loss or tragedy. 4. An abnormal emotional state characterized by exaggerated feelings of sadness, melancholy, dejection, worthlessness, emptiness, and hopelessness that are inappropriate and out of proportion to reality. The overt manifestations, which are extremely variable, range from a slight lack of motivation and inability to concentrate to severe physiologic alterations of body functions and may represent symptoms of a variety of mental and physical conditions, a syndrome of related symptoms associated with a particular disease, or a specific mental illness. The condition is neurotic when the precipitating cause is an intrapsychic conflict or a traumatic situation or event that is identifiable, even though the person is unable to explain the overreaction to it. The condition is psychotic when there is severe physical and mental functional impairment because of some unidentifiable intrapsychic conflict; it is often accompanied by hallucinations, delusions, and confusion concerning time, place, and identity. Depression may be expressed in a wide spectrum of affective, physiologic, cognitive, and behavioral manifestations. The varied behaviors represent the complex actions, reactions, and interactions of the depressed person to stimuli that may be either internal or external. Because the origin of depression can be genetic, pharmacologic, endocrinal, infectious, nutritional, neoplastic, or neurologic, the behavioral effects can appear as aggression or withdrawal, anorexia or overeating, anger or apathy, or any of a myriad of responses.

dermatitis

An inflammatory condition of the skin characterized by erythema and pain or pruritis. Various cutaneous eruptions occur and may be unique to a particular allergen, disease, or infection. The condition may be chronic or acute; treatment is specific to the cause. Types of dermatitis include actinic dermatitis, contact dermatitis, rhus dermatitis, and seborrheic dermatitis..

diplopia

Double vision caused by defective function of the extraocular muscles or a disorder of the nerves that innervate the muscles.

diverticulitis

Inflammation of one or more diverticula. The penetration of fecal matter through the thin-walled diverticula causes inflammation and abscess formation in the tissues surrounding the colon. With repeated inflammation, the lumen of the colon narrows and may become obstructed. During periods of inflammation, the patient will experience crampy pain, particularly over the sigmoid colon, fever, and leukocytosis. Barium enemas and proctoscopy are performed to rule out carcinoma of the colon, which exhibits some of the same symptoms. Conservative treatment includes bed rest, intravenous fluids, antibiotics, and nothing taken by mouth. In acute cases, bowel resection of the affected area greatly reduces mortality and morbidity.

diverticulosis

The presence of pouchlike herniations through the muscular layer of the colon, particularly the sigmoid colon. Diverticulosis affects increasing numbers of people over 50 years of age and may be the result of the modern, highly refined, low-residue diet. Most patients with this condition have few symptoms except for occasional bleeding from the rectum. Other reasons for bleeding, such as carcinoma and inflammatory bowel disease, must be ruled out. Barium enemas and proctoscopic examination are used in establishing diagnosis. An increase in the dietary fiber can aid in propelling the feces through the colon. Hemorrhage from bleeding diverticula can become quite severe, and the patient may require surgery. Diverticulosis may lead to diverticulitis.

DNH

Abbreviation for Do Not Hospitalize.

DNR

Abbreviation for do not resuscitate. This may also be referred to as "no code." The resident's status as "DNR" or "No Code" must be documented in the resident record by a physician. This documentation instructs the staff of a facility not to attempt to resuscitate a particular resident in the event of cardiac or respiratory failure. This decision needs to be made as part of a discussion involving the resident, family, and staff. The resident (or family member, if authorized) has a right to change their mind about this decision at any time.

drug exanthema

An inflammatory eruption of the skin caused by an allergic reaction to drugs.

dysarthria

Difficult, poorly articulated speech resulting from interference in the control over the muscles of speech, usually because of damage to a central or peripheral motor nerve.

dysesthesia

A common effect of spinal cord injury characterized by sensations of numbness, tingling, burning, or pain felt below the level of the lesion.

dyskinesia

An impairment of the ability to execute voluntary movements. Tardive dyskinesia is one type caused by an adverse effect of prolonged use of phenothiazine medications in elderly patients or those with brain injuries.

dyspnea

Shortness of breath or difficulty in breathing that may be caused by certain heart conditions, strenuous exercise, or anxiety.

dystonia

Any impairment of muscle tone. The condition commonly involves the head, neck, and tongue, and often occurs as an adverse effect of a medication.

ectropion

Eversion, most commonly of the eyelid, exposing the conjunctival membrane lining the eyelid and part of the eyeball. The condition may involve only the lower eyelid or both eyelids. The cause may be paralysis of the facial nerve or, in an older person, atrophy of the eyelid tissues.

electrodesiccation

A technique in electrosurgery in which tissue is destroyed by burning it with an electrical spark. It is used primarily for eliminating small superficial growths but may be used with curettage for eradicating abnormal tissue deeper in the skin. In the latter case, layers of skin may be burned, than successively scraped away. The procedure is performed with the patient under local anesthesia.

embolus

A foreign object, a quantity of air or gas, a bit of tissue or tumor, or a piece of a thrombus that circulates in the bloodstream until it becomes lodged in a vessel. Types of emboli include air embolus and fat embolus.

emphysema

An abnormal condition of the pulmonary system, characterized by overinflation and destructive changes of alveolar walls, resulting in a loss of lung elasticity and decreased gases. When emphysema occurs early in life, it is usually related to a rare genetic deficiency of serum alpha-1-antitrypsin, which inactivates the enzymes leukocyte collagenase and elastase. Acute emphysema may be caused by the rupture of alveoli by severe respiratory efforts, as in acute bronchopneumonia, suffocation, and whooping cough, and occasionally during labor. Chronic emphysema usually accompanies chronic bronchitis, a major cause of which is cigarette smoking. Emphysema is also seen after asthma or tuberculosis, conditions in which the lungs are overstretched until the elastic fibers of the alveolar walls are destroyed. In old age, the alveolar membranes atrophy and may collapse, resulting in large air-filled spaces with decreased total surface area of the pulmonary membranes.

entropion

Turning inward or turning toward, usually a condition in which the eyelid turns inward toward the eye.

erythema multiforme

A hypersensitivity syndrome characterized by polymorphous eruption of skin and mucous membranes. Macules, papules, nodules, vesicles or bullae, and target (bull's-eye-shaped) lesions are seen. Erythema multiforme has been associated with many infections, collagen diseases, drug sensitivities, allergies, and pregnancy. Definitive and preventive treatment depends on finding the specific cause, but topical or systemic corticosteroids are helpful in most cases.

exanthema

A skin eruption or rash that may have specific diagnostic features of an infectious disease, Chickenpox, measles, roseola infantum, and rubella are usually characterized by a particular type of exanthema. Also called exanthem.

fasciitis

1. An inflammation of the connective tissue, which may be caused by streptococcal or other types of infection, or an autoimmune reaction. 2. An abnormal, benign growth (Pseudosarcomatous fasciitis) resembling a tumor that develops in the subcutaneous oral

tissues, usually in the cheek. Commonly growing rapidly and then regressing, fasciitis consists of young fibroblasts and many capillaries and may be mistaken for fibrosarcoma. Also called fascitis.

flaccid

Weak, soft, and flabby; lacking normal muscle tone, such as flaccid muscles.

fluctuation

1. A wavelike motion of fluid in a body cavity after succussion. 2. A variation in a fixed value or mass.

fluent aphasia

Forms of aphasia in which the patient is able to say words easily even though the words may be unintelligible or not be related to a particular stimulus. Types of fluent aphasia include Wernicke's aphasia and conduction aphasia.

forced expiratory volume (FEV)

The volume of air that can be forcibly expelled in a fixed time period after full inspiration.

glenohumeral joint

The shoulder joint formed by the glenoid cavity of the scapula and the head of the humerus.

global aphasia

A loss of the ability to use any form of written or spoken language. The condition involves both sensory and motor nerve tracts. Communication is attempted through primitive gestures or the use of automatic words and phrases.

Heberden's node

An abnormal cartilaginous or bony enlargement of a distal interphalangeal joint of a finger, usually occurring in degenerative diseases of the joints. Compare Bouchard's node.

hemianopia

Defective vision or blindness in one half of the visual field. Also called hemiamblyopia.

hemiarthroplasty

A surgical procedure for repair of an injured or diseased hip joint that involves replacement of the head of the femur with a prosthesis without reconstruction of the acetabulum.

hemiopia

A condition involving only one eye or half the visual field.

hemiparesis

Muscular weakness of one half of the body.

hemiplegia

Paralysis of one side of the body. Types of hemiplegia include cerebral hemiplegia, facial hemiplegia, and spastic hemiplegia.

hemorrhage

A loss of a large amount of blood in a short period of time, either externally or internally. Hemorrhage may be arterial, venous, or capillary.

Observations: Symptoms of massive hemorrhage are related to hypovolemic shock: rapid, thready pulse; thirst; cold, clammy skin; sighing respirations; dizziness; syncope; pallor; apprehension; restlessness; and hypotension. If bleeding is contained within a cavity or joint, pain will develop as the capsule or cavity is stretched by the rapidly expanding volume of blood.

Interventions: Effort is directed toward stopping the hemorrhage. If the hemorrhage is external, pressure is applied directly to the wound or to the appropriate pressure points. Ice, applied directly to the wound, may slow bleeding by causing vasoconstriction. Body temperature may be maintained by keeping the person covered and flat. If an extremity is wounded, and if the bleeding is severe, a tourniquet may be applied proximal to the wound.

herpes zoster

An acute infection caused by reactivation of the latent varicella zoster virus, affecting mainly adults and characterized by the development of painful vesicular skin eruptions that follow the underlying route of cranial or spinal nerves inflamed by the virus. Also called shingles.

HIV (human immunodeficiency virus)

See human immunodeficiency virus

homonymous hemianopia

Blindness or defective vision in the right or left halves of the visual fields of both eyes.

Human immunodeficiency virus (HIV)

A type of retrovirus that causes AIDS. Retroviruses produce the enzyme reverse transcriptase, which allows transcription of the viral genome onto the DNA of the host cell. HIV is transmitted through contact with an infected individual's blood, semen, cervical secretions, cerebrospinal fluid, or synovial fluid. HIV infects T-helper cells of the immune system and results in infection with an incubation averaging 10 years. With the immune system destroyed, AIDS develops as Kaposi's sarcoma, pneumocystis carinii pneumonia, candidias, and tuberculosis, all of which attack organ systems throughout the body. Aside from the initial antibody tests that establish the diagnosis for HIV infection, the most important laboratory test for monitoring the infection is the CD4 lymphocyte test which determines the percentage of T lymphocytes that are CD4 positive; CD4 counts of greater than 500/mm^3 are considered most likely to respond to treatment of alpha-interferon α and/or zidovudine. A significant drop in the CD4 count is a signal for therapeutic intervention with antiretroviral therapy. Vaccines based on glycoprotein 120 and glycoprotein 160 are being investigated. These vaccines are designed to boost the immune system of people already infected with HIV. See also acquired immunodeficiency syndrome (AIDS).

hyperesthesia

An extreme sensitivity of one of the body's sense organs, such as pain or touch receptors in the skin.

hypertonic

Having a greater concentration of solute than another solution, hence exerting more osmotic pressure than that solution, such as a hypertonic saline solution that contains more salt than is found in intracellular and extracellular fluid. Cells shrink in a hypertonic solution. Compare isotonic.

hypodermoclysis

The injection of an isotonic or hypotonic solution into subcutaneous tissue to supply a patient with a continuous and large amount of fluid, electrolytes, and nutrients. The procedure is used to replace the loss or inadequate intake of water and salt during illness or surgery or after shock or hemorrhage and is performed only when the patient is unable to take fluids intravenously, orally, or rectally. The rate of absorption into the circulatory system is increased with the addition to the solution of the enzyme hyaluronidase. The most common sites of administration are the anterior thighs, the abdominal wall along the crest of the ilium, below the breasts in women, and directly over the scapula in children; sites should be changed when multiple infusions are given. The patient is placed in a comfortable position because the procedure takes a long time. The nurse observes for signs of circulatory collapse, respiratory difficulty, and edema at the site of injection.

hyponatremia

A less than normal concentration of sodium in the blood, caused by inadequate excretion of water or excessive water in the circulating bloodstream. In a severe case, the person may develop water intoxication, with confusion and lethargy, leading to muscle excitability, convulsions, and coma. Fluid and electrolyte balance may by restored by intravenous infusion of a balanced solution.

hypotonic

Having a smaller concentration of solute than another solution, hence exerting less osmotic pressure than that solution, such as a hypotonic saline solution that contains less salt than is found in intracellular or extracellular fluid. Cells expand in a hypotonic solution.

hypoventilation

An abnormal condition of the respiratory system, characterized by cyanosis, polycythemia, increased carbon dioxide arterial tension, and generalized decreased respiratory function. It occurs when the volume of air that enters the alveoli and takes part in gas exchanges is not adequate for the metabolic needs of the body. Hypoventilation may be caused by uneven distribution of inspired air (such as in bronchitis), obesity, neuromuscular or skeletal disease affecting the thorax, decreased response of the respiratory center to carbon dioxide, and reduced functional lung tissue, such as in atelectasis, emphysema, and pleural effusion. The result of hypoventilation is hypoxia, hypercapnia, pulmonary hypertension with cor pulmonale, and respiratory acidosis. Treatment includes weight reduction (in cases of obesity) artificial respiration, and possibly tracheostomy.

hypovolemia

An abnormally low circulating blood volume.

ichthyosis

Any of several inherited dermatologic conditions in which the skin is dry, hyperkeratotic, and fissured, resembling fish scales. It usually appears at or shortly after birth and may be part of one of several rare syndromes. Some types respond temporarily to bath oils, topical retinoic acid, or propylene glycol. A rare acquired variety occurs in adults accompanying a lymphoma or multiple myeloma.

impacted fracture

A bone break in which the adjacent fragmented ends of the fractured bone are wedged together.

incontinence

The inability to control urination or defecation. Urinary incontinence may be caused by cerebral clouding in the aged, infection, lesions in the brain or spinal cord, damage to peripheral nerves of the bladder, or injury to the sphincter or perineal structures, sometimes occurring in childbirth. Treatment includes bladder retraining, the implantation of an artificial sphincter, and the use of internal or external drainage devices. Stress incontinence precipitated by coughing, straining, or heavy lifting occurs more often in women than in men, and mild cases may be treated by exercises involving tightening and relaxing perineal and gluteal muscles, or they may respond to sympathomimetic drug therapy. Severe cases may require surgery to correct the underlying anatomic defect. Fecal incontinence may result from relaxation of the anal sphincter or by central nervous system or spinal cord disorders and may be treated by a program of bowel training. A Bradford frame with an opening for a bedpan or urinal may be used for bedridden incontinent patients.

infarction

1.The development and formation of an infarct. 2. An infarct. Types of infarction include myocardial infarction and pulmonary infarction.

infection

1. The invasion of the body by pathogenic microorganisms that reproduce and multiply, causing disease by local cellular injury, secretion of a toxin, or antigen-antibody reaction on the host. 2. A disease caused by the invasion of the body by pathogenic microorganisms.

ischemia

A decreased supply of oxygenated blood to a body organ or part, often marked by pain and organ dysfunction, as in ischemic heart disease. Some causes of ischemia are arterial embolism, atherosclerosis, thrombosis, and vasoconstriction. Compare infarction.

isotonic

Having the same concentration of solute as another solution, hence exerting the same amount of osmotic pressure as that solution, such as an isotonic saline solution that contains an amount of salt equal to that found in the intra- and extracellular fluid.

Kaposi's sarcoma (KS)

Begins as red or purple papules on the feet and slowly spreads in the skin, metastasizing to the lymph nodes and viscera. It is occasionally associated with diabetes, malignant lymphoma, AIDS, or other disorders.

KS (Kaposi's sarcoma)

See Kaposi's sarcoma.

lacuna

1. A small cavity within a structure, especially bony tissue. 2. A gap, as in the field of vision.

lacunar

Pertaining to or characterized by the presence of pits, depressions, hollows, or spaces.

lacunar state

A pseudobulbar disorder characterized by the appearance of small, smooth-walled cavities in the brain tissue. The condition usually follows a series of small strokes, particularly in older adults with arterial hypertension and arteriosclerosis.

laryngectomy

Surgical removal of the larynx, performed to treat cancer of the larynx. Before surgery, the patient is referred to a speech pathologist to discuss esophageal speech and prostheses. Antibiotics are usually administered to reduce the risk of infection. With the patient under regional or general anesthesia, the trachea is sutured to the skin, as in a tracheostomy, to ensure an adequate airway. In a partial laryngectomy only the vocal cords are removed, and the tracheostomy is closed within several days. If the malignancy is extensive, the entire larynx is removed, along with the thyroid cartilage and epiglottis; the tracheostomy is permanent, and a laryngectomy tube left in place. After surgery the patient is observed for excessive coughing or any vomiting of blood, and the laryngectomy tube is kept free of mucus. A humidifier or vaporizer is useful to decrease coughing and the production of mucus. Intravenous fluids are given, and liquid feedings may be given via nasogastric tube. A Magic Slate is useful for communication between patient, staff, and family. The laryngectomy tube is removed 3 to 6 weeks after surgery.

levodopa

An antiparkinsonian medication.

magnetic resonance imaging (MRI)

Medical imaging that uses nuclear magnetic resonance as its source of energy.

melanoma

Any of a group of malignant neoplasms, primarily of the skin, that are composed of melanocytes. Most melanomas develop from a pigmented nevus over a period of several months or years and occur most commonly in fair-skinned people with light-colored eyes. A previous sunburn also increases a person's risk. Any black or brown spot having an irregular border; pigment appearing to radiate beyond that border; a red, black, and blue coloration observable on close examination; or a nodular surface is suggestive of melanoma and is usually excised for biopsy. Prognosis depends on the kind of melanoma; its size, depth of invasion, and location; and the age and condition of the patient. Types of melanoma include amelanotic melanoma, benign juvenile melanoma, lentigo maligna melanoma, nodular melanoma, primary cutaneous melanoma, and superficial spreading melanoma.

Moh's micrographic surgery

Specialized surgical technique that minimizes tissue loss by using multiple frozen sections.

MRI (magnetic resonance imaging)

See magnetic resonance imaging.

multiinfarct dementia

A form of organic brain disease, caused by vascular disease that is characterized by the rapid deterioration of intellectual functioning. Symptoms include emotional lability, disturbances in memory, abstract thinking, judgment and impulse control, and focal neurologic impairment such as gait abnormalities, pseudobulbar palsy, and paresthesia.

multiple sclerosis

A progressive disease characterized by disseminated demyelination of nerve fibers of the brain and spinal cord. It begins slowly, usually in young adulthood, and continues throughout life with periods of exacerbation and remission. The first signs are paresthesias, or abnormal sensations in the extremities or on one side of the face. Other early signs are muscle weakness, vertigo, and visual disturbances, such as nystagmus, diplopia, and partial blindness. Later in the course of disease there may be extreme emotional lability, ataxia, abnormal reflexes, and difficulty in urination. Because many other conditions affect the nervous system and produce similar symptoms, the diagnosis of multiple sclerosis is difficult to make. A history of exacerbation and remission of symptoms and the presence of greater than normal amounts of protein in cerebrospinal fluid are characteristic. As the disease progresses, the intervals between exacerbations grow shorter and disability becomes greater. There is no specific treatment for the disease; corticosteroids and other drugs are used to treat the symptoms accompanying acute episodes. Physical therapy may help to postpone or prevent specific disabilities. The patient is encouraged to live as normal and active a life as possible.

Mycobacterium

A genus of rod-shaped, acid-fast bacteria having two significant pathogenic species: Mycobacterium leprae causes leprosy; M. tuberculosis causes tuberculosis.

myelopathy

Damage to the spinal cord nerves that causes extremity weakness, difficulty in walking, and
loss of bladder and bowel control.

myoclonus

A spasm of a muscle or a group of muscles.

neglect

A condition that occurs after a stroke in which a patient does not see on one side of the body, leading to a "neglect" of that area. During rehabilitation, patients are taught techniques to compensate for this loss.

nevus

A pigmented, congenital skin blemish that is usually benign but may become cancerous. Any change in color, size, or texture or any bleeding or itching of a nevus merits investigation. Also called birthmark, mole.

nonpressure ulcers

An open sore or lesion of the skin, with loss of substance, sometimes accompanied by the formation of pus. This can result from venous stasis ulceration, arterial ischemic ulcer, diabetic ulcer, vasculitic ulcer, embolic ulcer, and a malignancy.

Norwegian scabies

A severe infestation of human skin by an itch mite (Sarcoptes scabiei). The condition is associated with intense itching, crusting and scaling of the skin, and insect egg burrows that appear as discolored lines in the affected skin areas.

NREM

Abbreviation for Nonrapid Eye Movement.

NSAID

Abbreviation for Nonsteroidal Antiinflammatory Drug.

onychogryphosis

Thickened, curved, clawlike overgrowth of fingernails or toenails.

onychomycosis

Any fungal infection of the nails.

orthostatic hypotension

Abnormally low blood pressure occurring when an individual assumes the standing posture.

osmolarity

The osmotic pressure of a solution expressed in osmols or milliosmols per liter of the solution.

osteoarthritis

A form of arthritis in which one or many joints undergo degenerative changes, including subchondral bony sclerosis, loss of articular cartilage, and proliferation of bone and cartilage in the joint, forming osteophytes. Inflammation of the synovial membrane of the joint is common in late disease. The most common form of arthritis, its cause is unknown but may include chemical, mechanical, genetic, metabolic, and endocrine factors. Emotional stress often aggravates the condition. The condition usually begins with pain after exercise or use of the joint. Stiffness, tenderness to the touch, crepitus, and enlargement develop, and deformity, subluxation, and synovial effusion may eventually occur. Involvement of the hip, knee, or spine causes more disability than osteoarthritis of other areas. Treatment includes rest of the involved joints, heat, and antiinflammatory drugs. Systemic corticosteroids are contraindicated, but intraarticular injections of corticosteroids may give relief. Surgical treatment is sometimes necessary and may reduce pain and greatly improve the function of a joint. Hip replacement, joint debridement, fusion, and decompression laminectomy are some of the surgical procedures used in treating advanced osteoarthritis. Compare rheumatoid arthritis.

osteomyelitis

Local or generalized infection of bone and bone marrow, usually caused by bacteria introduced by trauma or surgery, by direct extension from a nearby infection, or via the bloodstream. Staphylococci are the most common causative agents.

Observations: The long bones in children and the vertebrae in adults are the most common sites of infection as a result of hematogenous spread. Persistent, severe, and increasing bone pain, tenderness, guarding on movement, regional muscle spasm, and fever suggest this diagnosis. Draining sinus tracts may accompany posttraumatic osteomyelitis or osteomyelitis from a contiguous infection. Specific diagnosis and selection of therapy depend on bacterial examination of bone, tissue, or pus.

Interventions: Treatment includes bed rest and parenteral antibiotics for several weeks. Surgery may be necessary to remove necrotic bone and tissue, to obliterate cavities, to remove infected prosthetic devices, and to apply prostheses to stabilize affected parts. Chronic osteomyelitis may persist for years with exacerbations and remissions despite treatment.

Nursing considerations: Any drainage is disposed of using usual precautions. Absolute rest of the affected part may be necessary, with careful positioning using pillows and sandbags for good alignment. During the early phase of infection, pain is extremely severe and extraordinary gentleness in moving and manipulating the infected part is essential.

otosclerosis

A hereditary condition of unknown cause in which irregular ossification in the bony labyrinth of the inner ear, especially of the stapes, occurs, causing tinnitus then deafness. The deafness is usually first noticed between 11 and 30 years of age. Women are affected twice as often as men. The condition may worsen in pregnancy. Stapedectomy is usually successful in restoring hearing permanently.

palilalia

An abnormal condition characterized by the increasingly rapid repetition of the same word or phrase, usually at the end of a sentence.

papilloma

A benign epithelial neoplasm characterized by a branching or lobular tumor.

paresthesia

Any subjective sensation, experienced as numbness, tingling, or a 'pins and needles' feeling. Paresthesias often fluctuate according to such influences as posture, activity, rest, edema, congestion, or underlying disease. When experienced in the extremities, it is sometimes identified as acroparesthesia.

Parkinson's disease

A slowly progressive, degenerative, neurologic disorder characterized by resting tremor, pill rolling of the fingers, a masklike facies, shuffling gait, forward flexion of the trunk, loss of postural reflexes, and muscle rigidity and weakness. It is usually an idiopathic disease of people over 60 years of age, although it may occur in younger people, especially after acute encephalitis or carbon monoxide or metallic poisoning, particularly by reserpine or phenothiazine drugs. Typical pathologic changes are destruction of neurons in basal ganglia, loss of pigmented cells in the substantia nigra, and depletion of dopamine in the caudate nucleus, putamen, and pallidum, structures in the neostriatum that normally contain high levels of the neurotransmitter dopamine. Signs and symptoms, which include resting tremor, bradykinesis, drooling, increased appetite, intolerance to heat, oily skin, emotional instability, and defective judgment, are increased by fatigue, excitement, and frustration. Palliative and symptomatic treatment of the disease focuses on correcting the imbalance between depleted dopamine and abundant acetylcholine in the striatum, because dopamine normally appears to inhibit excitatory cholinergic activity in this brain area. Levodopa, a dopamine precursor that crosses the blood-brain barrier, may be used, but many patients experience side effects such as nausea, vomiting, insomnia, orthostatic hypotension, and mental confusion. Carbidopa-levodopa, which contains an inhibitor of the enzyme dopa decarboxylase, limits peripheral metabolism of levodopa and thus causes fewer side effects. Anticholinergic drugs, such as benztropine mesylate, biperiden, procyclidine, and trihexyphenidyl, may be used as therapeutic agents but often cause ataxia, blurred vision, constipation, dryness of the mouth, mental disturbances, slurred speech, and urinary urgency or retention. Amantadine hydrochloride, an antiviral drug with antiparkinsonian activity, promotes the accumulation of dopamine in extracellular or synaptic sites, but the therapeutic effectiveness may not last more than 3 months in some patients; side effects, such as mental confusion, visual disturbances, and seizures, occur infrequently.

parkinsonism

A neurologic disorder characterized by tremor; muscle rigidity; hypokinesia; a slow, shuffling gait; and difficulty in chewing, swallowing, and speaking. It is caused by various lesions in the extrapyramidal motor system. Signs and symptoms resemble those of idiopathic Parkinson's disease and may develop during or after acute encephalitis and in syphilis, malaria, poliomyelitis, and carbon monoxide poisoning. Parkinsonism frequently occurs in patients treated with antipsychotic drugs, such as amitriptyline, chlorpromazine, fluphenazine, loxapine, thioridazine, and other phenothiazine derivatives.

periostitis

Inflammation of the periosteum. The condition is caused by chronic or acute infection or trauma and is characterized by tenderness and swelling of the affected bone, pain, fever, and chills. In severe cases blood or an albuminous serous exudate forms under the membrane. In syphilitic infections, periostitis may occur as an early symptom.

peripheral nervous system

The motor and sensory nerves and ganglia outside the brain and spinal cord. The system consists of 12 pairs of cranial nerves, 31 pairs of spinal nerves, and their various branches in body organs. Sensory, or afferent, peripheral nerves transmitting information to the central nervous system and motor, or efferent, peripheral nerves carrying impulses from the brain usually travel together but separate at the cord level into a posterior sensory root and an anterior motor root. Fibers innervating the body wall are designated somatic; those supplying internal organs are termed visceral. The autonomic system includes the peripheral nerves involved in regulating cardiovascular, respiratory, endocrine, and other automatic body functions. Nerves in the sympathetic or thoracolumbar division of the autonomic system secrete norepinephrine and cause peripheral vasoconstriction, cardiac acceleration, coronary artery dilation, bronchodilation, and inhibition of peristalsis. Parasympathetic nerves, which constitute the craniosacral division of the autonomic system, secrete acetylcholine, cause peripheral vasodilation, cardiac inhibition, and bronchoconstriction, and stimulate peristalsis. Injury to a peripheral nerve results in loss of movement and sensation in the area innervated distal to the lesion.

peripheral neuropathy

Any functional or organic disorder of the peripheral nervous system. Symptoms include a burning feeling, "pins and needles," and numbing or stabbing sensations in the extremities, particularly the feet. This condition is difficult to treat with conventional analgesics.

polyuria

The excretion of an abnormally large quantity of urine. Some causes of polyuria are diabetes insipidus, diabetes mellitus, diuretics, excessive fluid intake, and hypercalcemia.

PPD (purified protein derivative)

See purified protein derivative.

presbycusis

Loss of hearing sensitivity and speech intelligibility, associated with aging.

presbyopic

Pertaining to a decrease in accommodation as one grows older, and usually resulting in hyperopia or farsightedness.

pruritus

The symptom of itching, an uncomfortable sensation leading to the urge to scratch. Scratching often results in secondary infection. Some causes of pruritus are allergy, infection, jaundice, lymphoma, and skin irritation. Treatment is best directed at the cause; symptomatic relief may be obtained by antihistamines, starch baths, topical corticosteroids, cool water, or alcohol applications.

ptosis

An abnormal condition of one or both upper eyelids in which the eyelid droops because of a congenital or acquired weakness of the levator muscle or paralysis of the third cranial nerve. Partial ptosis and a small pupil may be caused by an unusual hematologic disorder of the sympathetic portion of the autonomic nervous system. The condition may be treated surgically by shortening the levator muscle.

purified protein derivative (PPD)

The material used in testing for tuberculin sensitivity. It is a dried form of tuberculin used in testing for past or present infection with tubercle bacilli. This product is usually introduced into the skin during such tests.

PWA

Abbreviation for Person with AIDS.

range of motion (ROM)

The range of movement of a joint, from maximum extension to maximum flexion, as measured in degrees of a circle.

REM

Abbreviation for Rapid Eye Movement.

residual volume

The amount of air remaining in the lungs at the end of a maximum expiration.

rheumatoid arthritis

A chronic, destructive, sometimes deforming collagen disease that has an autoimmune component. Rheumatoid arthritis is characterized by symmetric inflammation of the synovium and increased synovial exudate, leading to thickening of the synovium and swelling of the joint. Rheumatoid arthritis usually first appears in early middle age, between 36 and 50 years of age, and most commonly in women. The course of the disease is variable but is marked most frequently by remissions and exacerbation. Also called arthritis deformans, atrophic arthritis.

scabies

A contagious disease caused by Sarcoptes scabiei, the itch mite, characterized by intense itching of the skin and excoriation from scratching. The mite, transmitted by close contact with infected humans or domestic animals, burrows into outer layers of the skin, where the female lays eggs. Two to 4 months after the first infection, sensitization to the mites and their products begins, resulting in a pruritic papular rash most common on the webs of the fingers, flexor surfaces of the wrists and on the thighs. Secondary bacterial infection may occur. Diagnosis may be microscopic identification of adult mites, larvae, or eggs in scrapings of the burrows. All contacts are treated simultaneously with lindane (1 %), crotamiton (10 %), or other scabicide applied locally. Oral antihistamines and salicylates reduce itching.

sciatica

An inflammation of the sciatic nerve, usually marked by pain and tenderness along the course of the nerve through the thigh and leg. It may result in a wasting of the muscles of the lower leg.

seborrheic dermatitis

A common, chronic, inflammatory skin disease characterized by dry or moist, greasy scales and yellowish crusts. Common sites are the scalp, eyelids, face, external surfaces of the ears, axillae, breasts, groin, and gluteal folds. In acute stages there may be an exudate and infection resulting in secondary furunculosis. Occasionally generalized exfoliation results. In some people seborrheic dermatitis is associated with paralysis agitans, diabetes mellitus, malabsorption disorders, epilepsy, or an allergic reaction to gold or arsenic. Treatment includes selenium sulfide shampoos, topical and oral corticosteroids, topical antibiotics, proper therapy for any underlying systemic disorder, and avoidance of sweating and external irritants. Types of seborrheic dermatitis include cradle cap, dandruff, and seborrheic blepharitis.

sedative-hypnotic

A drug that reversibly depresses the activity of the central nervous system, used chiefly to induce sleep and to allay anxiety. Barbiturates and many nonbarbiturate sedative-hypnotics with diverse chemical and pharmacologic properties share the ability to depress the activity of all excitable tissue, but the arousal center in the brainstem is especially sensitive to their effects. Various sedative-hypnotics and minor tranquilizers with similar effects are used in the treatment of insomnia, acute convulsive conditions, and anxiety states, and to facilitate the induction of anesthesia. Although sedative-hypnotics have a soporific effect, they may interfere with the rapid eye movement sleep associated with dreaming and, when administered to patients with fever, may act paradoxically and cause excitement rather than relaxation. Sedative-hypnotics may interfere with temperature regulation, depress oxygen consumption in various tissues, and produce nausea and skin rashes; on elderly patients they may cause dizziness, confusion, and ataxia. Drugs in this group have a high potential for abuse that often results in physical and psychologic dependence; treatment of dependence involves gradual reduction of the dosage since abrupt withdrawal frequently causes serious disorders, including convulsions. Acute reactions to an overdose of a sedative-hypnotic may be treated with an emetic, activated charcoal, gastric lavage, and measures to maintain airway patency. Among nonbarbiturate sedative-hypnotics are chloral hydrate, ethchlorvynol, ethinamate, glutethimide, paraldehyde, triclofos sodium, minor tranquilizers (chlordiazepoxide, flurazepam, diazepam), diphenhydramine, and meprobamate.

sensorineural hearing loss

A form of hearing loss in which sound is conducted normally through the external and middle ear but a defect in the inner ear or auditory nerve results in hearing loss. Sound discrimination may or may not be affected. Amplification of the sound with a hearing aid will help many people with sensorineural hearing loss, but others have an intolerance to loud noises. Hearing aids must be adjusted properly to avoid discomfort.

sleep apnea

A sleep disorder characterized by periods of an absence of attempts to breathe. The apneic person is momentarily unable to move respiratory muscles or maintain airflow through the nose and mouth.

spastic

Of or pertaining to spasms or other uncontrolled contractions of the skeletal muscles.

spasticity

A form of muscular hypertonicity with increased resistance to stretch. It usually involves the flexors of the arms and the extensors of the legs. The hypertonicity is often associated with weakness, increased deep reflexes, and diminished superficial reflexes. Moderate spasticity is characterized by movements that require great effort and lack of normal coordination. Slight spasticity may be marked by gross movements that are coordinated smoothly, but combined selective patterns are incoordinated or impossible.

spectrometry

The procedure of measuring wavelengths of light and other electromagnetic waves.

squamous cell carcinoma

A slow-growing, malignant tumor of the squamous epithelium, frequently found in the lungs and skin and occurring also in the anus, cervix, larynx, nose, and bladder. The neoplastic cells characteristically resemble prickle cells and form keratin pearls on the surface of lesions. Also called epidermoid carcinoma.

status epilepticus

A medical emergency characterized by continual seizures occurring without interruptions. Status epilepticus can be precipitated by the sudden withdrawal of anticonvulsant drugs, inadequate body levels of glucose, a brain tumor, a head injury, a high fever, or poisoning. Therapy includes intravenous administration of anticonvulsant drugs, nutrients, and electrolytes. An adequate airway is usually maintained with an oral pharyngeal or endotracheal tube.

stereognosis

1. The faculty of perceiving and understanding the form and nature of objects by the sense of touch. 2. Perception by the senses of the solidity of objects.

stress incontinence

See incontinence.

sundowning

A condition in which elderly people tend to become confused or disoriented at the end of the day. Many of them have diminished visual acuity and varying degrees of sensorineural and conduction hearing loss. With less light, they lose visual cues that help them to compensate for their sensory impairments.

TEN (toxic epidermal necrosis)

See toxic epidermal necrosis.

thalamic syndrome

A vascular disorder involving the ventral and postlateral nuclei of the thalamus and related nerve fibers causing disturbances of sensation and partial or complete paralysis of one side of the body. A major effect is an increased threshold to all stimuli on the opposite side of the body so that any stimuli may cause an exaggerated response

TIA (transient ischemic attack)

See transient ischemic attack.

tophaceous gout

A form of purine metabolism disorder characterized by formation of chalky deposits of sodium biurate under the skin and joints. If untreated, the deposits may eventually destroy the involved joints.

total lung capacity (TLC)

The volume of gas in the lungs at the end of a maximum inspiration. It equals the vital capacity plus the residual capacity.

toxic epidermal necrolysis (TEN)

A rare skin disease characterized by epidermal erythema, superficial necrosis, and skin erosions. This condition, which affects mainly adults, makes the skin appear scalded, often leaving scars. Its cause is unknown, but it may result from toxic or hypersensitive reactions. It is commonly associated with drug reactions, such as those associated with butazones, sulfonamides, penicillins, barbiturates, and hydantoins. Other drugs may be involved, and the disease has also been associated with airborne toxins such as carbon monoxide. TEN also may indicate an immune response or it may be associated with severe physiologic stress. A similar skin disorder may be the result of staphylococcal infection.

transient ischemic attack (TIA)

An episode of cerebrovascular insufficiency, usually associated with a partial occlusion of an artery by an atherosclerotic plaque or embolism. The symptoms vary with the site and the degree of occlusion. Disturbance of normal vision in one or both eyes, dizziness, weakness, dysphasia, numbness, or unconsciousness may occur. The attack is usually brief, lasting a few minutes; rarely, symptoms continue for several hours.

Tzanck test

A microscopic examination of cellular material from skin lesions to help diagnose certain vesicular diseases. The tissue is scraped from the base of a vesicle, placed on a slide, and stained with Wright's or Giemsa's stain. Multinucleated giant cells are diagnostic of herpes virus or varicella. Typical pemphigus and other cells also can be identified.

urticaria

A pruritic skin eruption characterized by transient wheals of varying shapes and sizes with well-defined erythematous margins and pale centers. It is caused by capillary dilatation in the dermis that results from the release of vasoactive mediators, including histamine, kinin, and the slow, reactive substance of anaphylaxis associated with antigen-antibody reaction. Treatment includes antihistamines and removal of the stimulus or allergen. Cholinergic urticaria appears as wheals surrounded by a large axon flare. It may be caused by drugs, food, insect bites, inhalants, emotional stress, exposure to heat or cold, and exercise. Also called hives.

vital capacity (VC)

A measurement of the amount of air that can be expelled at the normal rate of exhalation after a maximum inspiration, representing the greatest possible breathing capacity. The vital capacity equals the inspiratory reserve volume plus the tidal volume plus the expiratory reserve volume. The average normal values of 4000 to 5000 ml are affected by age, physical dimensions of the chest sage, physical fitness, posture, and sex. The VC may be reduced by a decrease in functioning lung tissue, resulting from atelectasis, edema, fibrosis, pneumonia, pulmonary resection, or tumors; by limited chest expansion resulting from ascites, chest deformity, neuromuscular disease, pneumothorax, or pregnancy; or by airway obstruction.

Wernicke's encephalopathy

An inflammatory, hemorrhagic, degenerative condition of the brain, characterized by lesions in several parts of the brain, including the hypothalamus, mamillary bodies, and tissues surrounding ventricles and aqueducts. The condition is characterized by double vision, involuntary and rapid movements of the eyes, lack of muscular coordination, and decreased mental function, which may be mild or severe. Wernicke's encephalopathy is caused by a thiamine deficiency and is seen in association with chronic alcoholism. It also occurs as a complication of gastrointestinal tract disease and hyperemesis gravidarum associated with malabsorption and malnutrition. Also called Wernicke's syndrome.

written advance directive

A form of advance directive that allows a long-term care resident's expressed wishes and values to continue to guide treatment choices in the event that the resident cannot take part in the decision-making process.

xerosis

Epidermis lacking moisture or sebum, often characterized by a pattern of fine lines, scaling, and itching. Causes include too frequent bathing, low humidity, decreased production of sebum in aging skin, and ichthyosis. Treatment includes decreased frequency of bathing, increased humidity, bath oils, emollients such as lanolin and glycerine, and hydrophilic ointments.

Appendix A
Instructions for Completing the
Task Segmentation Protocol

Task segmentation refers to the breakdown of an activity of daily living (ADL) into a series of smaller subtasks. For example, choosing clean clothes is a subtask of dressing.

The Task Segmentation Protocol (TSP) is designed to be used in conjunction with the Health Care Financing Administration's Minimum Data Set (MDS) Self-Performance questions. Score each ADL in which the resident is receiving hands-on support or cueing to ensure task completion. Do not score for residents whose MDS ADL Self-Performance for the item is Independent (0) or Dependent (4).

Information will be obtained through resident observations and interviews with key staff caregivers. Be sure to question direct care staff (e.g., nurse assistants) since they are usually the most knowledgeable and reliable sources of information about a resident's actual performance in ADL.

PROCEDURE TO COMPLETE THE TSP

The TSP is a two-page inventory comprised of three sections. The first section consists of a checklist for three items that represent the cognitive tasks necessary to perform an ADL. This section describes these parts of the TSP.

KNOWS HOW TO USE OBJECTS

This section checks to determine whether a resident knows how to use an object (if one is needed to perform an activity).

AWARE OF NEED TO DO ACTIVITY

This section checks to determine whether a resident is aware of the need to perform an activity, or is aware of the need for devices or help. Devices that can be used for each activity are listed on the bottom of the second page of the TSP.

The middle section of the form consists of an 8-point rating scale (codes 0-7) for measuring the resident's Stepwise Performance of Activities. For each ADL task, record the level of resident function according to the code key. The following are examples of specific questions to use during the assessment to obtain detailed information about resident performance in each ADL area:

Example: Eating
fi Would the resident know it is mealtime or to ask for food if he or she were hungry?
fi How does the resident eat?
fi Can the resident use utensils, cups?

565

- Will the resident pick up a fork (or other utensil) and eat or does a staff member need to tell (cue) the resident to eat?
- Does the staff need to tell the resident to pick up a fork, or does the staff member need to pick up the fork and initiate the action for the resident to begin feeding him- or herself?
- Can the resident bring food and drink to the mouth?
- Does the resident need constant reminders to continue chewing and eating?
- Does the resident need to be reminded to clean him- or herself after eating?
- Does the staff perform the activity for the resident?

STEPWISE PERFORMANCE OF ACTIVITIES CODES

0   No help. Resident is not given any assistance such as verbal or physical cues or physical assistance.

1-2   Cueing. Can be verbal reminders or physical cues such   as modeling the activity, with no hands-on assistance.

Cueing is performed inconsistently, not always used

Cueing is performed consistently

3   Resident does part, without cueing. Resident does part of the activity or does the activity part of the time. Examples:

o Resident is independent in dressing, but resists care at times.When care is resisted, staff dress resident completely. Code 3.

o Resident brings food to mouth during most of the meal but stops before completing the meal. Staff feed the remainder to the resident. Code 4.

4-5   Resident does part, with cueing.

4   Cueing is performed inconsistently, or is not always used.

5   Cueing is performed consistently.

7   Activity is not done.

At the end of the middle section is an item, "Resident may be left alone safely?" Check this if the resident can be left alone while performing ADL tasks such as transfer, walking, wheelchair, and so forth.

The next section of the TSP form references "Items that May Enhance Resident's Self-Performance Equipment." After reviewing the resident's status in a particular ADL, ask the caregivers if they think the resident's performance in that area could be improved with any of the listed items. For example, is it possible that the resident could be more independent in transferring out of bed if the bed were lower in height? Check all that apply.

The last section of the TSP is an open box to be used to describe the nature of the encouragement and limit-setting procedures that appear to work with the resident. If there is a specific program in place, describe what has and has not worked. If there is no program, question (observe) direct care staff relative to these procedures.

COMPLETE TSP COLUMNS WHERE RECENT MDS SELF-PERFORMANCE SCORE = 1 TO 3 (Supervision to Extensive Assistance)

	TRANSFER (surface to surface)	WALKING	WHEEL-CHAIR	DRESSING	EATING	TOILET USE
Knows How to Use Objects needed to perform activity	Knows how transfer devices should be used bedside rails, chair arms	Knows how walking devices should be used cane, walks, hand rail	Knows how wheelchair should be used for locomotion	Knows how clothing items, closures should be used (e.g., sock, slip) closures (e.g., snaps)	Knows how eating utensils should be used	Knows how toilet, etc. should be used
	All ☐ Some ☐	All ☐ Some ☐	All ☐ Some ☐	All ☐ Some ☐	All ☐ Some ☐	All ☐ Some ☐
Aware of Own Needs	To transfer ☐ ---------------- For devices/ ☐ help	To walk ☐ ---------------- For devices/ ☐ help	To wheel ☐ ---------------- For devices/ ☐ help	To dress ☐ ---------------- For devices/ ☐ help	To eat ☐ ---------------- For devices/ ☐ help	To use toilet ☐ ---------------- For devices/ ☐ help
CODE FOR STEPWISE PERFORMANCE OF ACTIVITIES: 0 = No help 1 = Cueing inconsistent 2 = Cueing performed 3 = Resident does part without cueing 4 = Resident does part, with inconsistent cueing 5 = Resident does part, with consistent cueing 6 = Resident does none 7 = Activity not done						
Stepwise Performance of Activities	Positions in preparation to transfer ☐	Stand and maintains balance W/out devices ☐ With devices ☐ ☐	Repositions and arranges self in chair ☐	Chooses/ selects clean clothes ☐	Opens/pours, unwraps, cuts ☐	Aware of when to void/eliminate ☐
	Prepares chair/bed (locks pads, moves covers) ☐	Walks in room ☐	Propels self Uses arms ☐ Uses feet ☐	Obtains clothes ☐	Grasps food/ utensils/cup Food ☐ Utensils ☐ Cup ☐	Aware of need for privacy ☐
	Transfers (stands/ sits/lifts/ turns) ☐	Walks on unit ☐	Uses wheel-chair off the unit ☐	Grasps/puts on clothes: Upper body ☐ Lower body ☐	Scoops/ spears food ☐	Arranges clothes in preparation ☐

INDEX

A

Acquired immunodeficiency syndrome
 dementia and, 47
 prevalence in elderly, 47
Actinic keratoses, 299
 causes of, 299
 identification of treatment need, 299
 treatment protocol, 299
Activities of daily living
 clinical review, 419
 delirium and, 153
 evaluation, after hip fracture, 274
 infection and, 27
 overview, 419
 rehabilitation opportunities, 419
 reversible conditions, 419
Activities programming
 assessment, 446
 care plan development, 448
 crafts, 459
 evaluating program, 462
 games, 459
 gardening, 460
 hobby shop, 460
 holidays, 9
 music, 459
 overview, 445
 pets/children, 461
 problems/challenges, 449
 risk taking, 445
 toys, 460
 volunteers, 462
 wandering hallway, 461
ADL, see Activities of daily living
Advance directives, 472
 chart placement for, 476
 content of, 477
 effectiveness of, 476
 procedure for creating, 473
 staff objections to, 476
 type to use, 474
AIDS, see Acquired immunodeficiency syndrome
 care planning, 53
 care planning process, 48
 dementia and, 126
 drug therapy, 50
 etiology, 49
 health transitions, 53
 hospitalization frequency, 53
 overview, 48

 universal control precautions, 60
Airway clearance, 497
Akathisia, delirium and, 155
Alcohol, withdrawal, delirium and, 147
Alpha-adrenergic agents, urinary incontinence and, 383, 400
Alpha blockers, urinary incontinence and, 400
Alzheimer's disease, 121
 correlates of, 121
 delirium and, 146
 diagnostic standards, 122
 staffing training requirements, 140
 swallowing problems and, 316
 treating, 122
 troubleshooting, 141
Amphotericin, cryptococcus and, 58
Amsler Grid eye test, 242
Anemia, 2
Angiotensin-converting enzyme inhibitors, urinary incontinence and, 384
Anomia, 81
Antianxiety drugs, 198
 choosing/monitoring, 200
 side effects, 201
Anticholinergic medications
 drug therapy, 209
 falls and, 260
 psychotropic drugs and, 189
 urinary incontinence and, 399
Antidepressants, 181, 195
 choosing/monitoring, 195
 dementia and, 120
 falls and, 260
 hypothermia and, 11
 side effects, 195
Antihistamines, falls and, 260
Antipsychotic medications
 excessive use, 13
 inappropriate use, 20
Anxiety
 causes and pathophysiology, 173
 disorder, 162
 overview, 172
 risk factors, 173
Aphasia, 225
 after stroke, 79
 care plan, 231
 evaluation of, 79
Apnea, sleep, 69

Appearance
 assessment of, 1
 overall, 1
Appetite problems, 316
Artery, infarction of
 anterior cerebral, 77
 internal carotid, 76
 middle cerebral, 77
Arthritis
 assistive devices, 104
 chronic therapy, 103
 clinical features, 98
 crystal-induced, 98
 medical treatment, 102
 distraction/relaxation, 103
 evaluating involvement, 101
 exercise and, 103
 foot problems and, 283
 gait and, 101
 hip, 98
 knee, 99
 medications for, 101
 muscle strength, 101
 overview, 97
 pain levels, 101
 range of motion and, 101
 rest, 103
 rheumatoid, 98
 of the foot, 283
 shoulder pain, 99
 soft tissue disorders and, 100
 spine, 99
 thermal modalities, 103
Assessment, resident, vital signs and, 1
Asthma
 bronchodilator therapy and, 36
 forced expiratory volume in 1 second, 35
 swallowing problems and, 316
Atovaquone, *Pneumocystis carinii* pneumonia, 57
Atrophic urethritis, identification of, 380
Auscultatory gap, failure to recognize, 6
Azotemia, 2
AZT, 50

B

Balance
 assessment after a fall, 263
 falls and, 259

training, 440
Basal cell carcinoma, 299
    causes of, 299
    identification of treatment need,
        300
    treatment protocol, 300
Bathing, resident with respiratory
    problems, 44
Behavioral deficits, activities and, 450
Behavior changes, drug-induced, 208
Behavior management
    drug use and, 13
    strategies for, residents with de-
        mentia, 136
Behavior problems/symptoms
    causes of problems, 159
    disruptive behavior, 158
    environmental factors, 163
    frontal lobe dysfunction, 160
    identification of, 164
    impulse control, improving, 168
    medication side effects, 162
    nonpharmacologic interventions,
        165
    overview, 157
    personality disorders, 159
    physically abusive, 158
    psychosocial problems and, 216
    resistance to care, 158
    socially inappropriate, 158
    treatment of, 164
    verbally abusive, 158
    wandering, 158
Behavior therapy
    cognitive, 181
    urinary incontinence and, 393
Biologic therapy, 181
Bladder compliance, decreased, 385
Bladder emptying, improving, 397
Bladder retraining, 394
Blood flow, pedal, analysis, 279
Blood pressure, 1
    equipment application and use,
        6
    factors affecting, 2
    high, 2
    homeostasis, falls and, 259
    interpreting, 4
    low, 4
    measurement of, 4
        standardized procedure, 7
    measuring errors, expectation
        bias, 6
    possible measuring errors
        auscultatory gap, 6
        cardiac arrhythmia, 7
        pseudohypertension, 6
        terminal digit preference, 6
Blood transfusion
    HIV and AIDS screening, 48
    HIV risk factors, 50
Bowel disorders
    anorectal disease, 413
    cancer of colon/rectum/anus,
        415
    care plan development, 410
    constipation
        care plan for, 415
        patterns of, 407
    fecal incontinence
        causes of, 408
        identification of treatment
            need, 408
        persistent, care plan for, 415
    laboratory testing and, 409
    laxative use and, 413
    overview, 407
    physical examination and, 409
    rectal prolapse, 415
    stool production, 413
Braden scale, 309
Bradycardia, sinus, 8
Brain damage, dementia and, 130
Breathing, deep-breathing exercises,
    39
Bronchiectasis, chest physiotherapy
    and, 39
Bronchodilator therapy, 36
Burning mouth syndrome, 354

C
Caffeine, sleep disorders and, 67
Calcium-channel blockers
    pulse rate and, 8
    urinary incontinence and, 383,
        399
Cancer
    bladder, 385
    colon/rectum/anus, 415
    oral, 352
    prostate, 385
Candidiasis, 353
    HIV and, 54
Carbamazepine, 204
Carbon dioxide, 35
Cardiac arrhythmia, blood pressure
    monitoring and, 7
Cardiopulmonary disorders
    nutrition and, 46
    sleep and, 46
    symptoms of, 43
Cardiopulmonary rehabilitation, 41
    equipment for, 41
    exercise program, 41
    exercise screening, 41
Cardiovascular morbidity, high blood
    pressure and, 2
Cardiovascular problems, hip fracture
    and, 270
Cartilage, 97
Cataracts, 243
Catheters
    urinary incontinence and, 401
    urinary tract infection and, 271
Cerebral blood flow, hypertension
    and, 4
Cerebrovascular disease, overview, 74
Cheilitis/cheilosis, angular, 353

CHF, see Heart failure, congestive
Cholinergic medications, urinary in-
    continence and, 401
Clindamycin, central nervous system
    toxoplasmosis, 57
Cognitive assessment, 128
Cognitive deficits, 116
    activities and, 450
    identification of resident with,
        119
Combativeness, managing, 138
Communication
    aphasia and, 225
    dementia and, 130, 226
    depression and, 227
    dysarthria, 226
    hearing loss and, 225
    language barriers, 227
    overview, 224
    Parkinson's disease and, 112
    physiologic reserve, 227
    problems
        care planning, 229
        identification of resident,
            228
Complexion, assessment of, 1
Comprehension, 81
Computed tomography, stroke and, 86
Confusion, 1
    bradycardia and, 8
    inappropriate drug use and, 14
Conjunctival problems, 251
Constipation
    anticholinergic drugs and, 14
    causes of, 408
    identification of treatment need,
        408
    persistent, care plan for, 415
Corticosteroids, 37
    arthritis and, 101
Crixivan, 50
Cryptococcus, HIV and, 58
Cryptosporidiosis, HIV and, 56
Cyanosis, 9
Cytomegalovirus, HIV and, 58

D
Debridement, 311
Dehydration, 2
    caregiver observations, 335
    care plan for, 337, 342
    clinical consequences, 332
    decreased fluid intake, causes of,
        333
    determining reasons for, 338
    elderly predisposition to, 333
    fluid deficit
        causes of, 334
        estimating, 340
            formula weight compari-
                son, 340
            free water deficit formula,
                340
    high-risk patient care, 343

identification of treatment need, 334
intravenous fluid replacement, 341
laboratory testing, 335
maintenance therapy, 337
monitoring during therapy for, 338
oral rehydration therapy, 337
overview, 332
pathophysiology and terminology, 332
physical examination, 335
subcutaneous fluid administration, 341
terminal care and, 496
Delirium, 125
behavior problems and, 161
care planning, 151
diagnosing underlying cause, 149
emotional support, 152
health status review, 149
infection and, 27
laboratory studies, 151
overview, 145
physical examination, 151
predisposing factors, 146
recognizing, 147
resident, identifying, 146
signs/symptoms, 147
Delusion, 148
Dementia
activity options for residents with, 455
assessment of causal factors, 127
behavior problems and, 161
care plan, 234
cognitive assessment, 128
communication problems and, 226
delirium and, 146
depression and, 174
diagnosing, 119
diagnostic criteria, 116
diagnostic evaluation, 126
environmental settings, 457
HIV and, 59
interventions, 129
multiinfarct, 123
overview, 116
Parkinson's disease and, 110
sleep disorders and, 70
staffing training requirements, 140
treatment, 120
treatment strategies, 127
troubleshooting, 141
Dental care, see Oral health care
Dental referral, identification of need for, 347
Dental treatments, 349
Dentures, lack of, 348
Denture sore mouth, 353

Depression
activities and, 450
assessment, 177
care plan for, 235
causes and pathophysiology, 173
communication and, 227
dementia and, 174
drugs and, 175
irreversible dementia and, 124
laboratory studies, 179
medical history of resident, 177
medical illness and, 174
neurochemical abnormalities, 173
overview, 172
Parkinson's disease and, 111
prevention of, 183
resident with respiratory problems, 45
risk factors, 173
signs/symptoms of, 175
sleep and, 71
stroke and, 91
treatment plan, 179
underuse of antidepressants, 15
weight loss and, 11
Dermatitis
contact/irritant, 291
causes of, 292
pathophysiology and terminology, 291
treatment protocol, 292
seborrheic
causes of, 294
identification of treatment need, 294
treatment protocol, 294
Dermatologic examination, foot problems and, 280
Diabetes mellitus
bowel disorders and, 412
foot infection, diagnosing and treating, 284
foot problems and, 279
hip fracture and, 271
hypothermia and, 11
Diet, see under Nutrition
Digoxin, pulse rate and, 8
Dilantin hyperplasia, 354
Diphenhydramine, inappropriate use, 20
Discharge planning
overview, 512
postdischarge plan of care, 518
preadmission screening to prepare, 515
screening for, 514
targeting model, 516
targeting residents for, 512
Diuretics, urinary incontinence and, 383
Dizziness, bradycardia and, 8
Dopamine blocking effects, psycho-

tropic drugs and, 189
Dressing, resident with respiratory problems, 44
Drug metabolism, liver and, 16
Drug therapy, see also specific types
adverse reactions, 14
depression and, 175
preventing, 21
after hip fracture, 270
AIDS, protease inhibitors, 50
anticholinergic, side effects, 14
antidepressants, 181
underuse of, 15
antihypertensive, effects of, 3
antipsychotic, excessive use of, 13
antiviral therapy, 60
arthritis, 101
behavior problems, 167
candidiasis, 54
commonly prescribed, 14
corticosteroids, 101
cryptococcus, 58
cryptosporidiosis/isospora, 56
cytomegalovirus, 58
delirium, 154
elimination, 16
falls and, 260
guidelines for prescribing, 23
herpes simplex, 55
herpes zoster, 55
inappropriate use, defining, 20
inappropriate use of, 13
Kaposi's sarcoma, 60
lymphoma, central nervous system, 60
mood-stabilizing
choosing/monitoring, 202
monitoring, 205
side effects, 205
Mycobacterium avium complex, 58
nutritional status and, 319
optimal use of, 13
Parkinson's disease, 113
adverse reactions, 113
pharmacodynamics and, 18
pharmacokinetics and, 15
Pneumocystis carinii pneumonia, 57
pressure ulcers and, 309
progressive multifocal leukoencephalopathy, 59
psychoactive, 154
psychotropic drugs, 187
repeated drug dosing, 17
review of, 22
sedatives, excessive use of, 13
serum drug levels, 17
skin disorders and, 294
sleep disorders, 70
steady-state levels, 17
therapeutic untrial, 23

toxoplasmosis, 57
treatment response, inadequate, 209
tuberculosis, 56
urinary incontinence and, 381
vision disorders, 252
vision impairment and, 243
withdrawal from, delirium and, 147
Dry mouth, anticholinergic drugs and, 14
Dysarthria, 226
care plan for, 233
Dysphagia, 353
Dyspnea on exertion, 43

E
Electrocardiogram, bradycardia and, 8
Electroconvulsive therapy, 183
Embarrassment, activities and, 450
Emotional reactions, AIDS and HIV, 48
Emotional support, residents with delirium, 152
Emphysema, swallowing problems and, 316
Endurance training, 438
Energy, loss of, depression and, 176
Energy expenditure, basal, calculation of, 372
Enteritis, HIV and, 56
Environment, physical, dementia patients, 132
Environmental hazards, falls, eliminating, 264
Erythema multiforme, 295
Estrogen, urinary incontinence and, 400
Exanthema, drug, 295
Exercise
arthritis and, 103
program, cardiopulmonary rehabilitation, 41
vital sign changes, 43
rehabilitation and, 435
Expectation bias, 6
Eyedrops, 252

F
Falls
behavioral/cognitive factors, 261
blood pressure homeostasis, 259
disease-related factors, 260
environmental hazards, 261
eliminating, 264
evaluation after, 262
gait/balance, 259
high-risk resident, treating, 264
history taking after, 262
identification of problems, 261
inappropriate drug use and, 14
infection and, 27
laboratory studies, 263

muscle strength and, 259
overview, 258
physical examination after, 263
risk factors for, 262
training programs, 266
Family visits, psychosocial well-being and, 217
Fatigue, activities and, 450
Fecal impaction, 2, 413
Fecal incontinence, 407
causes of, 408
identification of treatment need, 408
persistent, care plan for, 415
Feeding tube
assessment, 359
basal energy expenditure, 372
care of tube site, 371
care plan development, 360
clinical considerations, 358
gastrostomy tube site, 371
identification of treatment need, 359
indications for, 359
overview, 358
protein requirement calculation, 374
tube blockage, 372
tube placement, 361
Femoral neck fractures, 269
Fever, 9, 10
Flexibility training, 442
Foot infection, diagnosing and treating, 284
Foot problems/disorders
arthritis and, 283
assessing, 279
bunions, 282
calluses, 282
care plan development, 279
corns, 281
dermatologic examination and, 280
diabetes mellitus and, 279
gout, 283
hallux valgus, 282
heel spurs, 283
nail disorders, 281
neurologic examination, 280
neuroma, 282
osteoarthritis and, 283
overview, 278
pedal ulcerations and, 279
peripheral arterial insufficiency and, 279
plantar fasciitis, 283
radiographic examination, 280
rheumatoid arthritis, 283
skin disorders, 281
treating, 281
Forced expiratory volume in 1 second, 35
Fractures, see specific type

Frontal lobe dysfunction, 160

G
Gait
abnormalities/disorder
antianxiety drug-induced, 201
antidepressant-induced, 198
mood-stabilizing drug-induced, 205
neuroleptic-induced, 194
abnormalities/disorders, psychotropic drugs and, 190
arthritis and, 101
assessment after a fall, 263
falls and, 259
Parkinson's disease and, 108
training, after hip fracture, 273
Games, 459
Ganciclovir, cytomegalovirus and, 58
Gastroenteritis, 413
Gastrointestinal disturbances, hip fracture and, 271
Gastrointestinal infection, prevalence of, 26
Genitourinary problems, hip fracture and, 271
Glasses, maintenance of, 256
Glaucoma, 245
Gout
crystal-induced, 102
foot problems and, 283

H
Hachinski ischemic scale, 123
Health-care costs, drugs, optimal use of, 13
Health status, review of, delirium and, 149
Hearing impairment, 225
activities and, 450
care plan, 229
Heart failure, congestive, 2
weight gain and, 11
Heart rate, response to stress, 9
Helplessness, depression and, 176
Hemiparesis, after stroke, 78
Hemiplegia, after stroke, 78
Hemorrhagic infarction, 75
Herpes simplex, 352
HIV and, 55
Herpes zoster, 297
causes of, 298
HIV and, 55
identification of treatment need, 298
ophthalmicus, 248
treatment protocol, 298
Hip, arthritis and, 98
Hip fracture
ADL evaluation, 274
concurrent illness and, 270
diabetes and, 271
femoral neck, 269

Hip fracture (*con't*)
  gait training, 273
  gastrointestinal disturbances and, 271
  hypotension and, 271
  identifying resident with, 268
  inappropriate drug use and, 14
  incontinence and, 272
  intertrochanteric, 270
  neurologic conditions and, 272
  nutrition and, 272
  overview, 268
  perioperative care, 270
  postoperative therapy, 273
  rehabilitative care plan, 274
  respiratory conditions and, 271
  steroid therapy and, 271
  surgical goals/treatment, 269
  thromboembolic disease and, 272
  urinary tract infection and, 271
  wheelchair use, 273
HIV, *see* Human immunodeficiency virus
  care planning, 53
  care planning process, 48
  classification system, 53
  drug therapy, 50
  etiology, 49
  major conditions associated with, 54
  overview, 48
  risk factors, 50
  transmission of, 50
  universal control precautions, 60
Hopelessness, depression and, 176
Human immunodeficiency virus, prevalence in elderly, 47
Hydrocephalus, 125
Hydronephrosis, urinary incontinence and, 385
Hypercalcemia, 412
Hyperglycemia, 2
Hypertension, 2
  systolic, treatment of, 3
Hypoglycemia, 2
Hypokalemia, 412
Hyponatremia, 2
Hypotension, 4
  antidepressant-associated, 197
  hip fracture and, 271
  neuroleptic-induced, 194
  psychotropic drugs and, 189
Hypothermia, 9
  causes of, 10
  signs of, 11
  treatment, 11
Hypothyroidism
  bowel disorders and, 412
  bradycardia and, 8
  hypothermia and, 11
I
Illness

acute, blood pressure elevation and, 4
depression and, 174
Impulse control, improving, 168
Incontinence
  anticholinergic drugs and, 14
  hip fracture and, 272
  stroke and, 92
  urinary
      absorbant garments and pads, 404
      atrophic urethritis, identification of, 380
      behavioral therapy, 393
      causes of, 377
      evaluation/treatment, 377
      excess urine production, 384
      identification of treatment need, 385
      medications for, 397
      mobility and, 384
      overview, 376
      physiology, 376
      psychological factors, 384
      therapy for men, 391
      therapy for women, 388
      treatment specifics, 393
      vaginitis, identification of, 380
  urinary/fecal, pressure ulcers and, 308
Indinavir, 50
Infarction, *see* specific types
  watershed, 78
Infection, *see also* specific types
  acute care hospitalization for, 28
  confirming presence of, 27
  control practices, residents, 60
  dehydration and, 338
  laboratory test results, 27
  nursing home treatment of, 28
  oral rehydration guidelines, 339
  overview, 26
  physical examination results, 27
  treating, 27
  universal precautions, 60
Inhalers, metered dose, 36
Insomnia, psychotropic drugs and, 189
Interpersonal difficulties, 163
Interpersonal therapy, 181
Ischemic infarction, 74
Isospora, HIV and, 56

K
Kaposi's sarcoma, HIV and, 59
Knee, arthritis and, 99

L
Laboratory testing
  bowel disorders and, 409
  dehydration, 335
  delirium, 151

depression, 179
falls and, 263
infection, 27
nutritional status and, 319
Lacunar syndromes, 78
Language barriers
  care plan for, 236
  communication and, 227
Language disorders, after stroke, 79
Lethargy, 1
Leukoencephalopathy, progressive multifocal, HIV and, 59
Levodopa
  Parkinson's disease and, 107
  side effects, 113
Lichen planus, 354
Lithium, 203
Liver, drug metabolism, 16
Living will, *see* Advance directives
Lungs, *see* entries under Pulmonary
  primary function of, 35
Lux, 65
Lymphoma, central nervous system, HIV and, 60

M
Macular degeneration, age-related, 246
Magnetic resonance imaging, stroke and, 86
Malignancy, occult, weight loss and, 11
Malnutrition, hypothermia and, 11
Manometer, equipment reliability, 5
Medical evaluation, nutritional status and, 319
Medicare, hospice benefits, 506
Medication regimen, review of, 22
Medications, *see* Drug therapy
Melanoma, malignant
  causes of, 302
  identification of treatment need, 302
  treatment protocol, 302
Mellaril, delirium and, 155
Mental disorders, behavior and, 160
Mental status
  drug-induced changes, 208
  examination, depression and, 178
Mercury, manometer levels, 4
Mobility, resident with respiratory problems, 45
Mood problems, psychosocial problems and, 216
Mortality, high blood pressure and, 2
Movement disorder
  antidepressant-induced, 197
  mood-stabilizing drug-induced, 205
  neuroleptic-induced, 194
  stimulant-induced, 207
Mucous plugging, chest physiotherapy

and, 39
Muscle, tone abnormalities, stroke
    and, 91
Muscle strength
    arthritis and, 101
    falls and, 259
Music, 459
Mycobacterium avium complex, HIV
    and, 58
Myocardial infarction
    silent, 2
    systolic hypertension and, 3

N
Necrolysis, toxic epidermal, 295
Neglect syndrome, 82
Neurochemical abnormalities, depres-
    sion and, 173
Neuroleptics, 192
    falls and, 260
    side effects, 194
Neurologic conditions, hip fracture
    and, 272
Neurologic examination, foot prob-
    lems and, 280
Neurologic problems/disorders, 2
Neuropsychological testing, 123
Norton scale, 309
Norvir, 50
Nursing home
    AIDS and HIV in, 49
    changing roles of, 513
    community hospice services, 505
    residents
        assessment, 1
        drugs, optimal use of, 13
        infection control practices,
            60
        resident education, 60
        stroke evaluation, 84
        vital signs, 1
    staff education
        AIDS and HIV, 49
        residents with dementia,
            137
Nutrition
    appetite problems, 316
        interventions for, 326
    cardiopulmonary problems and,
        46
    care plan establishment, 321
    chewing problems, interventions
        for, 325
    chewing problems and, 316
    clinical considerations, 317
    depression and, 180
    ethical considerations, 317
    feeding strategies, 328
    hip fracture and, 272
    increased nutrient requirements,
        316
    mechanical problems, 316
        interventions for, 325

medical evaluation results, 319
overview, 315
Parkinson's disease and, 110
physical factors and, 320
problems
    identification of treatment
        need, 318
    interventions for, 325
    laboratory testing, 319
psychosocial status and, 317
sense of taste loss, 329
sleep disorders and, 67
special diet adaptation, 316
    interventions for, 328
swallowing problems, 316
    interventions for, 325
treatment strategies, 323
Nutritional assessment, completing,
    321

O
Ocular disorders
    signs of, 242
    symptoms of, 241
Optic neuropathy, anterior ischemic,
    248
Oral health care
    angular cheilitis/cheilosis, 353
    aphthous stomatitis, 352
    burning mouth syndrome, 354
    candidiasis, 353
    canker sore, 352
    considerations, 350
    denture sore mouth, 353
    dilantin hyperplasia, 354
    drug reactions, 355
    dysphagia, 353
    herpes simplex, 352
    hygiene, 350
    lack of dentures, 348
    lesions/ulcers/inflammation, 348
    lichen planus, 354
    mouth pain/sensitivity, 347
    oral cancer, 352
    oral cavity treatments and diag-
        nostic conditions, 352
    overview, 347
    pemphigus/pemphigoid, 354
    periodontal disease, 354
    rampant tooth, 354
    tardive dyskinesia, 352
    taste disorders, 355
    teeth, broken or loose, 348
    xerostomia, 353
Oral hygiene, resident with respira-
    tory problems, 45
Oral intake, decreased, 358
Osteoarthritis, 97
    foot problems and, 283
Oxygen, 35
Oxygen therapy, resident with respi-
    ratory problems, 45

P
Pain
    activities and, 450
    arthritis and, 101
    Parkinson's disease and, 112
    syndromes, stroke and, 92
Palliative care, identification of treat-
    ment need, 483
Parkinsonism, delirium and, 155
Parkinson's disease
    bowel disorders and, 412
    clinical features, 108
    communication problems, 112
    dementia and, 110, 126
    depression and, 111
    gait disturbances, 108
    hypothermia and, 11
    interventions, 109
    levodopa, side effects, 113
    life expectancy, 107
    medications causing, 107
    nutrition, 110
    overview, 106
    pain and, 112
    recognition, 109
    sleep disturbance, 112
    visual problems and, 112
Pedal ulcerations, foot problems and,
    279
Pelvic muscles, strengthening, 396
Pemphigus/pemphigoid, 354
Periodontal disease, 354
Peripheral arterial insufficiency, foot
    problems and, 279
Personality disorders, 159
Pharmacodynamics, 18
Pharmacokinetics
    aging effects on, 15
    definition of, 15
    drug elimination, 16
Pharmacologic effects, delayed, 207
Pharmacology, *see* Drug therapy
Pharmacoreduction, 266
Physical abuse, 158
Physical disorders, behavior and, 160
Physical examination
    after fall, 263
    bowel disorders and, 409
    dehydration, 335
    depression and, 178
    infection, 27
Physical impairment, activities and,
    450
Physiologic reserve
    communication and, 227
    reduced, care plan for, 235
Physiotherapy, chest, 39
    technique for, 39
Plantar fasciitis, 283
Pneumonia, 2
    diagnostic criteria, 31
    management of, 31
    monitoring and follow-up, 32

Pneumonia (con't)
  Pneumocystic carinii, HIV and, 57
  treatment, 31
Polypharmacy, sleep disorders, 66
Prostate involutional agents, urinary incontinence and, 401
Protease inhibitors, AIDS and HIV and, 50
Protein requirement, calculation of, 374
Proteoglycan, 97
Pruritus, 296
  causes of, 296
Pseudogout, crystal-induced, 102
Pseudohypertension, failure to recognize, 6
Psychiatric illness, behavior problems and, 162
Psychodynamic therapy, 181
Psychosocial factors
  anxiety, terminally ill, 500
  nutrition and, 317
  terminally ill, 499
    grief and bereavement, 500
Psychosocial well-being
  assessment, 212
  behavior/mood problems and, 216
  care planning, 215
  long-standing problems, 214
  mental health consultation, 215
  monitoring, 222
  overview, 212
  situational factors, 214
  social history, 212
Psychotherapy, depression and, 180
Psychotropic drugs
  behavior problems and, 168
  choosing/assessing therapy, 191
  classes of, 192
  history of abuse of, 187
  identification of resident in need of, 187
  overview, 187
  patient current drug list, 189
  response to treatment, 188
  side effects, 191
  subjective impressions of effects, 191
  vital signs and, 190
Pulmonary disease, chronic obstructive
  forced expiratory volume in 1 second, 35
  swallowing problems and, 316
Pulmonary mechanics, see also Lungs
  age-related changes in, 35
  forced expiratory volume in 1 second, 35
  residual volume, 35
  tidal volume, 36
  total lung capacity, 35
  vital capacity, 35

Pulse, 1
  examination of, 9
  quality, 8
  rate, 8
  rhythm, 8
Pupillary changes, 240

R
Radiographic examination, foot problems and, 280
Range of motion, arthritis and, 101
Recognition, Parkinson's disease and, 109
Rehabilitation
  after hip fracture, 274
  care plan documentation, 442
  environmental modifications, 442
  equipment, 442
  exercise programs, 435
  intensive, 425
  nursing-based, 440
  resident involvement, 424
  watch group, 423
Residents, see Nursing home residents
Resistance training, 439
Respiratory illness/dysfunction
  activities of daily living, 44
  antibiotic use, 40
  bathing and dressing of resident, 44
  bronchodilator therapy and, 36
  causal factors, 36
  chest physiotherapy, 39
  chronic, hip fracture and, 271
  nursing care plan, 44
  nutritional treatment, 40
  oxygen effects, 40
  treating, 36
  treatment, 36
Respiratory rate, 1, 9
  measurement error, 9
Respiratory tract infection, prevalence of, 26
Restraint usage
  adverse effects, 465
  identification of treatment need, 467
  intervention strategies, 469
  intervention to remove, 469
  OBRA 1987 regulations, 467
  preventing, 467
  reduction of, overview, 464
  restraint-free care, 465
Retinal vein occlusion, 247
Retinopathy, diabetic, 246
Ritonavir, 50

S
Saquinavir, 50
Scabies, 292
  causes of, 293
  pathophysiology and terminology, 292
Secretion, clearing of, 40

Sedation, 189
Sedatives
  excessive use of, 13
  falls and, 260
Seizures, stroke and, 90
Self-harm, protecting resident from, 180
Sensory impairment, 147
Sensory modalities, alteration after stroke, 78
Sepsis, hypothermia and, 11
Shingles, HIV and, 55
Skin care, postoperative, after hip fracture, 270
Skin disorders
  actinic keratoses, 299
    causes of, 299
    identification of treatment need, 299
    treatment protocol, 299
  basal cell carcinoma
    causes of, 299
    identification of treatment need, 300
    treatment protocol, 300
  contact dermatitis, 291
  dermatitis
    contact/irritant
      causes of, 292
      pathophysiology and terminology, 291
    seborrheic, 294
      causes of, 294
      identification of treatment need, 294
      treatment protocol, 294
  drug reactions, 294
    drug exanthema, 295
    erythema multiforme, 295
    toxic epidermal necrolysis, 295
    urticaria, 295
  herpes zoster, 297
    causes of, 298
    identification of treatment need, 298
    treatment protocol, 298
  identification of treatment need, 291, 296
  irritant dermatitis, 291
  malignant melanoma, 301
    causes of, 302
    identification of treatment need, 302
    treatment protocol, 302
  nonpressure ulcers, 290
    causes of, 290
  overview, 289
  pathophysiology and terminology, 290
  pruritus, causes of, 296
  pruritus and, 296
  scabies, 292
    causes of, 293

identification of treatment need, 293
treatment protocol, 293
squamous cell carcinoma
  causes of, 300
  identification of treatment need, 301
  treatment protocol, 301
treatment protocol, 296
xerosis, 297
  causes of, 297
  treatment protocol, 297
Skin/soft tissue infection, prevalence of, 26
Sleep, cardiopulmonary problems and, 46
Sleep disorders, 64
  apnea, 66
  apnea with dementia, 66
  circadian rhythm disturbances, 69
  depression and, 71
  fragmentation, 65
  hygiene practices, 67
  medications for, 66
  Parkinson's disease and, 112
  sundowning, 67
  treatment for, 67
Sleep therapy, future directions in, 71
Smoking, cessation, 36
Social history, resident, 212
Soft tissue disorders, arthritis and, 100
Spinal cord lesion, 385
Spirometry, incentive, 39
Squamous cell carcinoma
  causes of, 300
  identification of treatment need, 301
  treatment protocol, 301
Steroid therapy, hip fracture and, 271
Stethoscope, 5
Stimulants, 205
  choosing/monitoring, 206
Stroke
  assessment scales, 88
  common syndromes of, 75
  depression and, 91
  diagnostic/therapeutic options, 84
    complications of, 89
  disabilities after, 78
  discharge plans, 82
  evaluating residents with, 84
  hypothermia and, 11
  identification of residents with, 83
  immobility effects, 93
  incontinence, 92
  muscle tone abnormalities, 91
  pain syndromes, 92
  preventing recurrence, 89
  prognostic indicators, 93
  rehabilitation, 87
  seizures and, 90
  swallowing problems and, 316

systolic hypertension and, 3
therapeutic modalities, 87
Sulfadiazine, central nervous system toxoplasmosis, 57
Syncope, bradycardia and, 8

T
Tabes dorsalis, 385
Tachycardia, 8
Tachypnea, 9
Tardive dyskinesia, delirium and, 155
3TC, 50
Teeth
  broken or loose, 348
  lack of dentures, 348
Temperature, 1
  infection and, 27
  measurement of, 9
Terminal care
  administrative issues, 504
  anorexia/cachexia, 496
  assessment, 490
  care planning, 486, 501
    family involvement, 486
  community hospice services, 505
  dehydration and, 496
  diarrhea, 495
  end-stage, 498
  facility preparedness, 485
  intervention, 491
  loss of taste, 495
  mouth care, 488
  nausea and vomiting, 493
  nerve blocks, 492
  nutrition and hydration, 488
  overview, 482
  pain management, 489
  palliative care and, identification of treatment need, 483
  psychosocial care, 499
  shortness of breath, 497
  sore mouth, 495
  spiritual care, 501
  symptom control, 489
Terminal digit preference, 6
Theophylline, oral, 37
Thermometers, low-reading, 11
Thioridazine, delirium and, 155
Thromboembolic disease, hip fracture and, 272
Toileting, resident with respiratory problems, 45
Tooth, rampant, 354
Toxoplasmosis, central nervous, HIV and, 57
Trimethoprim-sulfamethoxazole, Pneumocystis carinii pneumonia, 57
Tuberculosis, HIV and, 56, 61

U
Ulcers
  infected pressure
    diagnostic criteria, 32

managing, 32
monitoring and follow-up, 33
treatment, 32
nonpressure, 290
  causes of, 290
pressure
  assessment scales, 309
  clinical review, 304
  complicating conditions, 305
  diabetes mellitus, insulin-dependent and, 308
  friction and, 309
  history of previous, 309
  identification of treatment need, 304
  lower limb fracture and, 308
  malnutrition and, 308
  medication side effects, 309
  moisture and, 308
  overview, 303
  peripheral vascular disease and, 308
  preventive care plan, 305
  restraints and, 309
  tactile sensory perception, 309
  treatment strategies, 310
  urinary/fecal incontinence and, 308
  weight loss and, 308
  wound debridement/cleansing, 311
Urinary tract infection, 2
  diagnostic criteria, 29
  hip fracture and, 271
  managing, 29
  monitoring and follow-up, 30
  prevalence of, 26
  specimen collection, 29
  treatment, 29
Urticaria, 295
UTI, see Urinary tract infection

V
Vaginitis, identification of, 380
Valproate, 204
Varicella, HIV and, 61
Verbal abuse, 158
Vertebrobasilar system, infarction of, 77
Vision, screening tests, 242
Vision disorders
  activities and, 450
  Amsler Grip eye test, 242
  anterior ischemic optic neuropathy, 248
  blurred, anticholinergic drugs and, 14
  caring for resident with, 252
  cataracts, 243
  causes of, 243

Vision disorders (*con't*)
conjunctival problems, 251
corneal, 252
diabetic retinopathy, 246
disturbances after stroke, 79
dry eye, 249
examinations for, 242
eyedrops, 252
flashes, 250
floaters, 250
functional signs of, 240
glaucoma, 245
herpes zoster ophthalmicus, 248
identification of resident needing treatment, 240
lid disorders, 250
lid inflammation, 251
lid malpositions, 250
lid neoplasms, 251
macular degeneration, age-related, 246

medications and, 243
ocular
signs of, 242
symptoms of, 241
ointments, 255
overview, 239
Parkinson's disease and, 112
photopsias, 250
retinal vein occlusion, 247
topical medication administration, 252
vitreous opacities, 250
wet eye, 249
Visual appliances, maintenance of,
256
Vital signs, *see also* Blood pressure,
Pulse, Respiratory rate, and Temperature
cardiopulmonary rehabilitation,
acceptable changes in, 43
overview, 1

psychotropic drugs and, 189
Voiding, prompted, 395

W
Wandering, 158
Weight, body, 1
changes in, 11
measuring, 11
underlying cause for change in,
11
Wheelchair, after hip fracture, 273
Wound cleansing, 311
Wound debridement, 311

X
Xerosis, 297
causes of, 297
Xerostomia, 353

Y
Yeast infection, HIV and, 54